T0175475

THE WASHINGTON MANUAL®

Cardiology

Subspecialty Consult

FOURTH EDITION

THE WASHINGTON MANUAL®

Cardiology

FOURTH EDITION

Editors

Justin S. Sadhu, MD, MPHS, FACC

Associate Professor of Medicine
Department of Internal Medicine
Cardiovascular Division
Washington University School of
    Medicine
St. Louis, Missouri

Mustafa Husaini, MD, FACC

Assistant Professor of Medicine
Department of Internal Medicine
Cardiovascular Division
Washington University School of
    Medicine
St. Louis, Missouri

Dominique S. Williams, MD

Assistant Professor of Medicine
Department of Internal Medicine
Cardiovascular Division
Washington University School of
    Medicine
St. Louis, Missouri

Executive Editor

Thomas M. Ciesielski, MD

Associate Professor of Medicine
Department of Internal Medicine
Division of General Medicine
Washington University School of
    Medicine
St. Louis, Missouri

(⊞). Wolters Kluwer

Philadelphia • Baltimore • New York • London
Buenos Aires • Hong Kong • Sydney • Tokyo

Acquisitions Editor: Joe Cho
Development Editor: Ariel S. Winter
Editorial Coordinator: Anthony Gonzalez
Marketing Manager: Kirsten Watrud
Production Project Manager: Barton Dudlick/Alicia Jackson
Manager, Graphic Arts and Design: Stephen Druding
Senior Manufacturing Coordinator: Beth Welsh
Prepress Vendor: S4Carlisle Publishing Services

Fourth edition

9 8 7 6 5 4 3 2

Printed in the United States of America.

Library of Congress Cataloging-in-Publication Data

ISBN-13: 978-1-975113-36-0

ISBN-10: 1-975113-36-5

Cataloging in Publication data available on request from publisher.

---

shop.lww.com

SHER1023

Contributing Authors

Homaa Ahmad, MD
Assistant Professor of Medicine
Cardiovascular Division

Adefolakemi Babatunde, MD
Fellow (Graduated)
Cardiovascular Division

Richard G. Bach, MD, FACC
Professor of Medicine
Cardiovascular Division

Andrew E. Berdy, MD
Fellow (Graduated)
Cardiovascular Division

J. Ernesto Betancourt, MD
Fellow (Graduated)
Cardiovascular Division

Anita R. Bhandiwad, MD, FACC
Associate Professor of Medicine
Cardiovascular Division

Ankit K. Bhatia, MD
Fellow (Graduated)
Cardiovascular Division

Alan C. Braverman, MD, FACC
Professor of Medicine
Cardiovascular Division

Angela L. Brown, MD
Professor of Medicine
Cardiovascular Division

Murali M. Chakinala, MD
Professor of Medicine
Division of Pulmonary and Critical Care
  Medicine

Rahul A. Chhana, MD
Fellow (Graduated)
Cardiovascular Division

Courtney D. Chrisler, MD
Assistant Professor of Medicine
Division of Infectious Diseases

Daniel H. Cooper, MD
Associate Professor of Medicine
Cardiovascular Division

Sharon Cresci, MD, FACC
Associate Professor of Medicine
Cardiovascular Division

Brittany M. Dixon, MD
Fellow (Graduated)
Cardiovascular Division

Mitchell N. Faddis, MD, PhD, FACC
Professor of Medicine
Cardiovascular Division

Nathan L. Frogge, MD
Fellow (Graduated)
Cardiovascular Division

Amulya Gampa, MD
Fellow (Graduated)
Cardiovascular Division

Rugheed Ghadban, MD
Assistant Professor of Medicine
Cardiovascular Division

Marye J. Gleva, MD, FACC
Professor of Medicine
Cardiovascular Division

Mark Gdowski, MD
Fellow (Graduated)
Cardiovascular Division

Chirayu Gor, MD, FACC
Fellow (Graduated)
Cardiovascular Division

Robert J. Gropler, MD, FACC
Professor of Radiology and Medicine
Cardiovascular Division
Radiological Sciences Division

J. Gmerice Hammond, MD
Instructor in Medicine
Cardiovascular Division

Justin Hartupee, MD, PhD
Assistant Professor of Medicine
Cardiovascular Division

Mustafa Husaini, MD, FACC
Assistant Professor of Medicine
Cardiovascular Division

Sudhir K. Jain, MD, FACC
Associate Professor of Medicine
Cardiovascular Division

Andrew M. Kates, MD, FACC
Professor of Medicine
Cardiovascular Division

Benjamin Kopecky, MD, PhD
Instructor in Medicine
Cardiovascular Division

Anandita Agarwala Kulkarni, MD
Fellow (Graduated)
Cardiovascular Division

Howard I. Kurz, MD, MSE, FACC
Professor of Medicine
Cardiovascular Division

John Lasala, MD, PhD, FACC, MSCAI
Professor of Medicine
Cardiovascular Division

Kory J. Lavine, MD, PhD
Associate Professor of Medicine
Cardiovascular Division

Daniel J. Lenihan, MD, FACC
Professor of Medicine
Cardiovascular Division

Kathryn J. Lindley, MD, FACC
Associate Professor of Medicine
Cardiovascular Division

Zainab Mahmoud, MD
Instructor in Medicine
Cardiovascular Division

Majesh Makan, MD, FACC, FASE
Professor of Medicine
Cardiovascular Division

Sonakshi Manjunath, MD
Resident
Internal Medicine

Manuel Rivera Maza, MD
Fellow
Cardiovascular Division

Krasimira M. Mikhova, MD
Fellow
Cardiovascular Division

Joshua D. Mitchell, MD, FACC
Assistant Professor of Medicine
Cardiovascular Division

Jonathan D. Moreno, MD, PhD, FACC
Assistant Professor of Medicine
Cardiovascular Division

Michael E. Nassif, MD
Fellow (Graduated)
Cardiovascular Division

Amit Noheria, MD
Assistant Professor of Medicine
Cardiovascular Division

Geoffrey Joseph Orme, DO
Fellow (Graduated)
Cardiovascular Division

Jiafu Ou, MD
Associate Professor of Medicine
Cardiovascular Division

Nishath Quader, MD, FACC
Associate Professor of Medicine
Cardiovascular Division

Tarun Ramayya, MD
Fellow
Cardiovascular Division

Michael W. Rich, MD, FACC
Professor of Medicine
Cardiovascular Division

Elizabeth M. Riddell, MD
Fellow (Graduated)
Cardiovascular Division

Justin S. Sadhu, MD, MPHS, FACC
Associate Professor of Medicine
Cardiovascular Division

Joel D. Schilling, MD, PhD
Associate Professor of Medicine,
Immunology/Pathology
Cardiovascular Division

Thomas H. Schindler, MD
Professor of Radiology and Medicine
Cardiovascular Division
Nuclear Medicine Division

David B. Schwartz, MD, PhD, FACC
Associate Professor of Medicine
Cardiovascular Division

Lynne M. Seacord, MD, FACC
Associate Professor of Medicine
Cardiovascular Division

Adam Shpigel, MD, FACC
Fellow (Graduated)
Cardiovascular Division

Jasvindar Singh, MD, FACC
Associate Professor of Medicine
Cardiovascular Division

Marc Sintek, MD
Associate Professor of Medicine
Cardiovascular Division

Timothy W. Smith, DPhil, MD, FACC, FHRS
Professor of Medicine
Cardiovascular Division

Nishtha Sodhi, MD
Fellow (Graduated)
Cardiovascular Division

Sandeep S. Sodhi, MD, MBA
Assistant Professor of Medicine
Cardiovascular Division

Curtis M. Steyers III, MD
Fellow (Graduated)
Cardiovascular Division

Sangita Sudharshan, MD
Fellow (Graduated)
Cardiovascular Division

Suraj Sunder, MD
Fellow (Graduated)
Division of Pulmonology and Critical Care
   Medicine

Prashanth D. Thakker, MD
Assistant Professor of Medicine
Cardiovascular Division

Manoj Thangam, MD
Fellow (Graduated)
Cardiovascular Division

Justin M. Vader, MD, FACC
Associate Professor of Medicine
Cardiovascular Division

Hannah Wey, MD
Fellow
Cardiovascular Division

Dominique S. Williams, MD
Assistant Professor of Medicine
Cardiovascular Division

Jonathan D. Wolfe, MD
Fellow
Pulmonary and Critical Care Medicine

Natasha K. Wolfe, MD
Fellow (Graduated)
Cardiovascular Division

Erica Young, MD
Instructor in Medicine
Cardiovascular Division

Alan Zajarias, MD, FACC
Professor of Medicine
Cardiovascular Division

Kathleen W. Zhang, MD
Assistant Professor of Medicine
Cardiovascular Division

Department Chair's Note

It is a pleasure to present the latest edition of *The Washington Manual*® Subspecialty Consult Series: *Cardiology Subspecialty Consult*. This pocket-size book and online resource continues to be an excellent reference for medical students, interns, residents, and other practitioners who need ready access to practical clinical information to diagnose and treat patients with a wide variety of cardiovascular disorders. Medical knowledge continues to increase at an astounding rate, which creates a challenge for physicians to practice evidence-based medicine and keep up with new biomedical discoveries, novel therapeutics, and guidelines that can positively impact patient outcomes. *The Washington Manual*® Subspecialty Consult Series addresses this challenge by concisely and practically providing current scientific and clinical practice information to aid physicians and other clinical providers in the diagnosis, investigation, and treatment of cardiovascular diseases.

I want to personally thank the authors, who include house officers, fellows, and attendings at the Washington University School of Medicine and Barnes-Jewish Hospital. Their commitment to patient care and education is unsurpassed, and their efforts and skill in compiling this manual are evident in the quality of the final product. In particular, I would like to acknowledge our editors, Drs. Justin S. Sadhu, Mustafa Husaini, and Dominique S. Williams, and executive editor, Dr. Thomas M. Ciesielski, who have worked tirelessly to produce another outstanding edition of this manual. I believe this *Manual* will meet its desired goal of providing timely and practical knowledge that can be directly applied at the bedside and in outpatient settings to improve patient care.

Victoria J. Fraser, MD
Adolphus Busch Professor of Medicine
Chair, Department of Medicine
Washington University School of Medicine
St. Louis, Missouri

Preface

It is our great pleasure to present the fourth edition of *The Washington Manual™ Cardiology Subspecialty Consult*. Since the publication of the third edition of this text, the field of cardiovascular medicine has experienced rapid advances in many areas. The fourth edition has been thoroughly revised to reflect these updates and also includes new chapters on hypertension, cardio-oncology, cardiac amyloidosis, left ventricular assist devices and heart transplantation, and cardiovascular disease in women and pregnancy. This portable text is filled with high-impact information regarding the pathophysiology, evaluation, and management of common cardiovascular conditions, presented in a bulleted format with clear tables and figures to make it easy to find the information you need. We hope you will find this manual a very useful and trusted resource in the care of your patients and a valuable addition to your professional library.

We would like to extend special thanks to the editors of the prior editions, Drs. Peter Crawford, Phillip Cuculich, and Andy Kates. In addition, we express our deepest gratitude to the current and former Washington University School of Medicine faculty and fellows who generously contributed their expertise and enthusiasm to the present edition.

Finally, we thank you, the readers, for selecting our book. It is our sincere desire that this text will aid you in our common mission to heal, one heart at a time.

Justin S. Sadhu, MD, MPHS, FACC
Mustafa Husaini, MD, FACC
Dominique S. Williams, MD

Contents

Rating Scheme for the Strength of the Recommendations

Class I (Benefit >>> Risk): Recommendations are strong and indicate that the treatment, procedure, or intervention is useful and effective and should be performed or administered for most patients under most circumstances.

Class II: Recommendations are not as strong, denoting a lower degree of benefit in proportion to risk.

Class IIa (Benefit >> Risk): Benefit is generally greater than risk.

Class IIb (Benefit ≥ Risk): Benefit marginally exceeds risk. Implementation should be selective and based on careful consideration of individual patient factors and, for invasive procedures, available expertise.

Class III (Benefit = Risk or Risk > Benefit): Actions are specifically not recommended, either because studies have found no evidence of benefit or because the intervention causes harm.

Rating Scheme for the Strength of the Evidence

Level of Evidence A: High-quality, concordant evidence from more than one adequately powered randomized controlled trial, meta-analyses of high-quality trials, or randomized controlled trial data corroborated by high-quality registry or practice-based studies.

Level of Evidence B: Moderate-quality or less convincing evidence based on one or more trials, meta-analyses of moderate-quality studies, or data derived exclusively from registries or other sources that have not been externally validated.

Level of Evidence C: Firm scientific support for the recommendation is not available, with recommendation based on limited data or a consensus of expert opinion.

Reference

Halperin JL, Levine GN, Al-Khatib SM, et al. Further evolution of the ACC/AHA clinical practice guideline recommendation classification system: a report of the American College of Cardiology/American Heart Association Task Force on Clinical Practice Guidelines. *Circulation.* 2016;133:1426-28.

Approach to the Cardiovascular Consult

Amulya Gampa and Andrew M. Kates

GENERAL PRINCIPLES

- Consultative cardiology affords the opportunity to integrate physiology with physical examination skills in the setting of rapidly developing procedures and techniques, to practice evidence-based medicine in a constantly advancing technological environment, and, most importantly, to make a significant difference for the patient and the patient's family.
- In approaching the patient with potential cardiac issues, it is important to understand the role of the consultant in this process—that is, to know what makes a "good" and effective consultant.
- To help with this, we have taken the liberty to adapt Goldman's "Ten Commandments[1] for effective consultation" for the cardiologist:
  1. **Determine the question:** Establishing what question the referring physician wishes to be answered is critical when receiving a consult. Examples include: "What is this patient's perioperative risk for cardiac events?" "Does this patient require testing for ischemia?" "How should this elevated troponin be evaluated?" This will help the consultant give more appropriate and useful recommendations.
  2. **Establish urgency:** Understanding the patient acuity and the referring team's need for cardiology assistance will ultimately lead to the best care for the patient. It is the consultant's job to triage consults in this way and see critical patients as soon as possible, as these patients often require procedures such as cardiac catheterization or other urgent testing. Arranging procedures quickly and efficiently can help improve outcomes and avoid adverse events.
  3. **Review the data:** Obtaining pertinent information regarding the patient's course from the referring team is important. However, it is equally as vital for the consultant to review the data personally—the consultant may be able to pick up nuances in the history or objective data that may have otherwise been missed or not conveyed by the referring team. This means personally obtaining relevant patient history and examining the patient. One must also review the ECG, echocardiogram images, catheterization films, and other imaging studies if available. Oftentimes, there are subtleties in the primary images that are not detailed in the procedure report that may impact patient management.
  4. **Be brief:** Including the necessary detail about a patient's cardiac history and medical care is essential, but there is no need to repeat what the primary team already knows. Physicians are busy. Referring teams have a lot to do in caring for their multiple patients and will most benefit from succinct recommendations from the consultant. Short, but precise recommendations are best.
  5. **Be specific:** Providing recommendations that are easily readable, understandable, and unlikely to be misinterpreted is always appreciated. Just as recommendations should be short, they should also be specific. It is often helpful to include a problem list and/or differential diagnosis, followed by specific recommendations. For example, one should replace "start low-dose metoprolol" with "start metoprolol tartrate 12.5 mg twice daily." This can be extremely helpful, especially when the referring team is less familiar with cardiac medications and procedures.

6. **Provide a contingency plan:** Anticipating changes in status and providing a plan in case the initial recommendations do not work or no longer apply is important, as hospitalized patients often have cardiac conditions that are changing or unstable. The consultant's initial recommendations are, naturally, most applicable at the time the patient was seen, but things often change. For example, when providing recommendations for rate control in a patient with atrial fibrillation, a contingency plan explaining to increase the dose of β-blocker or switch to an IV drug can be immensely helpful. Such plans can decrease delays in care and save the consultant from repeat calls for additional recommendations.

7. **Understand your role:** Providing recommendations without actively managing the patient themselves is the commonly accepted convention for inpatient consultation. However, the referring team may at times prefer the consulting team place their own orders or may need help ordering tests when unsure how to do so. Surgical teams more often prefer this "co-management" approach to patient care.[2,3] The consultant's role should be specified and agreed upon by both sides during the initial discussion.

8. **Teach if possible:** Teaching when relaying recommendations can be helpful, when appropriate, for several reasons. What may seem obvious to the consultant may be new to the referring physician. This does not have to be teaching about a unique patient or presentation. This could be as simple as clarifying a normal or abnormal troponin level.

9. **Talk to the team:** Speaking with the team when relaying recommendations is a great way to answer any follow-up questions and discuss details that would have taken much longer to describe in a note. Moreover, a phone call or in-person conversation can help build professional relationships.

10. **Follow-up:** Making follow-up recommendations based on changes in patient status, providing clear communication when "signing off," and scheduling a follow-up appointment if necessary are important components to providing optimal consultative services.

- **Critical questions** that should be answered as quickly as possible, especially in assessing a patient who may be critically ill include:
  - Why is the patient being seen?
  - What is the patient's primary problem (often distinct from the previous)?
  - How stable is the patient, and what are their vital signs right now?
  - Where is the patient right now (home, clinic, patient testing, emergency department, ward, operating room, holding area, or intensive care unit [ICU])?
  - How long has the problem been present?
  - What are the important examination findings?
  - What does the ECG show?
  - The answers to these questions will help triage patients to be seen sooner rather than later. Unstable vital signs (hypotension, tachycardia, bradycardia, hypoxia), signs of cardiogenic shock (cool extremities, altered mental status, low urine output), and active chest pain not responding to medication are all signs of potential critical illness requiring rapid evaluation and treatment.
- **Next, start to collect relevant data:**
  - What is the patient's laboratory data?
  - What medications is the patient on?
  - What does the ECG show? The echo? The stress test or heart catheterization?
- Finally, consider the following issues when the patient is evaluated:
  - What diagnostic study, procedure, or therapeutic (medical or surgical) intervention is appropriate for this patient?
  - How soon does this patient need it?
  - Where does this patient need to be now (e.g., floor, ICU) to best receive care?

DIAGNOSIS

- After obtaining the relevant history, performing a focused examination, and reviewing available data, workup can begin. Often, this involves recommendations for diagnostic testing. As the consultant, one must make sure to specify the type of test as clearly as possible (if the consultant is not ordering the test themselves) and make sure to follow up the results to guide treatment.
- A diagnosis of the patient's cardiac pathology can often be made in the first few patient encounters.
- The consultant's ability to rapidly determine diagnosis and treatment will develop with knowledge and experience. We hope that this book will serve as a valuable resource for consultant physicians as they care for patients in the myriad clinical situations likely to be encountered.

TREATMENT

Once a diagnosis has been made, treatment can be recommended—in the form of lifestyle changes, medication, therapeutic procedures, or surgery. Once again, being as specific and succinct as possible, as well as closing the loop with the primary team, will ensure the patient receives the best care.

A BRIEF DISCLAIMER

Inherent in providing an opinion is an understanding of one's limitations. Although this book may serve as a thorough, useful review of several areas in cardiology—ranging from common clinical presentations, to acute coronary syndromes, to the many faces of heart failure, as well as issues in electrophysiology, valvular disease, and many places in between—it is by no means a substitute for reading the primary literature, reviewing published guidelines, amassing clinical experience, or undertaking advanced cardiology training. To quote Hippocrates: "As to diseases, make a habit of two things—to help, or at least to do no harm."

REFERENCES

1. Goldman L, Lee T, Rudd P. Ten commandments for effective consultations. *Arch Intern Med.* 1983;143:1753-5.
2. Pearson SD. Principles of generalist-specialist relationships. *J Gen Intern Med.* 1999;14(Suppl 1):S13-20.
3. Salerno SM, Hurst FP, Halvorson S, Mercado DL. Principles of effective consultation: an update for the 21st-century consultant. *Arch Intern Med.* 2007;167:271-5.

Cardiovascular Physical Examination

2

Ankit K. Bhatia and Justin M. Vader

GENERAL PRINCIPLES

- The physical examination is fundamental to the assessment and management of patients with known or suspected cardiovascular disease.
- Studies suggest that physicians' physical diagnostic skills have deteriorated over time as the scope of diagnostic technologies has increased.
- This chapter reviews the importance of physical examination findings in the diagnosis and management of cardiovascular disease and the context and evidence for their use.
- Physical examination findings are rapidly obtained data and may independently have modest effects on disease likelihood, but, in aggregate, strongly influence clinical diagnosis.

GENERAL PHYSICAL EXAMINATION AND CARDIOVASCULAR DISEASE

- Overall appearance
  - Age, sex, and body habitus are important variables impacting cardiovascular disease risk and significantly influence first impressions of disease likelihood.
  - Generalized distress findings such as agitation, diaphoresis, and nausea/vomiting may suggest states of high sympathetic or vagal tone, potentially portending worse pathology and prognosis.
  - Stigmata of past interventions such as sternotomy scars, pacemaker or implantable cardioverter-defibrillator, vascular access scars, and fistulae are useful, particularly in patients with limited ability to provide history.
  - Cardiovascular pathology is common in a variety of disease syndromes with characteristic examination findings (Table 2-1).
- Ophthalmologic examination
  - A variety of metabolic derangements manifest in corneal, palpebral, and retinal pathology that share associations with cardiovascular disease.
  - **Corneal arcus** is predictive of cardiovascular disease mainly due to association with increasing age.[1,2]
  - **Xanthelasma palpebrarum** suggests underlying hyperlipidemia.[3]
  - **Diabetic retinopathy**
    - Progression from mild disease (dot-blot hemorrhage, hard exudates, and microaneurysms) to moderate disease ("cotton-wool" spots) to severe disease (neovascularization)
    - Retinopathy, particularly advanced, is associated with increased cardiovascular events, stroke, and heart failure.[4-6]
  - **Hypertensive retinopathy** is predictive of coronary heart disease. However, routine fundoscopy does not appear to yield additional value in the management of chronic hypertension.[7]
- Skin and extremities
  - Edema
    - Common but nonspecific examination finding resulting from the net movement of fluid from the intravascular space to the interstitium

TABLE 2-1 SYNDROMIC PHYSICAL FINDINGS AND ASSOCIATED CARDIOVASCULAR DISEASE

Condition	Physical findings	Cardiovascular manifestations
Marfan syndrome	Pectus deformity, arm span > height, leg length > torso, pes planus, scoliosis, wrist sign, thumb sign	Bicuspid aortic valve, MVP, aortic aneurysm
Ehlers–Danlos syndrome	Hyperextensible skin, joint hypermobility, atrophic scars, velvety skin, high arching palate	Dysautonomia, MVP, aortic dissection (less than Marfan syndrome)
Loeys–Dietz syndrome	Similar to Marfan plus hypertelorism, bifid uvula	Bicuspid aortic valve, MVP, aortic aneurysm
Turner syndrome	Shield chest, webbed neck, short stature, female	Bicuspid aortic valve, aortic coarctation, anomalous pulmonary venous return
Noonan syndrome	Short stature, pectus excavatum, webbed neck	Pulmonic stenosis, ASD, VSD
LEOPARD syndrome	Multiple lentigines, hypertelorism, short stature, cryptorchidism	Left ventricular hypertrophy, PS, coronary artery dilatation
Fabry disease	Angiokeratomas, corneal clouding, anhidrosis/hyperhidrosis	Hypertension, cardiomyopathy
Down syndrome	Epicanthal fold, small chin, macroglossia, flat nasal bridge, single palmar crease, Brushfield spots	Endocardial cushion defects in 40%, VSD only in 30%

ASD, atrial septal defect; MVP, mitral valve prolapse; PS, pulmonic stenosis; VSD, ventricular septal defect.

- In addition to elevated venous pressures, low-oncotic states, capillary leak, or impaired lymphatic drainage may cause edema.
- The most common cause of bilateral leg edema is venous insufficiency, affecting 25% to 30% of the general population.[8]
- Assess jugular venous pulse (JVP) to determine if right atrial pressure is elevated
- Assess for stigmata of liver disease, nephrotic syndrome, and venous insufficiency. True anasarca is rare in heart failure.
  - Nail bed findings
    - **Capillary refill time and nail bed pallor** have limited reliability due to estimates of volume depletion and high interobserver variability in adults.[9]
    - **Digital clubbing** is present in a variety of disorders, including cyanotic congenital heart diseases.
      - Defined by nail fold angle >180 degrees, distal phalangeal depth > proximal depth, and Schamroth sign

□ Inspection of all digits for differential signs of clubbing and cyanosis may suggest the presence of vascular abnormalities, such as patent ductus arteriosus (PDA).
- Cutaneous manifestations of specific cardiovascular diseases include[10]:
  - Endocarditis: Janeway lesions, subungual splinter hemorrhages, and Osler nodes
  - Cholesterol emboli syndrome: livedo reticularis
  - Amyloidosis: waxy papular rash or "pinch purpura"
  - Family hyperlipidemia: Achilles tendon xanthoma
- **Pulmonary**
  - Respiratory rate and pattern
    - May reflect increased minute ventilation requirements to compensate for metabolic acidosis or a central response to physiologic stress or pain
    - **Respiratory failure** requiring positive pressure ventilation is a common presentation (3-5% of patients) in decompensated heart failure.[11]
    - **Cheyne–Stokes periodic breathing** during sleep is common in congestive heart failure (CHF), with a prevalence of 30% even in optimized outpatients.[12]
  - Auscultation
    - Most pertinently focused on crackles or wheezes
    - **Crackles** suggest pulmonary edema and are moderately predictive of heart failure in emergency department patients with dyspnea.[13]
    - Cardiogenic pulmonary edema implies a pulmonary capillary wedge pressure (PCWP) of >24 mm Hg in acute heart failure or >30 mm Hg in chronic heart failure.[14-16] Pulmonary edema requires higher pressures in chronic versus acute heart failure due to hypertrophy of lymphatics draining the lungs.[17]
    - **Wheezing** may result from pulmonary edema (cardiac asthma), in addition to its more common association with obstructive lung disease.[18]
  - Percussion, fremitus, and chest expansion
    - Asymmetry of percussion, tactile fremitus, and chest expansion are useful in detecting **pleural effusions**.[19]
    - Pleural effusions are a common finding in heart failure and may be bilateral or unilateral (more often right predominant).
    - Postcardiac injury syndrome with pleural and pericardial effusions may result from acute myocardial infarction (MI), cardiac surgery, or other cardiac trauma.
  - Positional breathlessness within 30 seconds bending forward (termed *bendopnea*) is suggestive of elevated cardiac filling pressures.[20]
- **Abdomen**: focused on the liver and intra-abdominal vascular structures
  - **Hepatomegaly** may be the result of chronically elevated right-sided cardiac and central venous pressures.
  - A pulsatile, enlarged liver suggests severe tricuspid regurgitation (TR).
  - **Ascites** may result from passive hepatic congestion in the setting of elevated right-sided pressures or right ventricular (RV) dysfunction. Restrictive or constrictive physiology should also be considered in the presence of cardiac ascites.

EXAMINATION OF THE ARTERIAL PULSES

- Pulse characterization
  - Assess pulse contour, timing, strength, volume, size, and symmetry, in addition to auscultation for bruits
  - A basic sequenced approach includes brachial, radial, femoral, popliteal, dorsalis pedis, and posterior tibialis.
  - Changes in the peripheral pulse contour may reflect aortic pathology, changes in cardiac output, or changes in arteriovenous (AV) synchrony (Figure 2-1).[21]

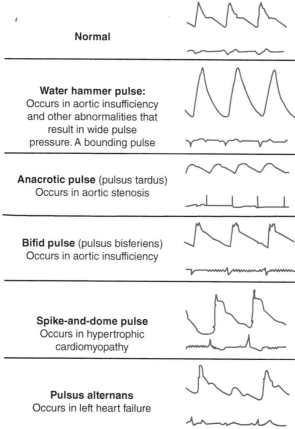

Normal

Water hammer pulse:
Occurs in aortic insufficiency
and other abnormalities that
result in wide pulse
pressure. A bounding pulse

Anacrotic pulse (pulsus tardus)
Occurs in aortic stenosis

Bifid pulse (pulsus bisferiens)
Occurs in aortic insufficiency

Spike-and-dome pulse
Occurs in hypertrophic
cardiomyopathy

Pulsus alternans
Occurs in left heart failure

FIGURE 2-1. Arterial pulse. (Adapted from Judge RD, Zuidema GD, Fitzgerald FT. *Clinical Diagnosis*. 5th ed. Little, Brown; 1989:258.)

○ **Pulse duration** reflects stroke volume in normal individuals and in patients with heart failure.
  ▪ In heart failure, pulse duration is abbreviated.
  ▪ In aortic stenosis (AS), prolonged ejection reflects worsening severity of stenosis.
  ▪ Slow-pulse rise (**pulsus tardus**) in either carotid[22] or radial[23] arteries is suggestive of severe AS.
○ **Pulsus alternans** is a common finding in severe left ventricular (LV) dysfunction.
○ **Bisferiens (biphasic) pulse** may suggest aortic regurgitation (AR), hypertrophic cardiomyopathy, or sepsis.
○ Pulse inequality or pulse delay may be important clues to aortic or large branch vessel pathology, such as aneurysm, dissection, or coarctation.
  ▪ Radial-to-radial delay suggests subclavian stenosis.
  ▪ Radial-to-femoral delay suggests aortic coarctation.
○ Dorsalis pedis pulses are absent in up to 3% of the population.[24]
○ **Allen test** for ulnar artery patency

- Routinely performed before radial artery cannulation or harvest
- Patient holds an elevated and clenched fist for 30 seconds with compression applied by examiner to the ulnar and radial pulses.
- After release of the ulnar pulse, this test is highly sensitive for a nonfunctional ulnar artery if color fails to return to digits at 3 seconds and is nearly 100% sensitive at 5 seconds.[25]
  - Abdominal palpation for the presence of an aortic aneurysm is a highly sensitive finding for large aneurysms (particularly if >4 cm in size) in patients at risk.[26]
- Arterial bruits
  - Best heard by examination in a quiet room with light pressure on the stethoscope using diaphragm or bell
  - Carotid bruit
    - Confers a fourfold increase in risk for transient ischemic attack (TIA) and doubles the risk for both stroke and cardiovascular death[27,28]
    - Absent in one-third of symptomatic carotid stenosis and is less common in critical carotid stenosis[29]
  - Abdominal bruits
    - May be present in patients with renovascular hypertension (e.g., renal artery stenosis, fibromuscular dysplasia)
    - Common in normal individuals of all ages[30]
    - Presence of both diastolic *and* systolic bruits is highly specific for renovascular disease.[31]
  - Iliac (periumbilical area), femoral, and popliteal arteries
    - May be detected in patients with known or suspected vascular disease
    - Even in an asymptomatic patient, femoral bruit is suggestive of peripheral vascular disease.[32]

BLOOD PRESSURE MEASUREMENT

- Use proper technique to avoid common errors (Table 2-2).
- Clinically significant blood pressure (BP) measurements
  - **Pulsus paradoxus**
    - >10 mm Hg inspiratory decrease in systolic blood pressure (SBP)
    - Inflate the cuff to 20 mm Hg above the measured SBP. Decrease pressure very gradually while watching the patient breathe.
      - Pulsus is the difference in SBP between where sounds are heard in expiration only and where sounds are heard in both inspiration and expiration.
      - Simultaneous evaluation of pulse oximeter waveform (on same arm as BP cuff) can reveal pulsus: pressure difference between seeing waveform in expiration only versus both inspiration/expiration.
    - May be observed in a variety of conditions, including cardiac tamponade, pericardial constriction (generally effusive-constrictive), myocardial restriction (rare), pulmonary embolism, cardiogenic shock, acute MI, and tension pneumothorax
    - Pulsus paradoxus >12 mm Hg is highly sensitive and moderately specific for **pericardial tamponade** in the setting of pericardial effusion.[33]
  - Pulse pressure (PP) and proportional pulse pressure (PPP)
    - PP reflects the interaction between stroke volume and arterial resistance.
    - $PP = SBP - \text{diastolic BP}$
    - $PPP = PP/SBP$
  - PP is narrow with low stroke volume and in AS.
  - PP is wide in high-output distributive states (e.g., sepsis, pregnancy, anemia, thyrotoxicosis, and AV fistula), chronic AR, aortic dissection, elevated intracranial pressure, and with increased vascular stiffness.

TABLE 2-2	NATIONAL KIDNEY FOUNDATION'S KIDNEY DISEASE OUTCOMES QUALITY INITIATIVE (NKF KDOQI) GUIDELINES FOR BP MEASUREMENT

1. Patient should rest 5 minutes in chair with back supported and bare arm at heart level.
2. Blood pressure bladder cuff should encircle at least 80% circumference of middle of upper arm. If arm >41 cm circumference, consider forearm.
3. Bell of stethoscope should be 2 cm above antecubital fossa.
4. Inflate the cuff to 30 mm Hg above palpated SBP. Deflate at 3 mm Hg per second.
5. Errors: cuff too small (overestimates BP), cuff too large (underestimates BP), incorrect patient position, rapid cuff deflation, monitor not kept at eye level, inadequate premeasurement rest

BP, blood pressure; SBP, systolic blood pressure.

- ○ Narrow PP is seen in heart failure and is associated with worse prognosis.[34]
- ○ PPP may be used to estimate cardiac index, with a PPP <25% indicating index <2.2 L/min/m^2.[35]
- ○ BP and pulse inequalities
  - Unequal upper extremity BPs are common in the general population with a 20% prevalence of SBP difference >10 mm Hg.[36]
  - Obstructive disease is unlikely unless differences are large (>40 mm Hg) and consistent.[37]
  - While marked arm–arm or arm–leg differences in BP may be useful in identifying acute aortic dissection, the prevalence in a large registry of dissection was quite low (<20%).[38]
  - Aortic coarctation is an uncommon secondary cause of hypertension in adults. Consider when >20 mm Hg differential between arm and leg SBP.

JUGULAR VENOUS PRESSURE ESTIMATES

- Proper technique is essential (Table 2-3).
- May be distinguished from carotid pulsation by the following:
  - ○ Biphasic contour
  - ○ Respiratory and positional variation
  - ○ Disappearance with proximal occlusion
- Distance from the sternal angle to mid-right atrium is 5 cm with the patient at 0 degree and increases to 8 to 9 cm with partial upright posture.
- JVP >3 cm above the sternal angle indicates elevated right atrial pressure.[39]
- External jugular vein examination can be highly reliable even in a critically ill population and may be superior to internal jugular vein observation.[40]
- Accurate measurement can be confounded in the setting of TR (prominent vs. waves).
- Conversion of cm H_2O to mm Hg is 1.36 to 1.

JUGULAR VENOUS WAVEFORMS

- Waveforms are presented in Figure 2-2.
- Clinically useful in the assessment of a number of conditions, including **constriction, tamponade, AV dyssynchrony, and RV infarction**
- The basic components of the waveform are as follows:
  - ○ A wave: atrial contraction—absent in atrial fibrillation, elevated with decreased RV compliance or tricuspid stenosis, "cannon" waves with AV dyssynchrony

TABLE 2-3 ASSESSING JUGULAR VENOUS PULSE

1. Observe the patient's right internal and external jugular veins by standing on patient's right with tangential light falling across the neck. Often easiest to observe looking along the surface of the sternocleidomastoid muscle.
2. Rotate patient neck to left 30–45 degrees and avoid over rotation.
3. Observe rise and fall of venous pulse throughout the respiratory cycle.
4. Occlude the venous pulse proximally to differentiate carotid and jugular contours.
5. Move the patient from 0- to 90-degree angle to discern maximal height of venous pulse. Traditionally, JVP estimate is conducted at 45-degree angle.
6. External jugular veins may be used if they show respiratory variation and expected venous contour.
7. Right atrial pressure in cm H_2O is estimated by adding 5 cm to vertical height of jugular pulse above the sternal angle of Lewis. Note: 1.36 cm H_2O = 1 mm Hg.

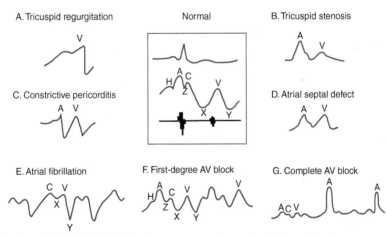

FIGURE 2-2. Pathologic jugular venous waveforms. AV, atrioventricular.

- ○ X descent: atrial relaxation—blunted in TR, prominent in tamponade
- ○ V wave: atrial venous filling against usually closed tricuspid valve—prominent in severe TR
- ○ Y descent: passive ventricular filling—prominent in constriction and restriction, blunted in tamponade

ABDOMINOJUGULAR (HEPATOJUGULAR) REFLUX

- Hold firm pressure on the right upper quadrant for 15 to 20 seconds while observing the jugular pulse wave.
- A positive test is defined as >3-cm rise in peak and trough of the wave sustained throughout the period of pressure.

- Manifests when RV cannot accommodate increased venous return, such as pericardial constriction, restriction, RV infarct, and LV failure with elevated PCWP
- Highly reproducible, and in dyspneic patients with heart failure, reliably suggests elevated PCWP and central venous pressure (CVP)[41]

CARDIAC PALPATION

- Place fingertips at the left second intercostal space (pulmonary artery), left sternal border (RV), and apex (LV).
- Normal finding: apical impulse is within 10 cm of midsternal line, <3 cm in diameter, and duration is <2/3 of systole.
- Noninvasive left ventricular ejection fraction (LVEF) estimate: sustained (2/3 systole) apical impulse palpation with nonpalpable S4 suggests LVEF <40%.[42]
- Left parasternal heave suggests RV hypertrophy.
- Palpable pulsation in the left second intercostal space suggests pulmonary hypertension.

CARDIAC AUSCULTATION

- Refer to Figure 2-3.
- Stethoscope
  - Diaphragm: High-pitched sounds: S1, S2, regurgitant murmurs, and pericardial rubs
  - Bell
    - Low-pitched sounds: S3, S4, and mitral stenosis (MS)
    - Firm pressure with the bell results in a functional change to a diaphragm.
- Normal heart sounds
  - S1 is produced by vibrations of mitral (M1) and tricuspid (T1) valve closure.
    - Intensity is increased in hypercontractile states, MS, with short PR interval.
    - Intensity is decreased in hypocontractile states, with long PR interval, and in acute AR.
    - Splitting results from late closure of tricuspid valve as in right bundle branch block and atrial septal defect (ASD).
  - S2 is produced by closure of aortic (A2) and pulmonic (P2) valve.
    - Aortic pressure normally exceeds pulmonary pressure; thus, A2 precedes P2 and is louder.
    - Increased intensity of A2 is heard in systemic hypertension.
    - Increased intensity of P2 is heard in pulmonary hypertension, accompanied by narrow inspiratory splitting.
    - Decreased S2 intensity seen in AS or pulmonic stenosis (PS).
  - Physiologic splitting of S2: as inspiration causes pulmonary capacitance to increase and LV preload to decrease, A2 occurs earlier and P2 occurs later.
  - Paradoxical splitting of S2 results when A2 occurs after P2 and inspiration, therefore, moves these sounds closer together.
    - Causes: left bundle branch block (LBBB), severe AS, or hypertrophic obstructive cardiomyopathy (HOCM) with LV outflow tract obstruction
    - Fixed splitting of S2 suggests the presence of an ASD or ventricular pacing.
- Gallops
  - S3 is produced by vibrations from the passive filling phase of ventricular diastole.
    - Left-sided S3 gallops are best heard at the apex using the bell with the patient in left lateral decubitus.
      - Specific for LV dysfunction/CHF in the acutely ill, dyspneic patient
      - Confers a worse prognosis in patients with a prior diagnosis of heart failure[13,43]
      - Indicative of severe regurgitation in the setting of AR, although an absent S3 does not exclude severe AR[44]

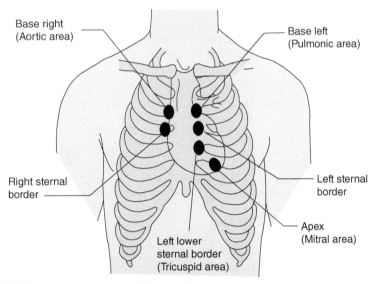

FIGURE 2-3. Cardinal auscultation positions.

- Right-sided S3 gallops are best heard at the lower left sternal border upon inspiration.
  - RV dysfunction with high RV filling pressures
  - May suggest acute pulmonary embolism in acutely ill patients
- **Physiologically normal S3 may be heard in young, athletic, or pregnant patients.**
  - S4 is produced by vibrations from the active filling phase of ventricular diastole.
    - Observed in conditions with decreased ventricular compliance in diastole, such as diastolic dysfunction
    - May indicate myocardial ischemia in the setting of acute chest pain
    - Will be absent in atrial fibrillation
- Ejection sounds
  - Heard around S1 and results from forceful LV ejection, rapid distension of either aorta or pulmonary artery, or with doming of either aortic or pulmonic valves
  - Heard in noncritical and noncalcific stenosis
  - Pulmonic ejection sounds are unique among right-sided heart sounds since they decrease in intensity during inspiration.
- Systolic clicks
  - Observed in valve prolapse—results from sudden tensing of elongated atrioventricular valve leaflets and chordae
  - Mitral valve prolapse (MVP)
    - High-pitched sound heard best with the diaphragm at apex or lower left sternal border in mid-to-late systole.
    - With the strain phase of Valsalva, the click of MVP intensifies and occurs earlier, then softens and occurs later with release.
    - This characteristic click is considered diagnostic for MVP.
    - The presence of a click in the absence of an MR murmur does not appear to be associated with a worse clinical outcome.[45]
- Murmurs
  - Systolic murmurs may be benign or pathologic. Diastolic murmurs are pathologic.

- Flow murmurs[46]
  - Grades 1 to 2 intensity
  - Left sternal border location
  - Follow a systolic ejection pattern
  - Associated with normal intensity, splitting of S2, and no other abnormal sounds or murmurs
  - Benign murmur for which echocardiographic evaluation is not indicated
- Early systolic murmurs
  - Related to ventricular ejection
  - Differential includes: AS, PS, MR, outflow tract obstruction
  - AS
    - Late peaking when associated with decreased intensity of S2 or slow rate of carotid rise[22]
    - Transmitted/radiation of sound to carotids
    - May also be heard as a musical apical (Gallavardin) murmur
    - Murmur intensity not necessarily associated with severity as it is deceptively reduced in patients with critical AS and decreased systolic function
  - PS
    - Left second intercostal space
    - Accentuated by inspiration
    - May be associated with a valve click or features of RV hypertrophy or failure
  - HOCM
    - Maneuvers that alter preload and afterload are useful in distinguishing HOCM from AS.
    - Murmur is less likely to radiate to carotids.
    - Murmur accentuates with Valsalva maneuver and with movement from squatting to standing (maneuvers that decrease preload).
- Holosystolic murmurs
  - Due to regurgitation across the atrioventricular valves or ventricular septal defect (VSD)
  - Mitral regurgitation
    - Holosystolic when ventricular pressure exceeds atrial pressure throughout systole
    - Radiation to the left axilla and back with anterior leaflet disruption and to the base with posterior leaflet disruption
    - Murmur intensity associated with severity of MR[47]
  - TR
    - Low pitched, sharply defined at the lower left sternal border
    - Difficult to detect with coincident MR
    - Inspiratory accentuation
  - VSD
    - Harsh, nonradiating, and associated with a palpable thrill
    - Louder at the left sternal border than at apex in acute VSD
    - Decreases in intensity and disappears in late systole as pulmonary hypertension develops, due to decreased left-to-right gradient[48]
- Diastolic clicks and murmurs
  - MS
  - Opening snap in early diastole
  - Brief high-pitched sound using diaphragm at the left sternal border
  - A2 to opening snap interval is not well correlated with valve area.[49]
- Early diastolic murmurs
  - AR
    - Blowing, decrescendo murmur at the sternal border

□ Accentuated by listening at end expiration with the patient sitting forward
□ Late diastolic rumbling murmur at the apex (Austin Flint murmur)
□ Often associated with systolic flow murmur due to increased stroke volume
- Pulmonic regurgitation
  □ Similar to the murmur of AR
  □ Distinguished by its accentuation with inspiration
○ Continuous murmurs
  - Most commonly systolic murmurs that carry over into diastole
  - The differential diagnosis includes PDA (pulmonic area), AV fistula, venous hum (e.g., jugular), and vascular stenotic lesions.
○ Pericardial rub
  - Suggestive of pericarditis
  - "Rough" sounding
  - Characteristically triphasic in patients who are in sinus rhythm, but either biphasic or monophasic in half of the cases[50]
  - Absence of a rub is not sufficient to exclude the diagnosis.[51]
○ Pericardial knock
  - Easily mistaken for the opening snap of MS
  - Best distinguished by the presence of the jugular venous findings of constrictive pericarditis

A SEQUENTIAL APPROACH

A systematic approach to the physical examination will improve diagnostic yield and accuracy. Such an approach is presented in Table 2-4.

TABLE 2-4	THE SEQUENTIAL APPROACH TO THE CARDIOVASCULAR EXAMINATION
1. Are right-sided cardiac pressures high?	Estimate jugular venous pressure
2. Can the right side handle volume?	Abdominojugular reflux Presence of right-sided S3
3. Is the right ventricle morphologically normal?	RV heave
4. Are pulmonary pressures high?	Loud P2 Narrowly split S2 TR murmur
5. Is left atrial pressure acutely high?	Crackles
6. Is LV function depressed?	Sustained apical impulse Nonpalpable S4 Short pulse duration Soft S1 Presence of S3
7. Is LV compliance impaired?	Presence of S4
8. Is systemic vascular resistance high?	Cool extremities

LV, left ventricular; RV, right ventricular; TR, tricuspid regurgitation.

REFERENCES

1. Fernandez AB, Keyes MJ, Penciana M, et al. Relation of corneal arcus to cardiovascular disease (from the Framingham Heart Study data set). *Am J Cardiol.* 2009;103(1):64-6.
2. Fernándeza A, Sorokina A, Thompson PD. Corneal arcus as coronary artery disease risk factor. *Atherosclerosis.* 2007;193:235-40.
3. Özdöl S, Sahin S, Tokgözoglu L. Xanthelasma palpebrarum and its relation to atherosclerotic risk factors and lipoprotein (a). *Int J Dermatol.* 2008;47:785-9.
4. Cheung N, Wang JJ, Klein R, et al. Diabetic retinopathy and the risk of coronary heart disease: the Atherosclerosis Risk in Communities Study. *Diabetes Care.* 2007;30:1742-6.
5. Cheung N, Rogers S, Couper DJ, et al. Is diabetic retinopathy an independent risk factor for ischemic stroke? *Stroke.* 2007;38:398-401.
6. Cheung N, Wang JJ, Rogers SL, et al. Diabetic retinopathy and risk of heart failure. *J Am Coll Cardiol.* 2008;51:1573-8.
7. van den Born BJ, Hulsman CA, Hoekstra JB, et al. Value of routine funduscopy in patients with hypertension: systematic review. *BMJ.* 2005;331:73-7.
8. Blankfield RP, Finkelhor RS, Alexander JJ, et al. Etiology and diagnosis of bilateral leg edema in primary care. *Am J Med.* 1998;105:192-7.
9. Lewin J, Maconochie I. Capillary refill time in adults. *Emerg Med J.* 2008;25:325-6.
10. Uliasz A, Lebwohl M. Cutaneous manifestations of cardiovascular diseases. *Clin Dermatol.* 2008;26:243-54.
11. Fonarow GC, Heywood JT, Heidenreich PA, et al. Temporal trends in clinical characteristics, treatments, and outcomes for heart failure hospitalizations, 2002 to 2004: findings from Acute Decompensated Heart Failure National Registry (ADHERE). *Am Heart J.* 2007;153:1021-8.
12. Hagenah G, Beil D. Prevalence of Cheyne–Stokes respiration in modern treated congestive heart failure. *Sleep Breath.* 2009;13:181-5.
13. Wang CS, FitzGerald JM, Schulzer M, et al. Does this dyspneic patient in the emergency department have congestive heart failure? *JAMA.* 2005;294:1944-56.
14. Mueller HS, Chatterjee K, Davis KB, et al. Present use of bedside right heart catheterization in patients with cardiac disease. *J Am Coll Cardiol.* 1998;32:P840-64.
15. Sprung CL, Rackow EC, Fein IA, et al. The spectrum of pulmonary edema: differentiation of cardiogenic, intermediate and non-cardiogenic forms of pulmonary edema. *Am Rev Respir Dis.* 1981;124:718-22.
16. McHugh TJ, Forrester J, Adler L, et al. Pulmonary vascular congestion in acute myocardial infarction: hemodynamic and radiologic correlations. *Ann Intern Med.* 1972;76:29-33.
17. Dumont AE, Clauss RH, Reed GE, et al. Lymph drainage in patients with congestive heart failure. Comparison with findings in hepatic cirrhosis. *N Engl J Med.* 1963;269:949-52.
18. Jorge S, Becquemin MH, Delerme S, et al. Cardiac asthma in elderly patients: incidence, clinical presentation and outcome. *BMC Cardiovasc Disord.* 2007;7:16.
19. Diaz-Guzman E, Budev MM. Accuracy of the physical examination in evaluating pleural effusion. *Clev Clin J Med.* 2008;75:297-303.
20. Thibodeau JT, Turer AT, Gualano SK, et al. Characterization of a novel symptom of advanced heart failure: bendopnea. *JACC Heart Fail.* 2014;2(1):24-31.
21. Judge RD, Zuidema GD, Fitzgerald FT. *Clinical Diagnosis.* 5th ed. Little, Brown; 1989:258.
22. Aronow WS, Kronzon I. Correlation of prevalence and severity of valvular aortic stenosis determined by continuous-wave Doppler echocardiography with physical signs of aortic stenosis in patients aged 62 to 100 years with aortic systolic ejection murmurs. *Am J Cardiol.* 1987;60:399-401.
23. Yoshioka N, Fujita Y, Yasukawa T, et al. Do radial arterial pressure curves have diagnostic validity for identify severe aortic stenosis? *J Anesth.* 2010;24:7-10.
24. Chavatzas D. Revision of the incidence of congenital absence of dorsalis pedis artery by an ultrasonic technique. *Anat Rec.* 1974;178:289-90.
25. Jarvis MA, Jarvis CL, Jones PR, et al. Reliability of Allen's test in selection of patients for radial artery harvest. *Ann Thorac Surg.* 2000;70:1362-5.
26. Lederle FA, Simel D. Does this patient have abdominal aortic aneurysm? *JAMA.* 1999;281:77-82.
27. Pickett CA, Jackson JL, Hemann BA, et al. Carotid bruits and cerebrovascular disease risk: a meta-analysis. *Stroke.* 2010;41:2295-302.
28. Pickett CA, Jackson JL, Hemann BA, et al. Carotid bruits as a prognostic indicator of cardiovascular death and myocardial infarction: a meta-analysis. *Lancet.* 2008;371:1587-94.

29. NASCET Collaborators. Beneficial effect of carotid endarterectomy in symptomatic patients with high-grade carotid stenosis. *N Engl J Med.* 1991;325:445-53.

30. Rivin AU. Abdominal vascular sounds. *JAMA.* 1972;221:688-90.

31. Grim CE, Luft FC, Weinberger MH, et al. Sensitivity and specificity of screening tests for renal vascular hypertension. *Ann Intern Med.* 1979;91:617-22.

32. Criqui MH, Fronek A, Klauber MR, et al. The sensitivity, specificity, and predictive value of traditional clinical evaluation of peripheral arterial disease: results from noninvasive testing in a defined population. *Circulation.* 1985;71:516-22.

33. Curtiss EI, Reddy PS, Uretsky BF, et al. Pulsus paradoxus: definition and relation to the severity of cardiac tamponade. *Am Heart J.* 1988;115:391-8.

34. Petrie CJ, Voors AA, van Veldhuisen DJ. Low pulse pressure is an independent predictor of mortality and morbidity in non ischaemic, but not in ischaemic advanced heart failure patients. *Int J Cardiol.* 2009;131:336-44.

35. Stevenson LW, Perloff JK. The limited reliability of physical signs for estimating hemodynamics in chronic heart failure. *JAMA.* 1989;261:884-8.

36. Clark CE, Campbell JL, Evans PH, et al. Prevalence and clinical implications of the inter-arm blood pressure difference: a systematic review. *J Hum Hypertens.* 2006;20:923-31.

37. Eguchi K, Yacoub M, Jhalani J, et al. Consistency of blood pressure differences between the left and right arms. *Arch Intern Med.* 2007;167:388-93.

38. Hagan PG, Nienaber CA, Isselbacher EM, et al. The International Registry of Acute Aortic Dissection (IRAD): new insights into an old disease. *JAMA.* 2000;283:897-903.

39. Seth R, Magner P, Matzinger F, et al. How far is the sternal angle from the mid-right atrium? *J Gen Intern Med.* 2002;17:852-6.

40. Vinayak AG, Levitt J, Gehlbach B, et al. Usefulness of the external jugular vein examination in detecting abnormal central venous pressure in critically ill patients. *Arch Intern Med.* 2006;166:2132-7.

41. Wiese J. The abdominojugular reflux sign. *Am J Med.* 2000;109:59-61.

42. Ranganathan N, Juma Z, Sivaciyan V. The apical impulse in coronary heart disease. *Clin Cardiol.* 1985;8:20-33.

43. Drazner MH, Rame JE, Stevenson LW, et al. Prognostic importance of elevated jugular venous pressure and a third heart sound in patients with heart failure. *N Engl J Med.* 2001;345:574-81.

44. Tribouilloy CM, Enriquez-Sarano M, Mohty D, et al. Pathophysiologic determinants of third heart sounds: a prospective clinical and Doppler echocardiographic study. *Am J Med.* 2001;111:96-102.

45. Etchells E, Bell C, Robb K. Does this patient have an abnormal systolic murmur? *JAMA.* 1997;277:564-71.

46. American College of Cardiology; American Heart Association Task Force on Practice Guidelines. ACC/AHA 2006 guidelines for the management of patients with valvular heart disease: a report of the American College of Cardiology/American Heart Association Task Force on Practice Guidelines. *J Am Coll Cardiol.* 2006;48:e1-148.

47. Desjardins VA, Enriquez-Sarano M, Tajik AJ, et al. Intensity of murmurs correlates with severity of valvular regurgitation. *Am J Med.* 1996;100:149-56.

48. Bleifer S, Donoso E, Grishman A. The auscultatory and phonocardiographic signs of ventricular septal defects. *Am J Cardiol.* 1960;5:191-8.

49. Ebringer R, Pitt A, Anderson ST. Haemodynamic factors influencing opening snap interval in mitral stenosis. *Br Heart J.* 1970;32:350-4.

50. Spodick DH. Pericardial rub. Prospective, multiple observer investigation of pericardial friction in 100 patients. *Am J Cardiol.* 1975;35:357-62.

51. Zayas R, Anguita M, Torres F, et al. Incidence of specific etiology and role of methods for specific etiologic diagnosis of primary acute pericarditis. *Am J Cardiol.* 1995;75:378-82.

Hypertension

3

Angela L. Brown, Anandita Agarwala Kulkarni, and J. Gmerice Hammond

GENERAL PRINCIPLES

Definition

- *Hypertension* is defined as the presence of a blood pressure (BP) elevation to a level that places patients at increased risk for end-organ damage in several vascular beds, including the retina, brain, heart, kidneys, and large conduit arteries.[1]
- Clinically, it is defined as systolic blood pressure (SBP) >130 mm Hg or a diastolic blood pressure (DBP) >80 mm Hg.[2]

Classification

- BP should be categorized as normal, elevated, or stage 1 or 2 hypertension to prevent and treat high BP (Table 3-1).[2]
- Individuals with SBP and DBP in two different categories should be classified using the higher BP category.

Epidemiology

- About 47%, or 116 million, of US adults have hypertension or are taking medications for hypertension.[3]
- Prevalence increases with age: 70% of older adults versus 32% of adults aged 40 to 59 years.[4]
- Hypertension is the leading risk factor for death and disability-adjusted life years worldwide,[5] and in the US, accounts for more cardiovascular disease (CVD)-related deaths than any other modifiable CVD risk factor.[6,7]
- The lifetime risk of developing hypertension (BP ≥ 140/90 mm Hg) is 90% for nonhypertensive adults aged 55 to 65 years.[8]
- Older adults (over age 65 years) account for the bulk of hypertension-related morbidity and mortality, which includes atherosclerotic cardiovascular disease (ASCVD), stroke,

TABLE 3-1	CLASSIFICATION OF BLOOD PRESSURE FOR ADULTS 18 YEARS AND OLDER[a]	
Category	**Systolic pressure (mm Hg)**	**Diastolic pressure (mm Hg)**
Normal	<120 and	<80
Elevated	120–129 and	<80
Stage 1 hypertension	130–139 or	80–89
Stage 2 hypertension	≥140 or	>90

[a]Not taking antihypertensive drugs and not acutely ill. Individuals with systolic blood pressure and diastolic blood pressure in two categories should be designated to the higher blood pressure (BP) category.

heart failure (HF), chronic kidney disease (CKD), left ventricular hypertrophy (LVH), atrial fibrillation, and peripheral arterial disease (PAD).[9] Incidence of these increases with higher levels of SBP and DBP.

- Hypertensive patients have an increase in cerebrovascular accidents and HF compared to normotensive subjects.
- BP control remains poor, with 56% of treated hypertensive patients having BP above target goal.[10]

Etiology

- Primary hypertension represents about 90% of all cases of hypertension. The cause of hypertension in these cases is not known but likely due to additive effects of genetics, race, age, gender, geographic location, socioeconomic status, and lifestyle factors.[2,11]
- Secondary hypertension comprises the remaining <10% of cases. Common causes include renal parenchymal disease, renovascular disease, primary hyperaldosteronism, pheochromocytoma, Cushing syndrome, coarctation of the aorta, and obstructive sleep apnea (Table 3-2).[2]
- BP typically increases with age.[2]
  ○ Growing evidence suggests a complex interplay between inflammation, oxidative stress, and endothelial dysfunction, leading to increased systemic vascular resistance as key mechanisms of biologic aging and the development of hypertension.[12]
  ○ Genetics, prenatal programming, and environmental factors may impact lifetime BP trajectory: children of mothers with hypertensive disorders of pregnancy have higher BP during adolescence, and young adults born preterm have higher rates of antihypertensive prescriptions.[13]
- Genetics of hypertension are complex, polygenic, and remain largely unknown.[11] Identified monogenic forms (Liddle syndrome, Gordon syndrome, glucocorticoid-remedial aldosteronism) that result in salt retention are rare.[14]
- Modifiable risk factors that contribute to the development of hypertension include overweight/obesity, insulin resistance, high dietary sodium intake, low physical activity, high alcohol consumption, low dietary intake of potassium, and stress.

DIAGNOSIS

Clinical Presentation

- Elevated BP is typically discovered in asymptomatic individuals during routine health visits.
- Hypertension diagnosis should be based on an average of two readings or more on two occasions or more.
- Proper techniques in measuring BP include:
  ○ Having the patient sit in a chair with feet flat on the floor, legs uncrossed, back supported, and arm resting at heart level for ≥5 minutes
  ○ Using a calibrated, appropriately fitting BP cuff (inflatable bladder encircling at least 80% of the arm)[15]
- BP should be measured in both arms, and the higher reading used.
- Out-of-office measurements of BP, either by ambulatory blood pressure monitoring (ABPM) or by home blood pressure monitoring (HBPM), are useful for confirmation and management of hypertension.[2]
  ○ The 2017 American College of Cardiology/American Heart Association (ACC/AHA) hypertension guidelines and the US Preventive Services Task Force (USPSTF) both recommend ABPM or HBPM to confirm the diagnosis of hypertension.[2,16]
  ○ ABPM was a better predictor of long-term CVD outcomes than office BPs.[16]

Causes of secondary hypertension	Clinical features	Screening tests
Renal parenchymal disease	UTIs, obstruction, hematuria, urinary frequency, nocturia, analgesic abuse, history of polycystic kidney disease, elevated serum creatinine	Renal ultrasound
Renovascular disease	Resistant hypertension or hypertension with abrupt onset, or that is worsening/difficult to control, known atherosclerotic disease, flash pulmonary edema, early-onset hypertension, young female	Renal duplex Doppler ultrasound, MRA, abdominal CT. Renal angiography is confirmatory test
Primary aldosteronism	Resistant hypertension with findings of hypokalemia, muscle cramps, weakness, adrenal mass	Plasma aldosterone/renin ratio (patients must stop aldosterone antagonists for 4–6 weeks before testing)
Obstructive sleep apnea	Resistant hypertension, snoring, daytime sleepiness, breathing pauses during sleep	Polysomnography
Drug or alcohol induced	Caffeine, nicotine, alcohol, NSAIDs, OCPs, cyclosporine, tacrolimus, sympathomimetics (decongestions, anorectics), cocaine, amphetamines, PCP, neuropsychiatric agents (TCAs, MAOIs), clonidine withdrawal, erythropoietin-stimulating agents, herbal medications	Drug screen and detailed history
Pheochromocytoma	Paroxysmal hypertension/hypertensive crisis, labile blood pressure, headaches, sweating, palpitations	Plasma and urine metanephrines
Cushing syndrome	Central weight gain, proximal muscle weakness, depression, hyperglycemia	Overnight 1-mg dexamethasone suppression test

(continued)

Causes of secondary hypertension	Clinical features	Screening tests
Hypothyroidism	Dry skin, cold intolerance, constipation, weight gain	TSH and free T4
Hyperthyroidism	Warm skin, heat intolerance, hyperdefecation, weight loss, proximal muscle weakness, insomnia, tremulousness	TSH and free T4
Aortic coarctation	Young patient with hypertension	Echocardiogram
Primary hyperparathyroidism	Hypercalcemia	Serum calcium; serum PTH level is confirmatory test
Congenital adrenal hyperplasia	Hypertension with hypokalemia; virilization	Low or normal aldosterone and renin. 11-β-OH, elevated deoxycorticosterone, 11-deoxycortisol, and androgens 17-α-OH
Mineralocorticoid excess (other than primary aldosteronism)	Early-onset hypertension that is resistant, hypokalemia or hyperkalemia	Low renin and low aldosterone
Acromegaly	Acral features/enlarging shoe, glove, or hat size; visual disturbances; diabetes mellitus	Serum growth hormone ≥1 ng/mL during oral glucose load and serum IGF-1 level. MRI of the pituitary is also confirmatory

IGF-1, insulin-like growth factor 1; MAOIs, monoamine oxidase inhibitors; MRA, magnetic resonance angiography; NSAIDs, nonsteroidal anti-inflammatory drugs; OCPs, oral contraceptive pills; PCP, phencyclidine; PTH, parathyroid hormone; TCAs, tricyclic antidepressants; TSH, thyroid-stimulating hormone; UTI, urinary tract infection.

Adapted from Whelton PK, Carey RM, Aronow WS, et al: 2017 ACC/AHA/AAPA/ABC/ACPM/AGS/APhA/ASH/ASPC/NMA/PCNA guideline for the prevention, detection, evaluation, and management of high blood pressure in adults. *Hypertension.* 2018;71(19):e13-115.

○ Importantly, ABPM and HBPM use different thresholds to categorize high BP than those previously indicated. Typically, a clinic BP of 140/90 mm Hg corresponds to home BP of 135/85 mm Hg and ABPM values of 135/85 mm Hg for daytime, 120/70 mm Hg for nighttime, and 130/80 mm Hg for 24-hour averages.[17]

Subtypes of Hypertension
* Isolated systolic hypertension
  ○ Defined as SBP ≥130 mm Hg and DBP <80 mm Hg
  ○ Occurs frequently in those aged 65 years and older
* White-coat hypertension is persistent elevation of BP in the office or presence of a health care worker, particularly a physician, though normal when measured with either ABPM or HBPM.[2,15]
* Masked hypertension
  ○ Controlled BP in the office, but elevated or uncontrolled elsewhere[2,15]
  ○ Often associated with target organ damage and increased risk of CVD compared to normotensives and those with white-coat hypertension
* Resistant hypertension
  ○ BP ≥130/80 mm Hg in hypertensive patients on three or more antihypertensive agents at maximum dose (or maximum tolerated dose), including a diuretic, or controlled BP on four or more antihypertensive agents at optimal doses[2]
  ○ Accounts for ~30% of uncontrolled and 10% of controlled US adults with treated hypertension[18] and is more prevalent in those of African descent
* Uncontrolled hypertension
  ○ Not synonymous with resistant hypertension
  ○ Includes patients with poor adherence and/or inadequate treatment regimen, as well as true resistant hypertension[19]
* Pseudohypertension
  ○ Caused by inflation of the BP cuff to higher pressures in order to compress very rigid arteries due to advanced (often calcified) arteriosclerosis[15]
  ○ Brachial and radial artery pulsations may still be palpable distal to the fully inflated cuff (Osler sign).
  ○ Potential for overprescribing antihypertensive medication resulting in orthostatic hypotension
* Hypertensive crisis[2]
  ○ Hypertensive urgencies
    ▪ Defined as substantial increase in BP, usually with a DBP >120 mm Hg, without acute or impending end-organ damage
    ▪ Often associated with patient withdrawal from or noncompliance with antihypertensive therapy
    ▪ Clinical presentation usually occurs in the upper levels of stage 2 hypertension and includes optic disc edema, progressive end-organ complications rather than damage, and severe perioperative hypertension.
  ○ Hypertensive emergencies
    ▪ Defined as BP >180/120 mm Hg with new or worsening end-organ damage
    ▪ Absolute BP level may not be as important as rate of BP rise (patients with chronic hypertension can often tolerate higher BP levels compared to those previously normotensive)[2] or evidence of end-organ damage.
    ▪ Accelerated–malignant hypertension is a subgroup of hypertensive emergency that refers to very high BP associated with retinopathy, papilledema, and rapidly progressing kidney or heart damage.

History

- In adults with new-onset or uncontrolled hypertension, a detailed history should seek to identify potential secondary causes of hypertension, including ingestion of over-the-counter medications, supplements, and prescription medications that can raise BP (Table 3-3).[2,19]
- A diagnosis of secondary hypertension should be considered in the following situations[2]:
  - Age of onset younger than 30 years
  - Onset of diastolic hypertension in adults older than 65 years
  - Stable hypertension that becomes difficult to control
  - Resistant hypertension
  - Accelerated/malignant hypertension

TABLE 3-3	MEDICATIONS AND SUBSTANCES THAT CAN INTERFERE WITH BLOOD PRESSURE CONTROL

Nonnarcotic analgesics
    Nonsteroidal anti-inflammatory agents, including aspirin
    Selective COX-2 inhibitors
Sympathomimetic agents
    Decongestants
    Diet pills
    Cocaine
    Caffeine
Antidepressants
    MAO inhibitors, SNRIs, TCAs
Atypical antipsychotics
    Clozapine, olanzapine
Stimulants
    Methylphenidate and dexmethylphenidate
    Dextroamphetamine, amphetamine, methamphetamine
    Modafinil
Alcohol
Oral contraceptives
Cyclosporine
Erythropoietin
Natural licorice
Herbal supplements
    Ephedra
    Ma huang
    St. John's wort
Systemic corticosteroids
Angiogenesis inhibitor or tyrosine kinase inhibitors

MAO, monoamine oxidase; SNRIs, serotonin–norepinephrine reuptake inhibitors; TCAs, tricyclic antidepressants.

Adapted from Whelton PK, Carey RM, Aronow WS, et al. 2017 ACC/AHA/AAPA/ABC/ACPM/AGS/APhA/ASH/ASPC/NMA/PCNA guideline for the prevention, detection, evaluation, and management of high blood pressure in adults. *Hypertension.* 2018;71(19):e13-115; Calhoun DA, Jones D, Textor S, et al. Resistant hypertension: diagnosis, evaluation, and treatment. A scientific statement from the American Heart Association Professional Educations Committee of the Council for High Blood Pressure Research. *Hypertension.* 2008;51(6):1403-19.

- ○ Abrupt onset of hypertension
- ○ Disproportionate end-organ damage for degree of hypertension
- ○ Unprovoked or excessive hypokalemia or metabolic alkalosis
- In patients who present with significant hypertension at a young age, a careful family history may suggest forms of hypertension that follow simple Mendelian inheritance.

Physical Examination

Should include investigation for end-organ damage or a secondary cause of hypertension by noting the presence of carotid bruits, an S_3 or S_4, cardiac murmurs, neurologic deficits, elevated jugular venous pressure, rales, retinopathy, unequal pulses, enlarged or small kidneys, Cushingoid features, and abdominal bruits.[1]

Differential Diagnosis

- Hypertension may be partly due to withdrawal from drugs, including alcohol, cocaine, and opioid analgesics.
- Rebound increases in BP may be seen in patients who abruptly discontinue antihypertensive therapy, particularly β-adrenergic antagonists and central α_2-agonists (see section Complications).
- Cocaine and other sympathomimetic drugs (e.g., amphetamines, phencyclidine hydrochloride) can produce hypertension in the setting of acute intoxication and when the agents are discontinued abruptly after chronic use.

Diagnostic Testing

- Goal: Identify patients with target organ damage, assess cardiovascular risk, and provide a baseline for monitoring for adverse effects of therapy.
- Basic laboratory data should include complete blood count, basic metabolic panel, estimated glomerular filtration rate (eGFR), lipid panel, fasting blood glucose, urinalysis, thyroid-stimulating hormone (TSH), and ECG.
- Additional diagnostic testing may include echocardiography to detect LVH and assess cardiac function, uric acid level, and urine albumin-to-creatinine ratio.
- ABPM may be indicated to[20]:
  - ○ Confirm diagnosis of hypertension
  - ○ Evaluate for suspected white-coat hypertension or masked hypertension
  - ○ Evaluate for nocturnal hypertension and overall BP lability in those with orthostatic-associated isolated systolic hypertension
  - ○ Evaluate for possible drug resistance

Screening for Secondary Hypertension

- Should occur based on clinical indications (see earlier), with suggestive physical examination findings, or in adults with resistant hypertension (Table 3-2)[2]
- If the screen is positive, refer to a physician with expertise in that form of hypertension.

TREATMENT

- Goal is to lower BP and prevent end-organ damage while controlling other modifiable cardiovascular risk factors.
- BP should be reduced to a goal of <130/80 mm Hg for most adults with hypertension.
- All patients with elevated BP or hypertension should engage in comprehensive nonpharmacologic therapy (lifestyle modifications). (See later for special considerations for older adults older than 75 to 80 years.)
- Patients with stage 1 hypertension should be managed based on their ASCVD risk score. Those with an estimated 10-year risk score of <10% can be managed with nonpharmacologic therapy, with reassessment in 3 to 6 months.

- Patients with stage 1 hypertension with a 10-year ASCVD risk score ≥10% and patients with stage 2 hypertension should be treated with a combination of pharmacologic and nonpharmacologic therapies, with reassessment in 1 month.
- In isolated systolic hypertension, the therapeutic goal should be to lower SBP to <130 mm Hg. Achieving this goal may be difficult as it is generally accepted (clinical trial data lacking) that DBP should be kept above 60 mm Hg to preserve myocardial perfusion.
- Patients with CKD, diabetes mellitus, CVD, stable ischemic heart disease, or heart failure with reduced ejection fraction (HFrEF) are considered high risk, and aggressive BP management should be pursued in these patients. (See section on Hypertension in the Setting of Comorbidities.)

Nonpharmacologic Therapy (Lifestyle Modifications) (Table 3-4)[2]

- Fundamental to prevention and management of high BP, either alone or in combination with drug therapy

TABLE 3-4	LIFESTYLE (NONPHARMACOLOGIC) MODIFICATIONS FOR TREATMENT OF HYPERTENSION	
Modification	**Dose**	**Approximate SBP reduction (mm Hg)**
Weight loss	Ideal body weight or at least 1 kg reduction (expect about 1 mm Hg for every 1 kg reduction in body weight)	5
Adoption of DASH eating plan	Rich in fruits, vegetables, whole grains, and low-fat dairy products with reduced content of saturated and trans fat	11
Dietary sodium reduction	<1500 mg/d—optimal; at least 1000 mg/d reduction	5–6
Dietary potassium increase	3500–5000 mg/d preferably by dietary consumption	4–5
Physical activity Aerobic	90–150 min/wk 65–75% heart rate reserve	5–8
Dynamic resistance	50–80% 1 rep maximum 6 exercises, 3 sets/exercise, 10 repetitions/set	4
Isometric resistance	4 × 2 minutes (hand grip), 1-minute rest between exercises, 30–40% max voluntary contraction, 3 sessions/wk	5
Limiting alcohol consumption	Men: ≤2 drinks daily[a] Women: ≤1 drink daily	4

[a]Typical standard drink in US: 12 oz of regular beer, 5 oz of wine, and 1.5 oz of spirits.

Adapted from Whelton PK, Carey RM, Aronow WS, et al. 2017 ACC/AHA/AAPA/ABC/ACPM/AGS/APhA/ASH/ASPC/NMA/PCNA guideline for the prevention, detection, evaluation, and management of high blood pressure in adults. *Hypertension.* 2018;71(19):e13-115.

- Effective interventions include weight loss, consuming a healthy diet, reduced dietary sodium intake, increased dietary potassium intake, increased physical activity, and moderation in alcohol intake.

Initial Drug Therapy

- Numerous oral agents in multiple classes are available to treat high BP (Table 3-5).[1]
- Special considerations based on patient characteristics (age, race), comorbid conditions (angina, HF, renal insufficiency, LVH, obesity, hyperlipidemia, gout, and bronchospasm), drug interactions, and cost may dictate initial drug choice.
- Thiazide/thiazide-type diuretics, calcium channel blockers (CCBs), angiotensin-converting enzyme inhibitors (ACEIs), and angiotensin-receptor blockers (ARBs) are all the first-line therapies for the general non-black population, including those with diabetes, based on multiple large randomized controlled trials (RCTs) showing comparable effects on decreasing overall cardiovascular and cerebrovascular mortality.[21]
- For black patients, thiazide diuretics and CCBs demonstrated decreased cardiovascular and cerebrovascular mortality compared with an ACEI and can be considered the first-line therapies (ALLHAT trial).[22-24] ARBs may be associated with less cough and angioedema compared to ACEIs, but offer no proven advantage for preventing CVD and stroke.
- In patients with CKD stage 3 or higher, or CKD with albuminuria ($\geq$300 mg/d), initial therapy or combination therapy including an ACEI or ARB is recommended.[2]
- Consider initiating two drugs from different classes for those with stage 2 hypertension and average BP $\geq$20/10 mm Hg above goal.

Combination Therapy

- Many patients will require two or more drugs to achieve optimal BP control.
- Regimens with complimentary mechanisms of actions should be used, starting with additional agents from one of the initial therapy drug classes. Exceptions include:
  - Concomitant use of a thiazide diuretic, K-sparing diuretic, and/or loop diuretic in various combinations may be considered in certain situations.
  - Dihydropyridine (DHP) and non-DHP CCBs can be combined, but not in the setting of concomitant β-blocker use.
- Simultaneous use of renin–angiotensin system (RAS) blockers (ACEI, ARB, direct renin inhibitor) increases cardiovascular and renal risk.[25,26]
- Use of fixed-dose combinations may improve medication adherence.

MONITORING/FOLLOW-UP

- Assess adherence, assess response to therapy, identify adverse responses to therapy, and monitor for target organ damage.
- Assessments should occur monthly until target BP is achieved.
- Includes home monitoring, team-based care, and telehealth strategies,[27] as adapted to local needs and resources

HYPERTENSION IN THE SETTING OF COMORBIDITIES[2]

Stable Ischemic Heart Disease

- Goal BP <130/80 mm Hg recommended.
- Initiate guideline-directed medical therapy (GDMT) with β-blockers, ACEIs, or ARBs as a first-line therapy.[28]
- DHP CCBs, thiazide diuretics, and mineralocorticoid-receptor blockers may be added if needed.

TABLE 3-5 COMMONLY USED ANTIHYPERTENSIVE AGENTS BY FUNCTIONAL CLASS

Drugs by class	Properties	Initial dose	Total daily dosage range (mg)
β-Adrenergic antagonists			
Atenolol[a]	Selective	50 mg PO daily	25–100
Betaxolol[a]	Selective	10 mg PO daily	5–40
Bisoprolol[a]	Selective	5 mg PO daily	2.5–20
Metoprolol	Selective	50 mg PO bid	50–450
Metoprolol XL	Selective	50–100 mg PO daily	50–400
Nebivolol[a,b]	Selective with vasodilatory properties	5 mg PO daily	5–40
Nadolol[a]	Nonselective	40 mg PO daily	20–240
Propranolol	Nonselective	40 mg PO bid	40–240
Propranolol LA	Nonselective	80 mg PO daily	60–240
Timolol	Nonselective	10 mg PO bid	20–40
Pindolol	ISA	5 mg PO daily	10–60
Labetalol	α- and β-antagonist properties	100 mg PO bid	200–1200
Carvedilol	α- and β-antagonist properties	6.25 mg PO bid	12.5–50[c]
Carvedilol CR[b]	α- and β-antagonist properties	10 mg PO daily	10–80
Acebutolol[a]	ISA, selective	200 mg PO bid, 400 mg PO daily	200–1200
Calcium channel antagonists			
Amlodipine	DHP	5 mg PO daily	2.5–10
Diltiazem		30 mg PO qid	90–360
Diltiazem LA		180 mg PO daily	120–540
Diltiazem CD		180 mg PO daily	120–480

Diltiazem XR	180 mg PO daily	120–540
Diltiazem XT	180 mg PO daily	120–480
Isradipine	DHP	2.5 mg PO bid	2.5–10
Nicardipine[b]	DHP	20 mg PO tid	60–120
Nifedipine	DHP	10 mg PO tid	30–120
Nifedipine XL (or CC)	DHP	30 mg PO daily	30–90
Nisoldipine	DHP	20 mg PO daily	20–40
Verapamil	80 mg PO tid	80–480
Verapamil SR	120 mg PO daily	120–480

Angiotensin-converting enzyme inhibitors[a]

Benazepril	10 mg PO bid	10–40
Captopril	25 mg PO bid–tid	50–450
Enalapril	5 mg PO daily	2.5–40
Fosinopril	10 mg PO daily	10–40
Lisinopril	10 mg PO daily	5–40
Moexipril	7.5 mg PO daily	7.5–30
Quinapril	10 mg PO daily	5–80
Ramipril	2.5 mg PO daily	1.25–20
Trandolapril	1–2 mg PO daily	1–4
Perindopril	4 mg PO daily	2–16

Angiotensin II receptor blockers[a]

Azilsartan[b]	40 mg PO daily	40–80
Candesartan	8 mg PO daily	8–32
Eprosartan	600 mg PO daily	600–800

(continued)

TABLE 3-5 COMMONLY USED ANTIHYPERTENSIVE AGENTS BY FUNCTIONAL CLASS (*continued*)

Drugs by class	Properties	Initial dose	Total daily dosage range (mg)
Irbesartan		150 mg PO daily	150–300
Olmesartan[b]		20 mg PO daily	20–40
Losartan		50 mg PO daily	25–100
Telmisartan		40 mg PO daily	20–80
Valsartan		80 mg PO daily	80–320
Direct renin inhibitor[d]			
Aliskiren[b]		150 mg PO daily	150–300
Diuretics[d]			
Chlorthalidone	Thiazide diuretic	25 mg PO daily	12.5–50
Hydrochlorothiazide	Thiazide diuretic	12.5 mg PO daily	12.5–50
Hydroflumethiazide[b]	Thiazide diuretic	50 mg PO daily	50–100
Indapamide	Thiazide diuretic	1.25 mg PO daily	2.5–5
Methyclothiazide	Thiazide diuretic	2.5 mg PO daily	2.5–5
Metolazone	Thiazide diuretic	2.5 mg PO daily	1.25–5
Bumetanide	Loop diuretic	0.5 mg PO daily (or IV)	0.5–5
Ethacrynic acid[b]	Loop diuretic	50 mg PO daily (or IV)	25–100
Furosemide	Loop diuretic	20 mg PO daily (or IV)	20–320
Torsemide	Loop diuretic	5 mg PO daily (or IV)	5–10
Amiloride	Potassium-sparing diuretic	5 mg PO daily	5–10
Triamterene[b]	Potassium-sparing diuretic	50 mg PO bid	50–200

Eplerenone	Aldosterone antagonist	25 mg PO daily	25–100
Spironolactone	Aldosterone antagonist	25 mg PO daily	25–100
α-Adrenergic antagonists			
Doxazosin		1 mg PO daily	1–16
Prazosin		1 mg PO bid–tid	1–20
Terazosin		1 mg PO at bedtime	1–20
Centrally acting adrenergic agents			
Clonidine		0.1 mg PO bid	0.1–1.2
Clonidine patch		TTS 1/wk (equivalent to 0.1 mg/d release)	0.1–0.3
Guanfacine		1 mg PO daily	1–3
Guanabenz		4 mg PO bid	4–64
Methyldopa[a]		250 mg PO bid–tid	250–2000
Direct-acting vasodilators			
Hydralazine[a]		10 mg PO qid	50–300
Minoxidil		5 mg PO daily	2.5–100
Miscellaneous			
Reserpine		0.5 mg PO daily	0.01–0.25

DHP, dihydropyridine; ISA, intrinsic sympathomimetic activity; TTS, transdermal therapeutic system.

[a]Adjusted in renal failure.

[b]Available only in brand name. Assume all drugs are available in generic form unless otherwise denoted by superscript "*b.*"

[c]Up to 100 mg total daily dosage for weight ≥85 kg.

[d]Renal function should be considered before initiation.

- In patients with stable ischemic heart disease and angina, DHP CCB may be added to β-blocker.
- β-Blockers and/or CCBs may be considered for hypertension control in patients with coronary artery disease (CAD) (without HFrEF) and have angina.[28]

Heart Failure with Reduced Ejection Fraction

- Goal BP <130/80 mm Hg
- Initiate GDMT with ACEIs or ARBs, angiotensin receptor neprilysin inhibitors, mineralocorticoid-receptor blockers, diuretics, and GDMT β-blockers.
- Non-DHP CCBs have not been shown to provide benefit and should be avoided.

Heart Failure with Preserved Ejection Fraction

- Hypertension is the most important cause of heart failure with preserved ejection fraction (HFpEF).
- Goal SBP <130 mm Hg
- ALLHAT showed that treatment of hypertension with chlorthalidone reduced the risk of HF compared with amlodipine, doxazosin, and lisinopril.[29]
- Diuretic therapy should be initiated as a first line for volume control in those with symptoms.
- ACEIs, ARBs, and β-blockers should be added to achieve BP goal.

Chronic Kidney Disease

- Goal BP <130/80 mm Hg
- ACEIs should be used as initial therapy in patients with CKD stage 3 or higher, or CKD stage 1 or 2 with albuminuria or albumin-to-creatinine ratio ≥300 mg/g and has been shown to slow progression of kidney disease.
- ARB may be used if intolerant of ACEI.

Postrenal Transplant

- Goal BP <130/80 mm Hg
- Initiate therapy with CCB, associated with improved GFR and survival.

Cerebrovascular Disease

- Management is complex and challenging.
- Important to recognize the type of stroke, acuity, and therapeutic options
- Studies are needed to define optimal BP reduction timing, target, and therapeutic agents.

Acute Intracranial Hemorrhage

- Consider continuous intravenous drug infusion (Table 3-6)[2,30] along with close monitoring if SBP >220 mm Hg.
- Immediate lowering of SBP <140 mm Hg for those presenting <6 hours after the acute event and with an SBP between 150 and 220 mm Hg has shown no benefit in reducing death or disability and can be harmful.

Acute Ischemic Stroke

- Patients presenting <72 hours after an acute event who qualify for thrombolytic therapy should have their BP lowered to <185/110 mm Hg before initiation of thrombolysis. BP should be maintained <180/105 mm Hg for 24 hours following thrombolysis.
- Patients presenting <72 hours after acute event who do not qualify for thrombolytic therapy and have a BP > 220/110 mm Hg should have their SBP/DBP lowered by 15% in the first 24 hours.

TABLE 3-6 INTRAVENOUS ANTIHYPERTENSIVE AGENTS TO TREAT HYPERTENSIVE EMERGENCIES

Drug	Administration and dosage	Onset	Duration of action	Dosage	Advantages	Disadvantages
Nitroglycerin	IV infusion 5–250 μg/min	1–2 minutes	3–5 minutes		Coronary perfusion, acute pulmonary edema	Headache, variable efficacy, tachyphylaxis; tolerance may develop with prolonged use. Do not use in volume-depleted patients
Sodium nitroprusside	IV infusion 0.5–10 μg/kg/min (initial dose, 0.25 μg/kg/min for eclampsia and renal insufficiency)	Immediate	2–3 minutes		Titration	Hypotension, nausea, vomiting, apprehension; risk of thiocyanate and cyanide toxicity is increased in renal and hepatic insufficiency, respectively; levels should be monitored; decrease dosage for elderly; must shield from light
Metoprolol	Loading dose: 5 mg IV (repeat every 10 minutes, up to 20 mg)	5–10 minutes	3–4 hours		Reduction in O₂ consumption	Bradycardia, heart block, bronchospasm
Fenoldopam	IV infusion 0.1–0.3 μg/kg/min	<5 minutes	30 minutes			Tachycardia, nausea, vomiting, increased intraocular pressure (glaucoma), sulfite allergy

(continued)

31

Drug	Administration and dosage	Onset	Duration of action	Dosage	Advantages	Disadvantages
Labetalol	IV bolus 20–80 mg q5–10 min, up to 300 mg IV infusion 0.5–2 mg/min	5–10 minutes	2–6 hours		β-Blocker and vasodilator	Hypotension/orthostasis, heart block, heart failure, bronchospasm, nausea, vomiting, scalp tingling, paradoxical pressor response; may not be effective in patients receiving α- or β-blockers
Esmolol	IV bolus 500 µg/kg/min for first 1 minute IV infusion 50–300 µg/kg/min	1–2 minutes	1–20 minutes		Selective β-blocker	Hypotension, heart block, heart failure, bronchospasm
Phentolamine	IV bolus 5–10 mg q5–15 min	1–2 minutes	3–10 minutes		Catecholamine excess	Hypotension, tachycardia, headache, angina, paradoxical pressor response
Hydralazine	IV bolus 10–20 mg q20 min (if no effect after 20 mg, try another agent)	10–20 minutes	3–6 hours		Eclampsia or impending eclampsia	Hypotension, fetal distress, tachycardia, headache, nausea, vomiting, local thrombophlebitis. Infusion site should be changed after 12 hours. Unpredictable response

Drug	Dose	Onset	Duration	Notes	Adverse effects / contraindications
Nicardipine	IV infusion 5 mg/h, increased by 2.5 mg/h q5 min up to 15 mg/h	1–5 minutes	3–6 hours	No dose adjustment for elderly	Hypotension, headache, tachycardia, nausea, vomiting; contraindicated in advanced aortic stenosis
Clevidipine	IV infusion 1–2 mg/h, double dose every 90 seconds until BP approaches target, then increasing less than double q5–10 min up to 32 mg/h; max duration 72 hours	2–4 minutes	5–15 minutes	Titration	Hypotension, reflex tachycardia; contraindicated in patients with soybean, soy product, egg, or egg product allergy and in those with deficient lipid metabolism; use low-end dose range for elderly
Enalaprilat	IV bolus 1.25 mg over 5 minutes, increase to 5 mg q6h	5–15 minutes	1–6 hours	Heart failure, acute LVF	Hypotension, relatively slow onset, dose not easily adjusted; do not use in acute myocardial infarction or bilateral renal artery stenosis; contraindicated in pregnancy

• For patients presenting <72 hours after acute event who do not qualify for thrombolytic therapy and have a BP ≤ 220/110 mm Hg, there is no benefit for preventing death or dependency to starting or resuming treatment for hypertension within the first 48 to 72 hours. Antihypertensive therapies may be resumed once the patient is neurologically stable.

Atrial Fibrillation
• Treatment of hypertension may prevent new-onset atrial fibrillation.
• ARB therapy may prevent recurrence.[31]

Peripheral Arterial Disease
• Treat similarly to hypertensive patients without PAD.
• No evidence that any class of drug is superior

Diabetes Mellitus
• Treatment should be initiated at a BP of ≥130/80 mm Hg and treated to goal of <130/80 mm Hg.
• Initiate therapy with diuretics, ACEIs, ARBs, or CCBs.
• May consider ACEIs or ARBs as initial therapy in the setting of albuminuria

Metabolic Syndrome
• Emphasis is on lifestyle modifications to improve insulin sensitivity, including healthy diet, weight loss, and increased exercise.
• Optimal pharmacologic therapy is not clear.

Valvular Heart Disease
Aortic Stenosis
• No specific trials comparing various agents for treating hypertension; however:
  ○ RAS blockade may improve LV fibrosis, reduce dyspnea, and improve exercise tolerance.
  ○ Use diuretics sparingly if small LV volumes present.
  ○ β-Blockers may be appropriate for those with LV dysfunction, prior MI, arrhythmias, or angina.
• Consider co-management with a valvular heart disease specialist.

Aortic Insufficiency
Avoid agents that slow heart rate.

Aortic Disease
• β-Blockers recommended as initial therapy for thoracic aortic disease.
• Although no RCTs are available, observational data suggest lower risk for operative repair with chronic aortic dissection and improved survival in those with type A and type B aortic dissections treated with β-blockers.
• Goal SBP ≤120 mm Hg and heart rate <60 bpm if tolerated[32]
• Antihypertensive agents with negative inotropic properties, including non-DHP calcium channel antagonists, β-adrenergic antagonists, methyldopa, clonidine, and reserpine, are preferred for the management in the postacute phase.

SPECIAL CONSIDERATIONS
Race and Ethnicity
• Hispanic Americans are a heterogeneous group with variable rates of hypertension and related outcomes based on the location of ancestral origin.[2]
  ○ Pooling RCT and epidemiologic data may not accurately reflect risk.

- BP control rates are low due to the lack of awareness and treatment.
- Higher prevalence of obesity and diabetes compared to other racial/ethnic groups
- Initial therapy in Hispanic Americans should follow recommendations for the general non-black population.
- Blacks have a higher prevalence of hypertension and lower control rates compared to other racial/ethnic groups.[33]
- Blacks have a 1.3-fold greater risk of nonfatal stroke, 1.8-fold greater risk of fatal strokes, 1.5-fold greater risk of HF, and 4.2-fold greater risk of end-stage renal disease (ESRD).[34]
- Apoprotein L1 (APOL1) genetic variant may account for the excess burden of CKD outcomes in some black patients and may cause the rate of renal decline to be unresponsive to BP lowering or RAS blockade.[35]
- Initial therapy in blacks should include a thiazide-type diuretic or CCB (see section Initial Drug Therapy). Chlorthalidone 12.5 to 25 mg/d or hydrochlorothiazide 25 to 50 mg/d.
- Most black adults will require two or more drugs to achieve goal BP.
  - Racial differences should not be the basis for excluding any class of antihypertensive agent in combination therapy.
  - Combination of ACEI or ARB with a thiazide diuretic or CCB results in similar BP reduction in blacks and other racial/ethnic groups.
- ACEIs or ARBs should be used in black patients with hypertension, diabetes, and nephropathy (albuminuria ≥300 mg/d, or ≥300 mg/g albumin-to-creatinine ratio), but offer no advantage in those without nephropathy.
- ACEIs, ARBs, and β-blockers should be used in black patients with HF, and β blockers should be used in patients with coronary heart disease (CHD) who have had an MI.
- Recognize that the adoption of lifestyle modifications may be challenging in ethnic minority patients due to the lack of access to healthy foods and safe spaces for exercise, poor social support, and financial considerations (social determinants of health).
- Consideration should be given to cultural preferences, beliefs, values, and learning styles.[35]

Women and Pregnancy
See Chapter 33.

Older Adults
General Concepts
- The definition of an older or elderly adult is an ever-moving target based on changes in demographics, culture, biomedical advances, and heterogeneity in functionality over the past few decades.[36]
- The 2017 ACC/AHA hypertension guideline defines older adults as those aged 65 years or older, whereas a widely accepted definition in recent clinical trials uses those older than 75 or those older than 80 years.[36]
- Isolated systolic hypertension is the most common form of hypertension in this age group.
  - Function of increased vascular stiffness, decreased vascular compliance, and increased salt sensitivity
  - Increased prevalence of orthostatic BP changes and labile BPs due to blunted baroreceptor responses
  - Characterized by widened pulse pressure
  - RCTs have demonstrated that lowering SBP in isolated systolic hypertension reduces risk of fatal and nonfatal stroke, cardiovascular events, and death.[37,38]

Evaluation Pearls[36]
- May need to use a child-size BP cuff for those with low body mass index
- Assess for orthostatic changes in BP.

- Use HBPM (or ABPM) to evaluate for white-coat hypertension.
- Query use of over-the-counter drugs, particularly NSAIDs, which are often not reported among active medications.
- Secondary causes of hypertension occur less frequently.
  - Renal artery stenosis is common but often difficult to determine whether it is responsible for BP elevation.
  - Consider intervention only if failure to respond to medical therapy.
- Calculate eGFR as patient's age strongly influences renal function for a given serum creatinine level.
- With resistant hypertension, consider nonadherence due to cognitive decline as a cause.
- Assess for frailty and functional status (decline of physical, cognitive, psychological, or social functioning).
- Adherence and safety are improved when patients are involved in the decision-making process.

Treatment Considerations
Goals
- Goal SBP should be <130 mm Hg for noninstitutionalized community-dwelling ambulatory older adults.[2]
  - RCTs have demonstrated that BP-lowering goals need not differ from those selected for persons younger than 65 years.[39]
  - No RCTs in persons older than 65 years have shown harm or less benefit compared to younger adults.
  - HYVET showed benefit of BP lowering on cardiac morbidity and mortality in octogenarians.[40]
  - SPRINT showed benefit of intensive therapy, SBP <120 mm Hg, in persons older than 75 years.[38]
  - Achieving this goal may be difficult in those with isolated systolic hypertension as it is generally accepted (clinical trial data lacking) that excess drops in DBP <60 mm Hg should be avoided in order to preserve myocardial perfusion.
- ASCVD risk assessment is recommended to guide therapy; however:
  - Analysis of NHANES (2011 to 2014) data set indicates that 88% of US adults aged 65 years or older have a 10-year ASCVD risk ≥10% or have a history of CVD.
  - For persons aged 75 years or older, 100% have either an ASCVD risk ≥10% or history of CVD.
- For those with high burden of disease or limited life expectancy, employ clinical judgment, patient preference, and a team-based approach to determine the intensity of BP lowering and choice of agents. These patients have not been represented in RCTs.

Lifestyle Modifications
- Little RCT evidence for a benefit with lifestyle modifications in those over age 80 years
- Weight reduction may cause loss of muscle mass.
- Excessive salt restriction may induce hyponatremia and orthostasis.
- Physical activity must be adapted to the person's functional capacity.

Pharmacologic Therapy
- Start with monotherapy.
- Diuretics, CCBs, ACEIs, and ARBs are all the first-line therapies and have been shown to reduce clinical events.
- Combination therapy may be used if BP not at goal.
- Monitor closely for drug-related adverse effects and for drug interactions related to polypharmacy.

Orthostatic Hypotension[41,42]
- Defined as an abnormal BP response to standing
- Clinically recognized as a decrease in SBP ≥20 mm Hg or absolute SBP ≤90 mm Hg and/or decrease in DBP ≥10 mm Hg within 3 minutes of standing
- Associated with increased risk of falls, syncope, cognitive impairment, and mortality
- Drug therapy is the most common cause and often overlaps with other risk factors:
  - Advanced age
  - Neurogenic autonomic dysfunction (Parkinson disease, multiple system atrophy, diabetes)
  - Dehydration
  - Prolonged bed rest
  - Other comorbidities
- May occur with or without symptoms of dizziness, lightheadedness, or fainting (syncope)
- Common cardiovascular and central nervous system drugs that may precipitate orthostatic hypotension are listed in Table 3-7.[42] Chronic use of ACEIs, ARBs, and β-blockers with intrinsic sympathomimetic activity does not appear to increase risk.
- Treatment strategies
  - Stop unnecessary medications.
  - Avoid warm environments due to increased vasodilation.
  - Avoid straining activities (e.g., due to constipation).
  - Use graduated movements from supine to seated to standing position.
  - Increase salt intake to increase volume.
  - Wear compression stockings, preferably waist-high.
  - Cross legs to increase preload.
  - Sleep in the head-up position.

Supine Hypertension and Orthostatic Hypotension[41]
- Often coexist in patients with autonomic nervous system disorders or chronic hypertension and characterized by baroreceptor dysfunction
- Consider evaluation with bedside postural test.
  - Measure BP after patient is supine for 5 to 10 minutes.
  - Repeat BP after patient stands motionless for 3 to 5 minutes with arms supported at heart level.
- Treatment strategies in addition to those mentioned earlier:
  - Avoid standing still for prolonged periods of time.
  - Avoid prolonged daytime recumbence; it is preferable to rest in a chair.

TABLE 3-7	COMMON CARDIOVASCULAR AND CENTRAL NERVOUS SYSTEM DRUGS THAT MAY PRECIPITATE ORTHOSTATIC HYPOTENSION

Cardiovascular drugs	Central nervous system drugs
Diuretics	Antidepressants
α-Blockers	Benzodiazepines
Nitrates	Antipsychotics
β-Blockers	Opioids
Calcium channel blockers	Trazodone

○ Avoid severe physical exertion.
○ Eat frequent low-carbohydrate meals.
○ Make use of portable chair during ambulation.
○ Wear abdominal binder.
○ Consider transdermal nitroglycerin during the nighttime.
○ Cautious use of short-acting pressor agents during the daytime (e.g., midodrine).

Obese Adults

- Mechanisms of obesity-induced hypertension are complex and include[43]:
  ○ Impaired sodium excretion
  ○ Increased sympathetic nervous system activity
  ○ Activation of the renin–angiotensin–aldosterone system
- Weight reduction should be the primary goal of therapy.
- Diuretic combinations and CCBs are often used a first-line therapy due to elevations in vascular resistance, higher cardiac output, expanded intravascular volume, and lower plasma renin activity in these patients.
- Add mineralocorticoid-receptor antagonists (MRAs) and dual α-/β-blockers as necessary.

Resistant Hypertension

Risk Factors
- Older age
- Obesity
- CKD
- Black race
- Diabetes

Prognosis
Risk of MI, stroke, ESRD, and death in those with resistant hypertension and CHD may be two- to sixfold higher than in those whose BP is more easily controlled.[44]

Evaluation[2]
- Confirm treatment resistance with office BP ≥130/80 mm Hg and patient on three or more antihypertensives at optimal doses of which one is a diuretic (if possible) or office BP < 130/80 mm Hg and patient requiring four or more antihypertensives.
- Exclude pseudoresistance
  ○ Inaccurate BP measurements
  ○ Nonadherence to prescribed medications
  ○ White-coat effect
- Optimize lifestyle factors: Address obesity, physical inactivity; and excess alcohol, high salt, and low fiber intake.
- Discontinue or reduce interfering substances.
  ○ NSAIDs, sympathomimetics, oral contraceptives, licorice, ephedra
  ○ See Table 3-3[2,19] for full list.
- Screen for secondary causes of hypertension (see earlier).

Pharmacologic Treatment Strategies[2,18,19]
- Maximize diuretic therapy.
  ○ Compared to hydrochlorothiazide 50 mg, chlorthalidone 25 mg provided greater 24-hour BP reduction by ABPM with the largest difference seen in nocturnal BP.
  ○ Chlorthalidone more likely to be effective than hydrochlorothiazide with eGFR 30 to 44 mL/min/1.73 m^2.

- Loop diuretic (furosemide bid, bumetanide or torsemide daily) if eGFR <30 mL/min/1.73 m^2 to improve volume control or if receiving potent vasodilator like minoxidil
- Add MRA as the fourth agent to the common three-drug regimen of thiazide diuretic, RAS blocker, and CCB.
  - Spironolactone 12.5 to 50 mg daily
  - Eplerenone 25 to 50 mg bid if intolerant of spironolactone
  - Consider amiloride 10 to 40 mg daily (potassium sparing) if intolerant of MRA.
- Add other agents with different mechanisms of action.
  - β-Blocker (may preferentially consider α-/β-blocker although no head-to-head studies available)
  - Peripheral α-1 blocker
  - Central sympatholytic (guanfacine, clonidine)
  - Direct vasodilator (hydralazine, minoxidil; beware of reflex tachycardia and fluid retention requiring concomitant use of β-blocker and loop diuretic)
- May consider renin-guided therapy
  - Low renin patients may respond better to diuretics, MRAs, α-1 blocker, and CCBs.
  - High renin patients may respond better to ACEIs, ARBs, β-blockers, and direct renin inhibitor.
- Refer to hypertension specialist if BP remains uncontrolled after 6 months of therapy.

Device Therapy[2]
- Remains investigational and not currently recommended for the management of resistant hypertension
- Interrupts sympathetic nerve activity
  - Carotid baroreceptor pacing
  - Renal nerve catheter ablation

Hypertensive Crisis
Clinical Assessment[30]
Distinguish between hypertensive emergencies and urgencies to guide therapy and prevent worsening of clinical condition.

History: Assess for Factors Triggering the Acute Rise in Blood Pressure
- Symptoms that simulate hypertensive crisis include headache, labyrinthitis, physical trauma, pain, and emotional distress.
- Duration of hypertension and medication adherence
- Prior similar episodes
- Medications that may interfere with BP control
- Use of alcohol or illicit substances
- Sudden discontinuation of adrenergic inhibitors (clonidine, methyldopa, β-blockers)

Physical Examination: Assess for End-Organ Damage
- Central nervous system: focal neurologic deficits, headache, dizziness, visual or speech disturbance, level of consciousness, confusion, agitation or apathy, neck stiffness, seizure
- Cardiovascular system: thoracic, precordial, abdominal, and back pain; gallop; dyspnea; peripheral pulses; oxygen saturation; presence of carotid murmur; pulsatile abdominal mass or abdominal murmur
- Renal and genitourinary system: changes in urinary volume or frequency, lower extremity edema, hematuria, dysuria
- Fundoscopy: vasospasm, arteriovenous nicking, copper or silver wiring, exudates, hemorrhages, papilledema

Testing According to Involvement of End Organs
- Central nervous system: CT, MRI, lumbar puncture
- Cardiovascular system: ECG, CXR, echocardiogram, cardiac enzymes, MRI
- Renal system: urinalysis, blood urea nitrogen (BUN), creatinine, electrolytes, blood gas

Hypertensive Emergencies[2,30,45]
- BP >180/120 mm Hg associated with new or worsening end-organ damage such as:
  - Hypertensive encephalopathy
  - Intracranial hemorrhage (ICH)
  - Ischemic stroke
  - Acute left ventricular failure (LVF) with pulmonary edema
  - Acute MI
  - Unstable angina
  - Dissecting aortic aneurysm
  - Progressive renal failure
  - Severe preeclampsia and eclampsia
- Actual BP may not be as important as rate of BP increase.
- Require immediate reduction of mean arterial BP by 20-25% within 1 to 2 hours and then to 160/100 to 110 mm Hg by 6 hours to prevent or minimize end-organ damage, and then a reduction to 130/80 mm Hg over the next 24 to 48 hours
- Exceptions to the BP-lowering strategy include:
  - Aortic dissection, eclampsia, and pheochromocytoma with hypertensive crisis require rapid lowering of SBP usually to <140 mm Hg in the first hour of treatment.[2]
  - Acute ICH and acute ischemic stroke—see section Cerebrovascular Disease.
- Use rapidly acting parenteral agents (Table 3-6)[2,30]; however, there are no high-quality randomized controlled data to inform decision-making regarding the first-line agent.
- Require frequent monitoring of BP response to therapy, usually in an intensive care unit
- A precipitous fall in BP may occur in patients who are elderly, volume depleted, or receiving other antihypertensive agents.

Hypertensive Urgencies[2,30,45]
- BP control can be accomplished gradually over 24 hours to several days with use of oral antihypertensives.
- Excessive or rapid decreases in BP should be avoided to minimize the risk of cerebral, renal, or coronary ischemia.

COMPLICATIONS

Withdrawal syndrome associated with discontinuation of antihypertensive therapy:
When substituting therapy in patients with moderate-to-severe hypertension, it is reasonable to increase doses of the new medication in small increments while tapering the previous medication to avoid excessive BP fluctuations. On occasion, an antihypertensive drug withdrawal syndrome develops, usually within the first 24 to 72 hours. Occasionally, BP rises to levels that are much higher than those of baseline values. The most severe complications of withdrawal syndrome include encephalopathy, stroke, MI, and sudden death. Withdrawal syndrome is associated most commonly with centrally acting adrenergic agents (particularly clonidine) and β-adrenergic antagonists but has been reported with other agents as well, including diuretics. Discontinuation of antihypertensive medications should be done with caution in patients with preexisting CVD or cardiac disease. Management of withdrawal syndrome by reinstitution of the previously administered drug is generally effective.[1]

REFERENCES

1. Brown AL, Williams DS, Parham JS, et al. Preventive cardiology. In: Crees Z, Fritz C, Heudebert, et al, eds. *The Washington Manual of Medical Therapeutics*. 36th ed. Wolters Kluwer; 2020:58-92.
2. Whelton PK, Carey RM, Aronow WS, et al. 2017 ACC/AHA/AAPA/ABC/ACPM/AGS/APhA/ASH/ASPC/NMA/PCNA guideline for the prevention, detection, evaluation, and management of high blood pressure in adults. *Hypertension*. 2018;71(19):e13-115.
3. Centers for Disease Control and Prevention. Hypertension cascade: hypertension prevalence, treatment and control estimates among US adults aged 18 years and older applying the criteria from the American College of Cardiology and American Heart Association's 2017 Hypertension Guideline—NHANES 2015-2018. US Department of Health and Human Services. 2021. Accessed 10/12/2021. https://millionhearts.hhs.gov/data-reports/hypertension-prevalence.html
4. Mozaffarian D, Benjamin EJ, Go AS, et al. Heart disease and stroke statistics—2015 update: a report from the American Heart Association. *Circulation*. 2015;131(4):e29-322.
5. Lim SS, Vos T, Flaxman AD, et al. A comparative risk assessment of burden of disease and injury attributable to 67 risk factors and risk factor clusters in 21 regions, 1990-2010: a systematic analysis for the Global Burden of Disease Study 2010. *Lancet*. 2012;380(9859):2224-60.
6. Forouzanfar MH, Liu P, Roth GA, et al. Global burden of hypertension and systolic blood pressure of at least 110 to 115 mm Hg, 1990-2015. *JAMA*. 2017;317:165-82.
7. Farley TA, Dalal MA, Mostashari F, Frieden TR. Deaths preventable in the US by improvements in use of clinical preventive services. *Am J Prev Med*. 2020;38:600-9.
8. Vasan RS, Beiser A, Seshadri S, et al. Residual lifetime risk for developing hypertension in middle-aged women and men: the Framingham Heart Study. *JAMA*. 2002;287(8):1003-10.
9. Weir MR, Cotton D, Rao JK, et al. In the clinic: hypertension. *Ann Intern Med*. 2014;161:ITC1-15.
10. Muntner P, Carey RM, Gidding S, et al. Potential U.S. population impact of the 2017 ACC/AHA high blood pressure guideline. *J Am Coll Cardiol*. 2018;71(2):109-18.
11. Carretero OA, Oparil S. Essential hypertension. *Circulation*. 2000;101:329-35.
12. Buford TW. Hypertension and aging. *Ageing Res Rev*. 2016;26:96-111.
13. Hinton TC, Adams ZH, Baker RP, et al. Investigation and treatment of high blood pressure in young people: too much medicine or appropriate risk reduction? *Hypertension*. 2020;75(1):16-22.
14. Lifton RP, Gharavi AG, Geller DS. Molecular mechanisms of human hypertension. *Cell*. 2001;104:545-56.
15. Pickering TG, Hall JE, Appel LJ, et al. Recommendations for blood pressure measurement in humans and experimental animals: Part 1: blood pressure measurement in humans: a statement for professionals from the Subcommittee of Professional and Public Educations of the American Heart Association Council on High Blood Pressure Research. *Circulation*. 2005;111:697-716.
16. Krist AH, Davidson KW, Mangione CM, et al; US Preventative Services Task Force. Screening for hypertension in adults: US Preventive Services Task Force reaffirmation recommendation statement. *JAMA*. 2021;325(16):1650-6.
17. Pickering TG, White WB; American Society of Hypertension Writing Group. ASH Position Paper: Home and ambulatory blood pressure monitoring. When and how to use self (home) and ambulatory blood pressure monitoring. *J Clin Hypertens (Greenwich)*. 2008;10(11):850-5.
18. Egan BM. Treatment resistant hypertension. *Ethn Dis*. 2015;25(4):495-8.
19. Calhoun DA, Jones D, Textor S, et al. Resistant hypertension: diagnosis, evaluation, and treatment. A scientific statement from the American Heart Association Professional Educations Committee of the Council for High Blood Pressure Research. *Hypertension*. 2008;51(6):1403-19.
20. Stergiou GS, Bliziotis IA. Home blood pressure monitoring in the diagnosis and treatment of hypertension: a systematic review. *Am J Hypertens*. 2011;24(2):123-34.
21. James PA, Oparil S, Carter BL, et al. 2014 Evidence-based guideline for the management of high blood pressure in adults: report from the panel members appointed to the Eighth Joint National Committee (JNC 8). *JAMA*. 2014;311(5):507-20.
22. ALLHAT Officers and Coordinators for the ALLHAT Collaborative Research Group. The Antihypertensive and Lipid-Lowering Treatment to Prevent Heart Attack Trial. Major outcomes in high-risk hypertensive patients randomized to angiotensin-converting enzyme inhibitor or calcium channel blocker vs diuretic the Antihypertensive and Lipid-Lowering Treatment to Prevent Heart Attack Trial (ALLHAT). *JAMA*. 2002;288:2981-97.
23. Ogedegbe G, Shah NR, Phillips C, et al. Comparative effectiveness of angiotensin-converting enzyme inhibitor-based treatment on cardiovascular outcomes in hypertensive blacks versus whites. *J Am Coll Cardiol*. 2015;65:1224-33.

24. Leenen FHH, Nwachuku CE, Black HR, et al. Clinical events in high-risk hypertensive patients randomly assigned to calcium channel blocker versus angiotensin-converting enzyme inhibitor in the Antihypertensive and Lipid-Lowering Treatment to Prevent Heart Attack Trial. *Hypertension.* 2006;48:374-84.

25. Yusuf S, Teo KK, Pogue J, et al; ONTARGET Investigators. Telmisartan, ramipril, or both in patients at high risk for vascular events. *N Engl J Med.* 2008;358:1547-59.

26. Parving H-H, Brenner BM, McMurray JJV, et al. Cardiorenal end points in a trial of aliskiren for type 2 diabetes. *N Engl J Med.* 2012;367:2204-13.

27. Green BB, Cook AJ, Ralston JD, et al. Effectiveness of home blood pressure monitoring. Web communication, and pharmacist care on hypertension control: a randomized controlled trial. *JAMA.* 2008;299:2857-67.

28. Fihn SD, Blankenship JC, Alexander KP, et al. 2014 ACC/AHA/AATS/PCNA/SCAI/STS focused update of the guideline for the diagnosis and management of patients with stable ischemic heart disease: a report of the American College of Cardiology/American Heart Association Task Force on Practice Guidelines, and the American Association for Thoracic Surgery, Preventive Cardiovascular Nurses Association, Society for Cardiovascular Angiography and Interventions, and Society of Thoracic Surgeons. *Circulation.* 2014;130:1749-67.

29. Piller LB, Baraniuk S, Simpson LM, et al. Long-term follow-up of participants with heart failure in the antihypertensive and lipid-lowering treatment to prevent heart attack trial (ALLHAT). *Circulation.* 2011;124:1811-18.

30. Vilela-Martin JF, Yugar-Toledo JC, Rodrigues M, et al. Luso-Brazilian position statement on hypertensive emergencies—2020. *Arq Bras Cardiol.* 2020;114(4):736-51.

31. Zhao D, Wang Z-M, Wang L-S. Prevention of atrial fibrillation with renin–angiotensin system inhibitors on essential hypertensive patients: a meta-analysis of randomized controlled trials. *J Biomed Res.* 2015;29:475-85.

32. Erbel R, Aboyans V, Boileau C, et al. 2014 ESC guidelines on the diagnosis and treatment of aortic diseases: document covering acute and chronic aortic diseases of the thoracic and abdominal aorta of the adult. The Task Force for the Diagnosis and Treatment of Aortic Diseases of the European Society of Cardiology (ESC). *Eur Heart J.* 2014;35(41):2873-926.

33. Kramer H, Han C, Post W, et al. Racial/ethnic differences in hypertension and hypertension treatment and control in the multi-ethnic study of atherosclerosis (MESA). *Am J Hypertens.* 2004;17:963-70.

34. Benjamin EJ, Blaha MJ, Chiuve SE, et al. Heart disease and stroke statistics—2017 update: a report from the American Heart Association. *Circulation.* 2017;135:e146-603.

35. Ferdinand KC. Management of high blood pressure in African Americans and the 2010 ISHIB consensus statement: meeting an unmet need. *J Clin Hypertens (Greenwich).* 2010;12:237-9.

36. Benetos A, Petrovic M, Strandberg T. Hypertension management in older and frail older patients. *Circ Res.* 2019;124(7):1045-60.

37. Prevention of stroke by antihypertensive drug treatment in older persons with isolated systolic hypertension. Final results of the Systolic Hypertension in the Elderly Program (SHEP). SHEP Cooperative Research Group. *JAMA.* 1991;265:3255-64.

38. Williamson JD, Supiano MA, Applegate WB, et al. Intensive vs standard blood pressure control and cardiovascular disease outcomes in adults aged ≥75 years: a randomized clinical trial. *JAMA.* 2016;315:2673-82.

39. Bavishi C, Bangalore S, Messerli FH. Outcomes of intensive blood pressure lowering in older hypertensive patients. *J Am Coll Cardiol.* 2017;69:486-93.

40. Beckett NS, Peters R, Fletcher AE, et al. Treatment of hypertension in patients 80 years of age or older. *N Engl J Med.* 2008;358:1887-98.

41. Naschitz JE, Slobodin G, Elias N, Rosner I. The patient with supine hypertension and orthostatic hypotension: a clinical dilemma. *Postgrad Med J.* 2006;82(966):246-53.

42. Rivasi G, Rafanelli M, Mossello E, Brignole M, Ungar A. Drug-related orthostatic hypotension: beyond anti-hypertensive medications. *Drugs Aging.* 2020;37(10):725-38.

43. Hall JE. The kidney, hypertension, and obesity. *Hypertension.* 2003;41(Pt 2):625-33.

44. Bangalore S, Fayyad R, Laskey R, et al. Prevalence, predictors, and outcomes in treatment-resistant hypertension in patients with coronary disease. *Am J Med.* 2014;127:71-81.e1.

45. Cherney D, Straus S. Management of patients with hypertensive urgencies and emergencies. *J Gen Intern Med.* 2002;17(12):937-45.

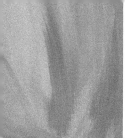

Primary and Secondary Prevention of Atherosclerotic Cardiovascular Disease

4

Amulya Gampa, Erica Young, and
Justin S. Sadhu

Primary Prevention

GENERAL PRINCIPLES

- Primary prevention of cardiovascular disease (CVD) refers to prevention of disease in a person without prior symptoms of CVD by optimizing risk factors with lifestyle modifications or medications.
- Prevention efforts at the population level include government warnings on cigarette use (beginning in the 1960s), efforts to reduce dietary fat intake (the 1960s and 1970s), the National High Blood Pressure Education Program (the 1970s and 1980s), and the National Cholesterol Education Program (the 1980s and 1990s).
- Prevention efforts at the level of the individual are targeted toward identifying patients at increased risk for CVD and optimizing risk factors.

RISK ASSESSMENT

- Much of a patient's overall health and cardiovascular risk is connected to nonmedical health-related social needs. Screening for and addressing these non–health-related measures that impact health outcomes can make a significant change in a patient's health.[1]
- Risk factors may be divided into nonmodifiable, modifiable (behavioral), and clinical (physiologic) factors.
- Routine risk factor screening commonly begins in childhood for at-risk individuals and continues into adulthood for all adults.[2]
- Blood pressure (BP), body mass index (BMI), waist circumference, and pulse should be recorded at each visit.
- Fasting or nonfasting serum lipoprotein profile and fasting blood glucose or hemoglobin A1C should be measured at least every 4 to 6 years starting at age 20 years.
- The American College of Cardiology (ACC) and American Heart Association (AHA) have published guidelines on cardiovascular risk assessment.[3]

Risk Assessment in Asymptomatic Patients Using Risk Scores

- The goal of risk assessment is to identify asymptomatic individuals without established CVD who may benefit from lifestyle changes and/or pharmacologic interventions.

- Risk scores combine traditional CVD risk factors to estimate the absolute risk of CVD for an individual over a specific time period, usually 10 years, as well as lifetime risk.
- The atherosclerotic cardiovascular disease (ASCVD) risk equation or pooled cohort equation (PCE) was developed to estimate the 10-year risk for ASCVD in non-Hispanic white and African American/Black individuals between 40 and 79 years of age.
- It is reasonable to estimate 10-year ASCVD risk every 4 to 6 years in adults without CVD who are 40 to 79 years of age.
- Race/ethnicity should be taken into account when estimating ASCVD risk. The PCEs can underestimate risk in certain populations, such as individuals of South Asian ancestry, and overestimate risk in others, such as those of East Asian ancestry.[4]
- In general, a 10-year ASCVD risk score of <5% is considered low risk, 5-<7.5% borderline risk, 7.5-<20% intermediate risk, and ≥20% high risk.
- In patients with intermediate ASCVD risk, it is reasonable to perform coronary artery calcium (CAC) scoring to reclassify risk and help guide the decision to use statin therapy.
  - A CAC score of 0, in the absence of risk factors such as diabetes, smoking, or family history of premature ASCVD, indicates low ASCVD risk for the following 10 years and likely low benefit from statin initiation.
  - A CAC score ≥100 or greater than the 75th percentile for age/sex/race is associated with increased ASCVD risk such that statin therapy would likely be beneficial.

Lifetime Risk Assessment

- Ten-year risk estimates greatly underestimate the risk of developing CVD in men <35 years and women <45 years.
- Patients should be encouraged to achieve or maintain an ideal risk factor profile from an early age to promote healthy aging.[5]
- Assessing 30-year or lifetime ASCVD risk based on traditional risk factors may be considered in adults who are 20 to 39 years of age, do not have CVD, and are not at high short-term risk.

Additional Risk Factors

- Several additional ASCVD risk factors are not included in the PCE.
- Lp(a) is a modified form of low-density lipoprotein (LDL) that is associated with increased ASCVD risk; it may be used for further risk stratification in patients with family history of premature ASCVD or personal history of ASCVD without other risk factors. Lp(a) should not be used as a target for therapy.
- The risk-enhancing factors listed in Figure 4-1[3,6] may be used to support the decision to initiate cholesterol-lowering therapy in intermediate-risk patients.
- Routine evaluation of carotid intima–media thickness is not recommended for individuals without CVD.

BEHAVIORAL RISK FACTORS

A healthy lifestyle is important in the prevention of CVD. The ACC/AHA Guideline on Lifestyle Management to Reduce CV Risk provides valuable assistance.

Diet

- A healthy diet offers one of the greatest potentials for reducing the risk of CVD.
- Dietary advice for reducing risk of CVD includes[7]:
  - Adopt a dietary pattern that emphasizes intake of vegetables, fruits, legumes, nuts, whole grains, and fish; and limits intake of sweets, sugar-sweetened beverages, and red meats.
  - Adapt this dietary pattern to appropriate calorie requirements, personal and cultural food preferences, and nutrition therapy for other medical conditions (including diabetes mellitus [DM]).

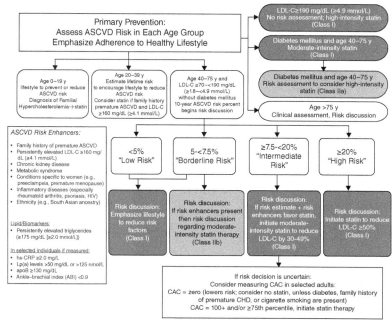

FIGURE 4-1. Major recommendations for the primary prevention of ASCVD. ASCVD, atherosclerotic cardiovascular disease; CAC, coronary artery calcium; hs-CRP, high-sensitivity C-reactive protein; LDL-C, low-density lipoprotein cholesterol. (Reprinted from Arnett DK, Blumenthal RS, Albert MA, et al. 2019 ACC/AHA guideline on the primary prevention of cardiovascular disease: Executive Summary: a report of the American College of Cardiology/American Heart Association Task Force on Clinical Practice Guidelines. *J Am Coll Cardiol.* 2019;74(10):1376-414. Copyright © 2019 by the American College of Cardiology Foundation and the American Heart Association, Inc. With permission.)

  ○ Achieve this pattern by following plans such as the Dietary Approach to Stop Hypertension (DASH) dietary pattern or the Mediterranean diet.
  ○ Plant-based diets can further decrease CVD risk.
  ○ Avoid *trans* fats and saturated fats, and replace them with unsaturated fats.
  ○ Reduce the percentage of calories from saturated fat.
• Dietary advice to those who would specifically benefit from BP lowering includes[8]:
  ○ Achieve a healthy diet by following the DASH dietary pattern, which recommends a diet rich in fruits, vegetables, whole grains, and low-fat dairy products, with reduced content of saturated and total fat.
  ○ Reduce dietary sodium by at least 1000 mg/day, with an optimal goal of <1500 mg/day.

Exercise

• Adults should engage in 150 minutes per week of moderate-intensity aerobic physical activity, or 75 minutes per week of vigorous-intensity aerobic physical activity, or an equivalent combination of moderate- and vigorous-intensity aerobic physical activity. Examples of moderate-intensity exercise include brisk walking, dancing, or biking on a flat surface. Examples of vigorous-intensity exercise include jogging, singles tennis, or bicycling uphill, see Table 4-1.[9]

TABLE 4-1	PHYSICAL ACTIVITY RECOMMENDATIONS FOR HEALTHY ADULTS

- In general, adults should move more and sit less throughout the day.
- Adults should perform 150–300 minutes of moderate-intensity activity, 75–150 minutes of vigorous-intensity activity, or an equivalent combination of moderate- and vigorous-intensity aerobic activity per week.
- Activity should ideally be spread throughout the week.
- Additional health benefits can be gained by performing more than the equivalent of 300 minutes of moderate-intensity activity per week.
- At least 2 days per week, adults should do muscle-strengthening activities of at least moderate intensity involving all major muscle groups.
- Activity is considered moderate intensity if a person can talk, but not sing while doing the activity.
- Activity is considered vigorous intensity if a person cannot say more than a few words without pausing to breathe.

Adapted from Piercy KL, Troiano RP, Ballard RM, et al. The physical activity guidelines for Americans. *JAMA.* 2018;320:2020-28.

- Adults should also perform muscle-strengthening activities that involve all major muscle groups 2 or more days a week.
- Sedentary or deconditioned adults should exercise at a lower intensity and duration and gradually increase exercise until they reach the recommended goal.
- Older adults should follow the adult guidelines if able or be as physically active as their condition allows.

Alcohol

- Moderate alcohol consumption (up to 2 drinks per day for men and 1 drink per day for women) appears to reduce total and cardiovascular mortality.[10,11] One drink is a 5-oz glass of wine, a 12-oz beer, or 1.5 oz of 80-proof spirit.
- The association of alcohol consumption with CVD follows a J-shaped curve. There is lower CVD death with moderate alcohol consumption, but an increase in all-cause and cardiovascular mortality with increasing consumption.
- In addition to increased mortality, increased alcohol consumption may result in hypertension, alcoholism, cirrhosis, accidents, suicide, and decreased economic productivity. Individuals should not be advised to increase alcohol consumption simply to improve their cardiovascular risk profile.

Tobacco Abuse

- Smoking is the leading cause of preventable disease and death among older adults.
- Adults should be screened for tobacco use at every healthcare visit and, if using, should be offered counseling and tools for cessation.[12]
- Recommendations to encourage smoking cessation include:
  ○ Ask patients about their tobacco use at every visit.
  ○ In a clear, strong, and personalized manner, advise every tobacco user to quit.
  ○ Assess the tobacco user's willingness to quit.
  ○ Assist by counseling and developing a plan for quitting.
  ○ Arrange follow-up and referral to special programs.
  ○ Urge avoidance of exposure to secondhand smoke at work and at home.
  ○ Consider the use of pharmacotherapy.

- Nicotine replacement therapy, including patches, gum, spray, lozenges, and inhalers, has been shown to significantly increase the rate of smoking cessation.[13]
- Bupropion, used alone or in combination with replacement therapy, has also been shown to increase smoking cessation rates.[14] Bupropion should not be used in patients with a history of seizures, anorexia, or bulimia.
- Varenicline, used for 12 to 24 weeks, has shown benefit in aiding in smoking cessation. Dosing should be adjusted for severe renal impairment.
- Dosing for smoking cessation therapies is detailed in Table 4-2.[14]
- E-cigarettes are not recommended for use as a cessation tool.
- E-cigarettes may worsen cardiovascular and pulmonary disease via emission of toxic gases, including nicotine and ultrafine particles.

TABLE 4-2	PHARMACOTHERAPY FOR SMOKING CESSATION
Medication	**Dosage/instructions**
Nicotine replacement therapy	
Gum	If first cigarette ≤30 minutes after waking: 4 mg If first cigarette >30 minutes after waking: 2 mg Weeks 1–6: 1 piece every 1–2 hours Weeks 7–9: 1 piece every 2–4 hours Weeks 10–12: 1 piece every 4–8 hours Maximum: 24 pieces/d Duration: up to 12 weeks
Lozenge	If first cigarette ≤30 minutes after waking: 4 mg If first cigarette >30 minutes after waking: 2 mg Weeks 1–6: 1 lozenge every 1–2 hours Weeks 7–9: 1 lozenge every 2–4 hours Weeks 10–12: 1 lozenge every 4–8 hours Maximum: 20 lozenges/d Duration: up to 12 weeks
Transdermal patch	If >10 cigarettes/d: 21 mg/d for 4–6 weeks, then 14 mg/d for 2 weeks, then 7 mg/d for 2 weeks If ≤10 cigarettes/d: 14 mg/d for 2 weeks, then 7 mg/d for 2 weeks Duration: 8–10 weeks
Nasal spray	1 dose = one spray in each nostril (0.5 mg nicotine/spray) 1–2 doses/h Maximum: 5 doses/h, 40 doses/d Duration: 3–6 months
Oral inhaler	6–16 cartridges/d (4 mg inhaled nicotine vapor/cartridge) Individualize dosing, starting with 1 cartridge every 1–2 hours Maximum: 16 cartridges/d Duration: 3–6 months

(*continued*)

TABLE 4-2	PHARMACOTHERAPY FOR SMOKING CESSATION (*continued*)
Medication	**Dosage/instructions**
Other medications	
Bupropion sustained release[a]	Start 1–2 weeks prior to quit date 150 mg every morning for 3 days, then 150 mg twice daily Duration: 7–12 weeks
Varenicline	Start 1 week prior to quit date Days 1–3: 0.5 mg every morning Days 4–7: 0.5 mg twice daily Weeks 2–12: 1 mg twice daily Duration: 12 weeks. Repeat 12-week course for selected patients

[a]May be used in combination with nicotine replacement therapy.

Adapted with permission of Annual Reviews, Inc. from Prochaska JJ, Benowitz NL. The past, present, and future of nicotine addiction therapy. *Annu Rev Med.* 2016;67:467-86; permission conveyed through Copyright Clearance Center, Inc.

Cannabis

- Cannabis or marijuana products are increasingly being used both medically and recreationally.
- Δ-9-Tetrahydrocannabinol (THC) and cannabidiol (CBD) are both found in cannabis and have been used for both their therapeutic and psychotropic properties.[15]
- To date, there is no strong evidence to suggest cardiovascular benefit with cannabis use, and it is not recommended for treatment or prevention of cardiovascular disorders.
- Chronic use also carries risks, including cannabinoid hyperemesis syndrome and increased chance of psychosis and schizophrenia in individuals with predisposition.[15]
- Smoked or vaporized cannabis products should be avoided as they contain many of the same carcinogens as smoked tobacco, though there is no strong evidence at this point linking cannabis smoke to cancers.

CLINICAL/PHYSIOLOGIC RISK FACTORS

Lipid Management

- The ACC/AHA have published recommendations for lipid management.[6]
- Lipid management for primary prevention of ASCVD starts with measurement of the lipid profile, including LDL cholesterol (LDL-C).
  - For most patients, a nonfasting lipid profile is sufficient.
  - For patients with very low LDL-C or triglyceride levels ≥400 mg/dL, LDL-C calculated by the Friedewald equation is not accurate. Direct LDL-C measurement should be used instead.
- Treatment involves use of moderate- or high-intensity statins (Table 4-3).
- Treatment is indicated based on a combination of clinical risk factors, lipid profile, and estimated ASCVD risk by the PCE (Figure 4-1).[3]
  - Patients with a history of clinical ASCVD should receive treatment (see section Secondary Prevention: Lipid Management).
  - Patients aged 20 to 75 years with severe hypercholesterolemia (LDL-C ≥190 mg/dL) should be treated with a maximally tolerated statin.

TABLE 4-3 HIGH-, MODERATE-, AND LOW-INTENSITY STATIN THERAPY

High-intensity statin therapy	Moderate-intensity statin therapy	Low-intensity statin therapy
Lowers LDL-C by ≥50%	Lowers LDL-C by 30–<50%	Lowers LDL-C by <30%
Atorvastatin 40–80 mg	Atorvastatin 10–20 mg	Simvastatin 10 mg
Rosuvastatin 20–40 mg	Rosuvastatin 5–10 mg	Pravastatin 10–20 mg
	Simvastatin 20–40 mg[a]	Lovastatin 20 mg
	Pravastatin 40–80 mg	Fluvastatin 20–40 mg
	Lovastatin 40 mg	
	Fluvastatin XL 80 mg	
	Fluvastatin 40 mg bid	
	Pitavastatin 1–4 mg	

bid, twice daily; FDA, Food and Drug Administration; LDL-C, low-density lipoprotein cholesterol; RCT, randomized controlled trial.

[a]Although simvastatin 80 mg was evaluated in RCTs, initiation of simvastatin 80 mg or titration to 80 mg is not recommended by the FDA due to the increased risk of myopathy, including rhabdomyolysis.

Adapted from Grundy SM, Stone NJ, Bailey AL, et al. 2018 AHA/ACC/AACVPR/AAPA/ABC/ACPM/ADA/AGS/APhA/ASPC/NLA/PCNA guideline on the management of blood cholesterol: a report of the American College of Cardiology/American Heart Association Task Force on Clinical Practice Guidelines. *J Am Coll Cardiol.* 2019;73(24):e285-350. Copyright © 2019 by the American College of Cardiology Foundation. With permission.

- Patients aged 40 to 75 years with DM should be treated with at least a moderate-intensity statin. High-intensity statin can be considered if additional risk-enhancing factors are present.
- Patients aged 40 to 75 years with LDL-C 70 to <190 mg/dL and without DM should have a 10-year ASCVD risk assessment by the PCE.
  - Moderate-intensity statin therapy is recommended if ASCVD risk is ≥20% (high risk) or if ASCVD risk is 7.5-<20% (intermediate risk) with risk-enhancing factors.
  - CAC score can assist in decision-making for patients with intermediate ASCVD risk (see section Risk Assessment in Asymptomatic Patients Using Risk Scores).
- The benefit of statins in older adults (>75 years) is less clear. The decision to continue or discontinue statin therapy should be made based on overall ASCVD risk, life expectancy, functional status, and patient preference.
- Adults with moderate (149 to 499 mg/dL) to severe (>500 mg/dL) hypertriglyceridemia should have risk factors such as lifestyle, comorbidities, and medications addressed to reduce triglycerides. It is reasonable to initiate a statin for adults aged 40 to 75 years with moderate or severe hypertriglyceridemia.
- When statin therapy is insufficient or not well tolerated, nonstatin therapies may be used in place of or in combination with statins (Table 4-4):
  - Ezetimibe, a cholesterol absorption inhibitor, is the most commonly used nonstatin therapy.
  - Bile acid sequestrants may also be used but can cause gastrointestinal side effects and hypertriglyceridemia.
  - PCSK9 inhibitors can significantly reduce LDL-C levels but are very expensive and generally have low cost-effectiveness at their current prices; cost-effectiveness remains uncertain for individuals with familial hyperlipidemia.

TABLE 4-4	NONSTATIN THERAPIES
Drug class	**Dosage[a]**
Cholesterol absorption inhibitors	Ezetimibe 10 mg
Bile acid sequestrants	Cholestyramine 4000–24,000 mg
	Colesevelam 3750 mg
	Colestipol 5000–30,000 mg
PCSK9 inhibitors[b]	Alirocumab 75–150 mg every 2 weeks
	Alirocumab 300 mg every 4 weeks
	Evolocumab 140 mg every 2 weeks
	Evolocumab 420 mg every 4 weeks
Omega-3 fatty acid	Icosapent ethyl 2 g twice daily

[a]Total daily dosage unless otherwise specified.
[b]PSCK9 inhibitors are administered by SC injection.
Adapted from Grundy SM, Stone NJ, Bailey AL, et al. 2018 AHA/ACC/AACVPR/AAPA/ABC/ACPM/ADA/AGS/APhA/ASPC/NLA/PCNA guideline on the management of blood cholesterol: a report of the American College of Cardiology/American Heart Association Task Force on Clinical Practice Guidelines. *Circulation.* 2019;139:e1082-143; and Orringer CE, Jacobson TA, Maki KC. National Lipid Association Scientific Statement on the use of icosapent ethyl in statin-treated patients with elevated triglycerides and high or very-high ASCVD risk. *J Clin Lipidol.* 2019;13(6):860-72.

- ○ Icosapent ethyl may be used to further decrease cardiovascular risk in patients ≥45 years of age with ASCVD or ≥50 years of age with DM requiring medication and at least one additional risk factor who are on maximally tolerated statin therapy and/or ezetimibe with fasting triglycerides 135 to 499 mg/dL.[16]
- • The addition of nonstatin therapies should be considered based on the following factors:
  - ○ Reduction in LDL-C and ASCVD risk with statin therapy and lifestyle modifications
  - ○ Potential drug–drug interactions or adverse events from addition of nonstatin therapy
  - ○ Convenience and cost of nonstatin therapy
  - ○ Anticipated life expectancy and comorbidities
  - ○ For primary prevention in individuals with LDL-C ≥190 mg/dL: if there is a <50% reduction in LDL-C and LDL-C ≥100 mg/dL on maximally tolerated statin therapy, the addition of ezetimibe can be beneficial. For patients with baseline LDL-C ≥220 mg/dL whose LDL-C level is ≥130 mg/dL despite maximally tolerated statin and ezetimibe therapy, a PCSK9 inhibitor can be considered.
  - ○ For primary prevention in patients with DM with LDL-C 70 to 189 mg/dL and 10-year ASCVD risk ≥20%: if there is a <50% reduction in LDL-C on maximally tolerated statin therapy, the addition of ezetimibe can be considered.
  - ○ For primary prevention in patients without DM with an LDL-C 70 to 189 mg/dL and 10-year ASCVD risk ≥7.5%: if there is a <30-50% reduction in LDL-C on maximally tolerated statin therapy, and additional risk factors are present, the addition of ezetimibe can be considered.
- • Statins are generally well tolerated though some patients may experience side effects.
  - ○ Statin-associated muscle symptoms are the most common side effects and include myalgias, myositis, and rhabdomyolysis, which is rare.
  - ○ Elevations in liver enzymes are infrequent, and liver failure is rare.

- There is a slightly increased risk of new-onset diabetes in patients with other risk factors for diabetes, such as impaired glucose tolerance or obesity.
- An effective approach to mild–moderate statin side effects is to stop the drug, openly discuss the risks and benefits of statins with the patient, and rechallenge with an alternate statin.

Hypertension

- Hypertension is the leading modifiable cause of ASCVD deaths in the US.
- The 2017 ACC/AHA Guideline for the Prevention, Detection, Evaluation, and Management of High Blood Pressure in Adults provides BP goals based on comorbidities and ASCVD risk.[8]
  - Lifestyle modification, including a healthy diet, exercise, weight loss, and decreased sodium intake, is recommended for all patients with hypertension.
  - Use of medication to lower BP is recommended for primary prevention of CVD in adults with:
    - estimated 10-year ASCVD risk ≥10% and an average systolic BP (SBP) ≥130 mm Hg or an average diastolic BP (DBP) ≥80 mm Hg
    - estimated 10-year ASCVD risk <10% and an SBP ≥140 mm Hg or a DBP ≥90 mm Hg
- First-line agents for antihypertensive therapy include thiazide/thiazide-like diuretics, calcium channel blockers, and angiotensin-converting enzyme (ACE) inhibitors or angiotensin receptor blockers (ARBs).
- Further recommendations may be found in Chapter 3.

Type 2 Diabetes Mellitus

- DM accelerates the progression of coronary artery disease (CAD) and increases the risk of acute coronary syndrome (ACS); it is a major ASCVD risk factor.
- Moderate- to high-intensity statins are recommended for those with diabetes (see section Lipid Management).
- A heart-healthy diet with a focus on whole grain intake and avoidance of refined carbohydrates is recommended for all patients with DM.
- Regular exercise is also recommended for all patients with DM for improved glycemic control and improved ASCVD risk.
- For patients who are at high risk for ASCVD (those with end-organ damage or who have multiple risk factors), initiation of a glucagon-like peptide 1 (GLP-1) agonist or sodium-glucose cotransporter 2 (SGLT-2) inhibitor is recommended, as these medications have been shown to decrease the risk of cardiovascular events.[17]
  - While metformin is generally the first-line drug of choice for patients with diabetes, GLP-1 agonists and SGLT-2 inhibitors may be considered as a first-line treatment in patients with established ASCVD or who are at high risk for ASCVD.[18]
  - For patients at high risk for ASCVD who are already taking metformin and require further medical therapy, addition of a GLP-1 agonist or SGLT-2 inhibitor is recommended.
  - Patient and clinician preferences should be considered when choosing between GLP-1 agonists and SGLT-2 inhibitors. While both classes reduce cardiovascular events, SGLT-2 inhibitors have benefit in the prevention of heart failure and kidney disease progression, while GLP-1 agonists can aid in weight loss.

Obesity

- Obesity is associated with hyperlipidemia, hypertension, and insulin resistance.
- Obesity increases risk of CVD, heart failure, and atrial fibrillation.

- BMI is the most commonly used and best validated tool for evaluating obesity. A BMI of 25 to 29.9 kg/m^2 is considered overweight, and BMI ≥30 kg/m^2 is considered obese.
- Increased waist circumference and waist–hip ratio have also been associated with increased CVD risk. Measuring waist circumference can be useful in patients with predominately central adiposity.
- Obese individuals with central adiposity are at particularly high risk for CVD.
- Although exercise is an important part of any weight loss program, dietary change is the mainstay of weight loss.
- Recommendations for weight loss include:
  ○ Initiation of a weight management program through caloric restriction and increased caloric expenditure
  ○ The goal is to reduce body weight by 5-10% in the first year of therapy.
  ○ Weight loss medications and/or bariatric surgery can be considered as an adjunct to lifestyle and behavioral modification.
- Bariatric surgery is associated with reduced CAD risk when compared with nonsurgical weight management.[19]

Aspirin

- In the current era of statin use and stricter BP control, aspirin for primary prevention of ASCVD appears to confer less overall benefit than previously considered, while still increasing bleeding risk. The use of aspirin for primary prevention and age at which potential harm exceeds benefit for the general population remain areas of active discussion and vary between guidelines.[3,20]
- Both ASCVD risk and bleeding risk should be taken into consideration when discussing aspirin for primary prevention.
  ○ In adults aged 40 to 70 years, low-dose aspirin (75 to 100 mg daily) might be considered if there is a high ASCVD risk and low bleeding risk.[3]
  ○ Aspirin is not recommended for patients with high bleeding risk or a history of bleeding.
  ○ Routine use of aspirin for primary prevention is not recommended for adults over 70 years of age.[3]

Secondary Prevention

GENERAL PRINCIPLES

- Secondary prevention is the prevention of disease progression or death in patients who are symptomatic or have previously been diagnosed with CVD.
- Aggressive risk factor management improves survival and quality of life and reduces recurrent events and need for interventional procedures.[21] Please see Table 4-5 for a summary of secondary recommendations.[6,21-23]

SPECIAL TOPICS IN SECONDARY PREVENTION

Lipid Management

- High-intensity statins are generally recommended for all individuals aged 20 to 75 years with CVD.

TABLE 4-5	ASCVD SECONDARY PREVENTION RECOMMENDATIONS
Factor	**Goal**
Smoking	Complete cessation
	Avoidance of exposure to environmental tobacco smoke
Blood pressure	See Chapter 3
Cholesterol	High-intensity statin therapy
Physical activity	At least 30 minutes of moderate-intensity activity 5–7 days/wk
Weight	BMI 18.5–24.9 kg/m^2 (initial goal 5-10% weight loss from baseline if overweight/obese)
	Waist circumference men <40″
	Waist circumference women <35″
Diabetes	HbA1C ≤7%
Antiplatelet agents/ anticoagulants	Aspirin 75–162 mg daily indefinitely
	If intolerant/allergic to aspirin: clopidogrel 75 mg daily
	Aspirin + P2Y12 receptor antagonist after ACS (12 months) or PCI with stent (generally at least 6 months), potentially up to 30 months (duration to be individualized based on assessment of bleeding vs. thrombotic risk)
ACE inhibitors	Recommended for all who have heart failure or SIHD or MI with LVEF ≤40%
	Also recommended in those with hypertension, diabetes, or chronic kidney disease
	ARBs recommended for those who are intolerant of ACE inhibitors
	Reasonable for patients who have had ACS or SIHD and other vascular disease
Aldosterone blockers	Recommended for post-MI patients without significant renal impairment or hyperkalemia who are already on therapeutic doses of ACE inhibitor and β-blocker, who have LVEF ≤40%, and who have either diabetes or heart failure
β-Blockers	Recommended to be continued for 3 years in patients who have had an MI/ACS
	Recommended in all patients with LVEF ≤40% and prior MI or heart failure
	Consider chronic therapy for all patients with coronary or other vascular disease
Influenza vaccine	Recommended for all patients with CVD
Depression	Screen for depression in patients with recent CABG or MI. Reasonable to consider screening for depression in patients with SIHD

(continued)

TABLE 4-5	ASCVD SECONDARY PREVENTION RECOMMENDATIONS (*continued*)
Factor	**Goal**
Cardiac rehabilitation	Recommended for all patients with ACS, CABG, PCI, chronic angina, and/or peripheral artery disease (either immediately post or within the past year) Can also be considered for those with SIHD at high risk

ACE, angiotensin-converting enzyme; ACS, acute coronary syndrome; ARB, angiotensin receptor blocker; ASCVD, atherosclerotic cardiovascular disease; BMI, body mass index; CABG, coronary artery bypass grafting; HbA1C, hemoglobin A1C; LVEF, left ventricular ejection fraction; MI, myocardial infarction; PCI, percutaneous coronary intervention; SIHD, stable ischemic heart disease.

Data from Grundy SM, Stone NJ, Bailey AL, et al. 2018 AHA/ACC/AACVPR/AAPA/ABC/ACPM/ADA/AGS/APhA/ASPC/NLA/PCNA guideline on the management of blood cholesterol: a report of the American College of Cardiology/American Heart Association Task Force on Clinical Practice Guidelines. *Circulation.* 2019;139:e1082-143; Smith SC Jr, Benjamin EJ, Bonow RO, et al. AHA/ACCF secondary prevention and risk reduction therapy for patients with coronary and other atherosclerotic vascular disease: 2011 update: a guideline from the American Heart Association and American College of Cardiology Foundation. *Circulation.* 2011;124:2458-73; Amsterdam EA, Wenger NK, Brindis RG, et al. 2014 AHA/ACC guideline for the management of patients with non-ST-elevation acute coronary syndromes: a report of the American College of Cardiology/American Heart Association Task Force on Practice Guidelines. *Circulation.* 2014;130:e344-426; and Fihn SD, Gardin JM, Abrams J, et al. 2012 ACCF/AHA/ACP/AATS/PCNA/SCAI/STS guideline for the diagnosis and management of patients with stable ischemic heart disease: a report of the American College of Cardiology Foundation/American Heart Association Task Force on Practice Guidelines, and the American College of Physicians, American Association for Thoracic Surgery, Preventive Cardiovascular Nurses Association, Society for Cardiovascular Angiography and Interventions, and Society of Thoracic Surgeons. *Circulation.* 2012;126:e354-471.

- Recommendations for initiating statin therapy in patients with ASCVD are shown in Figure 4-2.[6]
- The addition of nonstatin therapies can be considered for secondary prevention.
  - For individuals with LDL-C >70 mg/dL or non–high-density lipoprotein cholesterol (HDL-C) >100 mg/dL on maximally tolerated statin therapy, the addition of ezetimibe can be considered. A PCSK9 inhibitor can be considered next for those at very high risk. Icosapent ethyl may be considered in patients with elevated fasting triglycerides despite maximally tolerated statin therapy.
  - See the Primary Prevention: Lipid Management section for details on nonstatin therapies and management of statin-associated side effects.
- Bempedoic acid is a novel agent that lowers LDL-C by inhibiting ATP-citrate lyase, upstream of β-hydroxy β-methylglutaryl coenzyme A (HMG-CoA) reductase in the cholesterol synthesis pathway.
  - Bempedoic acid has been approved by the Food and Drug Administration (FDA) for use in patients with clinical ASCVD who have not achieved goal LDL-C lowering despite changes in diet and maximally tolerated statin therapy, as well as in patients with familial hypercholesterolemia.[24]
  - Although bempedoic acid has been shown to reduce LDL, its effects on cardiovascular outcomes are currently being studied.[25]

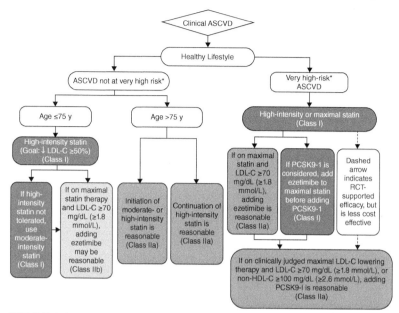

FIGURE 4-2. Initiating statin therapy in individuals with clinical ASCVD. ASCVD, atherosclerotic cardiovascular disease; LDL-C, low-density lipoprotein cholesterol; RCT, randomized controlled trial. (Reprinted from Grundy SM, Stone NJ, Bailey AL, et al. 2018 AHA/ACC/AACVPR/AAPA/ABC/ACPM/ADA/AGS/APhA/ASPC/ NLA/PCNA guideline on the management of blood cholesterol: a report of the American College of Cardiology/American Heart Association Task Force on Clinical Practice Guidelines. *J Am Coll Cardiol.* 2019;73(24):e285-350. Copyright © 2019 by the American College of Cardiology Foundation. With permission.)
*10-year ASCVD risk score of <5% is considered low risk, 5-<7.5% borderline risk, 7.5-<20% intermediate risk, and ≥20% high risk.

Hypertension

- Use of BP lowering medication is recommended for secondary prevention of recurrent CVD in patients with clinical CVD and an average SBP ≥130 mm Hg or an average DBP ≥80 mm Hg.[8]
- Further recommendations can be found in Chapter 3.

Diabetes Mellitus

In individuals with established ASCVD and DM, treatment with a GLP-1 agonist or SGLT-2 inhibitor is recommended.

Antiplatelet Therapy

- Low-dose aspirin (75 to 100 mg daily) is indicated in most patients with a history of CVD to reduce mortality and cardiovascular events.
- In patients with an allergy to or intolerance of aspirin, or coronary stents, other antiplatelet agents (e.g., clopidogrel) can be considered.

Cardiac Rehabilitation

- Comprehensive cardiac rehabilitation services include long-term, multidisciplinary programs involving medical evaluation, prescribed exercise, cardiac risk factor modification, and education.[26]
- Patients receive counseling related to nutrition, smoking cessation, psychosocial issues, and management of diabetes, hypertension, and hyperlipidemia.
- Cardiac rehabilitation has been shown to improve mortality, functional capacity, depression, and medication adherence.
- Cardiac rehabilitation is recommended and covered by Medicare for patients with a history of coronary artery bypass surgery, percutaneous coronary intervention, current stable angina, heart transplantation, heart valve repair or replacement, myocardial infarction in the previous 12 months, stable chronic heart failure with reduced left ventricular ejection fraction, or recent cerebrovascular accident (women only).
- Patients should be referred for cardiac rehabilitation prior to hospital discharge or at the first outpatient visit for any of the above diagnoses or procedures. If not hospitalized, patients should be referred within 12 months of the condition.[27]
- Aerobic exercise training can generally begin within 1 to 2 weeks after unstable angina/non–ST-segment elevation myocardial infarction treated with percutaneous coronary intervention or coronary artery bypass grafting.[22]
- A physical activity history or exercise testing can be considered in patients with stable CAD before referral to an exercise program to guide prognosis and exercise prescription.[23]
- Patients are encouraged to engage in moderate-intensity activity five times a week for 30 to 60 minutes and perform resistance training at least 2 days per week.[28]

REFERENCES

1. Billioux A, Verlander K, Anthony S, Alley D. Standardized screening for health-related social needs in clinical settings: the Accountable Health Communities Screening Tool. Presented at: National Academy of Medicine Perspectives; 2017; Washington, DC.
2. de Ferranti SD, Steinberger J, Ameduri R, et al. Cardiovascular risk reduction in high-risk pediatric patients: a scientific statement from the American Heart Association. *Circulation.* 2019;139:e603-34.
3. Arnett DK, Blumenthal RS, Albert MA, et al. 2019 ACC/AHA guideline on the primary prevention of cardiovascular disease: a report of the American College of Cardiology/American Heart Association Task Force on Clinical Practice Guidelines. *J Am Coll Cardiol.* 2019;74:e177-232.
4. Kandula NR, Kanaya AM, Liu K, et al. Association of 10-year and lifetime predicted cardiovascular disease risk with subclinical atherosclerosis in South Asians: findings from the Mediators of Atherosclerosis in South Asians Living in America (MASALA) study. *J Am Heart Assoc.* 2014;3:e001117.
5. Lichtenstein AH, Appel LJ, Brands M, et al. Diet and lifestyle recommendations revision 2006: a scientific statement from the American Heart Association Nutrition Committee. *Circulation.* 2006;114:82-96.
6. Grundy SM, Stone NJ, Bailey AL, et al. 2018 AHA/ACC/AACVPR/AAPA/ABC/ACPM/ADA/AGS/AphA/ASPC/NLA/PCNA guideline on the management of blood cholesterol: a report of the American College of Cardiology/American Heart Association Task Force on Clinical Practice Guidelines. *Circulation.* 2019;139:e1082-143.
7. American Heart Association. The American Heart Association diet and lifestyle recommendations. Accessed 7/21/21. https://www.heart.org/en/healthy-living/healthy-eating/eat-smart/nutrition-basics/aha-diet-and-lifestyle-recommendations
8. Whelton PK, Carey RM, Aronow WS, et al. 2017 ACC/AHA/AAPA/ABC/ACPM/AGS/AphA/ASH/ASPC/NMA/PCNA guideline for the prevention, detection, evaluation, and management of high blood pressure in adults: a report of the American College of Cardiology/American Heart Association Task Force on Clinical Practice Guidelines. *J Am Coll Cardiol.* 2018;71:e127-248.
9. Piercy KL, Troiano RP, Ballard RM, et al. The physical activity guidelines for Americans. *JAMA.* 2018;320:2020-8.

10. Ronksley PE, Brien SE, Turner BJ, Mukamal KJ, Ghali WA. Association of alcohol consumption with selected cardiovascular disease outcomes: a systematic review and meta-analysis. *BMJ.* 2011;342:d671.

11. O'Keefe JH, Bybee KA, Lavie CJ. Alcohol and cardiovascular health: the razor-sharp double-edged sword. *J Am Coll Cardiol.* 2007;50:1009-14.

12. Patnode CD, Henderson JT, Thompson JH, Senger CA, Fortmann SP, Whitlock EP. Behavioral counseling and pharmacotherapy interventions for tobacco cessation in adults, including pregnant women: a review of reviews for the U.S. Preventive Services Task Force. *Ann Intern Med.* 2015;163:608-21.

13. Stead LF, Perera R, Bullen C, et al. Nicotine replacement therapy for smoking cessation. *Cochrane Database Syst Rev.* 2012;11:CD000146.

14. Prochaska JJ, Benowitz NL. The past, present, and future of nicotine addiction therapy. *Annu Rev Med.* 2016;67:467-86.

15. Page RL, Allen LA, Kloner RA, et al. Medical marijuana, recreational cannabis, and cardiovascular health: a scientific statement from the American Heart Association. *Circulation.* 2020;142:e131-52.

16. Orringer CE, Jacobson TA, Maki KC. National Lipid Association Scientific Statement on the use of icosapent ethyl in statin-treated patients with elevated triglycerides and high or very-high ASCVD risk. *J Clin Lipidol.* 2019;13(6):860-72.

17. Das SR, Everett BM, Birtcher KK, et al. 2020 Expert consensus decision pathway on novel therapies for cardiovascular risk reduction in patients with type 2 diabetes: a report of the American College of Cardiology Solution Set Oversight Committee. *J Am Coll Cardiol.* 2020;76:1117-45.

18. Cosentino F, Grant PJ, Aboyans V, et al. 2019 ESC Guidelines on diabetes, pre-diabetes, and cardiovascular diseases developed in collaboration with the EASD. *Eur Heart J.* 2020;41:255-323.

19. Powell-Wiley TM, Poirier P, Burke LE, et al. Obesity and cardiovascular disease: a scientific statement from the American Heart Association. *Circulation.* 2021;143:e984-1010.

20. USPSTF. Aspirin use to prevent cardiovascular disease: preventive medication. 2021. Accessed 12/22/21. https://www.uspreventiveservicestaskforce.org/uspstf/draft-recommendation/aspirin-use-to-prevent-cardiovascular-disease-preventive-medication

21. Smith SC Jr, Benjamin EJ, Bonow RO, et al. AHA/ACCF secondary prevention and risk reduction therapy for patients with coronary and other atherosclerotic vascular disease: 2011 update: a guideline from the American Heart Association and American College of Cardiology Foundation. *Circulation.* 2011;124:2458-73.

22. Amsterdam EA, Wenger NK, Brindis RG, et al. 2014 AHA/ACC guideline for the management of patients with non-ST-elevation acute coronary syndromes: a report of the American College of Cardiology/American Heart Association Task Force on Practice Guidelines. *Circulation.* 2014;130:e344-426.

23. Fihn SD, Gardin JM, Abrams J, et al. 2012 ACCF/AHA/ACP/AATS/PCNA/SCAI/STS guideline for the diagnosis and management of patients with stable ischemic heart disease: a report of the American College of Cardiology Foundation/American Heart Association Task Force on Practice Guidelines, and the American College of Physicians, American Association for Thoracic Surgery, Preventive Cardiovascular Nurses Association, Society for Cardiovascular Angiography and Interventions, and Society of Thoracic Surgeons. *Circulation.* 2012;126:e354-471.

24. Markham A. Bempedoic acid: first approval. *Drugs.* 2020;80:747-53.

25. Nicholls S, Lincoff AM, Bays HE, et al. Rationale and design of the CLEAR-outcomes trial: evaluating the effect of bempedoic acid on cardiovascular events in patients with statin intolerance. *Am Heart J.* 2021;235:104-12.

26. Servey JT, Stephens M. Cardiac rehabilitation: improving function and reducing risk. *Am Fam Physician.* 2016;94:37-43.

27. Thomas RJ, Balady G, Banka G, et al. 2018 ACC/AHA clinical performance and quality measures for cardiac rehabilitation: a report of the American College of Cardiology/American Heart Association Task Force on Performance Measures. *Circ Cardiovasc Qual Outcomes.* 2018;11:e000037.

28. Squires RW, Kaminsky LA, Porcari JP, et al. Progression of exercise training in early outpatient cardiac rehabilitation: an official statement from the American Association of Cardiovascular and Pulmonary Rehabilitation. *J Cardiopulm Rehabil Prev.* 2018;38:139-46.

The Cardiac Patient Undergoing Noncardiac Surgery

Brittany M. Dixon and Lynne M. Seacord

5

GENERAL PRINCIPLES

- Preoperative evaluation of the patient with known or suspected cardiovascular disease undergoing noncardiac surgery is one of the most common reasons for cardiac consultation.
- The role of the consultant is to determine the stability of the patient's cardiovascular status and whether the patient is in the best medical condition within the context of the surgical illness.
- **The term "cardiac clearance" is strongly discouraged. Rather, the purpose of the evaluation is to determine cardiovascular risk assessment and provide medical optimization.** The evaluation may include discussions with the surgeon, anesthesiologist, and other physicians, when appropriate.
- In 2014, the American College of Cardiology (ACC) and the American Heart Association (AHA) published joint guidelines that provide updated recommendations for this purpose.[1]
  - Perioperative cardiac evaluation considers both the nature of the surgery and the clinical characteristics of the patient. Risk for specific types of surgery is indicated in Table 5-1.[2]
  - Patients undergoing low-risk procedures do not generally require further preoperative cardiac testing.

Emergent Surgery

- In the setting of a surgical emergency, preoperative evaluation should be limited to a rapid assessment, including vital signs, volume status, labs (hemoglobin, electrolytes, renal function), and ECG. Only the most essential tests and interventions are appropriate until the acute surgical emergency is resolved.
- The consultation should include recommendations about perioperative and postoperative cardiac management (e.g., need for telemetry, medications while NPO), and the consulting team should see the patient in postoperative follow-up.

Nonemergent Surgery

- Under less urgent circumstances, perioperative cardiac evaluation may involve temporary postponement or cancellation of an elective procedure. The algorithm for perioperative cardiac evaluation and management is shown in Figure 5-1.[1]
- For any nonemergent surgery, the first step is to assess whether the patient has an active high-risk cardiac condition (Figure 5-1).[1] **If such an active high-risk cardiac condition is present, elective surgery is postponed until diagnosis and treatment of this condition is complete.** These conditions include:
  - Acute coronary syndrome (ACS) (ST-segment elevation myocardial infarction, non–ST-segment elevation myocardial infarction, unstable angina)

TABLE 5-1	RISK STRATIFICATION BASED ON THE TYPE OF SURGERY
Risk stratification[a]	**Procedure examples**
High risk (>5%)	Aortic and major vascular surgery Open lower limb revascularization/related procedures Pneumonectomy Duodeno-pancreatic surgery or liver resection Pulmonary or liver transplant
Intermediate risk (1–5%)	Other intraperitoneal surgery (splenectomy, cholecystectomy, hiatal hernia repair, etc.) Symptomatic carotid surgery Peripheral arterial angioplasty Head and neck surgery Major neurologic and orthopedic surgery (hip and spine) Major urologic/gynecologic surgery Renal transplant
Low risk (<1%)[b]	Endoscopic procedures Eye surgery Breast surgery Dental procedures Minor gynecologic/urologic/orthopedic surgery Other ambulatory procedures

[a]Surgical risk estimate reflects 30-day risk of cardiovascular death and myocardial infarction based on specific surgical intervention only. It does not include additional risk based on patient comorbidities.

[b]These procedures do not generally require further preoperative cardiac testing.

Modified from Kristensen SD, Knuuti J, Saraste A, et al. 2014 ESC/ESA guidelines on noncardiac surgery: cardiovascular assessment and management: The Joint Task Force on non-cardiac surgery: cardiovascular assessment and management of the European Society of Cardiology (ESC) and the European Society of Anaesthesiology (ESA). *Eur Heart J.* 2014;35(35):2383-431. Reproduced by permission of The European Society of Cardiology..

- ○ Severe stable angina
- ○ Decompensated heart failure
- ○ Significant arrhythmias, including symptomatic bradycardia, Mobitz type II or complete atrioventricular (AV) block, atrial fibrillation with uncontrolled ventricular rates, and ventricular tachycardia
- ○ Symptomatic/severe valvular disease, including severe aortic stenosis and severe mitral stenosis
- The next step is to determine the combined clinical–surgical risk of a patient. Several risk-prediction tools have been validated for predicting perioperative major cardiac events in patients undergoing noncardiac surgery, including the Goldman Revised Cardiac Risk Index (RCRI), American College of Surgeons National Surgical Quality Improvement Program Myocardial Infarction and Cardiac Arrest (NSQIP MICA), and American College of Surgeons NSQIP Surgical Risk Calculator.[3-6]
- The RCRI (shown in Table 5-2) is a simple, validated tool that is most often used to assess perioperative risk of major cardiac complications.[3,4]
- **Patients at low cardiac risk may proceed to surgery with no further cardiac testing.**

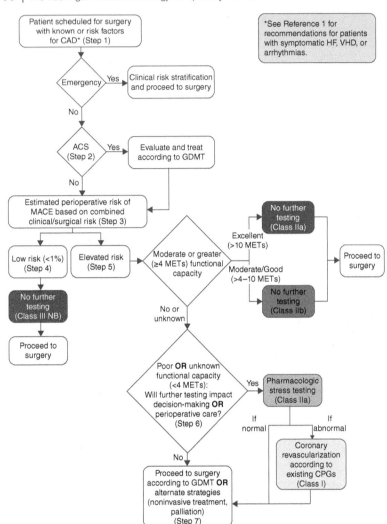

FIGURE 5-1. Algorithm for cardiac evaluation and management. ACS, acute coronary syndrome; CAD, coronary artery disease; GDMT, guideline-directed medical therapy; HF, heart failure; MACE, major adverse cardiac event; MET, metabolic equivalent of task; NSTEMI, non–ST-segment elevation myocardial infarction; STEMI, ST-segment elevation myocardial infarction; UA, unstable angina; VHD, valvular heart disease. (Reprinted from Fleisher LA, Fleischmann KE, Auerbach AD, et al. 2014 ACC/AHA guideline on perioperative cardiovascular evaluation and management of patients undergoing noncardiac surgery: Executive Summary: a report of the American College of Cardiology/American Heart Association Task Force on Practice Guidelines. *J Am Coll Cardiol.* 2014;64(22):2373-405. Copyright © 2014 American College of Cardiology Foundation and the American Heart Association, Inc. With permission.)

TABLE 5-2 GOLDMAN REVISED CARDIAC RISK INDEX (RCRI)

Six independent predictors of cardiac complications

1. High-risk type of surgery
2. History of ischemic heart disease[a]
3. History of heart failure
4. History of cerebrovascular disease
5. Diabetes mellitus requiring insulin
6. Preoperative serum creatinine >2 mg/dL (177 µmol/L)

Estimated rate of complications according to number of predictors[b]

No risk factors—0.4% (95% CI: 0.1–0.8)

One risk factor—1.0% (95% CI 0.5–1.4)

Two risk factors—2.4% (95% CI 1.3–3.5)

Three or more risk factors—5.4% (95% CI 2.8–7.9)

[a]History of myocardial infarction or abnormal stress test, active chest pain, ECG with ischemic changes including Q waves.

[b]Cardiac complications include cardiac death, nonfatal myocardial infarction, and nonfatal cardiac arrest.

Adapted from Goldman L, Caldera DL, Nussbaum SR, et al. Multifactorial index of cardiac risk in noncardiac surgical procedures. *N Engl J Med*. 1977;297:845-50, and Lee TH, Marcantonio ER, Mangione CM, et al. Derivation and prospective validation of a simple index for prediction of cardiac risk of major noncardiac surgery. *Circulation*. 1999;100:1043-9.

Functional Assessment

- If no active cardiac condition is present and the patient is at intermediate or high cardiac risk, the patient's functional capacity must be carefully assessed (Figure 5-1).[1]
- The patient's functional status is a reliable predictor of both perioperative and long-term cardiac risks. Functional status—often expressed in metabolic equivalents of task (METs)—is based on the ability to perform different activities (Table 5-3).[2]

TABLE 5-3 ESTIMATION OF FUNCTIONAL STATUS

Energy	Activity
1 MET	Basic activities of daily living (eat, dress, use the toilet) Walk short distances at slower speeds
4 METs	Climb a flight of stairs or walk up a hill Run a short distance Do heavy work around the house (scrubbing floors, lifting, or moving heavy furniture)
>10 METs	Strenuous sports like swimming, singles tennis, football, basketball, or skiing

MET, metabolic equivalent of task.

Modified from Kristensen SD, Knuuti J, Saraste A, et al. 2014 ESC/ESA guidelines on noncardiac surgery: cardiovascular assessment and management. *Eur Heart J*. 2014;35:2383-431.

- **Patients who can complete 4 METs or greater generally require no further cardiac testing before proceeding with surgery.**
- If a patient has a poor or unknown functional capacity, the clinician may consider further diagnostic testing before surgery (Figure 5-1).[1]

DIAGNOSTIC TESTING

- Before pursuing preoperative diagnostic testing, one must consider the consequences of positive study results. As stressed in the guidelines, **preoperative tests should be recommended only if the information obtained will result in a change in the surgical procedure performed, a change in medical therapy or monitoring during or after surgery, or a postponement of surgery until the cardiac condition can be corrected or stabilized.**[1,2]
- For patients with elevated risk and poor or unknown functional capacity, it may be reasonable to perform exercise testing with cardiac imaging or noninvasive pharmacologic testing to assess for myocardial ischemia, if it will change management.
- Routine screening with noninvasive stress testing is not useful for low-risk patients or patients undergoing low-risk noncardiac surgery.

TREATMENT

Medications

β-Blocker Therapy

- The role of perioperative β-blockade has been the subject of ongoing debate. Randomized controlled trials have shown that perioperative β-blockade started within 1 day or less before noncardiac surgery prevents nonfatal myocardial infarction (MI) but increases the risks of stroke, death, hypotension, and bradycardia.[7,8]
- **Current guidelines recommend that β-blockers should be continued in patients undergoing surgery who have been on β-blockers chronically.**[1]
- In patients in whom β-blocker therapy is indicated to treat a cardiac condition, it is reasonable to begin the β-blocker in the preoperative setting to assess its safety and tolerability, preferably days to weeks before surgery.[1]
- **β-Blocker therapy should NOT be started on the day of the surgery.**[1]

Antiplatelet Therapy

- Antiplatelet management in patients undergoing elective noncardiac surgery is summarized in Figure 5-2.[9]
- Management of perioperative antiplatelet therapy should be determined by a consensus of the surgeon, anesthesiologist, cardiologist, and patient. The relative risk of stent thrombosis—a rare but highly morbid condition—should be weighed against that of perioperative bleeding.[1]
- **Current guidelines recommend continuing aspirin throughout the perioperative period** in patients being treated with dual antiplatelet therapy (DAPT) for previous coronary stenting, unless there is a major contraindication.[9]
- **The recommended minimum duration of dual antiplatelet therapy (DAPT) using aspirin and a P2Y12 inhibitor (typically clopidogrel, prasugrel, or ticagrelor) after stent placement is an area of active investigation.**[9-11]
  - With earlier-generation stents, rates of stent thrombosis, MI, and death were highest in the first 4 to 6 weeks after stent placement. Risk of stent thrombosis is lower with newer-generation drug-eluting stents.[9]
  - Per current guidelines, DAPT should be continued for **at least 3 to 6 months after drug-eluting stent** and 30 days after bare metal stent implantation.[9]

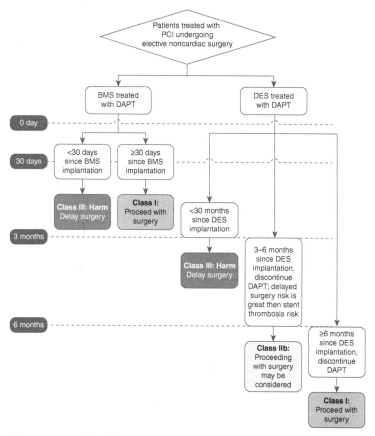

Colors correspond to Class of Recommendation in Table 1. BMS indicates bare metal stent; DAPT, dual antiplatelet therapy; DES, drug-eluting stent; and PCI, percutaneous coronary intervention.

FIGURE 5-2. Treatment algorithm for the timing of elective noncardiac surgery in patients with coronary stents. BMS, bare metal stent; DAPT, dual antiplatelet therapy; DES, drug-eluting stent; PCI, percutaneous coronary intervention. (Reprinted from Levine GN, Bates ER, Bittl JA, et al. 2016 ACC/AHA guideline focused update on duration of dual antiplatelet therapy in patients with coronary artery disease: a report of the American College of Cardiology/American Heart Association Task Force on Clinical Practice Guidelines. *J Am Coll Cardiol.* 2016;68(10):1082-115. Copyright © 2016 by the American College of Cardiology Foundation and the American Heart Association, Inc. With permission.)

- To minimize bleeding risk, when applicable, discontinuation of P2Y12 inhibitors for a minimum of 5 to 7 days is recommended before noncardiac surgery.
  - DAPT should be resumed as soon as possible following surgery.[1,9]
  - Use of "bridging" medications in place of P2Y12 inhibitors should not be routinely recommended.

Other Medical Therapy

- Statins should be continued in patients currently taking statins and scheduled for noncardiac surgery.[1] Initiation of statin in patients undergoing vascular surgery is reasonable.[1]

- Continuation of angiotensin-converting enzyme (ACE) inhibitors or angiotensin-receptor blockers (ARBs) perioperatively is reasonable.[1]
- The use of nitrates perioperatively has not been shown to reduce the incidence of perioperative MI or death and is not recommended.[2]
- For patients taking vitamin K antagonists or direct-acting oral anticoagulants (DOACs), risks of bleeding must be carefully weighed against benefits of remaining on anticoagulation.

Choice of Anesthetic Route

There is no evidence that anesthesia employing a neuraxial route (spinal or epidural) reduces MI or death when compared to an intravenous or volatile anesthetic.[2]

Preoperative Revascularization

- Routine preoperative coronary angiography is not recommended.[1]
- In the Coronary Artery Revascularization Prophylaxis (CARP) trial, over 500 patients were randomized to revascularization or no revascularization before elective vascular surgery.[12] All patients were considered to have elevated risk for a perioperative cardiac complication on the basis of risk factor profile, symptoms, or abnormal stress test. Of those with a nuclear stress test, over 70% had moderate-to-large ischemic burden on stress imaging. Of note, all patients underwent coronary angiography; patients with left main stenosis of at least 50%, LV ejection fraction <20%, and severe aortic stenosis were excluded. Results showed no significant difference between groups in regard to the primary composite end point of death or MI at either 30-day or 2.7-year follow-up.

MONITORING/FOLLOW-UP

- Despite advances in preoperative risk assessment, medical therapy, and surgical and anesthetic techniques, cardiovascular complications continue to be among the most common and treatable adverse consequences of noncardiac surgery. Patients who have a symptomatic MI after surgery have a marked increase in their risk of death.[12] Thus, the consultant's role should continue after risk assessment to the postoperative setting for all but the lowest risk patients.
- Perioperative MI can be documented by assessing clinical symptoms, serial ECGs, and cardiac-specific biomarkers when indicated before and after surgery. In patients with clinically suspected ischemia or those with ECG evidence of ischemia or infarction, serial ECGs and troponin measurements are indicated.
- Many perioperative conditions including heart failure, hypotension, sepsis, and pulmonary embolism may be associated with troponin elevation in the absence of acute MI. For this reason, **routine serial measurement of troponin in the absence of clinical symptoms or ECG changes is discouraged**.

REFERENCES

1. Fleisher LA, Fleischmann KE, Auerbach AD, et al. 2014 ACC/AHA guideline on perioperative cardiovascular evaluation and management of patient undergoing noncardiac surgery. *J Am Coll Cardiol.* 2014;64:e77-137.
2. Kristensen SD, Knuuti J, Saraste A, et al. 2014 ESC/ESA guidelines on noncardiac surgery: cardiovascular assessment and management. *Eur Heart J. 2014*;35:2383-431.
3. Goldman L, Caldera DL, Nussbaum SR, et al. Multifactorial index of cardiac risk in noncardiac surgical procedures. *N Engl J Med.* 1977;297:845-50.
4. Lee TH, Marcantonio ER, Mangione CM, et al. Derivation and prospective validation of a simple index for prediction of cardiac risk of major noncardiac surgery. *Circulation.* 1999;100:1043-9.
5. Davenport DL, Ferraris VA, Hosokawa P, Henderson WG, Khuri SF, Mentzer RM Jr. Multivariable predictors of postoperative cardiac adverse events after general and vascular surgery: results from the patient safety in surgery study. *J Am Coll Surg.* 2007;204:1199-210.

6. Gupta PK, Gupta H, Sundaram A, et al. Development and validation of a risk calculator for prediction of cardiac risk after surgery. *Circulation*. 2011;124:381-7.

7. Wijeysundera DN, Duncan D, Nkonde-Price C, et al. Perioperative beta-blockade in noncardiac surgery: a systematic review for the 2014 ACC/AHA guideline on perioperative cardiovascular evaluation and management of patients undergoing noncardiac surgery: a report of the American College of Cardiology/American Heart Association Task Force on Practice Guidelines. *J Am Coll Cardiol*. 2014;130:2246-64.

8. POISE Study Group. Effects of extended-release metoprolol succinate in patients undergoing non-cardiac surgery (POISE trial): a randomised controlled trial. *Lancet*. 2008;371:1839-47.

9. Levine GN, Bates ER, Bittle JA, et al. 2016 ACC/AHA guideline focused update on duration of dual antiplatelet therapy in patients with coronary artery disease. *J Am Coll Cardiol*. 2016;68:1082-1115.

10. Riddell JW, Chiche L, Plaud B, Hamon M. Coronary stents and noncardiac surgery. *Circulation*. 2007;116:e378-82.

11. Capodanno D, Alfonso F, Levine GN, Valgimigli M, Angiolillo DJ. ACC/AHA versus ESC guidelines on dual antiplatelet therapy: JACC guideline comparison. *J Am Coll Cardiol*. 2018;72(23 Pt A):2915-31.

12. McFalls EO, Ward HB, Moritz TE, et al. Coronary-artery revascularization before elective major vascular surgery. *N Engl J Med*. 2004;351:2795-804.

Evaluation of Acute Chest Pain

Adam Shpigel and Justin S. Sadhu

GENERAL PRINCIPLES

- Acute chest pain is the second most common presenting complaint among patients presenting to the emergency department (ED), with 6.5 million annual visits.[1]
- The etiology of acute chest pain ranges from benign and self-resolving to life-threatening conditions.
- Patients may present to an outpatient clinic or to the ED with chest pain. Serious cardiac or pulmonary pathology is more likely in the ED but may still be present in the outpatient setting.
- The initial assessment of acute chest pain should include rapid evaluation for life-threatening pathology. The following entities demand rapid identification and treatment to avoid death or disability:
  - Acute coronary syndrome (ACS) (ST-elevation myocardial infarction [STEMI], non–ST-elevation myocardial infarction [NSTEMI], or unstable angina [UA])
  - Aortic dissection
  - Pulmonary embolism
  - Cardiac tamponade
  - Tension pneumothorax
- Other causes of chest pain can be investigated if the abovementioned entities are excluded.

DIAGNOSIS

Clinical Presentation

History

- The history is paramount in arriving at the correct diagnosis without delay.
- The extent of the history will vary based on clinical urgency and the patient's hemodynamic status. For instance, if STEMI is identified, there may only be time for a focused history pending transfer to the cardiac catheterization lab. If the patient is unstable, resuscitation should be performed concurrently with obtaining history.
- Important historical questions for the patient include:
  - Location (Ask the patient to point to the affected area. Sometimes, chest pathology can be felt in the upper abdomen.)
  - Onset (When did it start? Suddenly or gradually? What were you doing at the time?)
  - Timing (Is the pain steady or waxing/waning? If the latter, how long does each episode last?)
  - Have you had this pain before?
  - Describe the pain. (Is it pressure like or squeezing? Sharp/stabbing? Tearing? Burning? Aching? Does it feel like heartburn?)
  - Provoking factors (Worse with exertion, deep breathing, position, or touching the area?)

- ○ Palliating factors (Better with rest, position, or nitroglycerin?)
- ○ Radiation (To arms, jaw, neck, or back?)
- Symptoms associated with the pain (Nausea/vomiting? Dyspnea? Diaphoresis? Neurological symptoms? Syncope or presyncope?)
- Patients may not describe their symptoms as "chest pain." The provider should be alert to other descriptions they may use, including "pressure" and "discomfort."
- Relevant comorbidities should be assessed, including cardiac risk factors (hypertension, hyperlipidemia, diabetes mellitus, family history, smoking), as well as known cardiac disease. Other major organ system pathology should be elicited. This may be available on chart review, as well.
- Prior testing should be reviewed, if results are available in the medical record or known to the patient (including prior stress testing, cardiac catheterization, or thoracic imaging).
- Drug use, in particular cocaine and other stimulants, is important to query.
- If there is concern for pulmonary embolism (PE), ask about relevant risk factors (history of known deep vein thrombosis, immobilization, oral contraceptive use, pregnancy or recent delivery, recent surgery, malignancy, or trauma).

Physical Examination

- Vital signs should be assessed immediately on presentation. Hypotension, severe hypertension, tachycardia, tachypnea, and hypoxia are ominous signs and suggest possible life-threatening pathology.
- Blood pressure should be checked in both arms.
- A general assessment of the patient should be made. Patients who appear uncomfortable, in distress, or diaphoretic should be assumed to have serious pathology.
- A targeted physical examination should be performed, focusing on likely etiologies of the patient's chest pain.
- Notable findings on cardiac examination that may suggest causes of chest pain are detailed in Tables 6-1 and 6-2.

Diagnostic Testing

- An electrocardiogram (ECG) should be obtained on all patients presenting with acute chest pain. The American College of Cardiology/American Heart Association (ACC/AHA) Joint Committee on Clinical Practice guidelines recommend obtaining and interpreting the ECG within 10 minutes of ED arrival.[2,3]
  - ○ ECG findings in acute causes of chest pain are presented in Table 6-1.
  - ○ Serial ECGs should be obtained in patients with persistent or worsening symptoms or an adverse change in clinical condition.
- Cardiac troponin (cTn) should be obtained in all patients with suspicion of ACS.
  - ○ cTn I and cTn T are highly specific for myocardial injury and are the preferred biomarkers for use in evaluating suspected myocardial infarction (MI). Creatine kinase (CK) and CK-MB are no longer recommended for this purpose and have been eliminated at many centers.
  - ○ High-sensitivity cardiac troponin (hs-cTn) assays are extremely sensitive for the detection of cTn and may be used to detect or exclude cardiac injury more rapidly than conventional cTn assays.
  - ○ *Acute myocardial injury* is defined as a serum troponin above the 99th percentile for the assay being used. A pattern of rise and fall should be observed with ACS. The initial rise in troponin generally starts 2 to 3 hours following the onset of myocardial ischemia.

TABLE 6-1	CAUSES OF ACUTE CHEST PAIN					
Cause of chest pain	History	Physical examination	Laboratory	ECG	Imaging	Treatment options
Acute Coronary Syndrome	Most commonly substernal chest pain or pressure often with dyspnea, diaphoresis, nausea, and radiation to the arms, neck, or jaw. Unlikely to last for only a few seconds or to be constant for >24 hours. Presentation can be highly variable, with some patients presenting with just dyspnea or primarily abdominal symptoms. Associated symptoms are particularly common in women, the elderly, and patients with diabetes.	Frequently normal. Patient may appear uncomfortable and diaphoretic. If heart failure is present, rales and elevated JVP may be present. In cardiogenic shock, hypotension, diaphoresis, altered mentation, and cool extremities.	Troponin elevation in myocardial infarction. CK-MB no longer recommended.	ST-segment elevation, ST-segment depression, T-wave inversion, hyperacute T waves, new left bundle branch block, tachyarrhythmias and bradyarrhythmias, De Winter criteria, Wellens waves; posterior MI may show prominent R wave and ST depression in lead V1 and can be identified more reliably by posterior ECG.	Generally no significant findings unless heart failure is present.	Reperfusion, medical therapy depending on clinical features

| Pulmonary Embolism | Dyspnea, chest pain (often sharp, pleuritic but can be variable), cough with or without hemoptysis, lightheadedness, or syncope. Swelling of an extremity may be suggestive of deep vein thrombosis. Assess for VTE risk factors. | Tachypnea, tachycardia, and hypoxia common. RV heave may be present. If patient is in shock, hypotension, diaphoresis, altered mentation, and cool extremities. | D-Dimer elevation. Troponin, BNP elevated when right heart strain is present. | Tachycardia common. Other findings variable and often not present; can include incomplete RBBB, RV strain pattern with T-wave inversion V1-4 ± inferior leads, dominant R wave in V1, P pulmonale (>2.5 mm in lead II). The classic "S1Q3T3" is seen in only 20% of patients. | PE CTA, V/Q scan. Usually silent on CXR, but occasionally can see Hampton hump (wedge-shaped opacity adjacent to pleura) or Westermark sign (distal oligemia). TTE useful for findings of right heart strain, including McConnell and 60/60 signs | Anticoagulation, thrombolysis, invasive management depending on clinical stability |

(continued)

TABLE 6-1 CAUSES OF ACUTE CHEST PAIN (continued)

Cause of chest pain	History	Physical examination	Laboratory	ECG	Imaging	Treatment options
Aortic Dissection	Tearing/ripping severe chest pain often radiating to the back. Can have additional symptoms depending on complications (e.g., severe aortic regurgitation, cardiac tamponade, neurological findings if dissection has extended to carotid arteries or spinal circulation).	Severe hypertension is common. Hypotension is an ominous sign potentially representing tamponade or rupture. Interarm blood pressure difference ≥20 mm Hg may be seen, but is not sensitive or specific. Wide pulse pressure if aortic regurgitation is present. Physical examination signs of aortic regurgitation and cardiac tamponade should be sought. Potential neurologic deficits.	In some studies, D-dimer <500 ng/mL had high negative predictive value, but elevated D-dimer is nonspecific. Troponin may be elevated, especially if involves coronary ostium.	Can cause coronary ischemia if involves aortic root. Otherwise, frequently silent.	CTA, TEE, MRA. CXR will sometimes show widened mediastinum	Type A: emergent surgery Type B: generally medical management unless high-risk features present

Condition	History	Exam	Labs	ECG	Imaging	Management
Pericarditis, tamponade	Often pleuritic central chest pain, sometimes with relief on leaning forward and exacerbation in supine position.	Pericardial friction rub, may be transient.	Variable. In pericarditis, frequently elevated WBC and inflammatory markers (e.g., ESR, CRP).	Pericarditis: diffuse ST-elevation spanning multiple coronary distributions and PR depression; opposite pattern in aVR. Large effusion can be associated with diminished QRS voltages and electrical alternans.	TTE	Pericardiocentesis, pericardial window
Tension Pneumothorax	Often iatrogenic or in setting of trauma. Severe dyspnea and chest pain (often sharp, pleuritic). Lightheadedness or syncope.	Respiratory distress, tachypnea, tachycardia, hypotension, asymmetric lung excursion, absent breath sounds on side of pneumothorax, hyperresonance to percussion over affected side, jugular venous distention	No lab work is sensitive or specific.	Generally silent.	CXR will show pneumothorax often with mediastinal shift	Needle decompression, chest tube

BNP, brain natriuretic peptide; CXR, chest x-ray; MRA, magnetic resonance angiography; PE CTA, pulmonary embolism computed tomography angiography; RBBB, right bundle branch block; RV, right ventricle; TTE, transthoracic echo; TEE, transesophageal echo; V/Q, ventilation/perfusion; VTE, venous thromboembolism.

TABLE 6-2	CHEST PAIN–DIRECTED PHYSICAL EXAMINATION WITH SPECIFIC CLINICAL PEARLS
Blood pressure	• Check both arms, especially if considering aortic dissection
	• Severe hypertension and hypotension require urgent intervention
	• Pulsus paradoxus: inspiratory drop of >10 mm Hg in SBP (may be seen with cardiac tamponade)
Jugular veins	• Start with patient reclined at 45 degrees. Patients with significantly elevated JVP may need to be sitting up at 90 degrees before the jugular venous pulse can be seen
	• Hepatojugular reflux: sustained distention of jugular veins with pressure on abdomen (heart failure)
	• Kussmaul sign: elevation (or lack of decrease) in JVP with inspiration (pericardial constriction)
Carotid arteries	• Palpation for stroke volume: normal carotid upstroke unlikely in severe LV dysfunction or AS
	• Pulsus parvus et tardus: weak and late pulse (AS)
Palpation	• Laterally displaced PMI (dilated LV)
	• RV heave (right-sided heart failure)
Heart sounds	• S3 (heart failure)
	• S4 (hypertension and/or heart failure; never heard with atrial fibrillation)
	• Friction rub (pericarditis)
Murmurs	• Acute AR or MR may not have a murmur
	• AS: crescendo–decrescendo systolic murmur, loudest at RUSB, commonly with radiation to the carotids when severe
	• AR: diastolic murmur; always pathologic (aortic root dilation, endocarditis, dissection)
	• MR: systolic blowing murmur loudest at apex (ischemia, LV dilation, prolapse, HCM)
	• VSD: harsh, loud holosystolic murmur (3–8 days after septal MI)
Pulmonary	• Crackles/rales (atelectasis, pneumonia, pulmonary edema)
	• Wheezing (usually bronchospasm, but can occur with heart failure)
	• Absent breath sounds with tracheal deviation away from affected side (tension pneumothorax)
	• Decreased breath sounds, dullness to percussion (pneumonia and/or pleural effusion)
Musculoskeletal	• Pain that is reproducible on examination is rarely cardiac in nature
	• Dermatomal rash with pain (herpes zoster)

TABLE 6-2	CHEST PAIN–DIRECTED PHYSICAL EXAMINATION WITH SPECIFIC CLINICAL PEARLS (*continued*)
Abdominal	• Hepatomegaly, pulsatile liver, and ascites (heart failure)
	• Epigastric pain with palpation (PUD or pancreatitis)
	• RUQ pain (cholecystitis)
Extremities	• Cool extremities (poor cardiac output or occlusive ischemic event if unilateral; also PVD indicates systemic atherosclerosis)
	• Pitting edema (volume overload)

AR, aortic regurgitation; AS, aortic stenosis; HCM, hypertrophic cardiomyopathy; JVP, jugular venous pressure; LV, left ventricle; MI, myocardial infarction; MR, mitral regurgitation; PUD, peptic ulcer disease; PVD, peripheral vascular disease; RUQ, right upper quadrant; VSD, ventricular septal defect.

- D-Dimer is useful in patients being evaluated for PE who are assessed to be at low-to-intermediate risk. In these patients, a negative D-dimer effectively rules out PE. In patients at higher risk, imaging is generally also required.
- Other lab work is sometimes useful but rarely helps establish the diagnosis. This includes complete blood count, basic metabolic profile (particularly for assessment of renal function), brain natriuretic peptide (BNP) or N-terminal (NT)-pro hormone BNP (NT-proBNP), and arterial blood gas.
- A CXR should be obtained in most patients presenting with acute chest pain. This is particularly helpful in identifying pneumothorax and pneumonia. ACS is generally radiographically silent unless congestive heart failure is present. PE can cause certain findings (see Table 6-1) but is most commonly not apparent on CXR. CXR may show a widened mediastinum but is not sensitive for the diagnosis of aortic dissection.

Acute Coronary Syndrome: Diagnostic Considerations

- High-risk features for acute myocardial infarction (AMI) include exertional chest pressure radiating to shoulders/arms, with associated nausea, vomiting, or diaphoresis, or symptoms worse than the patient's typical angina (or similar to prior AMI pain). The absence of these features does not reduce the likelihood of AMI.
- Findings that suggest a lower risk for AMI include pain that is "sharp" (stabbing), pleuritic, positional, or reproducible on palpation. These features do not, however, exclude ACS.
- Women, the elderly, and patients with diabetes are more likely to present with accompanying symptoms such as shortness of breath, nausea, vomiting, abdominal discomfort, or syncope.[3]
- If STEMI is identified on initial ECG, the goal should be to achieve rapid reperfusion (see Chapter 9). In percutaneous coronary intervention (PCI)-capable centers, the goal door-to-balloon time for primary PCI is <90 minutes. If PCI is not available, decision should be made rapidly regarding thrombolysis (within 30 minutes of arrival) and/or transfer to a PCI-capable center.
- If STEMI is not identified, the ECG should be evaluated for other high-risk findings that may warrant immediate or early angiography. These include new (or presumed new) left bundle branch block, posterior MI, De Winter pattern (1 to 3 mm upsloping ST-segment depression at the J point in the precordial leads with associated tall,

symmetric T waves—associated with proximal left anterior descending [LAD] occlusion),[4] or Wellens syndrome. Posterior or right-sided leads may be necessary if there is suspicion for acute posterior or right ventricular infarction, respectively.

- Given the time constraints imposed by an STEMI diagnosis, a targeted history should be obtained, with particular care given to those aspects of the history that could affect the reperfusion strategy. Of particular note:
  - Rapid assessment of symptoms to exclude potential alternate diagnoses (e.g., aortic dissection masquerading as ACS)
  - Known prior cardiac history, including prior coronary assessment (and bypass graft anatomy if applicable), if this can be done in a timely manner
  - Medications, especially anticoagulants and antiplatelet agents, as well as metformin
  - Allergies (in particular to contrast dye)
  - Active or recent bleeding
  - Hemodynamic instability requiring resuscitative measures including possible mechanical circulatory support at the time of intervention
  - Tachyarrhythmias or bradyarrhythmias requiring active management (e.g., cardioversion, insertion of a temporary pacemaker)
- If the diagnosis of STEMI is established, reperfusion should not be delayed for additional testing (lab draws, echocardiography, imaging). These, however, may be helpful if the diagnosis is unclear.
- Initial medications should be given immediately or en route to the catheterization lab. These include aspirin 162 to 325 mg (if not yet given) and heparin. Loading of a P2Y12 inhibitor upstream of intervention is generally appropriate, as well, although it is sometimes deferred until the patient arrives in the cardiac catheterization lab.
- When ACS is suspected but STEMI is not initially identified, further evaluation is indicated.
- Immediate attempts at reperfusion are indicated for patients with NSTEMI or UA if signs of clinical instability are present (acute heart failure, cardiogenic shock, arrhythmias, refractory angina).
- Patients with suspected NSTEMI/UA should be risk stratified. There are several available clinical prediction rules used for this purpose, including the thrombolysis in myocardial infarction and global registry of acute coronary events scores, which are available as online calculators. In general, higher scores favor an early invasive strategy for reperfusion (see Chapter 8).
- In addition, various clinical decision pathways have been developed to help triage patients, including the HEART (history, ECG, age, risk factors, and troponin)[5] pathway and emergency department acute coronary syndrome (EDACS).[3] These pathways incorporate troponin values and other clinical features and may identify patients at low risk who do not require hospital admission or further cardiac testing.
- For patients with suspected NSTEMI/UA, serial cardiac biomarkers should be obtained. Several different algorithms have been established for monitoring biomarkers in this setting.
- In common practice, if the first cTn is negative, a second is drawn 6 to 8 hours later. Two negative tests 6 to 8 hours apart are usually sufficient to rule out an MI.
- With hs-cTn, two negative tests obtained 1 to 3 hours apart (depending on the individual assay) or a single negative test after at least 3 hours of symptoms usually excludes myocardial injury. A study of 14,600 patients found that an initial negative hs-cTn T with no ischemic ECG changes was associated with 99.8% negative predictive value for MI within 30 days.[6]
- Conversely, a single positive troponin in the appropriate clinical setting is sufficient to make the diagnosis of AMI.[7] Treatment should then proceed according to guidelines for NSTEMI management (see Chapter 8).

- Patients at low risk (30-day risk of death or major adverse cardiovascular event <1%) and with negative serial biomarkers can generally be safely discharged, provided no other dangerous etiology has been identified for the chest pain.
- If the patient is assessed to be high risk for UA, consideration may be given to proceeding with coronary computed tomography angiography (CTA). If the risk is intermediate, stress testing or coronary CTA may be pursued during the same ED visit or hospital admission.

Other Etiologies of Chest Pain

Additional diagnostic testing is tailored to the pathology suspected to be present.

- Aortic dissection (see Chapter 20)
  - When acute aortic dissection is strongly suspected, the tests of choice are the following[8]:
    - CT aortogram. This has a sensitivity of 98% for aortic dissection and excellent anatomic definition. This requires that the patient be stable enough to transfer to the CT scanner.
    - Transesophageal echocardiogram (TEE). This has a sensitivity of 94% for aortic dissection, with a small "blind spot" caused by air in the trachea. This can be done rapidly at bedside without the need to transport the patient.
    - Magnetic resonance aortogram (MRA). High sensitivity for aortic dissection (98%) and excellent anatomic definition. This requires a relatively stable patient, given the time required for transport and scanning.
    - Aortography. Seldom used today, given invasive nature and availability of excellent alternatives.
  - Identification of ascending (Stanford type A) dissection is a surgical emergency with high early mortality and role for immediate transfer to the operating room.
- PE
  - The diagnostic strategy for PE depends on the pretest likelihood based on the history and physical examination. In patients with moderate or high pretest probability, imaging is warranted.
  - The pretest probability of PE should be determined based on validated clinical prediction rules, which include the Wells/modified Wells criteria and the Pulmonary Embolism Rule-Out Criteria (PERC).[9]
  - The imaging test of choice is PE protocol CTA. In patients with strong reasons to avoid contrast exposure (impaired renal function and/or anaphylactic reaction), nuclear ventilation–perfusion scanning is an option, but with the downside of frequent intermediate probability results requiring further testing.
- Pericarditis and myocarditis
  - Pericarditis should be suspected based on compatible symptoms, examination, and ECG findings (see Chapter 17).
  - Pericarditis can be life-threatening when accompanied by myocarditis, which can be identified by elevated biomarkers, the presence of heart failure signs and symptoms, and myocardial dysfunction on echocardiography.
  - Cardiac MRI with gadolinium enhancement is useful in assessing for myocardial and/or pericardial inflammation and fibrosis.
  - Pericarditis can also be acutely life-threatening when accompanied by pericardial effusion, resulting in cardiac tamponade.
- Pericardial effusion and tamponade
  - The causes of pericardial effusion are numerous and include acute pericarditis, malignancy, infection, and autoimmune etiologies. The hemodynamic consequences of a pericardial effusion depend on the size of the effusion and the rate of accumulation.

- Cardiac tamponade can be suspected based on history and physical examination, with classic findings including Beck triad (hypotension, jugular venous distension, and muffled heart sounds). Hypotension, in particular, is a late and ominous finding.
- In all cases of suspected tamponade, the clinician should assess for pulsus paradoxus. Pulsus paradoxus is an exaggerated drop in systolic pressure during inspiration. This can be assessed using a manual blood pressure cuff, either by auscultation or by bedside Doppler ultrasound of a distal pulse. A fall of 10 mm Hg or greater is consistent with pulsus paradoxus and should prompt concern for a hemodynamically significant effusion.
- Transthoracic echocardiography should be rapidly obtained for all suspected tamponade. Of note, tamponade is a clinical diagnosis, with findings on echocardiography playing a supporting role.
- Tension pneumothorax is life-threatening and can result from trauma, iatrogenic injury during central line placement, or other causes of pneumothorax. CXR is the imaging modality of choice.
- Severe valvular heart disease, including aortic stenosis, mitral stenosis, and acute severe mitral regurgitation (MR), may also present with chest pain.[3]

TREATMENT

- Initial management of chest pain should consist of the following:
  - Assessment of airway, breathing, and circulation and immediate attention to compromise of any of these (basic life support [BLS]/advanced cardiac life support [ACLS])
  - Establishing intravenous (IV) access and cardiac monitoring
  - Drawing blood for initial labs
  - Supplemental oxygen if hypoxic
- ACS should be managed according to guidelines, with treatment options described in the corresponding chapters in this book (see Chapters 8 and 9). This may include immediate catheterization lab activation (in the case of STEMI or other unstable ACS), delayed invasive strategy, or medical management.
- Treatment of PE generally consists of anticoagulation. Patients with hemodynamic instability may require additional therapies, including systemic thrombolysis, catheter-directed thrombolysis, or surgical embolectomy depending on circumstances.
- Pericardial effusion with cardiac tamponade is treated with pericardiocentesis, often with pericardial drain placement. This may need to be done at the bedside in cases of profound hemodynamic compromise or cardiac arrest. For recurrent, malignant, or loculated effusion, surgical drainage with pericardial window may be indicated.
- Treatment of tension pneumothorax is by decompression of the affected hemithorax, needle decompression, and/or chest tube placement.
- Proximal (type A) aortic dissection requires immediate surgery, with mortality increasing if surgery is delayed (see Chapter 20). Distal (type B) dissection can generally be managed with aggressive IV β-blockade and blood pressure lowering, though surgery may be required in certain clinical settings (e.g., end-organ ischemia or refractory pain).

REFERENCES

1. Rui P, Kang K. National Hospital Ambulatory Medical Care Survey: 2017 emergency department summary tables. National Center for Health Statistics. Accessed 12/11/21. https://www.cdc.gov/nchs/data/nhamcs/web_tables/2017_ed_web_tables-508.pdf
2. Amsterdam EA, Wenger NK, Brindis RG, et al. 2014 ACC/AHA guidelines for the management of patients with non-ST-elevation acute coronary syndromes. *Circulation.* 2014;130:344-426.

3. Gulati M, Levy PD, Mukherjee D, et al. 2021 AHA/ACC/ASE/CHEST/SAEM/SCCT/SCMR guideline for the evaluation and diagnosis of chest pain: a report of the American College of Cardiology/American Heart Association Joint Committee on Clinical Practice Guidelines. *J Am Coll Cardiol.* 2021;78:e187-285.

4. De Winter RJ, Wellens HJJ, Wilde AAM. A new ECG sign of proximal LAD occlusion. *N Engl J Med.* 2008;359:2071-3.

5. Six AJ, Backus BE, Kelder JC. Chest pain in the emergency room: value of the HEART score. *Neth Heart J.* 2008;16:191–196.

6. Bandstein N, Ljung R, Johansson M, Holzmann MJ. Undetectable high-sensitivity cardiac troponin T level in the emergency department and risk of myocardial infarction. *J Am Coll Cardiol.* 2014;63:2569-78.

7. Thygesen K, Alpert JS, Jaffe AS, et al.; Executive Group on behalf of the Joint European Society of Cardiology (ESC)/American College of Cardiology (ACC)/American Heart Association (AHA)/World Heart Federation (WHF) Task Force for the Universal Definition of Myocardial Infarction. Fourth universal definition of myocardial infarction (2018). *J Am Coll Cardiol.* 2018;72:2231-64.

8. Moore AG, Eagle KA, Bruckman D. Choice of computed tomography, transesophageal echocardiography, magnetic resonance imaging, and aortography in acute aortic dissection: International Registry of Acute Aortic Dissection (IRAD). *Am J Cardiol.* 2002;89:1235-8.

9. Kline JA, Courtney DM, Kabrhel C, et al. Prospective multicenter evaluation of the pulmonary embolism rule-out criteria. *J Thromb Haemost.* 2008;6:772-80.

Stable Angina

Prashanth D. Thakker and David B. Schwartz

GENERAL PRINCIPLES

Definition

- Angina is a symptom of myocardial ischemia, most commonly caused by coronary artery disease (CAD).
  - "Typical angina" is (1) substernal chest discomfort with a characteristic quality and duration that is (2) precipitated by stress and (3) relieved by rest or nitroglycerin.
  - "Atypical angina" meets two of the abovementioned criteria.
  - "Noncardiac chest pain" meets one or none of the abovementioned criteria.
- Angina is often described as a pressure or heaviness in the chest. Anginal equivalent symptoms vary from patient to patient but may include exertional dyspnea, fatigue or weakness, diaphoresis, dizziness, nausea, and syncope.
- Women (more often than men) and patients with diabetes mellitus may experience "atypical" symptoms such as epigastric discomfort or other symptoms as their anginal equivalent.

Classification

- The Canadian Cardiovascular Society (CCS) Angina Classification Scale is commonly employed to stratify patients in terms of severity. Anginal symptoms are precipitated by the following:
  - Class I: Strenuous activity
  - Class II: Moderate activity, such as walking more than one flight of stairs
  - Class III: Mild activity, such as walking less than one flight of stairs
  - Class IV: Any activity. Symptoms may also occur at rest.
- The severity of angina is **not** directly proportional to the degree of angiographic stenosis of the diseased coronary artery (or arteries).
- More severe angina does correlate with an increased short-term risk of death or nonfatal myocardial infarction (MI).

Epidemiology[1]

- Approximately 15.5 million Americans have coronary heart disease (CHD).
- Despite the well-documented decline in cardiovascular mortality in the United States, ischemic heart disease remains the leading single cause of death.
- In the United States, CHD is responsible for nearly one-third of all deaths in patients over the age of 35 years.

Pathophysiology

- Stable angina most often results from fixed coronary lesions that produce a mismatch of myocardial oxygen supply and demand with increasing cardiac workload.
- Determinants of myocardial oxygen demand include heart rate (HR), afterload or systemic vascular resistance, myocardial wall stress (measured by preload), and myocardial contractility.

- A fixed stenosis of an epicardial coronary artery, usually >70% of the original luminal diameter of the vessel, is sufficient to limit blood flow distal to the lesion.
- The presence of CAD can predispose patients to heart failure, arrhythmias, and sudden cardiac death.

Risk Factors for Coronary Artery Disease

- Tobacco use
- Hypertension
- Diabetes mellitus
- Dyslipidemia
- Metabolic syndrome
- Family history of CAD
- Age

DIAGNOSIS

Clinical Presentation

History

- A thorough history can often yield an accurate diagnosis in a patient presenting with chest discomfort.[1-3] See Table 7-1 for pretest likelihood of CAD.
- Evaluating the nature of symptoms, risk factors, and history will help risk-stratify the patient and provide a pretest probability of CAD.
- Pertinent information about the chest discomfort includes location, character/quality of the discomfort, setting, duration, severity, associated symptoms, and exacerbating and attenuating factors.
- Patients with diabetes may not experience any anginal symptoms despite having ischemic heart disease.
- Important social history includes total past and present tobacco use as well as drug use (cocaine or other stimulants).
- Assessment of functional status
  ○ Sedentary patient may not exert themselves enough to experience angina.
  ○ Alternatively, patients who are relatively inactive may be limiting their activity due to anginal symptoms.

TABLE 7-1	PRETEST LIKELIHOOD (%) OF CORONARY ARTERY DISEASE IN SYMPTOMATIC PATIENTS ACCORDING TO AGE AND SEX					
	Nonanginal chest pain		Atypical angina		Typical angina	
Age (years)	Men	Women	Men	Women	Men	Women
30–39	4	2	34	12	76	26
40–49	13	3	51	22	87	55
50–59	20	7	65	31	93	73
60–69	27	14	72	51	94	86

Reprinted from Fihn SD, Gardin JM, Abrams J, et al. 2012 ACCF/AHA/ACP/AATS/PCNA/SCAI/STS guideline for the diagnosis and management of patients with stable ischemic heart disease: a report of the American College of Cardiology Foundation/American Heart Association Task Force on Practice Guidelines, and the American College of Physicians, American Association for Thoracic Surgery, Preventive Cardiovascular Nurses Association, Society for Cardiovascular Angiography and Interventions, and Society of Thoracic Surgeons. *J Am Coll Cardiol.* 2012;60(24):e44-164. Copyright © 2012 American College of Cardiology Foundation and the American Heart Association, Inc. With permission.

Physical Examination

As with the history, the physical examination is a key component in the evaluation of the patient with suspected coronary disease. A focused examination must include:

- Vital signs (including blood pressure readings in both arms, HR, and oxygen saturation)
- Head, ears, eyes, nose, and throat: corneal arcus senilis, xanthelasma, and diagonal earlobe crease (Frank sign)
- Neck: carotid artery bruits
- Lungs: rales (if present during an episode of chest pain may suggest pulmonary edema secondary to ischemia)
- Cardiac: murmurs (suggestive of stenotic or regurgitant valvular disease), S3 or S4 gallops, and friction rubs. Assess the position, size, and characteristics of the precordial impulse.
- Abdomen: listen for bruits (aortic or renal arteries), pulsatile mass (abdominal aortic aneurysm).
- Extremities: strength of the peripheral pulses (femoral, dorsalis pedis, posterior tibialis, etc.); listen for femoral artery bruits, peripheral edema, or signs of vascular insufficiency.

Differential Diagnosis

- Congenital cardiac anomalies
- Myocardial bridge
- Coronary arteritis
- Coronary artery ectasia
- Radiation arteriopathy
- Cocaine
- Aortic stenosis
- Hypertrophic cardiomyopathy
- Prinzmetal (variant) angina. Coronary artery spasm may be provoked during cardiac catheterization by the infusion of dopamine, acetylcholine, or ergonovine.
- Microvascular angina
- Other cardiac causes
  - Myocardial disease—chronic heart failure (thought secondary to myocardial stretch), myocarditis, reversible left ventricular (LV) dysfunction related to stress (Takotsubo cardiomyopathy)
  - Pericardial disease: pericarditis
  - Vasculature: aortic dissection
- Other noncardiac causes (Table 7-2)

Diagnostic Testing

The initial evaluation should be tailored to the level of clinical suspicion for CHD and the degree of symptoms experienced by the patient.

Laboratories

- Biochemical markers including a CBC, fasting glucose, and lipid profile should be obtained in all patients with suspected CHD, with an added troponin in acute coronary syndrome (ACS) presentations.
- Elevated baseline C-reactive protein, lipoprotein(a), and homocysteine levels are associated with an increased risk of CAD and can be evaluated in those patients in whom standard cardiac risk factors are absent and an alternative explanation for CAD is sought.

TABLE 7-2 NONCARDIAC CAUSES OF CHEST PAIN

Pulmonary:
Pulmonary embolism or pulmonary hypertension
Lung parenchyma: pneumonia or pneumothorax
Pleural tissue: pleuritis or pleural effusion
Gastrointestinal:
Gastroesophageal reflux disease
Esophageal spasm or abnormal motility
Achalasia
Esophagitis
Esophageal rupture (Boerhaave syndrome)
Peptic ulcer disease
Pancreatitis
Cholecystitis

Urologic:
Nephrolithiasis
Pyelonephritis
Dermatologic:
Herpes zoster
Musculoskeletal:
Costochondritis
Rib fractures
Rheumatoid arthritis
Psoriatic arthritis
Fibromyalgia
Psychiatric:
Anxiety disorder
Panic disorder
Somatoform disorders
Delusional disorder

Electrocardiography
- **A normal rest electrocardiogram (ECG) does not exclude the presence of CAD.**
- The presence of the following ECG abnormalities increases the likelihood of a cardiac etiology in patients with chest discomfort:
  - Pathologic Q waves (>0.4 mV and >25% of the corresponding R wave) consistent with a prior MI
  - Resting ST-segment depression
  - T-wave inversion
  - LV hypertrophy (LVH)

Imaging
A CXR should be obtained if there is an evidence of congestive heart failure, valvular disease, or aortic disease, or if an abnormal cardiac impulse is noted on physical examination.

Diagnostic Procedures
Exercise Stress Testing
- Exercise stress testing (without imaging) provides functional information and allows risk stratification in patients with suspected angina.
- The Bruce protocol is most commonly used, consisting of 3-minute stages of increasing treadmill speed and incline.
- Monitor for appropriate physiologic response to exercise with blood pressure and HR measurements during the exercise and recovery periods.
- Question for the presence of anginal symptoms.
- Monitor throughout the study to evaluate for ischemic ECG changes.
- The **Duke treadmill score** (DTS) provides prognostic information.
  - DTS = (minutes of exercise − [5 × maximum ST-segment deviation (mm)] − [4 × angina score]).
  - Angina score is defined as 0 (no angina), 1 (nonlimiting anginal symptoms), or 2 (angina requiring termination of the test).
  - Scores of >5, −10 to 4, and <−11 are associated with low, moderate, and high risk, respectively, of subsequent cardiovascular events (Table 7-3).[4]

TABLE 7-3	SURVIVAL ACCORDING TO RISK GROUPS BASED ON DUKE TREADMILL SCORE		
Risk group (score)	Percentage of total	4-year survival (%)	Annual mortality (%)
Low (≥+5)	62	99	0.25
Moderate (−10 to +4)	34	95	1.25
High (<−11)	4	79	5.0

Modified from Mark DB, Shaw L, Harrell FE Jr, et al. Prognostic value of a treadmill exercise score in outpatients with suspected coronary artery disease. *N Engl J Med*. 1991;325:849-53.

- Exercise sufficient to increase the HR to 85% of maximum predicted heart rate (MPHR = 220 − age) is necessary for optimal sensitivity.
- Medications such as β-blockers, calcium channel blockers (CCBs) (verapamil and diltiazem), and nitrates should be discontinued in patients before performing stress tests when evaluating for new ischemia. These medications can be continued if the stress test is performed to optimize medical therapy.
- Exercise stress testing has a sensitivity and specificity of ~75%.
- The specificity of the test is adversely affected by the presence of resting ECG abnormalities, inability to exercise, or medication use, which may prohibit attaining 85% of the MPHR (e.g., β-blockers).
- A positive stress test indicative of severe CHD is defined by presence of any of the following:
  ○ New ST-segment depression at the start of exercise
  ○ New ST-segment depression >2 mm in multiple leads
  ○ Hypotensive response to exercise
  ○ Development of heart failure or sustained ventricular arrhythmia during the study
  ○ Prolonged interval after exercise (>5 minutes) before ischemic changes return to baseline
- Patients with a markedly positive stress test should undergo cardiac catheterization to be evaluated for coronary revascularization options.
- Exercise stress testing is **contraindicated** for patients with the following:
  ○ Acute MI:
    ▪ A submaximal or symptom-limited stress test may be performed in stabilized patients after 48 hours.
    ▪ A standard stress test may be performed after 4 to 6 weeks.
  ○ Unstable angina not previously stabilized by medical therapy
  ○ Cardiac arrhythmias causing symptoms or hemodynamic compromise
  ○ Symptomatic severe aortic stenosis
  ○ Symptomatic heart failure
  ○ Acute pulmonary embolism, myocarditis, pericarditis, and aortic dissection

Cardiac Stress Testing with Imaging
- Stress testing with imaging is an appropriate initial diagnostic study in patients with the following:
  ○ Evidence of preexcitation (Wolff–Parkinson–White syndrome)
  ○ LVH
  ○ Left bundle branch block (LBBB)

- ○ Ventricular pacing
- ○ Resting ST- and T-wave changes (intrinsic or due to digoxin therapy)
- **Stress myocardial perfusion imaging** (see Chapter 37)
  - ○ Imaging with thallium-201 (^{201}Tl) or technetium-99m (^{99}mTc) sestamibi increases sensitivity for the detection of CAD to 80% and specificity to 80-90%.
  - ○ Stress perfusion imaging allows the diagnosis and localization of areas of ischemia, determination of ejection fraction, and distinction between ischemic and infarcted tissue (viability).
- **Pharmacologic stress testing**
  - ○ There are three vasodilator agents used in stress testing: dipyridamole, adenosine, and regadenoson.
  - ○ **Regadenoson** is a coronary vasodilator with a high avidity for the A2A receptor and less so for the A1, A2B, and A3 receptors.
  - ○ **Adenosine** causes coronary vasodilation through A2A receptors, with greater dilation of normal coronary vessels than stenotic vessels. Undesirable effects of adenosine are mediated through activation of the A1 (atrioventricular [AV] block), A2B (peripheral vasodilation), and A3 (bronchospasm) receptors.
  - ○ **Dipyridamole** inhibits adenosine deaminase and phosphodiesterase, resulting in an increase in adenosine, which, in turn, causes coronary vasodilation through A2A receptors. The response and potential side effects are similar to those of adenosine.
  - ○ Methylxanthines (i.e., caffeine, theophylline, and theobromine) are competitive inhibitors of adenosine and should be withheld before testing.
  - ○ Aminophylline 50 to 250 mg IV is used to reverse the bronchospastic effect of the vasodilator agents.
  - ○ **Indications** for adenosine stress testing include those for exercise stress testing AND in the following conditions:
    - ▪ Inability to perform adequate exercise (i.e., due to pulmonary disease, peripheral vascular disease, or musculoskeletal or mental conditions)
    - ▪ Baseline ECG abnormalities such as LBBB, ventricular preexcitation, and permanent ventricular pacing
    - ▪ Risk stratification of clinically stable patients into low- and high-risk groups very early after acute MI (>1 day) or presentation with a presumptive ACS
  - ○ **Contraindications** for adenosine stress testing include:
    - ▪ Patients with asthma with active wheezing (adequately controlled asthma is not a contraindication)
    - ▪ Bronchospasm
    - ▪ Second- or third-degree AV block without a pacemaker or sick sinus syndrome
    - ▪ Systolic blood pressure <90 mm Hg
    - ▪ Recent use of dipyridamole and dipyridamole-containing medications (e.g., Aggrenox)
    - ▪ Methylxanthine use (such as aminophylline, caffeine, and theobromine) within 12 hours of testing
    - ▪ Known hypersensitivity to adenosine
    - ▪ Acute MI or ACS
  - ○ Profound sinus bradycardia (HR <40 bpm) is a relative contraindications for adenosine stress testing.
  - ○ Common side effects of adenosine include[5]:
    - ▪ Flushing (35-40%)
    - ▪ Chest pain (25-30%), which is not specific for CHD
    - ▪ Dyspnea (20%)
    - ▪ Dizziness (7%)
    - ▪ Nausea (5%)
    - ▪ Symptomatic hypotension (5%)

- Indications and contraindications for regadenoson stress testing are the same as that for adenosine.
  - Common side effects of regadenoson include shortness of breath, flushing, and headache.
  - Less common side effects include chest pain, dizziness, nausea, and abdominal discomfort.
  - Selectivity for the A2A receptor would suggest that regadenoson would have a lower rate of side effects than adenosine (and dipyridamole), but limited available data do not support this assumption.[6]
- **Exercise stress echocardiography**
  - Compared with standard exercise treadmill testing, stress echocardiography provides additional clinical value for detecting and localizing myocardial ischemia and visualizing cardiac structure and function.
  - Pharmacologic stress testing with dobutamine may be preferable in patients who cannot exercise to the optimal level (>85% MPHR) or in other specified circumstances (see earlier).
- Stress testing with cardiac magnetic resonance imaging and positron emission tomography: These newer imaging modalities have shown promise in the noninvasive evaluation of CAD (see Chapters 36 and 38).

Stress Testing in Specific Populations
- Stress testing **after MI**
  - A submaximal study performed 2 to 7 days after acute MI or a maximal exercise stress test 4 to 6 weeks after MI aids in determining the patient's ischemic burden and provides prognostic information.
  - A treadmill stress test after acute MI, either with or without revascularization, helps guide recommendations for a cardiac rehabilitation program.
  - Vasodilator-mediated stress testing with ^{201}Tl or ^{99}mTc sestamibi imaging may be performed within 48 hours of an acute MI in clinically stable patients.
- Stress testing in patients with **established CHD**
  - The routine use of stress testing in asymptomatic patients after percutaneous or surgical revascularization remains controversial.
  - Stress testing in patients older than 5 years from coronary artery bypass grafting (CABG) and/or those older than 2 years from percutaneous coronary intervention (PCI) in whom revascularization is reasonable.
  - Stress testing should be performed in conjunction with an imaging modality (nuclear or echocardiographic) to increase test sensitivity and localize any ischemia.
- Stress testing in the **elderly**
  - Exercise testing poses additional challenges in the elderly as their functional capacity is often compromised by muscle weakness and deconditioning (see Chapter 34).
  - Pharmacologic testing is encouraged in these settings.

Coronary Angiography
- Coronary angiography or cardiac catheterization is considered the "gold standard" technique for diagnosing CAD (see Chapter 39).
- **Indications**
  - Known or suspected angina with a markedly positive stress test
  - Survived sudden cardiac death (e.g., ventricular tachycardia)
  - High pretest probability of left main or three-vessel CAD or for patients whose occupation requires a definitive diagnosis
  - Recent nondiagnostic stress test and for individuals who are unable to undergo noninvasive testing

- In selected patients with recurrent hospitalizations for chest pain or those with an overriding desire for a definite diagnosis and an intermediate or high pretest probability of CAD
- Patients with angina who are suspected of having a nonatherosclerotic cause of ischemia (e.g., coronary anomaly, coronary dissection, and radiation vasculopathy)
- **Coronary angiography is not indicated (class III indication) for stable angina responding to medical therapy or patients with asymptomatic disease.**

TREATMENT

- The goal of treatment of patients with stable angina is to reduce symptoms of ischemia.
- Both pharmacologic therapy and revascularization are important options that should be considered in addition to diet and lifestyle modifications.[7-9]
- One approach to guide the treatment of patients with ischemic heart disease is the "AB-CDE" mnemonic: **A**ntiplatelet therapy, **B**lood pressure control/β-blocker, **C**holesterol lowering/**C**igarette cessation, **D**iabetes control/**D**iet and weight loss, **E**xercise/**E**jection fraction.

Medication

- The purpose of medication therapy is to:
  - Reduce myocardial oxygen demand
  - Improve myocardial oxygen supply
  - Treat cardiac risk factors (e.g., hypertension, diabetes, and obesity)
  - Control exacerbating factors (valvular stenosis and anemia) that may precipitate ischemia
- **Aspirin**
  - The use of aspirin in patients with stable angina has been shown to reduce cardiovascular events by 33%.
  - Clopidogrel (75 mg/day) can be used in patients who are allergic to or intolerant of aspirin.[10]
  - Both aspirin and clopidogrel can be used in patients with severe CAD, although with an increased risk of bleeding.[11]
  - Consultation with an allergist should be considered for the patient suspected of having an aspirin allergy.
- **β-Blockers**
  - β-Blockers should be considered an initial therapy for symptomatic patients with a history of prior MI.
  - Effective in controlling angina by decreasing HR, contractility, and blood pressure. In addition, the reduction in HR also allows for increased diastolic filling time and may increase coronary perfusion.
    - The dose can be adjusted to result in a resting HR of 50 to 60 beats per minute (bpm).
    - In patients with persistent angina, a target HR <50 bpm is warranted, provided that no symptoms are associated with the bradycardia and that heart block does not develop.
    - With moderate exercise (climbing two flights of stairs), the HR should be <90 bpm.
  - Use is contraindicated in patients with severe bronchospasm, significant AV block, marked resting bradycardia, or decompensated heart failure.
  - β-Blocking agents with β-1 selectivity (such as metoprolol and atenolol) are preferable in patients with asthma, chronic obstructive pulmonary disease (COPD), insulin-dependent diabetes mellitus, or peripheral vascular disease.

- Permanent pacemaker placement may be indicated in patients for whom β-blockade results in symptomatic bradycardia but is otherwise warranted.
- Titration of β-blocker dosing should occur over 6 to 12 weeks.
- β-Blockers should be weaned over a 2- to 3-week period (to prevent worsening angina or precipitation of an ischemic event) if side effects warrant discontinuation of the medication.

- **CCBs**
  - CCB may be used in lieu of β-blockers when contraindicated or not tolerated.
  - CCBs are also used in conjunction with β-blockers if the latter alone are not fully effective at relieving anginal symptoms.
  - CCBs decrease systemic vascular resistance and blood pressure, resulting in a decrease in myocardial oxygen demand.
  - They reduce the transmembrane flux of calcium, decreasing coronary vascular resistance and increasing coronary blood flow, thus increasing myocardial oxygen supply. This is the principal mechanism of benefit in vasospastic angina.
  - CCBs may also decrease contractility (negative inotropic effects), which can decrease myocardial oxygen demand.
  - Some CCBs (nondihydropyridines) also decrease HR (negative chronotropy) or decrease conduction through the AV node, thereby reducing myocardial oxygen demand.
  - Use of short-acting dihydropyridines (e.g., nifedipine) should be avoided because of their risk of adverse cardiac events.

- **Nitrates**
  - Nitrates are endothelium-independent vasodilators.
  - They reduce myocardial oxygen demand by decreasing preload through venodilation and afterload by effects on blood pressure.
  - They dilate epicardial coronary arteries and increase myocardial oxygen supply.
  - Long-acting formulations for chronic use or sublingual preparations for acute anginal symptoms can be used as adjuncts to baseline therapy with β-blockers and/or CCBs.
  - Sublingual preparations can be used at the first indication of angina or prophylactically before engaging in activities that are known to precipitate angina.
    - Patients should seek prompt medical attention if angina occurs at rest or fails to respond to the third sublingual dose.
    - The patient should take the medication while seated because of possible side effects of hypotension.
  - Nitrate tolerance, resulting in reduced therapeutic response, may occur with all nitrate preparations. Maintaining a nitrate-free period of 10 to 12 hours can enhance treatment efficacy.
  - The benefits of nitrate therapy may be offset by the detrimental long-term effects of reactive oxygen species generated by these agents.

- **Ranolazine**
  - The mechanism of action providing angina relief is unclear; however, ranolazine appears to have an effect on the function of cardiac myocyte sodium ion channels.[12,13]
  - Its benefits in relieving angina are independent of effects on HR or blood pressure.[14-16]

- **Angiotensin-converting enzyme (ACE) inhibitors**
  - A reduction in exercise-induced myocardial ischemia has been reported with the addition of an ACE inhibitor in patients with stable angina with optimal β-blockade and normal LV function.[17-20] However, not all trials have shown a benefit.[21]
  - The potential benefit is thought to be independent of blood pressure effects.

- **Cholesterol-lowering agents**
  - Multiple agents including statins, proprotein convertase subtilisin/kexin type 9 (PCSK9) inhibitors, fibrates, bile acid sequestrants, and niacin have been shown to reduce recurrent events and improve overall outcome in patients with established CAD.

○ The most studied of these agents are the 3-hydroxy-3-methyl-glutaryl-CoA reductase or HMG Co-A reductase inhibitors (statins). Some evidence suggests that statins exert beneficial (pleiotropic) effects on endothelial function, independent of their effects on low-density lipoprotein (LDL) levels.

- Miscellaneous include:
  ○ There is an association between influenza infection and acute MI. Current guidelines advocate the use of the influenza and pneumococcal vaccines in high-risk patients with CAD.[22]
  ○ Chelation therapy and acupuncture have not been found to be effective in relieving symptoms and are not recommended for the treatment of chronic stable angina according to current guidelines.[23]
  ○ There are new data emerging that anti-inflammatory therapies (e.g., canakinumab) may reduce cardiovascular events, independent of lipid-lowering agents.[24]

Nonpharmacologic Therapies

- Medical therapy with at least two and preferably three classes of antianginal agents should be attempted before the treatment is considered a failure.
- Patients who are refractory to medical therapy should be assessed with coronary angiography if the anatomy has not already been defined.
- **PCI**
  ○ Catheter-based revascularization is ideal for candidates for PCI who have angina, have single- or two-vessel CAD, have normal LV function, and do not have diabetes.
  ○ Stents are deployed after percutaneous transluminal coronary angioplasty (PTCA) for most lesions warranting percutaneous revascularization as long-term patency rates and overall outcomes are improved compared with PTCA alone.
  ○ Patients enrolled in the COURAGE trial had stable angina and were randomized to either PCI with optimal medical therapy or optimal medical therapy alone and followed for a median of 4.6 years.[9,25]
    ■ PCI did not reduce the risk of death, MI, or other major cardiovascular events over the course of the trial.
    ■ Of note, <10% of screened patients were enrolled, a substantial number of patients assigned to initial medical therapy alone crossed over into the PCI arm, and a relatively small percentage of patients received drug-eluting stents.
    ■ A discussion of relevant data is appropriate in the setting of shared decision-making for PCI versus medical management alone.
  ○ The risks of elective PCI include <1% mortality, a 2-5% rate of nonfatal MI, and <1% need for emergent CABG for an unsuccessful procedure.
  ○ Coronary artery dissection often can be repaired with stent placement but may necessitate bypass surgery.
- **CABG**
  ○ CABG is optimal for patients at a high risk for cardiac mortality, including those with (1) left main disease, (2) two- or three-vessel disease involving the proximal left anterior descending artery and LV dysfunction, and (3) diabetes and multivessel coronary disease with LV dysfunction.[25-27]
  ○ The risk of surgery includes 1-3% mortality, a 5-10% incidence of perioperative MI, a small risk of perioperative stroke or cognitive dysfunction, and a 10-20% risk of vein graft failure in the first year, along with added mortality and complications from comorbid factors.
  ○ Approximately 75% of patients remain free of recurrent angina or adverse cardiac events at 5 years of follow-up.
  ○ The use of internal mammary artery grafts is associated with >95% graft patency at 10 years, compared with 60% for saphenous vein grafts.[28]

- The 1-year patency of radial artery grafts has not been shown to be superior to saphenous vein grafts; however, medium-term (1 to 5 years) patency and long-term (>5 years) patency were superior to radial grafts in a meta-analysis.[29,30]
- After 10 years of follow-up, 50% of patients develop recurrent angina or other adverse cardiac events related to late vein graft failure or progression of native CAD.
- Two U.S. trials (the multicenter BARI[31] and the single-center EAST[32]) evaluated PTCA versus CABG in patients with multivessel disease. The 5-year results of these trials showed that early and late survival rates are equivalent for both PTCA and CABG groups. However, **subgroup analysis showed a clear survival benefit with CABG for patients with diabetes and with severe multivessel disease.**

- Alternative therapies
  - Transmyocardial laser revascularization has been delivered by percutaneous technique (yttrium–aluminum–garnet [YAG] laser) and by epicardial surgical techniques (CO_2 or YAG laser).
    - A thoracotomy approach is used to deliver a series of transmural endomyocardial channels.
    - Surgical transmyocardial laser revascularization has been shown to improve symptoms in patients with stable angina. The mechanism responsible is controversial and may be related more to denervation effects than an improvement in myocardial perfusion.[33-38] Not all trials, however, have shown a benefit.[39-41]
    - There are conflicting data on whether this improves exercise capacity, and no benefit has been demonstrated in terms of increasing myocardial perfusion or reducing mortality.
  - Enhanced external counterpulsation (EECP) performed 1 to 2 hours/day, five times a week for 7 weeks of treatment in patients with chronic stable angina, and a positive stress test was shown to decrease the frequency of angina and increase the time to exercise-induced ischemia.
    - Treatment improves anginal symptoms in approximately 75-80% of patients.[42,43]
    - Current guidelines give a class IIB recommendation for EECP as a consideration for relief of refractory angina.[23]

MONITORING/FOLLOW-UP

- Slight changes in a patient's anginal complaints can often be treated with titration or adjustment of the antianginal regimen.
- Reassessment with a stress test (likely in conjunction with an imaging modality) or a cardiac catheterization is warranted for a patient with significant change in anginal complaints (frequency, severity, or time to onset with activity), or in whom the symptoms are not sufficiently responsive to adjustments in medical therapy. Revascularization (either percutaneous or surgical) should be considered if the anatomy is amenable.

REFERENCES

1. Sanchis-Gomar F, Perez-Quilis C, Leischik R, Lucia A. Epidemiology of coronary heart disease and acute coronary syndrome. *Ann Transl Med.* 2016;4:256.
2. Diamond GA, Forrester JS. Analysis of probability as an aid in the clinical diagnosis of coronary artery disease. *N Engl J Med.* 1979;300:1350-8.
3. Chaitman BR, Bourassa MG, Davis K, et al. Angiographic prevalence of high-risk coronary artery disease in patient subsets (CASS). *Circulation.* 1981;64:360-7.
4. Fihn SD, Gardin JM, Abrams J, et al. 2012 ACCF/AHA/ACP/AATS/PCNA/SCAI/STS guideline for the diagnosis and management of patients with stable ischemic heart disease. *Circulation.* 2012;126:e354-471.

5. Mark DB, Shaw L, Harrell FE Jr, et al. Prognostic value of a treadmill exercise score in outpatients with suspected coronary artery disease. *N Engl J Med.* 1991;325:849-53.

6. Henzlova MJ, Cerqueira MD, Mahmarian JJ, et al. Stress protocols and tracers. *J Nucl Cardiol.* 2006;13:e80-90.

7. Brink HL, Dickerson JA, Stephens JA, Pickworth KK. Comparison of the safety of adenosine and Regadenoson in patients undergoing outpatient cardiac stress testing. *Pharmacotherapy.* 2015;35:1117-23.

8. Abrams J. Chronic stable angina. *N Engl J Med.* 2005;352:2524-33.

9. Boden WE, O'Rourke RA, Teo KK, et al. Optimal medical therapy with or without PCI for stable coronary disease. *N Engl J Med.* 2007;356:1503-16.

10. CAPRIE Steering Committee. A randomized, blinded trial of clopidogrel versus aspirin in patients at risk of ischemic events. *Lancet.* 1996;348:1329-39.

11. Squizzato A, Keller T, Romualdi E, et al. Clopidogrel plus aspirin versus aspirin alone for preventing cardiovascular disease. *Cochrane Database Syst Rev.* 2011;1:CD005158.

12. Beyder A, Strege PR, Reyes S, et al. Ranolazine decreases mechanosensitivity of the voltage-gated sodium ion channel Na(v)1.5: a novel mechanism of drug action. *Circulation.* 2012;125:2698-706.

13. Stone PH, Chaitman BR, Stocke K, et al. The anti-ischemic mechanism of action of ranolazine in stable ischemic heart disease. *J Am Coll Cardiol.* 2010;56:934-42.

14. Chaitman BR, Pepine CJ, Parker JO, et al. Effects of ranolazine with atenolol, amlodipine, or diltiazem on exercise tolerance and angina frequency in patients with severe chronic angina: a randomized controlled trial. *JAMA.* 2004;291:309-16.

15. Chaitman BR, Skettino SL, Parker JO, et al. Anti-ischemic effects and long-term survival during ranolazine monotherapy in patients with chronic severe angina. *J Am Coll Cardiol.* 2004;43:1375-82.

16. Stone PH, Gratsiansky NA, Blokhin A, et al. Antianginal efficacy of ranolazine when added to treatment with amlodipine: the ERICA (Efficacy of Ranolazine in Chronic Angina) trial. *J Am Coll Cardiol.* 2006;48:566-75.

17. van den Heuvel AF, Dunselman PH, Kingma T, et al. Reduction of exercise-induced myocardial ischemia during add-on treatment with the angiotensin-converting enzyme inhibitor enalapril in patients with normal left ventricular function and optimal beta blockade. *J Am Coll Cardiol.* 2001;37:470-4.

18. Kaski JC, Rosano G, Gavrielides S, et al. Effects of angiotensin-converting enzyme inhibition on exercise-induced angina and ST segment depression in patients with microvascular angina. *J Am Coll Cardiol.* 1994;23:652-7.

19. Fox KM, Bertrand M, Ferrari R, et al. Efficacy of perindopril, in reduction of cardiovascular events among patients with stable coronary artery disease: randomized, double-blind, placebo-controlled, multicentre trial (the EUROPA study). *Lancet.* 2003;362:782-8.

20. Yusuf S, Sleight P, Pogue J, et al. Effects of an angiotensin-converting-enzyme inhibitor, ramipril, on cardiovascular events in high-risk patients (HOPE). *N Engl J Med.* 2000;342:145-53.

21. Braunwald E, Domanski M, Fowler S, et al. Angiotensin-converting-enzyme inhibition in stable coronary artery disease. *N Engl J Med.* 2004;351:2058-68.

22. Centers for Disease Control and Prevention. Vaccine information for adults. Accessed 22/07/21. https://www.cdc.gov/vaccines/adults/rec-vac/health-conditions/heart-disease.html

23. Fihn SD, Blankenship JC, Alexander KP, et al. ACC/AHA/AATS/PCNA/SCAI/STS focused update of the guideline for the diagnosis and management of patients with stable ischemic heart disease. *Circulation.* 2014;130:1749-67.

24. Ridker PM, Everett BM, Thuren T, et al. Antiinflammatory therapy with Canakinumab for atherosclerotic disease. *N Engl J Med.* 2017;377:1119-31.

25. Weintraub WS, Spertus JA, Kolm P, et al. Effect of PCI on quality of life in patients with stable coronary disease. *N Engl J Med.* 2008;359:677-87.

26. Yusuf S, Zucker D, Peduzzi P, et al. Effect of coronary artery bypass graft surgery on survival: overview of 10-year results from randomized trials by the Coronary Artery Bypass Graft Surgery Trialists Collaboration. *Lancet.* 1994;344:563-70.

27. Hannan EL, Racz MJ, Walford G, et al. Long-term outcomes of coronary-artery bypass grafting versus stent implantation. *N Engl J Med.* 2005;352:2174-83.

28. Goldman S, Zadina K, Moritz T, et al. Long-term patency of saphenous vein and left internal mammary artery grafts after coronary artery bypass surgery: results from a Department of Veterans Affairs Cooperative Study. *J Am Coll Cardiol.* 2004;44:2149-56.

29. Athanasiou T, Saso S, Rao C, et al. Radial artery versus saphenous vein conduits for coronary artery bypass surgery: forty years of competition—which conduit offers better patency? A systematic review and meta-analysis. *Eur J Cardiothorac Surg.* 2011;40:208-20.

30. Goldman S, Sethi GK, Holman W, et al. Radial artery grafts vs saphenous vein grafts in coronary artery bypass surgery: a randomized trial. *JAMA.* 2011;305:167-74.
31. The Bypass Angioplasty Revascularization Investigators (BARI). Comparison of coronary bypass surgery with angioplasty in patients with multi-vessel disease. *N Engl J Med.* 1996;335:217-225.
32. King SB 3rd, Kosinski AS, Guyton RA, et al. Eight-year mortality in the Emory Angioplasty versus Surgery Trial (EAST). *J Am Coll Cardiol.* 2000;35:1116-21.
33. Allen KB, Dowling RD, Angell WW, et al. Transmyocardial revascularization: 5-year follow-up of a prospective, randomized multicenter trial. *Ann Throc Surg.* 2004;77:1228-34.
34. Allen KB, Dowling RD, Schuch DR, et al. Adjunctive transmyocardial revascularization: five-year follow-up of a prospective, randomized trial. *Ann Thorac Surg.* 2004;78:458-65.
35. Aaberge L, Rootwelt K, Blomhoff S, et al. Continued symptomatic improvement three to five years after transmyocardial revascularization with CO_2 laser: a late clinical follow-up of the Norwegian Randomized trial with transmyocardial revascularization. *J Am Coll Cardiol.* 2005;39:1588-93.
36. Allen KB, Dowling RD, Fudge TL, et al. Comparison of transmyocardial revascularization with medical therapy in patients with refractory angina. *N Engl J Med.* 1999;341:1029-36.
37. Beek JF, van der Sloot JA, Huikeshoven M, et al. Cardiac denervation after clinical transmyocardial laser revascularization: short-term and long-term iodine123-labeled meta-iodobenzylguanide scintigraphic evidence. *J Thorac Cardiovasc Surg.* 2004;127:517-24.
38. Burkhoff D, Schmidt S, Schulman SP, et al. Transmyocardial laser revascularisation compared with continued medical therapy for treatment of refractory angina pectoris: a prospective randomised trial. ATLANTIC Investigators. Angina Treatments-Lasers and Normal Therapies in Comparison. *Lancet.* 1999;354:885-90.
39. Schofield PM, Sharples LD, Caine N, et al. Transmyocardial laser revascularisation in patients with refractory angina: a randomised controlled trial. *Lancet.* 1999;353:519-24.
40. Nägele H, Stubbe HM, Nienaber C, Rödiger W. Results of transmyocardial laser revascularization in non-revascularizable coronary artery disease after 3 years follow-up. *Eur Heart J.* 1998;19:1525-30.
41. Iwanski J, Knapp SM, Avery R, et al. Clinical outcomes meta-analysis: measuring subendocardial perfusion and efficacy of transmyocardial laser revascularization with nuclear imaging. *J Cardiothorac Surg.* 2017;12:37.
42. Lawson WE, Hui JC, Lang G. Treatment benefit in the enhanced external counterpulsation consortium. *Cardiology.* 2000;94:31-5.
43. Soran O, Kennard ED, Kfoury AG, Kelsey SF; IEPR Investigators. Two-year clinical outcomes after enhanced external counterpulsation (EECP) therapy in patients with refractory angina pectoris and left ventricular dysfunction (report from the International EECP Patient Registry). *Am J Cardiol.* 2006;97:17-20.
44. Ernst E. Chelation therapy for coronary heart disease: an overview of all clinical investigations. *Am Heart J.* 2000;140:139-41.
45. Lamas GA, Goertz C, Boineau R, et al. Effect of disodium EDTA chelation regimen on cardiovascular events in patients with previous myocardial infarction: the TACT randomized trial. *JAMA.* 2013;309:1241-50.
46. Nissen SE. Concerns about reliability in the Trial to Assess Chelation Therapy (TACT). *JAMA.* 2013;309:1293-4.
47. Andraws R, Berger JS, Brown DL. Effects of antibiotic therapy on outcomes of patients with coronary artery disease: a meta-analysis of randomized controlled trials. *JAMA.* 2005;293:2641-7.

Non–ST-Segment Elevation Acute Coronary Syndromes

8

Richard G. Bach

Acute Coronary Syndromes

GENERAL PRINCIPLES

- Acute coronary syndromes (ACSs) represent a group of specific clinical conditions resulting from myocardial ischemia or myocardial infarction (MI), related most often to atherothrombotic coronary obstruction (Figure 8-1).[1]
- For practical purposes, ACS can be divided into ST-segment elevation ACS (STE-ACS, or more commonly, ST-segment elevation MI [STEMI]) and non–ST-segment elevation ACS (NSTE-ACS), which includes both non–ST-segment elevation MI (NSTEMI) and unstable angina (UA). Notably, the clinical presentation and symptoms may be similar for these syndromes.
- The primary goals of treatment in NSTE-ACS are to relieve and/or limit ischemia, prevent infarction or reinfarction, and improve outcomes.
- Rapid identification of ACS allows for timely risk stratification and initiation of appropriate therapies.

Definitions

- STEMI (see Chapter 9) is diagnosed in an appropriate clinical setting with the finding of ≥1 mm (0.1 mV) ST elevation in at least two contiguous leads of an ECG, associated with cardiac biomarker elevation.
- NSTE-ACS is diagnosed in an appropriate clinical setting when such an event is associated with an ECG that does not show ST-segment elevation. The ECG may show ST depression or T-wave abnormalities, but may also be normal, with (NSTEMI) or without (UA) myocardial necrosis demonstrated by cardiac biomarker elevation.[1]
- The current universal definition for acute myocardial infarction (AMI)[2] defines AMI as acute myocardial injury with clinical evidence of acute myocardial ischemia and with detection of a rise and/or fall of cardiac troponin (cTn) values with at least one value above the 99th percentile of upper reference limit and at least one of the following:
  - Symptoms of myocardial ischemia
  - New ischemic ECG changes
  - Development of pathologic Q waves
  - Imaging evidence of new loss of viable myocardium or new regional wall motion abnormality in a pattern consistent with an ischemic etiology
  - Identification of a coronary thrombus by angiography or autopsy (not for type 2 or type 3 MIs)

Classification

NSTE-ACS can be subdivided into UA and NSTEMI based on the absence or presence, respectively, of myocardial necrosis (i.e., elevated cardiac biomarkers).

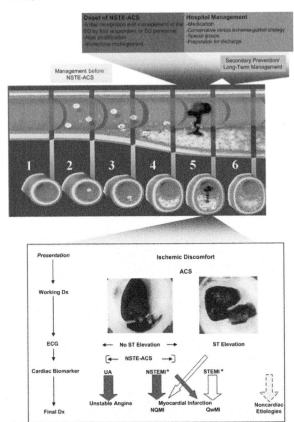

FIGURE 8-1. Common pathophysiology of acute coronary syndromes (ACSs). The top half of the figure illustrates the progression of plaque formation and development of ACS. The numbered sections of the artery depict the process of atherogenesis from (1) normal artery to (2) extracellular lipid in the subintima to (3) fibrofatty stage to (4) procoagulant expression and weakening of the fibrous cap. ACS develops with (5) disruption of the fibrous cap, which is the stimulus for thrombosis. Thrombus formation and possible coronary vasospasm can reduce blood flow in the affected coronary artery and cause ischemic chest pain. (6) Thrombus resorption may be followed by collagen accumulation and smooth muscle cell growth, resulting in plaque stabilization and healing. The bottom half illustrates the clinical correlates in ACS. Flow reduction may be related to a completely occlusive thrombus (bottom half, right side) or subtotally occlusive thrombus (bottom half, left side). Most patients with ST elevation (thick white arrow in bottom panel) develop Q-wave MI (QwMI), and a few (thin white arrow) develop non-Q-wave MI (NQMI). Those without ST elevation have either UA or NSTEMI (thick red arrows), based on the absence or presence of elevated cardiac biomarkers, respectively. Most patients presenting with NSTEMI develop NQMI; a few may develop QwMI. The spectrum of clinical presentations including UA, NSTEMI, and STEMI is referred to as ACS. *Elevated cardiac biomarker (e.g., troponin). Dx, diagnosis; ED, emergency department; MI, myocardial infarction; NSTE-ACS, non–ST-elevation acute coronary syndromes; NSTEMI, non–ST-elevation myocardial infarction; STEMI, ST-elevation myocardial infarction; UA, unstable angina. (Reprinted from Amsterdam EA, Wenger NK, Brindis RG, et al. 2014 AHA/ACC guideline for the management of patients with non-ST-elevation acute coronary syndromes: a report of the American College of Cardiology/American Heart Association Task Force on Practice Guidelines. *J Am Coll Cardiol.* 2014;64(24):e139-228. Copyright © 2014 American Heart Association, Inc., and the American College of Cardiology Foundation. With permission.)

Epidemiology

- The estimated annual incidence of MI is >600,000 new attacks and >200,000 recurrent attacks.[3]
- The average age at first AMI for men is 65.6 years and for women is 72.0 years.[3]
- Approximately every 40 seconds, an American will suffer from an AMI.[3]
- One out of every six deaths in the US is attributable to ACS.[3]
- In-hospital mortality is similar between STEMI and NSTEMI patients.[4]
- A 1-year mortality is higher for NSTEMI patients compared with STEMI patients.[4]
- Mortality from ACS has declined dramatically with the advent of evidence-based therapies, but up to 25% of patients do not receive optimal medical therapy for ACS, resulting in a significant increase in mortality in those patients.[5]

Etiology

Myocardial ischemia in NSTE-ACS results from a mismatch between myocardial oxygen supply and demand. Several mechanisms responsible, but not mutually exclusive, for this mismatch include[1]:

- **Coronary atherothrombosis** associated with coronary artery plaque rupture or erosion (Figure 8-1) (see section on Pathophysiology)
- **Coronary vasospasm** resulting from focal vasoconstriction of an epicardial coronary vessel related to hypercontractility of vascular smooth muscle with or without microvascular derangement (e.g., endothelial dysfunction)
- Other mechanical obstructions to coronary blood flow (e.g., thromboembolism and spontaneous coronary dissection)
- Secondary NSTE-ACS resulting from
  - Reduced coronary blood flow (e.g., hypotension)
  - Increased myocardial oxygen demand (e.g., tachycardia and thyrotoxicosis)
  - Reduced myocardial oxygen delivery (e.g., anemia and hypoxia)

Pathophysiology

- NSTE-ACS/UA typically results from severe narrowing and/or transient occlusion of a coronary artery:
  - The majority of cases of NSTE-ACS are due to a **critical decrease in coronary blood supply via partial occlusion of the affected vessel**.
  - This is distinct from most STEMI, which is due to a sudden obstruction of coronary blood supply due to total occlusion of the affected vessel.
- Coronary occlusion typically results from atherothrombosis at vulnerable plaques, which may involve a ruptured atherosclerotic plaque, or plaque erosion/ulceration.
- Coronary atherothrombosis involves platelet-mediated thrombosis at sites of plaque rupture, ulceration, or erosion; exposure of the subendothelium to the bloodstream initiates a cascade of events culminating in local thrombus formation.

Risk Factors

- The traditional major risk factors for the development of coronary artery disease (CAD) include hypertension, hyperlipidemia, smoking, diabetes, and a family history of premature CAD.
- Each patient presenting with NSTE-ACS should undergo a thorough assessment of CAD risk factors to initiate appropriate secondary prevention.

DIAGNOSIS

Clinical Presentation

History
- The symptoms associated with NSTE-ACS are highly variable and can include:
  - Chest pressure or heaviness with or without radiation to the arm(s), back, shoulder(s), neck, or jaw; at times, discomfort may be located solely in these areas outside the chest.
  - Indigestion or heartburn
  - Nausea and/or vomiting with or without epigastric discomfort
  - Shortness of breath or dyspnea on exertion
  - Weakness, dizziness, lightheadedness, or loss of consciousness
- Physicians should recognize that **up to half of the MIs may be silent**.[6]
- Symptoms that typically differentiate NSTE-ACS from chronic stable angina include:
  - Chest discomfort that occurs at rest lasting >20 minutes
  - Chest discomfort developing with increased severity, frequency, or duration
  - Chest discomfort occurring with less exertion
  - New-onset exertional angina of <2-month duration that limits physical activity
  - Angina that severely limits normal physical activity (i.e., angina with walking 1 to 2 blocks or a single flight of stairs)
- Symptoms that are **unlikely to be associated with NSTE-ACS** include[1]:
  - Pleuritic pain
  - Pain localized to the middle or lower abdominal region
  - Pain localized with one finger
  - Reproducible pain with movement or palpation
  - Pain lasting a few seconds
  - Pain radiating to the lower extremities
  - However, the **presence of atypical symptoms does not exclude the possibility of ACS**.

Physical Examination
- The physical examination in patients with NSTE-ACS is rarely specific or sensitive.
- May be helpful to support considering alternative diagnoses
- Assess for signs/symptoms of heart failure and/or shock, including:
  - Extra heart sounds (S_3)
  - Elevated jugular venous pressure
  - Pulmonary rales
  - Peripheral edema
  - Hypotension
  - Cyanosis
  - Cool or clammy extremities
- Awareness of the complications of AMI is important, as certain physical examination finding may be present at the time of diagnosis or complicate the course of NSTE-ACS (see Chapter 9).

Diagnostic Criteria

NSTE-ACS is a clinical diagnosis that is based on:
- History of symptoms compatible with myocardial ischemia, as described earlier
- An ECG that may be supportive if showing ST-segment depression and/or T-wave inversion or transient nondiagnostic ST elevation (but that may also be within normal limits)
- Assessment of cardiac biomarkers

Differential Diagnosis

- Cardiovascular (CV): acute pericarditis, myocarditis, cardiac tamponade, aortic dissection, aortic stenosis, hypertrophic cardiomyopathy (HCM), or congestive heart failure

- Pulmonary: pulmonary embolism, pneumothorax, pneumonia, asthma, or chronic obstructive pulmonary disease
- Gastrointestinal (GI): esophageal spasm, esophagitis, reflux disease, peptic ulcer disease, gastritis, or cholecystitis
- Psychiatric: anxiety disorders
- Musculoskeletal: muscle sprain/strain, costochondritis, rib fracture, painful lower rib syndrome, fibromyalgia, inflammatory arthropathies, SAPHO syndrome (i.e., synovitis, acne, pustulosis, hyperostosis, and osteitis), sickle cell disease, and malignancy

Diagnostic Testing

Laboratories

- **Cardiac biomarkers** should be measured on presentation and repeated serially over several hours.
- **cTns** (troponins T and I) measured in serum are highly specific and sensitive markers of myocardial necrosis and are essential for the diagnosis of ACS and for risk stratification in patients with ACS. Newer **high sensitivity troponin** assays are even more highly sensitive and analytically precise and allow determination of the 99th percentile of cTn concentration in reference subjects that serves as the upper reference limit (URL). Their high precision allows measurement of small differences in cTn over time. They are recommended for routine clinical use for the diagnosis of myocardial injury.[2]
  - Detected **as early as 2 hours** after myocardial damage
  - Peak levels occur 8 to 12 hours after the event and **can remain elevated for up to 14 days**.
  - cTn may be elevated in several other cardiac and noncardiac conditions, where myocardial injury may occur in the absence of MI[2]:
    - After direct cardiac injury (e.g., defibrillator discharges, cardiac surgery or ablation, cardiac contusion, and myopericarditis), stress-induced (takotsubo) cardiomyopathy, or hypertensive urgency/emergency
    - Noncardiac conditions (e.g., pulmonary embolism, acute and chronic renal disease)
    - Healthy subjects after extreme endurance events (e.g., marathons)
- Creatine kinase (CK-MB) is present in both skeletal and myocardial muscle cells.
  - No longer considered as sensitive or specific a test for diagnosing ACS as cTns
  - Can aid in the timing of myocardial injury when symptoms are ambiguous
  - CK-MB isoenzyme is readily detectable in the blood of normal subjects at low levels, and elevated levels can occur with damage to both skeletal and cardiac muscle cells.
  - Usually increases within 4 to 6 hours after injury, with peak level attained in ~10 to 18 hours
  - Due to its short half-life, CK-MB, if available, can be useful for assessing recurrent postinfarct ischemic events, because a fall and subsequent rise suggest reinfarction.
- **B-type natriuretic peptide** is another biomarker that has been shown to predict subsequent mortality in the setting of NSTE-ACS.[7]

Electrocardiography

Approximately 50% of patients with NSTE-ACS present with significant ECG abnormalities, including[2]:

- ST-segment depression ≥0.5 mm in two contiguous leads
- T-wave inversion ≥1 mm in two contiguous leads with prominent R wave or R/S ratio >1
- Symmetric T-wave inversions of >2 mm across the precordium are fairly specific for myocardial ischemia and worrisome for a lesion located in the proximal left anterior descending (LAD) artery
- Nonspecific ST-segment changes or T-wave inversions
  Note: **A normal ECG does not exclude the presence of ACS.**

Imaging
- Noninvasive stress testing: Exercise or pharmacologic stress testing with an imaging modality (either echocardiography or myocardial perfusion) can be used to risk stratify patients with relatively low-risk ACS.
- Cardiac computed tomographic angiography (CCTA) and cardiac magnetic resonance imaging (CMR) have been used to assess low-risk populations, although their precise roles in patients with ACS remain under study (see Chapter 36).
  - CCTA may be useful in excluding obstructive CAD in symptomatic patients with a low pretest probability for disease, especially patients with a negative ECG and normal cardiac biomarkers.
  - CMR can allow cardiac functional assessment, perfusion imaging (adenosine or dobutamine), and myocardial viability testing at the expense of prolonged study times, patient claustrophobia, and problems with certain metallic implants (e.g., pacemakers/defibrillators).

Coronary Angiography
- **Coronary angiography** is useful in providing detailed diagnostic information about the presence of coronary artery lesions among patients with symptoms of NSTE-ACS.
- **Indicated for patients who undergo the initial invasive strategy** (see section on Early Invasive versus Initial Conservative Strategy)
- Women and non-white patients are less likely to have significant angiographic epicardial CAD (see Chapter 33). *MI with nonobstructive coronary artery* (MINOCA) is a recently coined term used to describe patients with a diagnosis of MI who are found to have nonobstructive or normal coronary arteries by coronary angiography. The pathophysiology of ACS in these patients is incompletely understood but may involve plaque disruption not detectable by angiography, coronary vasospasm, or microvascular disease. Some patients may have a nonischemic process mimicking an MI presentation, such as myocarditis.[8]

TREATMENT

Risk Stratification
- Risk stratification allows tailoring of evidence-based diagnostic and therapeutic interventions based on the patient's risk for adverse outcomes. Guidelines strongly recommend (class I) the use of risk scores (see later) to assess prognosis in patients with NSTE-ACS.[1]
- These tools can help rapidly assess the risk for adverse ischemic and bleeding outcomes.
- The Thrombolysis In Myocardial Infarction (TIMI) risk score can differentiate patients' risk based on criteria that predict the likelihood of death, MI, or urgent revascularization (Table 8-1).[9]
- Higher TIMI risk score has been shown to correlate with poorer outcomes (Table 8-2).[9]
- The Global Registry of Acute Coronary Events (GRACE) risk model predicts in-hospital and postdischarge mortality or MI. The GRACE clinical application tool is a web-based downloadable application available at http://www.outcomes-umassmed.org/grace/.[1]

Bleeding Risk Assessment
- Bleeding in the setting of NSTE-ACS is associated with worse clinical outcomes.[10]
- All patients with NSTE-ACS should be assessed for their risk of bleeding when deciding therapeutic strategies.

TABLE 8-1 CALCULATING TIMI RISK SCORE

Each positive risk factor is worth 1 point. Points are added together to determine the TIMI risk score (maximum 7).

Risk factors:
- Age >65 years (1 point)
- Known CAD (>50% stenosis) (1 point)
- Severe anginal symptoms (>2 episodes of chest pain in the past 24 hours) (1 point)
- ST deviation on admission ECG (1 point)
- Elevated serum cardiac markers (1 point)
- Use of ASA in the 7 days before presentation (1 point)
- ≥3 risk factors for CAD (1 point):
  - Family history
  - Diabetes
  - Hypertension
  - Dyslipidemia
  - Current smoker

ASA, aspirin; CAD, coronary artery disease; TIMI, thrombolysis in myocardial infarction.

Data from Antman EM, Cohen M, Bernink PJ, et al. The TIMI risk score for unstable angina/non-ST elevation MI: a method for prognostication and therapeutic decision making. *JAMA* 2000;284:835–42.

TABLE 8-2 CARDIOVASCULAR OUTCOMES ACCORDING TO TIMI RISK SCORE. RATE OF DEATH, MI, OR URGENT REVASCULARIZATION AT 14 DAYS FROM THE TIMI 11B AND ESSENCE TRIALS ACCORDING TO TIMI RISK SCORE

TIMI Risk Score	Number (%) of patients	Rate of composite end point (%)
0/1	85 (4.3)	4.7
2	339 (17.3)	8.3
3	627 (32.0)	13.2
4	573 (29.3)	19.9
5	267 (13.6)	26.2
6/7	66 (3.4)	40.9

TIMI, thrombolysis in myocardial infarction.

Data from Antman EM, Cohen M, Bernink PJ, et al. The TIMI risk score for unstable angina/non-ST elevation MI: a method for prognostication and therapeutic decision making. *JAMA*. 2000;284:835-42.

- The CRUSADE bleeding score (ranges from 1 to 100) is a validated risk score for NSTE-ACS that determines a patient's baseline risk of in-hospital bleeding, ranging from 3.1% to 19.5% in the lowest and highest quintiles, respectively.[10]
- A simplified score calculator is available online (http://www.crusadebleedingscore.org).[10]

Early Invasive versus Initial Ischemia-Guided Strategy

- For NSTE-ACS, evidence-based initial management involves selection of an early invasive or initial conservative (ischemia-guided) strategy (Figure 8-2).[1]
- In the early invasive strategy, patients undergo diagnostic coronary angiography with intent to revascularize significant CAD when indicated.
- **Patients for whom the invasive strategy is preferred**[1]:
  - Recurrent chest pain despite maximal medical therapy
  - Elevated cardiac biomarkers
  - New ST-segment depression
  - Signs of heart failure
  - New or worsening mitral regurgitation
  - Hemodynamic instability
  - Sustained ventricular tachycardia
  - Prior coronary artery bypass grafting (CABG)
  - High-risk score (e.g., TIMI 5 to 7)
  - Percutaneous coronary intervention (PCI) within 6 months
  - Reduced left ventricular ejection fraction (LVEF)
- Patients with refractory rest angina despite maximal medical therapy, hemodynamic compromise, or unstable rhythm should be referred for immediate angiography.
- **In the ischemia-guided strategy, the patient may be treated with medical therapy followed by diagnostic testing** (stress testing with or without imaging) performed before discharge.
- **Patients for whom the conservative strategy is preferred**[1]:
  - Low-risk score (e.g., TIMI 0 to 2)
  - Patient or physician preference
  - Risk of revascularization outweighs benefits.
- For patients who undergo noninvasive diagnostic testing, coronary angiography should be performed in patients with LVEF <40% or intermediate- or high-risk stress test results.[1]

Medications

- All patients should receive medical management directed at relieving ischemia and reducing the risk for adverse cardiac events.
- The primary goals of pharmacotherapy in NSTE-ACS are:
  - To rapidly limit ischemia and control chest pain with anti-ischemic and analgesic medications
  - To reduce further thrombus formation and disease progression with an appropriate antithrombotic therapy using antiplatelet and anticoagulation therapies

Anti-ischemic Therapy

- Anti-ischemic therapy focuses on improving the balance of oxygen supply and demand.
- Bed rest/monitoring:
  - Limit activity to bed/chair rest to reduce myocardial oxygen demand
  - Continuous ECG/telemetry monitoring
- **Oxygen** is indicated during the acute phase of NSTE-ACS among patients with an arterial oxygen saturation <90% or presenting with cyanosis or respiratory distress.
- **Nitrates**:
  - Nitroglycerine acts as a vasodilator on both the systemic (i.e., reducing myocardial oxygen demand) and coronary circulation (i.e., increasing coronary blood flow).
  - Initial dose is sublingual (SL) nitroglycerine 0.4-mg tablets or spray every 5 minutes, up to 3 doses. IV nitroglycerine initiated at a dose of at least 10 μg/minute for:
    - Chest pain that is refractory to SL nitroglycerine
    - Elevated blood pressure (BP)
    - Heart failure symptoms

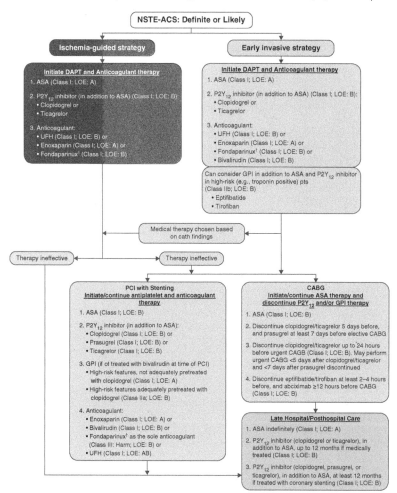

FIGURE 8-2. Management of patients with definite or likely NSTE-ACS. Schematic algorithm depicting key steps in the management of patients with suspected NSTE-ACS. †In patients who have been treated with fondaparinux (as upfront therapy) who are undergoing PCI, an additional anticoagulant with anti-IIa activity should be administered at the time of PCI because of the risk of catheter thrombosis. ASA, aspirin; CABG, coronary artery bypass graft; cath, catheter; COR, Class of Recommendation; DAPT, dual-antiplatelet therapy; GPI, glycoprotein IIb/IIIa inhibitor; LOE, Level of Evidence; NSTE-ACS, non–ST-elevation acute coronary syndrome; PCI, percutaneous coronary intervention; pts, patients; UFH, unfractionated heparin. Class of recommendations: Class I, should be performed; Class IIa, reasonable; Class IIb, may be considered; Class III: should not be performed and may be harmful. LOE grading: LOE A, multiple populations evaluated; data derived from multiple RCTs or meta-analyses; LOE B, limited populations evaluated; data derived from a single RCT or nonrandomized studies; LOE C, very limited populations evaluated; data consensus opinion of experts, case studies, or standard of care. (Reprinted from Amsterdam EA, Wenger NK, Brindis RG, et al. 2014 AHA/ACC guideline for the management of patients with non-ST-elevation acute coronary syndromes: a report of the American College of Cardiology/American Heart Association Task Force on Practice Guidelines. *J Am Coll Cardiol.* 2014;64(24):e139-228. Copyright © 2014 American Heart Association, Inc., and the American College of Cardiology Foundation. With permission.)

- Titrate by 10 μg/minute or greater increments every 5 minutes until the patient is chest pain free or hypotension (systolic blood pressure [SBP] <100 mm Hg) prevents further increases in dose.
- There is no maximum dose, but 200 μg/minute may be considered high enough to warrant additional therapy.
- Nitrates are generally contraindicated with:
  - SBP <90 mm Hg *or* heart rate (HR) <50 or >100 beats per minute (bpm)
  - Recent phosphodiesterase inhibitor use: within 24 hours of sildenafil or 48 hours of tadalafil
  - Timing for administration of nitrates with vardenafil is unknown, and thus, nitrates should be avoided.
- Nitrates should be used with caution in certain cardiac conditions that may be highly preload dependent:
  - Inferior MI with right ventricular infarct physiology
  - Severe aortic stenosis
  - HCM with significant left ventricular (LV) outflow tract obstruction
  - Cardiac tamponade
  - Restrictive cardiomyopathy
- Patients should generally be discharged with either SL or spray nitroglycerine for PRN use for anginal symptoms.
- **β-Blockers:**
  - β-Blockers have a proven benefit on mortality for patients with AMI.[1]
  - **Oral β-blocker therapy should be initiated within the first 24 hours** for patients who do not have contraindications (see later).
  - For appropriate patients, treatment may be initiated with metoprolol 5 mg IV every 5 minutes times 3 doses to a target HR of 50 to 60 bpm while maintaining SBP >100 mm Hg.
  - After the IV bolus(es) or in patients without active chest pain, start oral (PO) metoprolol, 25 to 50 mg every 6 hours, or atenolol, 50 to 100 mg daily.
  - PRN, IV bolus(es) may be repeated for patients with recurrent chest pain.
  - β-Blockers are contraindicated and may be harmful in patients with[1]:
    - Signs of heart failure
    - Evidence of a low cardiac output
    - Increased risk of cardiogenic shock (age >70 years, SBP <120 mm Hg, HR <60 bpm, or sinus tachycardia >120 bpm)
    - PR interval >0.24 seconds
    - Second- or third-degree heart block
    - Active asthma or reactive airway disease
- **Calcium channel blockers** (CCBs):
  - Considered for use in patients who have a contraindication to β-blockers.[1] However, no data have shown significant mortality benefit with the use of CCB.
  - Nondihydropyridines (e.g., verapamil or diltiazem) may be used in the absence of severe heart failure.
  - Nondihydropyridine CCB can be used as a third-line agent in patients continuing to have chest pain in the setting of adequate β-blockade and nitrates.
  - Extended-release dihydropyridines (e.g., amlodipine) may be used when clinically indicated.
  - Short-acting dihydropyridines, such as nifedipine, are associated with an increased risk of death when used without β-blockade in the setting of NSTE-ACS and are **contraindicated**.
- **Morphine:**
  - May be considered for patients with persistent chest pain despite nitrates[1]

○ Improves myocardial oxygen demand by reducing preload and sympathetic drive, due to its analgesic and anxiolytic properties

○ Dosed in 2- to 4-mg IV boluses with repeated doses PRN

○ Care should be exercised as morphine can mask symptoms that may indicate a need for intervention and can also lead to hypotension, respiratory depression, and delayed absorption of oral medications, such as antiplatelet agents. No clinical trial data have documented a reduction in adverse outcomes with morphine in the setting of NSTE-ACS.

○ Naloxone 0.4 to 2 mg IV in 2- to 3-minute intervals (maximum 10 mg) can be given to acutely reverse morphine's effects in the setting of overdosage.

Antithrombotic Therapy

• Antithrombotic therapy is essential to reduce further thrombus formation and major adverse cardiac events (MACEs), including death, MI, and stroke.

• Therapy may be tailored to each patient's individual risk.

• **All patients without contraindications should receive anticoagulation plus antiplatelet therapy**.

• Anticoagulation:

○ Anticoagulant therapy should be initiated as soon as possible after presentation for patients without contraindications.

○ Agents may act at different levels of the coagulation cascade to prevent thrombin generation.

○ Currently, the following four antithrombin agents can be considered with variable selection potentially based on the type of management strategy and considerations regarding bleeding risk[1]:

  ▪ Early invasive: unfractionated heparin (UFH), enoxaparin, fondaparinux, or bivalirudin[1]

  ▪ Initial conservative: UFH, enoxaparin, and fondaparinux

○ **UFH**:

○ UFH acts by binding antithrombin III (ATIII), which, in turn, binds to and inactivates thrombin (factor II), factor IXa, and factor Xa.

○ IV UFH should be administered with a recommended loading bolus of 60 units/kg (maximum 4000 units) followed by a continuous infusion of 12 units/kg (maximum 1000 units/hour).

○ The dose should be adjusted to maintain activated partial thromboplastin time of 1.5 times to bid the URL.

○ The duration of therapy may be determined by the management strategy[1]:

  ▪ Uncomplicated PCI: typically discontinue therapy after PCI

  ▪ Complicated PCI: at the discretion of the interventional cardiologist

  ▪ Conservative therapy: 48-hour duration

○ In cases of overdosage or refractory, life-threatening bleeding, protamine sulfate can be given to reverse the anticoagulant action of UFH (1 mg protamine sulfate IV for every 100 units of active heparin).

○ Except for rare situations, protamine sulfate should be avoided in patients with NSTE-ACS.

○ Heparin-induced thrombocytopenia (HIT) is a serious complication of heparin (unfractionated and less frequently low molecular weight) therapy.

○ **Low-molecular-weight heparins** (LMWHs):

  ▪ LMWHs are obtained by shortening the polysaccharide tail on the heparin molecule.

  ▪ Advantages over UFH include better bioavailability, SC dosing, predictable anticoagulant activity that does not require laboratory monitoring, less frequent type II HIT ($<1\%$), and lower overall cost.

- Disadvantages include a long half-life that can make emergent catheterization or PCI more complicated and an inability to effectively reverse its effects in the setting of refractory bleeding (i.e., only partly reversed with protamine sulfate).
- For patients with NSTE-ACS of age <75 years, enoxaparin may be administered at a dose of 30 mg IV bolus followed 15 minutes later by 1 mg/kg SC q12h (or q24h if creatinine clearance [CrCl] <30 mL/minute).[1]
- For patients aged 75 years or older, omit the IV bolus and administer 0.75 mg/kg SC q12h (or 1 mg/kg SC q24h if CrCl <30 mL/minute).
- Enoxaparin is typically discontinued after uncomplicated PCI. For patients managed conservatively, there may be benefit to continued treatment for the duration of hospitalization.[1]

○ **Fondaparinux**:
- Synthetic polysaccharide that contains the same pentasaccharide sequence found in UFH and LMWH
- Binds ATIII to predictably inhibit factor Xa without inhibiting thrombin
- Lacks the necessary domain to complex with PF4, which decreases the risk of HIT
- Administered as 2.5 mg SC daily
- Discontinued after uncomplicated PCI or may be continued for the duration of the hospitalization in patients managed conservatively
- Based on OASIS trials, compared with enoxaparin, fondaparinux appeared to reduce the risk of bleeding but **should not be the sole anticoagulant to support PCI** due to an increased risk of catheter-related thrombosis.[11,12]

○ **Bivalirudin**:
- Bivalirudin is a direct thrombin inhibitor with a class I recommendation for NSTE-ACS in the American College of Cardiology/American Heart Association (ACC/AHA) practice guidelines.
- Acts by directly binding to and inactivating thrombin
- If chosen as an initial medical therapy, bivalirudin is administered as 0.1 mg/kg IV bolus and then 0.25 mg/kg/hour infusion.
- For patients undergoing PCI, bivalirudin is administered as 0.75 mg/kg IV bolus followed by 1.75 mg/kg/hour infusion to continue for 4 hours after PCI.
- Dosage adjustment is required in patients with CrCl <30 mL/minute or on dialysis.
- Bivalirudin may be considered for patients at an increased risk for bleeding undergoing invasive management—based on the results of the ACUITY trial that showed a significant reduction in major bleeding with similar efficacy in ACS patients compared with heparin combined with a glycoprotein (GP) IIb/IIIa inhibitor.[13]

Antiplatelet Therapy
- Antiplatelet therapy is essential in the management of ACS.
- Aspirin (ASA) inhibits the production of thromboxane A2 and has been shown to reduce adverse ischemic events.
- Antagonists of the platelet P2Y$_{12}$ receptor have been shown to further reduce adverse ischemic events when added to ASA, and the combination is commonly termed **dual-antiplatelet therapy (DAPT)**.
- Additional parenteral antiplatelet agents, the GP IIb/IIIa receptor antagonists, have also been shown to reduce adverse ischemic events among patients with high-risk ACS, but may be associated with significantly increased bleeding risk, and their use has declined. GP IIb/IIIa antagonists can be considered especially as a bail-out option during PCI in the setting of no-reflow or a thrombotic complication.

- **ASA**:
  ○ A loading dose of non-enteric-coated ASA 162 to 325 mg should be given immediately— by emergency medical services or on arrival to the emergency department (ED)—unless there is a history of serious intolerance or contraindication.

○ ASA at 81 to 325 mg daily should be continued indefinitely; compared with higher doses, doses <100 mg daily have been associated with lower bleeding risk and are generally preferred for long-term therapy.

○ For patients unable to take ASA, a loading dose of a $P2Y_{12}$ inhibitor, clopidogrel, should be administered followed by a daily maintenance dose.

○ If a patient is allergic to ASA, then consultation with an allergist for possible desensitization is recommended, if feasible.

- **Adenosine diphosphate (ADP) $P2Y_{12}$ receptor antagonists**:

  ○ Patients with ACS should also be treated with an oral antagonist of the $P2Y_{12}$ receptor as part of **DAPT**. Currently available indicated choices include clopidogrel, prasugrel, and ticagrelor.

  ○ Among patients with ACS undergoing PCI who have not been adequately pretreated with an oral $P2Y_{12}$ inhibitor, the short-half-life IV $P2Y_{12}$ inhibitor, cangrelor, may be considered for acute use to support the PCI procedure.

  ○ An oral $P2Y_{12}$ inhibitor in addition to ASA (i.e., DAPT) is recommended for up to 12 months to all patients with NSTE-ACS without contraindications or an excessive bleeding risk.[1,14]

  ○ Clopidogrel and ticagrelor are indicated for patients with ACS, regardless of management strategy.

  ○ Prasugrel is indicated for ACS patients undergoing invasive management and PCI.

  ○ The timing of initial administration of a $P2Y_{12}$ inhibitor to patients with NSTE-ACS has been debated and should be considered in the context of ischemic and bleeding risk. Randomized trials have shown benefit of early administration (on presentation), which is endorsed in ACC/AHA guidelines.[1] Early administration before coronary angiography may delay revascularization or contribute to bleeding for patients requiring surgical revascularization. The recently updated European Society of Cardiology (ESC) guidelines[14] recommend not administering routine pretreatment with a $P2Y_{12}$ receptor inhibitor in NSTE-ACS patients in whom coronary anatomy is not known and an early invasive management is planned. In such a strategy, initiation of a $P2Y_{12}$ inhibitor may be delayed until after coronary angiography. For patients undergoing an ischemia-guided strategy, early treatment may be considered.[14]

  ○ ACC/AHA guidelines state that it is reasonable to prescribe ticagrelor over clopidogrel for NSTE-ACS and that it is reasonable to prescribe prasugrel over clopidogrel for patients with NSTE-ACS undergoing PCI not at high risk for bleeding.[1] Based on the results of the ISAR-REACT 5 trial,[15] recently updated ESC guidelines[14] endorse prasugrel over ticagrelor for NSTE-ACS patients undergoing PCI.

  ○ Variations on the antiplatelet agents, combinations, and duration of treatment following PCI among patients with ACS have been subject to intensive study over the past several years, and determining the optimal strategy for an individual ACS patient remains a work-in-progress but may be considered in the context of differing patient bleeding and ischemic risks. Among patients with ACS and high ischemic risk who tolerate DAPT for 12 months without bleeding, continuing DAPT beyond 12 months using clopidogrel or ticagrelor may reduce ischemic events.[16,17] Among patients at high bleeding risk, shortened duration of DAPT by discontinuation of the $P2Y_{12}$ inhibitor after 3 to 6 months can reduce bleeding events and may be considered.[18] In the TWILIGHT study, patients at higher bleeding risk after PCI who were treated with ASA and ticagrelor and without a bleeding or ischemic event at 3 months who had ASA discontinued while continuing to take ticagrelor alone had significantly reduced bleeding without a significant increase in adverse ischemic events at 12 months.[19] These observations suggest an individualized approach to the choice of antiplatelet agents and duration of DAPT may favorably affect bleeding and ischemic outcomes.

  ○ **Clopidogrel**:

    ▪ Clopidogrel is given as a loading dose of 600 mg PO followed by 75 mg PO daily.[1]

- Prodrug that requires metabolic conversion to its active metabolite via cytochrome P450 (CYP) isoenzymes in the liver; genetic variability in certain isoenzymes (e.g., CYP2C19) and drug–drug interactions that affect isoenzyme activity can affect the degree of platelet inhibition by clopidogrel. The clinical implications of these observations remain under study.
- Clopidogrel is generally well tolerated, but rare cases of thrombotic thrombocytopenic purpura (TTP) have been observed.
- The CURRENT-OASIS-7 trial demonstrated a reduction in MACE at 30 days with a slight increase in major bleeding in higher risk NSTE-ACS patients who underwent PCI and received a 600-mg loading dose of clopidogrel followed by 150 mg daily for 1 week and then 75 mg daily compared with patients receiving a 300-mg loading dose of clopidogrel and then 75 mg daily.[20]
- For patients undergoing PCI, a loading dose of 600 mg is preferred before or at the time of PCI. As mentioned previously, for select patients, this may be followed by 150 mg daily for 6 days and then 75 mg daily for at least 1 year.[1]
- Routine platelet function and genetic testing to determine the platelet inhibitory response to clopidogrel are not recommended and should only be considered in patients at a high risk for poor clinical outcomes and if the results will alter management.[1]
- In patients with established high on-treatment platelet reactivity, alternative agents such as prasugrel and ticagrelor should be considered.[21]
- Of note, it is recommended that clopidogrel be withheld for at least 5 days before surgery for patients requiring CABG for revascularization.[1]
- Clopidogrel is the preferred $P2Y_{12}$ inhibitor for patients with high or very high bleeding risk.[14]
  - **Prasugrel**:
    - Prasugrel is a more potent and rapid inhibitor of the $P2Y_{12}$ receptor compared with clopidogrel.[22]
    - Prasugrel should be restricted to patients undergoing PCI.[1]
    - It is administered as a 60-mg PO loading dose for patients at the time of or up to 1 hour after PCI and then 10 mg PO daily thereafter.[1]
    - In the TRITON-TIMI-38 trial, prasugrel reduced MACE by 19% in ACS patients undergoing PCI who received prasugrel compared with clopidogrel (300-mg loading dose followed by 75 mg daily) at the expense of increasing the risk of major bleeding.[23]
    - Prasugrel is **absolutely contraindicated in patients with a history of stroke/transient ischemic accident (TIA)**.[1]
    - It should be used with caution in patients whose body weight is <60 kg or who have an increased risk of bleeding, where a maintenance dose of 5 mg daily may be considered.[1]
    - In patients aged 75 years or older, prasugrel is generally not recommended, except in high-risk situations (e.g., diabetes or prior MI).[1]
    - Of note, it is recommended that prasugrel be withheld for at least 7 days before surgery for patients requiring CABG for revascularization.[1]
  - **Ticagrelor**:
    - Ticagrelor is a nonthienopyridine antagonist of the platelet $P2Y_{12}$ receptor.
    - It is reversible and a short-acting agent, with a half-life of 7 to 9 hours.
    - It is administered as a 180-mg PO loading dose followed 12 hours later by 90 mg PO bid.
    - The PLATO trial demonstrated a 16% reduction in major cardiac events with ticagrelor compared with clopidogrel in ACS patients; however, it was associated with a slightly increased rate of non-CABG major bleeding.[24]

- Given its shorter half-life, it may be theoretically useful regarding concerns for delaying CABG in patients whose coronary anatomy has not yet been defined, but the Food and Drug Administration (FDA) and package insert recommend withholding ticagrelor for 5 days before major surgery.
- When ticagrelor is used, the recommended daily maintenance dose of ASA is 81 mg.[1]
○ **GP IIb/IIIa inhibitors**:
  - GP IIb/IIIa platelet receptors bind fibrinogen and other ligands, mediating the final common pathway for platelet aggregation.
  - Available GP IIb/IIIa inhibitors include eptifibatide and tirofiban.
  - **Addition of a GP IIb/IIIa inhibitor to DAPT** (i.e., ASA and ADP P2Y$_{12}$ antagonist) **may be considered in patients who are not at high risk for bleeding** who have[1,14]:
    □ High-risk features including positive troponins, diabetes mellitus, and significant ST-segment depression
    □ Refractory ischemia despite maximal medical therapy
    □ Delay to angiography >48 hours
  - GP IIb/IIIa inhibitors may be omitted if a patient does not have high-risk features and has received a loading dose of P2Y$_{12}$ antagonist.[1,14]
  - GP IIb/IIIa inhibitors should not be initiated before PCI in patients on DAPT who are at low risk (TIMI risk score <2) or at high risk for bleeding.[1]
  - Thrombocytopenia, which can be severe, is an uncommon, but well-described complication of these agents and should prompt discontinuation of the drug.
  - **Eptifibatide** mimics a peptide sequence on fibrinogen that has a high affinity for the fibrinogen-binding sites for the GP IIb/IIIa receptor.
  - **Tirofiban** is a nonpeptide synthetic derivative of tyrosine that also has a high affinity for the fibrinogen-binding sites for the GP IIb/IIIa receptor.
    □ Eptifibatide is given with a loading bolus of 180 μg/kg (maximum 22.6 mg) over 2 minutes, followed by a maintenance infusion at 2 μg/kg/minute (maximum 15 mg/hour). If a patient's CrCl is <50 mL/minute, then the maintenance infusion is decreased to 1 μg/kg/minute (maximum 7.5 mg/hour).
    □ Tirofiban is administered with a loading bolus of 0.4 μg/kg per minute over 30 minutes, followed by a maintenance infusion of 0.1 μg/kg per minute. Both bolus and infusion doses should be decreased by 50% in patients with a CrCl of <30 mL/minute.
    □ Eptifibatide and tirofiban are renally eliminated, dosages should be renally adjusted, and both are contraindicated in patients with severe renal insufficiency or on dialysis.
    □ The half-lives of both are 2 to 3 hours, and platelet aggregation returns to normal within 8 to 12 hours after discontinuation of either drug.
    □ The duration of therapy in NSTE-ACS is variable and may continue until 18 to 24 hours after PCI.

Additional Secondary Prevention
- Secondary prevention is discussed in detail in Chapter 4.
- **Angiotensin-converting enzyme (ACE) inhibitors and angiotensin-receptor blockers (ARBs)**:
  ○ **Should be initiated within the first 24 hours in patients with an LVEF <40% or with signs of heart failure**[1]
  ○ ARB may be used in ACE inhibitor–intolerant patients.
  ○ Also consider for patients with LVEF >40% or without signs of heart failure, especially for those patients with preexisting hypertension
  ○ Because of the potential for harm, an IV ACE inhibitor should be used with caution in the first 24 hours, except in cases of uncontrolled hypertension.

- Aldosterone-receptor blockers:
  - May be considered in the early recovery phase after ACS in patients who are tolerating therapeutic doses of an ACE inhibitor and have[1]:
    - Diabetes mellitus
    - Signs of congestive heart failure
    - LVEF <40%
  - In the absence of renal dysfunction (CrCl <30 mL/minute) or hyperkalemia, spironolactone or eplerenone may be considered.
  - When initiating therapy, it is important to follow potassium levels and renal function closely.
- **Lipid-lowering therapy**:
  - If lipid profile is unknown, patients should have a fasting lipid panel within 24 hours of presentation.
  - High-intensity hydroxymethylglutaryl-coenzyme A reductase inhibitors **(statins),** defined as those that can reduce low-density lipoprotein (LDL) cholesterol by >50%, which include high-dose atorvastatin or rosuvastatin, **should be initiated in all patients who do not have a contraindication, regardless of a patient's baseline** LDL.[25]
  - Per recent ACC/AHA guidelines, goal LDL is <70 mg/dL, while more recent ESC guidelines recommend an LDL goal of <55 mg/dL. In the PROVE IT-TIMI 22 trial, high-dose statin therapy (atorvastatin 80 mg daily) decreased MACE in ACS patients compared with moderate-dose statin therapy (pravastatin 40 mg daily).[26] In IMPROVE-IT, the addition of the nonstatin lipid-lowering agent ezetimibe to statin therapy reduced LDL levels significantly <70 mg/dL and resulted in reduced ischemic outcomes.[27]
  - Clinical trials have demonstrated that the proprotein convertase subtilisin kexin 9 (PCSK9) inhibitors (evolocumab and alirocumab) are highly effective at reducing cholesterol and reducing CV events for patients after ACS or with established congenital heart disease (CHD).[28,29] For patients following ACS who do not tolerate a statin or who do not reach goal LDL levels with statin therapy, the use of a PCSK9 inhibitor should be considered to reduce LDL levels and ischemic events.
- Proton-pump inhibitors (PPIs):
  - PPIs should be considered in patients requiring DAPT who have an indication for therapy, a history of GI bleeding, or a risk of GI bleeding.[30]
  - In observational studies, an association between PPI use and increased adverse CV events for patients receiving clopidogrel has raised concerns regarding an interaction between PPIs and clopidogrel, resulting from reduced platelet inhibition due to an effect of PPIs on CYP enzyme activity.
  - This observation was not confirmed in the prospective, randomized COGENT trial where PPIs did show significant benefit in reducing GI-related adverse events for patients receiving clopidogrel.[31]
- Oral anticoagulation:
  - For patients with NSTE-ACS undergoing PCI who have indications for oral anticoagulation, prolonged triple antithrombotic therapy (TAT) with ASA, an ADP $P2Y_{12}$ antagonist, and warfarin is associated with a significantly **increased risk of serious bleeding**.[32]
  - For such patients, after a short period (~1 week) of triple therapy, dual antithrombotic therapy (DAT) with warfarin or a novel oral anticoagulant (NOAC) and single-antiplatelet therapy using a $P2Y_{12}$ antagonist, typically clopidogrel, is recommended for 12 months. Among patients at high bleeding risk, DAT may be shortened to 6 months by discontinuation of the $P2Y_{12}$ antagonist, and for patients at high ischemic risk, TAT may be prolonged for up to 1 month.[14]
  - For patients requiring TAT with warfarin and DAPT, the dosage of ASA should not exceed 75 to 81 mg daily, and the therapeutic range of warfarin should be maintained to a goal international normalized ratio of no >2 to 2.5.[1]

- Fibrinolytics (thrombolytics): There has been no benefit observed and even a possibility of increased risk of adverse outcome for patients with NSTE-ACS treated with fibrinolytic therapy; therefore, they are contraindicated in this setting.[1]
- NSAIDs:
  - Among patients with ACS, both nonselective cyclooxygenase (COX) inhibitors and COX-2 inhibitors (except ASA) are associated with an increased risk of death, reinfarction, myocardial rupture, hypertension, and heart failure in large meta-analyses.[1]
  - They are contraindicated during hospitalization for NSTE-ACS.
  - Acetaminophen, low-dose opiates, and nonacetylated salicylates are acceptable alternatives for treating chronic musculoskeletal pain in patients with NSTE-ACS.
  - A nonselective COX inhibitor (e.g., naproxen) is reasonable if the abovementioned therapies are insufficient.
- Glucose-lowering medications and diabetes mellitus:
  - The recently published ESC ACS guidelines recommended that all patients with NSTE-ACS have their glycemic status evaluated and carefully managed.[14]
  - Data from recent randomized trials have shown reduced CV events from the use of two newer classes of glucose-lowering agents, the glucagon-like peptide-1-receptor antagonists[33] and the sodium-glucose cotransporter-2 inhibitors,[34] and strongly suggest that these agents should be recommended in patients with type 2 diabetes mellitus and CV disease, including those following ACS.[14]

Nonpharmacologic Therapies

- Hemodynamic support:
  - Intra-aortic balloon counterpulsation (IABP) or percutaneous left ventricular assist devices (LVADs, e.g., Impella catheters) may be considered in patients with ACS with[1]:
    - Refractory ischemic symptoms despite maximal medical therapy
    - Hemodynamic compromise
    - Mechanical complications of MI (e.g., acute mitral regurgitation)
  - Percutaneous LVADs have superior hemodynamic support compared with IABP in patients with cardiogenic shock secondary to AMI, but may be associated with a higher rate of complication; added clinical benefit has not yet been adequately demonstrated in large-scale prospective randomized clinical trials of ACS patients[35] but is the topic of ongoing study.
- Blood transfusion:
  - Theoretically, increasing blood hemoglobin concentration in patients who are anemic should improve oxygen-carrying capacity and improve myocardial oxygen supply.
  - However, observational studies have linked transfusion of stored blood to future adverse outcomes, and there remains uncertainty regarding the appropriate indications or threshold hemoglobin value that should trigger transfusion therapy.
  - Transfusion of patients with ACS to a hemoglobin >8 or >10 g/dL or to a hematocrit $>30\%$ has been recommended but based on limited data regarding benefit, and the optimal threshold for transfusion of patients with ACS remains uncertain and the topic of ongoing study.

Surgical Management

- When considering potential revascularization strategies, patients with left main or multivessel disease may be risk stratified using the **SYNTAX score** (Society of Thoracic Surgeons and Synergy between Percutaneous Coronary Intervention with TAXUS and Cardiac Surgery).[12]
- Revascularization by CABG may be indicated for ACS patients with[1]:
  - Unprotected left main disease, although PCI is now considered an acceptable alternative in uncomplicated left main disease, especially in patients with a SYNTAX score <22[12]
  - Three-vessel disease (CABG may be preferred if SYNTAX >22 and good surgical candidate), especially in the setting of impaired LV function

- Two-vessel disease with proximal LAD involvement
- Diabetic patients with multivessel CAD, including LAD disease

Lifestyle/Risk Modification

- Secondary prevention is discussed in detail in Chapter 4.
- Smoking cessation:
  - All patients should be assessed for current use and desire to quit.
  - Cessation and reduction of environmental exposure is advised for all patients.
  - Pharmacotherapy is useful and should be considered for any patient starting cessation.
- BP control:
  - Patients should be aggressively treated to a goal BP of <130/80 mm Hg.
  - Medications with BP-lowering activity that are used to treat NSTE-ACS should be maximized before adding additional BP-lowering agents.
- Weight management:
  - Body mass index (BMI) should be assessed during the hospitalization and at each subsequent visit.
  - Goal BMI is 18.6 to 24.9 kg/m^2.
  - For patients who initiate weight loss therapy, a reasonable goal is reduction in weight by 10% over a period of several months.
- Physical activity:
  - All patients should be encouraged to perform moderate aerobic activity for 30 to 60 minutes five to seven times per week.[1]
  - Weight training can be incorporated 2 days out of each week.
  - **Daily walking can begin immediately upon discharge**.
  - Sexual activity can be resumed 7 to 10 days after discharge.
- Cardiac rehabilitation:
  - **All patients should be referred for cardiac rehabilitation**.[1,14]
  - Cardiac rehabilitation can reduce mortality following ACS by as much as 27%, but as few as 16% of patients are referred for rehabilitation.

Cocaine-/Methamphetamine-Associated Myocardial Infarction

GENERAL PRINCIPLES

- An estimated 25 million Americans have used cocaine.[36]
- Cocaine-induced angina is likely secondary to increased myocardial oxygen demand from:
  - Increased BP, HR, and contractility
  - Vasoconstriction/vasospasm of epicardial vessels
  - Increased platelet aggregation
  - Accelerated atherosclerosis, thereby increasing the risk of coronary thrombosis
- The risk of MI is increased by a factor of 24 immediately after cocaine use.[36]
- The incidence of ACS after methamphetamines is unclear, but the pathophysiology is considered likely similar to that of cocaine abuse.

DIAGNOSIS

- Patients with cocaine-induced chest pain should undergo the same diagnostic considerations as other patients with symptoms of NSTE-ACS.
- Diagnostic angiography with intent to perform PCI should be considered for all patients with persistent new ST-elevation or new ST-depression or T-wave changes despite nitroglycerine and CCB therapy.[1]

TREATMENT

- Treatment algorithm is modified:
  - All patients should still receive **ASA**.
  - SL or IV **nitrates** should also be given, especially in those with ST-segment or T-wave changes.[1]
  - **CCB**, such as IV diltiazem, can be used to reduce myocardial oxygen demand.
  - β-**Blockers are relatively contraindicated**, as they can lead to unopposed α-mediated vasoconstriction and worsen myocardial ischemia. **Potential exceptions are carvedilol and labetalol**, which have both β- and α-blocking properties and may be administered to patients with SBP >100 mm Hg or HR >100 bpm, provided they have been given nitroglycerine or CCB 1 hour before administration.
  - **Benzodiazepines** are also used as an anxiolytic to reduce ischemia.
  - Even in the setting of vasospasm, many patients may still have luminal thrombosis or plaque rupture requiring PCI.
- Patients with methamphetamine-induced ACS should be treated similar to patients with cocaine-induced angina.

REFERENCES

1. Amsterdam EA, Wenger NK, Brindis RG, et al. 2014 AHA/ACC guideline for the management of patients with non-ST-elevation acute coronary syndromes: a report of the American College of Cardiology/American Heart Association Task Force on Practice Guidelines. *J Am Coll Cardiol.* 2014;64(24):e139-228.
2. Thygesen K, Alpert JS, Jaffe AS, et al. Fourth universal definition of myocardial infarction (2018). *Circulation.* 2018;138:e618-51.
3. Virani SS, Alonso A, Aparicio HJ, et al. Heart disease and stroke statistics-2021 update a report from the American Heart Association. *Circulation.* 2021;143:e254-743.
4. Montalescot G, Dallongeville J, Belle E, et al. STEMI and NSTEMI: are they so different? 1 year outcomes in acute myocardial infarction as defined by the ESC/ACC definition (the OPERA registry). *Eur Heart J.* 2007;28:1409-17.
5. Peterson ED, Roe MT, Mulgund J, et al. Association between hospital process performance and outcomes among patients with acute coronary syndromes. *JAMA.* 2006;295:1912-20.
6. Kannel WB. Silent myocardial ischemia and infarction: insights from the Framingham Study. *Cardiol Clin.* 1986;4:583-91.
7. Galvani M, Ottani F, Oltrona L, et al. N-terminal pro-brain natriuretic peptide on admission has prognostic value across the whole spectrum of acute coronary syndromes. *Circulation.* 2004;110:128-34.
8. Reynolds HR, Maehara A, Kwong RY, et al. Coronary optical coherence tomography and cardiac magnetic resonance imaging to determine underlying causes of myocardial infarction with nonobstructive coronary arteries in women. *Circulation.* 2021;143:624-40.
9. Antman EM, Cohen M, Bernink PJ, et al. The TIMI risk score for unstable angina/non-ST elevation MI: a method for prognostication and therapeutic decision making. *JAMA.* 2000;284:835-42.
10. Subherwal S, Bach RG, Chen AY, et al. Baseline risk of major bleeding in non-ST-segment-elevation myocardial infarction: the CRUSADE (Can Rapid risk stratification of Unstable angina patients Suppress ADverse outcomes with Early implementation of the ACC/AHA Guidelines) bleeding score. *Circulation.* 2009;119:1873-82.
11. Fifth Organization to Assess Strategies in Acute Ischemic Syndromes; Yusuf S, Mehta SR, Chrolavicius S, et al. Comparison of fondaparinux and enoxaparin in acute coronary syndromes. *N Engl J Med.* 2006;354:1464-76.
12. Levine GN, Bates ER, Blankenship JC, et al. 2011 ACCF/AHA/SCAI guideline for percutaneous coronary intervention: a report of the American College of Cardiology Foundation/American Heart Association Task Force on Practice Guidelines and the Society for Cardiovascular Angiography and Interventions. *Circulation.* 2011;124:e574-651.
13. Stone GW, White HD, Ohman EM, et al. Bivalirudin in patients with acute coronary syndromes undergoing percutaneous coronary intervention: a subgroup analysis from the Acute Catheterization and Urgent Intervention Triage strategy (ACUITY) trial. *Lancet.* 2007;369:907-19.

14. Collet JP, Thiele H, Barbato E, et al. 2020 ESC guidelines for the management of acute coronary syndromes in patients presenting without persistent ST-segment elevation. *Eur Heart J.* 2021;42:1289-367.

15. Schupke S, Neumann FJ, Menichelli M, et al. Ticagrelor or prasugrel in patients with acute coronary syndromes. *N Engl J Med.* 2019;381:1524-34.

16. Mauri L, Kereiakes DJ, Yeh RW, et al. Twelve or 30 months of dual antiplatelet therapy after drug-eluting stents. *N Engl J Med.* 2014;371:2155-66.

17. Bonaca MP, Braunwald E, Sabatine MS. Long-term use of ticagrelor in patients with prior myocardial infarction. *N Engl J Med.* 2015;373:1274-5.

18. Costa F, van Klaveren D, James S, et al. Derivation and validation of the predicting bleeding complications in patients undergoing stent implantation and subsequent dual antiplatelet therapy (PRECISE-DAPT) score: a pooled analysis of individual-patient datasets from clinical trials. *Lancet.* 2017;389:1025-34.

19. Mehran R, Baber U, Sharma SK, et al. Ticagrelor with or without aspirin in high-risk patients after PCI. *N Engl J Med.* 2019;381:2032-42.

20. The Current-Oasis Investigators 7; Mehta SR, Bassand JP, et al. Dose comparisons of clopidogrel and aspirin in acute coronary syndromes. *N Engl J Med.* 2010;363:930-42.

21. Levine GN, Bates ER, Bittl JA, et al. 2016 ACC/AHA focused update on duration of dual antiplatelet therapy in patients with coronary artery disease: a report of the American College of Cardiology/American Heart Association Task Force on Clinical Practice Guidelines. *J Am Coll Cardiol.* 2016;68:1082-115.

22. Depta JP, Bhatt DL. Aspirin and platelet adenosine diphosphate receptor antagonists in acute coronary syndromes and percutaneous coronary intervention: role in therapy and strategies to overcome resistance. *Am J Cardiovasc Drugs.* 2008;8:91-112.

23. Wiviott SD, Braunwald E, McCabe CH, et al. Prasugrel versus clopidogrel in patients with acute coronary syndromes. *N Engl J Med.* 2007;357:2001-15.

24. Wallentin L, Becker RC, Budaj A, et al. Ticagrelor versus clopidogrel in patients with acute coronary syndromes. *N Engl J Med.* 2009;361:1045-57.

25. Grundy SM, Stone NJ, Bailey AL, et al. 2018 AHA/ACC/AACVPR/AAPA/ABC/ACPM/ADA/AGS/APhA/ASPC/NLA/PCNA guideline on the management of blood cholesterol: executive summary: a report of the American College of Cardiology/American Heart Association Task Force on Clinical Practice Guidelines. *J Am Coll Cardiol.* 2019;73:3168-209.

26. Cannon CP, Braunwald E, McCabe CH, et al. Intensive versus moderate lipid lowering with statins after acute coronary syndromes. *N Engl J Med.* 2004;350:1495-504.

27. Cannon CP, Blazing MA, Giugliano RP, et al. Ezetimibe added to statin therapy after acute coronary syndromes. *N Engl J Med.* 2015;372:2387-97.

28. Schwartz GG, Steg PG, Szarek M, et al. Alirocumab and cardiovascular outcomes after acute coronary syndrome. *N Engl J Med.* 2018;379:2097-107.

29. Gencer B, Mach F, Murphy SA, et al. Efficacy of evolocumab on cardiovascular outcomes in patients with recent myocardial infarction: a prespecified secondary analysis from the FOURIER trial. *JAMA Cardiol.* 2020;5:952-7.

30. Abraham NS, Hlatky MA, Antman EM, et al. ACCF/ACG/AHA 2010 Expert Consensus Document on the concomitant use of proton pump inhibitors and thienopyridines: a focused update of the ACCF/ACG/AHA 2008 expert consensus document on reducing the gastrointestinal risks of antiplatelet therapy and NSAID use. A report of the American College of Cardiology Foundation Task Force on Expert Consensus Documents. *J Am Coll Cardiol.* 2010;56:2051-66.

31. Bhatt DL, Cryer BL, Contant CF, et al. Clopidogrel with or without omeprazole in coronary artery disease. *N Engl J Med.* 2010;363:1909-17.

32. Dewilde WJ, Oirbans T, Verheugt FW, et al. Use of clopidogrel with or without aspirin in patients taking oral anticoagulant therapy and undergoing percutaneous coronary intervention: an open-label, randomised, controlled trial. *Lancet.* 2013;381:1107-15.

33. Marso SP, Bain SC, Consoli A, et al. Semaglutide and cardiovascular outcomes in patients with type 2 diabetes. *N Engl J Med.* 2016;375:1834-44.

34. Zinman B, Wanner C, Lachin JM, et al. Empagliflozin, cardiovascular outcomes, and mortality in type 2 diabetes. *N Engl J Med.* 2015;373:2117-28.

35. Seyfarth M, Sibbing D, Bauer I, et al. A randomized clinical trial to evaluate the safety and efficacy of a percutaneous left ventricular assist device versus intra-aortic balloon pumping for treatment of cardiogenic shock caused by myocardial infarction. *J Am Coll Cardiol.* 2008;52:1584-8.

36. Lange RA, Hillis LD. Cardiovascular complications of cocaine use. *N Engl J Med.* 2001;345:351-8.

Acute ST-Segment Elevation Myocardial Infarction

9

Mark Gdowski, Nishtha Sodhi, and Howard I. Kurz

GENERAL PRINCIPLES

- **The pathophysiology of** ST-segment elevation myocardial infarction **(STEMI) is different from that of the other acute coronary syndromes (ACSs): unstable angina and non–ST-segment elevation myocardial infarction** (UA/NSTEMI).
- STEMI is a medical emergency. Treatment requires rapid recognition/diagnosis, coordination of health care resources, and rapid decision-making regarding reperfusion.
- Reducing time to reperfusion (i.e., "door-to-balloon" or "door-to-needle") has become a major benchmark for institutional quality of cardiovascular care.

Definition

- The clinical definition of myocardial infarction (MI)[1] requires **the rise and/or fall of cardiac biomarkers of myocardial necrosis IN ADDITION to at least one of the following**:
  - Ischemic symptoms
  - Electrocardiogram (ECG) changes consistent with ischemia or pathologic Q waves
  - Confirmation of infarction on imaging
  - Coronary thrombus identified on angiography or by autopsy
- ST-segment elevation myocardial infarction (STEMI) is defined as a clinical syndrome of myocardial ischemia in association with persistent ST-segment elevations (STEs) on ECG and subsequent release of biomarkers of necrosis.[2]

Epidemiology

- An estimated 500,000 patients in the United States suffer an STEMI annually.
- A significant proportion of these patients die from sudden cardiac death due to ventricular arrhythmia before arriving to the hospital.
- In-hospital and 1-year mortality rates from STEMI have decreased significantly with advances in goal-directed medical therapy and interventions.[2]
- Current overall survival rates across the majority of U.S. centers are >90%.
- However, the death rate remains high (>50%) among the subgroup of patients who develop cardiogenic shock or other mechanical complications of STEMI.

Etiology

- Any condition that interrupts coronary flow sufficiently to cause myocardial cell death can lead to MI.
- This usually results from an **acute change in a preexisting coronary plaque** with subsequent activation of thrombotic mediators and clot formation.
- There is a spectrum of the degree of coronary artery obstruction and cell death. STEMI results from complete coronary artery occlusion.
- Other conditions that may result in STEMI include:
  - Severe coronary vasospasm
  - Coronary artery embolization
  - Spontaneous coronary artery dissection

Pathophysiology

- STEMI is caused by an acute occlusion of an epicardial coronary artery, most often due to atherosclerotic plaque rupture/erosion and subsequent thrombus formation.
- The mechanisms involved vary by age and gender:
  - **Plaque rupture** causes the majority of STEMI events in men and older women.
  - **Plaque erosion** (with no disruption of the fibrous cap) is more common in younger women.
- With **plaque rupture**, mild-to-moderate immature plaques (i.e., those that do not significantly impede coronary flow at baseline) with thin fibrous caps and lipid-rich cores rupture in the acute setting of inflammation, shear forces, and local rheologic factors.
- This initiates a sequence of platelet aggregation, fibrin deposition, and vasoconstriction, forming the classic **fibrin-rich red thrombus**, which completely occludes the involved artery, predisposing to STEMI, with total transmural ischemia/infarction.
- Left untreated, the mortality rate of an uncomplicated STEMI can exceed 30%.
- Mechanical complications are more common when an STEMI is untreated.
- In addition, the heart may undergo detrimental remodeling.

DIAGNOSIS

Clinical Presentation

Patients presenting with a suspected ACS should undergo rapid evaluation. A focused history, physical examination, and ECG interpretation should be performed within 10 minutes of arrival in the emergency department to allow for timely reperfusion when appropriate.

History

- Chest discomfort is the most common symptom.
  - Progressive, substernal to left sided, and often similar in quality to typical angina (including chest heaviness, tightness, squeezing, pressure, or burning)
  - Usually intense and prolonged, lasting >20 to 30 minutes
  - **Unlike UA/NSTEMI, rest and nitroglycerin usually do not provide significant relief.**
  - **Severe, tearing chest pain that radiates to the back or focal neurologic deficits should raise concern for aortic dissection**, which can mimic ACS; in addition, dissections of the ascending aorta more commonly involve the right coronary artery (RCA) and may cause STEs on ECG.
- The initial history should include timing of symptom onset as well as prior history of cardiac procedures or surgery.
- The clinician should review potential issues complicating primary percutaneous coronary intervention (PCI), including allergy to contrast agents, use of anticoagulants, issues related to vascular access (peripheral vascular disease or previous peripheral revascularization procedures), previous cardiac catheterizations and complications, history of renal dysfunction, central nervous system disease, pregnancy, bleeding diathesis, and/or active recreational drug use (e.g., cocaine).
- If fibrinolytic therapy is being considered, relevant absolute and relative contraindications should be reviewed (Table 9-1).[2]

Physical Examination

- Important in determining other potential sources of chest pain, assessing prognosis, and establishing a baseline to aid the early recognition of complications

TABLE 9-1 CONTRAINDICATIONS TO FIBRINOLYTIC THERAPY

Absolute contraindications

Any prior intracranial hemorrhage or hemorrhagic stroke

Known structural cerebral vascular lesion (e.g., arteriovenous malformation)

Known intracranial malignancy (primary or metastatic)

Ischemic stroke within 3 months

Suspected aortic dissection

Active bleeding or bleeding diathesis (excludes menstruation)

Significant closed-head or facial trauma within 3 months

Severe uncontrolled hypertension (SBP > 180 mm Hg or DBP > 110 mm Hg)

Relative contraindications

History of severe, poorly controlled chronic hypertension

History of prior ischemic stroke >3 months; dementia or known intracranial pathology not covered in absolute contraindications

Traumatic or prolonged (>10 minutes) CPR or major surgery within 3 weeks

Recent internal bleeding (within 2–4 weeks)

Noncompressible vascular punctures

Pregnancy

Active peptic ulcer

Oral anticoagulant use

Allergy or previous use of streptokinase (>5 days ago)

CPR, cardiopulmonary resuscitation; DBP, diastolic blood pressure; SBP, systolic blood pressure.

Modified from O'Gara PT, Kushner FG, Ascheim DD, et al. 2013 ACCF/AHA guideline for the management of ST-elevation myocardial infarction: a report of the American College of Cardiology Foundation/American Heart Association Task Force on Practice Guidelines. *J Am Coll Cardiol*. 2013;61(4):e78-140. Copyright © 2013 American College of Cardiology Foundation and the American Heart Association, Inc. With permission.

- The goal is to determine hemodynamic stability, the presence of cardiogenic pulmonary edema, or mechanical complications of MI (papillary muscle dysfunction, free wall rupture, and ventricular septal defect [VSD]) and exclude other etiologies of acute chest discomfort.
- Should include assessment of vital signs including bilateral brachial blood pressures and oxygenation as well as jugular venous pressure; pulmonary examination for pulmonary edema; cardiac examination for arrhythmia, murmurs, gallops, or friction rub; vascular examination for evidence of peripheral vascular disease and pulse deficits; and neurologic examination (especially before the administration of fibrinolytics)

Differential Diagnosis

- Given the risks of both fibrinolytic therapy and primary PCI, alternative diagnoses must be considered in patients presenting with chest pain.
- In particular, administration of fibrinolytic agents in certain conditions, such as aortic dissection, may lead to death.
- Differential diagnosis of chest pain:
  - Life-threatening: aortic dissection, pulmonary embolus, perforated ulcer, tension pneumothorax, and Boerhaave syndrome (esophageal rupture with mediastinitis)
  - Other cardiac and noncardiac causes: pericarditis, myocarditis, vasospastic angina, gastroesophageal reflux disease, esophageal spasm, costochondritis, pleurisy, peptic ulcer disease, panic attack, biliary or pancreatic pain, cervical disc or neuropathic pain, and somatization and psychogenic pain disorder

- Differential diagnosis of STE on ECG: pericarditis, pulmonary embolism, aortic dissection with coronary artery involvement, normal variant, early repolarization, left ventricular (LV) hypertrophy with strain, Brugada syndrome, myocarditis, hyperkalemia, bundle branch block, Prinzmetal angina, and hypertrophic cardiomyopathy

Risk Stratification

- Multiple risk assessment tools utilize information from the history, physical examination, and diagnostic evaluation to provide an estimate of 30-day mortality following acute MI (AMI).
- The **Killip classification** (Table 9-2) uses bedside physical examination findings, including an S3 gallop, pulmonary congestion, and cardiogenic shock.[3]
- The **Forrester classification** (Table 9-3) uses hemodynamic monitoring variables of cardiac index and pulmonary capillary wedge pressure (PCWP).[4]
- The **Thrombolysis in Myocardial Infarction (TIMI) risk score** (Figure 9-1), in combination with history and examination findings in patients with STEMI treated with fibrinolytics.[5] This is a different risk score than the TIMI risk score used in the setting of UA/NSTEMI.

Diagnostic Testing

Laboratories

- **Cardiac biomarkers** are important in the diagnosis and prognosis of STEMI but are often not yet available/resulted for the initial decision-making process.
- These markers of myocardial necrosis are discussed in detail in Chapter 8.
- Standard laboratory evaluation should include a basic metabolic profile, magnesium level, liver function tests, lipid profile, complete blood count, and coagulation studies.

Electrocardiogram

- The ECG should be performed and interpreted within 10 minutes of presentation (Table 9-4).
- The ECG should be repeated every 20 to 30 minutes for up to 4 hours if the patient has persistent symptoms with clinical suspicion for AMI but the ECG is nondiagnostic.
- Hyperacute T waves, either tall or deeply inverted, may be an early sign of AMI that warrants close monitoring.
- Importantly, **up to 10% of patients with an acute complete coronary occlusion may have a normal ECG.** Certain LV myocardial segments are not adequately represented by the standard 12-lead ECG, particularly the posterior and lateral walls, which are supplied by the left circumflex (LCx) artery.
- **ECG criteria for diagnosis of STEMI**: New STE at the J point (junction between the end of the QRS complex and the beginning of the ST segment) in two anatomically contiguous leads using the following diagnostic thresholds: ≥0.1 mV (1 mm) in all leads other than V2 and V3, where the following diagnostic thresholds apply: ≥0.2 mV (2 mm) in men aged 40 years or older, ≥0.25 mV (2.5 mm) in men younger than 40 years, or ≥0.15 mV (1.5 mm) in women.
- The location (Table 9-4) and degree of STE suggest the involved coronary artery, indicate prognosis, and can alert the physician to potential complications of MI.
- Special considerations:
  - A **new left bundle branch block (LBBB)** in the setting of acute chest symptoms suggests occlusion of the proximal left anterior descending (LAD).
  - Patients presenting with this finding should be managed in the same manner as those with a classic STEMI.
  - In the setting of an old LBBB or a right ventricular (RV)-paced rhythm, an acute injury pattern may be supported by the **Sgarbossa criteria**[6]:
    - STE ≥1 mm in the presence of a positive QRS complex (STE is concordant with QRS)

TABLE 9-2 KILLIP CLASSIFICATION IN ACUTE MI

Class	Definition	Mortality (%)
I	No CHF	6
II	S3 and/or basilar rales	17
III	Pulmonary edema	30–40
IV	Cardiogenic shock	60–80

CHF, congestive heart failure; MI, myocardial infarction.

Modified from Killip T III, Kimball JT. Treatment of myocardial infarction in a coronary care unit. A two-year experience with 250 patients. *Am J Cardiol.* 1967;20(4):457-64. Copyright © 1967 Elsevier. With permission.

TABLE 9-3 FORRESTER CLASSIFICATION SYSTEM FOR ACUTE MI

Class	Cardiac index (L/min/m^2)	PCWP (mm Hg)	Mortality (%)
I	≥2.2	<18	3
II	≥2.2	≥18	9
III	<2.2	<18	23
IV	<2.2	≥18	51

MI, myocardial infarction; PCWP, pulmonary capillary wedge pressure.

Data from Forrester JS, Diamond G, Chatterjee K, Swan HJ. Medical therapy of acute myocardial infarction by application of hemodynamic subsets (first of two parts). *N Engl J Med.* 1976;295:1356-62.

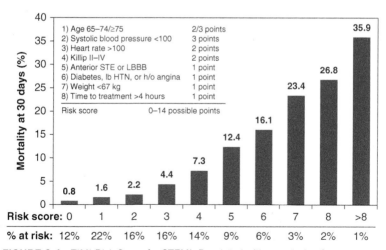

FIGURE 9-1. TIMI Risk Score for STEMI. Reprinted with permission from Morrow DA, Antman EM, Charlesworth A, et al. TIMI risk score for ST-elevation myocardial infarction: a convenient, bedside, clinical score for risk assessment at presentation. *Circulation.* 2000;102(17):2031-37. Copyright © 2000 by American Heart Association.

TABLE 9-4 ANATOMIC DISTRIBUTION BASED ON ECG LEADS

Leads with STE	Myocardium	Coronary artery
I, aVL	High lateral wall	Diagonal or proximal LCx
V5, V6	Lateral wall	LCx
V1, V2	Septal	Proximal LAD
V2–V4	Anterior wall	LAD
II, III, aVF	Inferior	RCA or LCx

ECG, electrocardiogram; LAD, left anterior descending; LCx, left circumflex; RCA, right coronary artery.

- ST-segment depression ≥1 mm in lead V1, V2, or V3
- STE ≥5 mm in the presence of a negative QRS complex (STE is discordant with QRS)
  ○ **Posterior MI** is often unrecognized and **should be suspected in the setting of inferior or lateral wall infarct**. Isolated posterior MI is uncommon.
  - ST-segment depression in leads V1 to V3 represents STEs in the posterior wall.
  - Prominent R waves in these anterior precordial leads represent posterior Q waves.
  - Inferoposterior and posterolateral MIs typically involve the RCA or obtuse marginal branch of the LCx coronary artery, respectively.
  - An ECG utilizing **posterior leads (V7 to V9)** placed on the back may help distinguish posterior MI from anterior ischemia or reciprocal depression in patients presenting with ST depression in leads V1 to V3.
  ○ **STE in the inferior leads should always prompt a right-sided ECG** to assess for **RV infarction**. STE in leads V3R and V4R suggests RV involvement.
  - RV infarction should also be suspected on a standard 12-lead ECG when there is STE in V1 along with changes indicating inferior MI.
  - The finding of STE in lead III greater than in lead II also suggests RV infarct.
  - Proximal RCA lesions typically involve the RV, as RV marginal branches arise early from the RCA.
  - RV infarcts undergo revascularization using the same guiding principles as other STEMIs, but certain aspects of treatment are unique, including the importance of maintaining adequate preload and the cautious use of nitrate and β-blocker therapy to avoid hypotension.
  ○ Pericarditis versus STEMI:
  - With pericarditis, ST segments normalize before the onset of T-wave inversion, whereas T waves invert before ST normalization in STEMI.
  - STE in pericarditis is typically diffuse, does not correlate with a particular vascular territory, and does not exhibit reciprocal ST depressions.
  - PR-segment depression in acute pericarditis may also differentiate these two conditions (see Chapter 26).
  - Pericarditis may present later in the course of AMI and should be differentiated from recurrent ischemia or stent thrombosis.

Imaging
- A portable **chest radiograph** (CXR) should be performed during the initial evaluation.
  ○ Pulmonary edema on CXR has important prognostic and therapeutic implications.

- Before initiating fibrinolytic therapy, review for mediastinal widening, which may suggest aortic dissection. Of note, normal mediastinal width does not exclude dissection.
- A **transthoracic echocardiogram** (TTE) may aid in evaluation of a patient with chest pain and nondiagnostic ECG (i.e., LBBB of unknown duration, paced rhythm). Segmental wall motion abnormalities suggest myocardial ischemia or MI, assuming no baseline wall motion abnormalities, and can help localize the territory at risk.

TREATMENT

- Prompt treatment is important as soon as STEMI is suspected, as the risks of morbidity and mortality are related to ischemic time.
- All medical centers should establish the American College of Cardiology/American Heart Association (ACC/AHA) guideline-based STEMI protocol.
- These should address the use of fibrinolytic therapy versus rapid transport to a primary PCI facility when primary PCI is unavailable.[2]
- In the emergency department, an STEMI protocol should be activated and should include a history, physical examination, and 12-lead ECG within 10 minutes of arrival.
- The goal of immediate management is to identify appropriate candidates for reperfusion therapy, either by primary PCI or by fibrinolytics, and to immediately initiate this process.
- Two peripheral IVs should be inserted upon arrival.
- Telemetry should be placed to monitor for arrhythmias.
- Supplemental oxygen should be administered if saturations are <90%. Mechanical ventilation should be considered, if necessary, as this decreases the work of breathing and reduces myocardial oxygen demand.

Medications

- Medications used for the treatment of patients with STEMI are similar to those with NSTEMI/UA. See Chapter 8 for a detailed discussion of these agents.
- Medical therapy should include administration of antiplatelet and anticoagulant agents that reduce myocardial ischemia.
  - Chewable **aspirin (ASA)** 162 to 325 mg should be given to all patients with suspected STEMI; after PCI, ASA 81 mg/day should be given indefinitely.[7]
  - A loading dose of a **P2Y12 inhibitor** should be given to all patients when STEMI is suspected.
    - If the patient is going for PCI, one of the following agents should be used in addition to ASA and anticoagulation:
      - **Clopidogrel** 600 mg loading dose followed by 75 mg/day
      - **Prasugrel** 60 mg loading followed by 10 mg/day (contraindicated in patients with prior cerebrovascular accident [CVA], weight <60 kg, and older than 75 years of age)
      - **Ticagrelor** 180 mg loading dose followed by 90 mg bid (maintenance dose of ASA should be 81 mg/day)
      - **IV cangrelor** may be considered in patients who cannot take oral medications (e.g., the patient is vomiting or sedated) and may also be used as an adjunct during primary PCI at the discretion of the operator.
    - If the patient is to receive fibrinolytic therapy along with ASA and an anticoagulant, patients should receive: clopidogrel 300 mg loading dose if given during the first 24 hours of fibrinolytic therapy; if started 24 hours after administration, a 600-mg loading dose is preferred. The maintenance dose of clopidogrel is 75 mg/day.
  - **Anticoagulant** therapy should be given on presentation for all patients.

- **Unfractionated heparin (UFH)** is used by many operators due to availability and real-time monitoring using activating clotting times (ACTs). If the patient has received fibrinolytic therapy, UFH should be continued for at least 48 hours.
- **Enoxaparin (low-molecular-weight heparin/LMWH):**
  - Enoxaparin with full-dose tenecteplase significantly improved the composite end point of mortality, in-hospital reinfarction, and in-hospital refractory ischemia, with a similar safety profile as heparin with full-dose tenecteplase in the ASSENT-3 trial.[8]
  - Patients on therapeutic enoxaparin should not be given UFH.
- **Bivalirudin** is an alternative to UFH during PCI for STEMI.
  - Bivalirudin is associated with decreased bleeding rates but higher rate of stent thrombosis compared to the combination of UFH and glycoprotein IIb/IIIa inhibitors during PCI.[9]
  - Bivalirudin is the agent of choice in patients with known heparin-induced thrombocytopenia (HIT).
- **Glycoprotein IIb/IIIa inhibitors** should not be used routinely in patients presenting with STEMI.
  - They are not recommended in conjunction with fibrinolytic therapy.
  - They may be considered as adjunct therapy at the time of PCI, at the discretion of the operator.
- **Supplemental oxygen** administration should be guided by pulse oximetry and is indicated for the first 6 hours or longer following AMI if the oxygen saturation is <92%.
- **Morphine:**
  - Provides analgesia for ischemic cardiac pain, produces a favorable hemodynamic effect, and reduces myocardial oxygen consumption
  - Can be given as doses of 2 to 4 mg IV and repeated every 10 minutes until pain is relieved or hypotension occurs
  - Of note, pharmacokinetic studies suggest morphine delays the antiplatelet effect of oral P2Y12 inhibitors.[10] There is conflicting evidence whether this influences mortality or infarct size.[11]
- **Magnesium:** indicated when plasma magnesium level is documented to be <2 mg/dL or in the setting of torsades de pointes.
- **β-Blockers** reduce major cardiac events, including mortality, recurrent ischemia, and malignant arrhythmias.
  - Oral β-blockers should be started within the first 24 hours following STEMI in patients who do not exhibit evidence of new heart failure (HF) or cardiogenic shock.[12]
  - IV β-blockers should be used with caution in the setting of STEMI. Sinus tachycardia can be a compensatory response to maintain cardiac output and should not prompt IV β-blocker use.
- **Angiotensin-converting enzyme (ACE) inhibitors** reduce short-term mortality, incidence of HF, and recurrent MI and should be administered within the first 24 hours following STEMI.[13]
  - Patients with HF, left ventricular ejection fraction (LVEF) <40%, and large anterior MI benefit most from this therapy.
  - **Angiotensin-receptor blockers** should be given to patients with indication for, but intolerance of, ACE inhibitors.
- **Aldosterone-receptor antagonists** should be considered in patients post-MI with LVEF <40% and either symptomatic HF or diabetes mellitus.[14]
- **High-intensity statin** therapy should be initiated in all patients in the absence of contraindications.

Reperfusion

- Reperfusion is most beneficial when performed early in the course of AMI.
- The optimal reperfusion strategy should be center specific, with consideration of available resources. An algorithm to aid in the decision-making process is shown in Figure 9-2.[2] Although most protocols are based on door-to-balloon time, symptom-to-balloon time is the most important predictor of myocardial salvage.
- **Primary PCI is the preferred reperfusion strategy when door-to-balloon time is** <90 minutes and is most important for myocardial salvage when symptoms are ongoing for <90 minutes.[2]
  - The opportunity for myocardial salvage is the greatest in the first 3 hours following vessel occlusion.

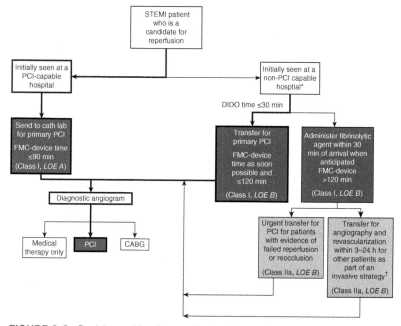

FIGURE 9-2. Decision making for reperfusion therapy. Bold arrows and boxes are the preferred strategies. Performance of PCI is dictated by an anatomically appropriate culprit stenosis. *Patients with cardiogenic shock or severe heart failure initially seen at a non–PCI-capable hospital should be transferred for cardiac catheterization and revascularization as soon as possible, irrespective of time delay from MI onset. †Angiography and revascularization should not be performed within the first 2 to 3 hours after administration of fibrinolytic therapy. CABG, coronary artery bypass graft; DIDO, door-in–door-out; FMC, first medical contact; LOE, level of evidence; MI, myocardial infarction; PCI, percutaneous coronary intervention; STEMI, ST-elevation myocardial infarction. (Reprinted from O'Gara PT, Kushner FG, Ascheim DD, et al. 2013 ACCF/AHA guideline for the management of ST-elevation myocardial infarction: a report of the American College of Cardiology Foundation/American Heart Association Task Force on Practice Guidelines. *J Am Coll Cardiol.* 2013;61(4):e78-e140. Copyright © 2013 American College of Cardiology Foundation and the American Heart Association, Inc. With permission.)

- ○ Patients who present with MI symptoms >12 and <24 hours after pain onset should be considered for reperfusion, particularly in the setting of continued ischemia suggested by STE, persistent symptoms, recurrent ischemia, LV dysfunction, and widespread ECG changes. Patients with prior MI, percutaneous revascularization, or coronary artery bypass grafting (CABG) may also be considered.
  - ○ In facilities without PCI capability, the choice of whether to give fibrinolytics or transport is based on the duration of symptoms, the time needed to transport, and the clinical condition.

Primary Percutaneous Coronary Intervention
- Primary PCI is the preferred therapy if performed in a timely manner (door-to-balloon time <90 minutes) by individuals skilled in the procedure (>75 PCIs per year, of which 11 are STEMIs) and in high-volume centers (>400 PCIs per year, of which >36 are primary PCIs for STEMI per year).[15]
- It has superior efficacy in opening occluded arteries with less reinfarction, lower risk of intracranial hemorrhage, and improved survival when compared with fibrinolytics.
- Transradial approach in STEMI reduces the incidence of major bleeding and may have a mortality benefit compared to transfemoral access,[16] although this was not confirmed by a more recent trial that incorporated bleeding avoidance strategies.[17]
- Drug-eluting stents reduce the need for target vessel revascularization without increasing the incidence of stent thrombosis.
- Percutaneous intervention on the noninfarct-related artery in the setting of STEMI had previously been reserved for cardiogenic shock. However, a recent trial showed a mortality advantage for infarct-related–only PCI in this setting.[18] Several other recent trials have suggested a clinical benefit for complete revascularization for patients who present with STEMI who are not in cardiogenic shock.[19-21]

Fibrinolytic Therapy
- **Fibrinolytic therapy** is indicated when primary PCI is not available in a timely manner (anticipated delay of >120 minutes).
- If primary PCI is not available, fibrinolytic therapy should be administered to patients presenting with up to 12 to 24 hours of ongoing symptoms if no contraindications are present. Fibrinolytic therapy should be administered within 30 minutes of initial patient contact.
- Patients who present to a facility without PCI capability should be transferred immediately for primary PCI if time from first medical contact to PCI will be <120 minutes; these patients should not be given fibrinolytics.
- The benefits of early (<12 hours) fibrinolytic therapy are well established, with pooled data from the Thrombolytic Therapy Trialists' (FTT) Collaborative Group displaying an 18% relative reduction in mortality.[22]
- The greatest potential for significant myocardial salvage is within the first 3 hours of symptom onset. Fibrinolytic therapy is contraindicated in patients presenting >24 hours after symptom onset.
- Absolute and relative contraindications for fibrinolytic therapy are shown in Table 9-1.[2]
- Various fibrinolytic agents are available and have similar efficacy. These medications vary in the rate of administration. Details are shown in Table 9-5.[2]
- **Bleeding risk:**
  - ○ The most common and potentially serious side effect of fibrinolytic therapy is bleeding, with intracranial hemorrhage being the most severe.
  - ○ Risks associated with intracerebral hemorrhage (ICH) include age 75 years or older, female sex, African American race, prior stroke, systolic blood pressure (SBP) ≥160 mm Hg, use of tissue plasminogen activator (tPA) rather than other agents, International Normalized Ratio (INR) >4, and Prothrombin time (PT) >24 seconds.[23,24]

TABLE 9-5 **FIBRINOLYTIC AGENTS**

Medication	Streptokinase	Alteplase (tPA)	Reteplase (rPA)	Tenecteplase (TNK-tPA)
Dose	1.5 MU over 30–60 minutes	Up to 100 mg in 90 minutes (based on weight)[a]	10 units × 2 each over 2 minutes	30–50 mg based on weight[b]
Bolus administration	No	No	Yes	Yes
Antigenic	Yes	No	No	No
Allergic reactions (hypotension most common)	Yes	No	No	No
Systemic fibrinogen depletion	Marked	Mild	Moderate	Minimal
Patency rates (90-minute TIMI grades 2–3 flow)	60–68%	73–84%	84%	85%

[a]Bolus 15 mg, infusion 0.75 mg/kg times 30 minutes (maximum 50 mg), then 0.5 mg/kg not to exceed 35 mg over the next 60 minutes to an overall maximum of 100 mg.

[b]Thirty milligrams for weight <60 kg; 35 mg for 60–69 kg; 40 mg for 70–79 mg; 45 mg for 80–89 kg; 50 mg for 90 kg or more.

Modified from O'Gara PT, Kushner FG, Ascheim DD, et al. 2013 ACCF/AHA guideline for the management of ST-elevation myocardial infarction: a report of the American College of Cardiology Foundation/American Heart Association Task Force on Practice Guidelines. *J Am Coll Cardiol.* 2013;61(4):e78-140. Copyright © 2013 American College of Cardiology Foundation and the American Heart Association, Inc. With permission.

- Fibrinolytic therapy is not effective in patients with hypotension. Patients in cardiogenic shock should be transferred for primary PCI if at all feasible. If fibrinolytic therapy is given in the setting of cardiogenic shock, hypotension should be aggressively treated with mechanical support devices, such as intra-aortic balloon pump (IABP) and vasopressors.

Rescue Percutaneous Coronary Intervention
- Fibrinolytic therapy fails to achieve coronary artery patency in 15-50% of patients. Rescue (salvage) PCI is appropriate for patients who have received fibrinolytic therapy but have:
  ○ Ongoing symptoms and persistent STE (>50% of original degree of elevation) 90 minutes after administration.
  ○ Cardiogenic shock, congestive HF, refractory arrhythmias, or particularly those with large anterior MIs.
- CABG is indicated in the setting of failed PCI in patients with ongoing signs and symptoms of ischemia or in patients whose coronary anatomy is not suitable for PCI.
- Routine PCI early after successful fibrinolytic therapy should be avoided. Early trials of routine PCI after fibrinolysis did not show an improvement in mortality or reinfarction when compared to conservative, ischemia-driven management, primarily because benefits were offset by a higher rate of bleeding complications.

Later Evaluation and Treatment

- Currently, all patients are monitored in the intensive care unit (ICU) for at least 24 hours following STEMI. However, certain very low-risk patients (single-vessel disease with successful PCI, normal ejection fraction (EF), young age without other comorbidities) may be considered for admission to a monitored bed without ICU admission.
- Continuous telemetry monitoring, preferably with display of one of the leads involved in STE, to monitor for recurrent ischemia and arrhythmias
- Daily evaluation should include assessment for recurrent anginal and HF symptoms, physical examination for new murmurs or evidence of HF, and an ECG.

COMPLICATIONS

Cardiogenic Shock

- Cardiogenic shock is an infrequent but serious complication of STEMI and is defined as hypotension in the setting of ventricular dysfunction that results in organ hypoperfusion (e.g., renal failure, mental status changes, dyspnea).
- It typically occurs within the first 48 hours after symptom onset, particularly with large anterior infarcts.
- The associated mortality rate is ~50%. These patients frequently require invasive hemodynamic monitoring and inotropic and/or mechanical support.
- The SHOCK trial demonstrated a significant benefit of revascularization over medical therapy in patients with cardiogenic shock in whom revascularization could be performed within 18 hours of the onset of shock.[25]
- Mechanical circulatory support devices including IABP, percutaneous LV assist device (e.g., Impella pump), or extracorporeal membrane oxygenation can be used as a bridge to recovery or bridge to a long-term durable mechanical support (LV assist device).

Free Wall Rupture

- Free wall rupture generally occurs 2 to 6 days after AMI.
- It occurs most commonly in patients without prior angina or MI and with large infarcts by enzyme criteria.
- It may present as hypotension, cardiac tamponade, or pulseless electrical activity. Mortality is very high, and management consists of volume resuscitation, inotropes, pericardiocentesis, and surgical repair.

Ventricular Pseudoaneurysm

- A cardiac pseudoaneurysm consists of a contained rupture sealed by thrombus and pericardium.
- It is often found incidentally and may be associated with a to-and-fro murmur or a hemodynamically significant pericardial effusion.
- Diagnosis is by echocardiography, which can often differentiate from a true aneurysm.
- Surgical intervention is frequently advised due to the risk of complete rupture.

Ventricular Septal Rupture

- Ventricular septal rupture typically occurs 2 to 5 days after AMI.
- It is more common in anterior MIs.
- It presents with a new harsh holosystolic murmur with or without hemodynamic compromise.
- Diagnosis is usually by echocardiography, with color Doppler demonstrating a communication between the LV and RV. Pulmonary artery (PA) catheterization reveals a step-up in oxygen saturation in PA and RV blood samples compared with samples taken from the right artery (RA).
- Management involves an IABP, inotropes, vasodilators, and surgical versus catheter-based closure.

Mitral Valve Papillary Muscle Rupture

- Papillary muscle rupture usually occurs 2 to 7 days after AMI.
- It most frequently involves the posteromedial papillary muscle due to its single blood supply from the posterior descending artery.
- It usually associated with inferior MI and presents with a new holosystolic murmur (heard only 50% of the time), cardiogenic shock, and pulmonary edema. Diagnosis can be made by echocardiography or PA catheter waveforms with prominent V waves due to severe mitral regurgitation.
- Treatment involves afterload reduction with IABP or vasodilators, revascularization, and surgical repair.

Right Ventricular Infarct

- RV infarct occurs in the setting of inferior MI and presents with the triad of hypotension, elevated jugular venous pressure with Kussmaul sign, and clear lung fields.
- It is diagnosed by right-sided ECG with STE in V3R and V4R or by RV dysfunction on echocardiography.
- Treatment includes volume loading to PCWP of 18 to 20 mm Hg, avoidance of nitrates, and inotropic support if needed to treat hypotension.

Arrhythmias

- Many arrhythmias are associated with STEMI.
- Accelerated idioventricular rhythm should not be treated unless there is hemodynamic disturbance.
- Ventricular arrhythmias are common early after the onset of STEMI.
- Prophylactic antiarrhythmic infusion after AMI to suppress ventricular tachycardia/ventricular fibrillation (VT/VF) does not improve mortality and is not indicated.
- Bradycardias may warrant a temporary transvenous pacer if associated with significant atrioventricular (AV) block.
  - AV block in association with an **inferior MI** usually portends a **good prognosis**, as the mechanism is ischemia of the AV node (the AV nodal branch derives from the RCA) and a compensatory Bezold–Jarisch reflex, which stimulates vagal tone. This may persist up to 1 to 2 weeks.
  - AV block in association with an **anterior MI** usually portends a **poor prognosis** (permanent pacemaker likely required), as the mechanism is infarction of part of the distal conduction system.
- Implantable cardioverter-defibrillator (ICD) should not be routinely implanted in patients with significant LV systolic dysfunction following MI or those with ventricular arrhythmias in the setting of ischemia or immediately following reperfusion.
  - ICD therapy is indicated for patients who develop sustained VT/VF >48 hours after STEMI despite coronary reperfusion.
  - Patients with persistent depressed LV systolic function (EF ≤35%) and New York Heart Association (HYHA) class II or III symptoms or LVEF ≤30% regardless of HF symptoms ≥40 days after STEMI should be considered for ICD placement.[2]
  - A wearable cardioverter-defibrillator should be considered, especially in high-risk patients, for the first 6 weeks after STEMI.

Acute Pericarditis

- Acute pericarditis after STEMI typically occurs 1 to 4 days after MI.
- It may cause recurrent chest discomfort and widespread STE.
- PR depression may occur on ECGs but is uncommon; pericardial rub may be heard on examination.
- ASA is recommended for the treatment of pericarditis after STEMI.
- NSAIDs and glucocorticoids should be avoided in patients with acute pericarditis early after AMI.

- Colchicine along with ASA should also be considered, though there is no direct evidence in its efficacy in peri-infarction pericarditis.
- Heparin should be avoided in these patients owing to the risk of hemorrhagic transformation and only used if necessary.

Dressler Syndrome

- Dressler syndrome presents 2 to 10 weeks after MI with fever, malaise, and pleuritic chest discomfort.
- Patients have an elevated erythrocyte sedimentation rate, and echocardiography may demonstrate pericardial effusion.
- First-line treatment is with high-dose NSAIDs and colchicine.

Left Ventricular Thrombus

- An LV thrombus may occur with large anteroapical MIs with resulting akinetic or dyskinetic segments on echocardiogram or left ventriculogram.
- Treatment consists of anticoagulation for 3 to 6 months.

Ventricular Aneurysm

- After an STEMI, the myocardium may undergo expansion and thinning, resulting in an aneurysm.
- Persistent STE >4 weeks after AMI is suggestive, but not diagnostic, of an aneurysm.
- Echocardiography establishes the diagnosis and provides information regarding LV function and the presence of thrombus.
- Patients may present with HF, ventricular arrhythmias, or an embolic event.
- Prevention involves timely reperfusion and afterload reduction, preferably with an ACE inhibitor, to help reduce adverse LV remodeling and subsequent aneurysm formation.
- Once an aneurysm has formed, additional treatment may include anticoagulation and potentially surgical resection in selected cases.

MONITORING/FOLLOW-UP

- Patients should be seen in the office ~1 month after discharge and every 3 to 12 months thereafter.
- Cardiac rehabilitation is indicated 2 weeks after AMI. Participation in cardiac rehabilitation after an MI is associated with decreased mortality and recurrent MI as well as improvements in quality of life, functional capacity, and social support.

OUTCOME/PROGNOSIS

- Late risk stratification is primarily determined by LV function and residual ischemia. Patients with LVEF <30% are at particularly high risk.
- Other factors including age, the presence of renal insufficiency, and HF have been used in a variety of risk scores to further define prognosis.

REFERENCES

1. Thygesen K, Alpert JS, Jaffe AS, et al; Executive Group on behalf of the Joint European Society of Cardiology (ESC)/American College of Cardiology (ACC)/American Heart Association (AHA)/World Heart Federation (WHF) Task Force for the Universal Definition of Myocardial Infarction. Fourth universal definition of myocardial infarction (2018). *J Am Coll Cardiol*. 2018;72:2231-64.
2. O'Gara PT, Kushner FG, Ascheim DD, et al. 2013 ACCF/AHA guideline for the management of ST-elevation myocardial infarction: executive summary. *J Am Coll Cardiol*. 2013;61:485-510.

3. Killip T III, Kimball JT. Treatment of myocardial infarction in a coronary care unit. A two-year experience with 250 patients. *Am J Cardiol.* 1967;20:457-64.

4. Forrester JS, Diamond G, Chatterjee K, Swan HJ. Medical therapy of acute myocardial infarction by application of hemodynamic subsets (first of two parts). *N Engl J Med.* 1976;295:1356-62.

5. Morrow DA, Antman EM, Charlesworth A, et al. TIMI risk score for ST-elevation myocardial infarction: a convenient, bedside, clinical score for risk assessment at presentation. *Circulation.* 2000;102:2031-7.

6. Sgarbossa EB, Pinski SL, Barbagelata A, et al. Electrocardiographic diagnosis of evolving acute myocardial infarction in the presence of left bundle-branch block. *N Engl J Med.* 1996;334:481-7.

7. Jolly SS, Pogue J, Haladyn K, et al. Effects of aspirin dose on ischaemic events and bleeding after percutaneous coronary intervention: insights from the PCI-CURE study. *Eur Heart J.* 2009;30:900-7.

8. The Assessment of the Safety and Efficacy of a New Thrombolytic Regimen (ASSENT)-3 Investigators. Efficacy and safety of tenecteplase in combination with enoxaparin, abciximab, or unfractionated heparin: the ASSENT-3 randomised trial in acute myocardial infarction. *Lancet.* 2001;358:605-13.

9. Stone GW, Witzenbichler B, Guagliumi G, et al. Bivalirudin during primary PCI in acute myocardial infarction. *N Engl J Med.* 2008;358:2218-30.

10. Hobl EL, Stimpfl T, Ebner J, et al. Morphine decreases clopidogrel concentrations and effects a randomized, double-blind, placebo-controlled trial. *J Am Coll Cardiol.* 2014;63:630-5.

11. Vaidya GN, Khan A, Ghafghazi S. Effect of morphine use on oral P2Y12 platelet inhibitors in acute myocardial infarction: meta-analysis. *Indian Heart J.* 2019;71:126-35.

12. Chen ZM, Pan HC, Chen YP, et al. Early intravenous then oral metoprolol in 45,852 patients with acute myocardial infarction: randomized placebo-controlled trial. *Lancet.* 2005;366:1622-32.

13. GISSI-3: effects of lisinopril and transdermal glyceryl trinitrate singly and together on 6-week mortality and ventricular function after acute myocardial infarction. *Lancet.* 1994;343:1115-22.

14. Pitt B, Zannad F, Remme W, et al. The effect of spironolactone on morbidity and mortality in patients with severe heart failure. *N Engl J Med.* 1999;341:709-17.

15. Levine GN, Bates ER, Blankenship JC, et al. 2011 ACCF/AHA/SCAI guideline for percutaneous coronary intervention: a report of the American College of Cardiology Foundation/American Heart Association Task Force on Practice Guidelines and the Society for Cardiovascular Angiography and Interventions. *Circulation.* 2011;124:e574-651.

16. Romagnoli E, Biondi-Zoccai G, Sciahbasi A, et al. Radial versus femoral randomized investigation in ST-segment elevation acute coronary syndrome: the RIFLE-STEACS study. *J Am Coll Cardiol.* 2012;60:2481-90.

17. Le May M, George W, Derek S. Safety and efficacy of femoral access vs radial access in ST-segment elevation myocardial infarction: the SAFARI Randomized Clinical Trial. *JAMA.* 2020;5(2):126-34.

18. Thiele H, Akin I, Sandri M, et al. PCI strategies in patients with acute myocardial infarction and cardiogenic shock. *N Engl J Med.* 2017;377:2419-32.

19. Engstrom T, Kelbaek H, Helqvist S, et al. Complete revascularisation versus treatment of the culprit lesion only in patients with ST-segment elevation myocardial infarction and multivessel disease (DANAMI-3-PRIMULTI): an open-label, randomised controlled trial. *Lancet.* 2015;386:665-71.

20. Wald D, Morris JK, Wald NJ, et al. Randomized trial of preventive angioplasty in myocardial infarction. *N Engl J Med.* 2013;369:1115-23.

21. Gershlick AH, Khan JN, Kelly DJ, et al. Randomized trial of complete versus lesion-only revascularization in patients undergoing primary percutaneous coronary intervention for STEMI and multivessel disease: the CvLPRIT trial. *J Am Coll Cardiol.* 2015;65:963-72.

22. Thrombolytic Therapy Trialists' (FTT) Collaborative Group. Indications for thrombolytic therapy in suspected acute myocardial infarction: collaborative overview of early mortality and major morbidity results from all randomised trials of more than 1000 patients. *Lancet.* 1994;343:311-22.

23. Brass LM, Lichtman JH, Wang Y, et al. Intracranial hemorrhage associated with thrombolytic therapy for elderly patients with acute myocardial infarction: results from the Cooperative Cardiovascular Project. *Stroke.* 2000;31:1802-11.

24. Huynh T, Cox JL, Massel D, et al. Predictors of intracranial hemorrhage with fibrinolytic therapy in unselected community patients: a report from the FASTRAK II project. *Am Heart J.* 2004;148:86-91.

25. Hochman JS, Sleeper LA, Webb JG, et al. Early revascularization in acute myocardial infarction complicated by cardiogenic shock. *N Engl J Med.* 1999;341:625-34.

Evaluation of Acute Heart Failure

10

Sangita Sudharshan and Joel D. Schilling

GENERAL PRINCIPLES

- Heart failure (HF) is a common clinical syndrome with significant morbidity and mortality. Early detection can lead to initiation of appropriate lifesaving and symptom-reducing therapies.
- Ischemic cardiomyopathy (ICM) is the most common cause of HF with reduced left ventricular (LV) ejection fraction (HFrEF). Hypertension (HTN), diabetes mellitus (DM), obesity, and coronary artery disease (CAD) play a contributory role in HF with preserved ejection fraction (HFpEF).
- The three primary objectives of the history and physical examination are to (1) identify the cause of HF, (2) assess the progression and severity of the illness, and (3) assess the volume status.
- To guide treatment decisions, the physician's goal is to classify the patient as having one of the three common clinical phenotypes: (1) "flash" pulmonary edema with HTN, (2) slowly progressive fluid accumulation, or (3) a low cardiac output state.

Definition

- HF is a clinical syndrome characterized by dyspnea, exercise intolerance, and fluid retention in the setting of abnormal cardiac function. Diagnosis is based on history and physical examination.
- Pathophysiologically, HF is defined by the combination of symptoms, biomarkers, and evidence of cardiac dysfunction.
- Patients with HF require higher intracardiac filling pressures to successfully maintain cardiac output. Overactivation of compensatory mechanisms leads to excessive fluid retention and manifests clinically with pulmonary and/or peripheral edema.

Classification

- Patients with HF can be broadly classified into four groups based on their clinical presentation:
  - Warm and dry (well-compensated HF)
  - Warm and wet (congested without evidence of low cardiac output)
  - Cold and dry (low cardiac output without congestion)
  - Cold and wet (low cardiac output with congestion, highest risk population)
- Patients can also be classified by whether their signs and symptoms are predominantly left HF (dyspnea, orthopnea, pulmonary edema), right HF (venous distention, abdominal distention/ascites, edema), or a combination of both.
- LV failure can be further subdivided based on ejection fraction (EF) (i.e., HFrEF vs. HFpEF).
- Patients who present with HF should be categorized as new-onset cardiomyopathy or an exacerbation of chronic LV dysfunction, with the latter being more common.
- Chronic HF is further categorized based on the New York Heart Association (NYHA) functional class and the American Heart Association (AHA) disease stage (see Chapters 11 and 12).
- Figure 10-1 depicts the relationships between three classification systems for patients with HF.[1]

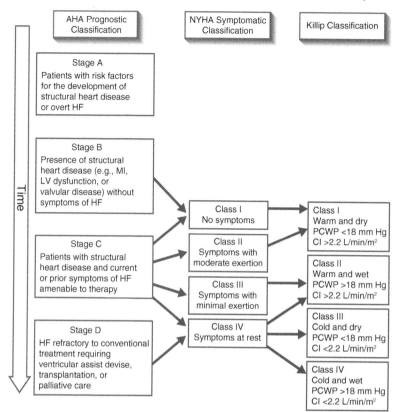

FIGURE 10-1. Classification of heart failure. AHA, American Heart Association; CI, cardiac index; HF, heart failure; LV, left ventricular; MI, myocardial infarction; NYHA, New York Heart Association; PCWP, pulmonary capillary wedge pressure. (From McBride BF, White CM. Acute decompensated heart failure: a contemporary approach to pharmacotherapeutic management. *Pharmacotherapy.* 2003;23(8):997-1020. Reprinted by permission of John Wiley & Sons, Inc.)

Epidemiology

- HF is one of the fastest growing cardiovascular diagnoses in the United States.
- More than 5 million people in the United States currently have HF, with an estimated 550,000 new diagnoses each year. There are over 1 million hospitalizations for HF annually, at a cost exceeding $33 billion.[2,3]
- Despite significant advancements in the management of HF, the mortality remains high; once a patient is hospitalized for HF, the 1- and 5-year death rates are approximately 30% and 50%, respectively.
- About 50% of patients who are hospitalized for HF have HFpEF.[4]
- Approximately 75% of patients with acute decompensated HF have a prior history of HF.

Etiology

- It is useful to subdivide patients into two groups: (1) patients with HFrEF and (2) patients with HFpEF.
- These two patient populations represent distinct disease processes, often with differing underlying pathophysiology and clinical presentations.
  - Among patients with HFrEF (EF ≤ 40%), approximately two-thirds will have an ICM. This generally results from prior myocardial infarction (MI).
  - The causes of non-ICM in patients with systolic dysfunction are more varied and are shown in Table 10-1.
- HFpEF is commonly associated with older age, HTN, DM, obesity, and, occasionally, CAD (about 25%). Less common causes of HFpEF include infiltrative cardiomyopathies, hypertrophic cardiomyopathy, and Fabry disease.
  - HFpEF is more common in females and patients >65 years of age.
  - Atrial fibrillation (AF) and chronic renal insufficiency are frequent comorbidities in this patient population.
  - **Cardiac amyloidosis**, particularly associated with transthyretin (TTR) accumulation, **is likely more common than previously recognized among patients with HFpEF.** Further evaluation for this should be considered in those with increased LV wall thickness in the absence of HTN, low voltage on ECG with increased wall thickness on transthoracic echocardiogram (TTE), the "bull's-eye" sign on strain imaging, carpal tunnel syndrome, neuropathy, or other neurologic symptoms.

TABLE 10-1	COMMON ETIOLOGIES OF HF
Heart failure with reduced EF	**Heart failure with preserved EF**
CAD	HTN
HTN	Diabetes
Myocarditis:	CAD
Infectious	
Autoimmune	
Toxin induced:	Infiltrative:
Alcohol	Amyloid
Cocaine	Sarcoid
Amphetamines	Hemochromatosis
Chemotherapies	Hypertrophic cardiomyopathy
Genetic	High output:
Cardiac specific:	Arteriovenous malformation
ARVC/D	Arteriovenous fistula
Generalized myopathies:	Hyperthyroidism
Duchenne or Becker muscular dystrophy	Anemia
Diabetes	Constrictive
Peripartum	Idiopathic cardiac fibrosis
Tachycardia induced	
Dilated cardiomyopathy: familial, idiopathic	
hemochromatosis	

ARVC/D, arrhythmogenic right ventricular cardiomyopathy/dysplasia; CAD, coronary artery disease; EF, ejection fraction; HF, heart failure; HTN, hypertension; PSF, preserved systolic function.

Pathophysiology

- HF is associated with **compensatory activation of the renin–angiotensin and sympathetic nervous systems** as a means of maintaining cardiac output in the setting of abnormal myocardial function.
- Although initially adaptive, over time, **these neurohumoral responses lead to excessive fluid retention and elevated vascular resistance**. Together, these processes raise intracardiac filling pressures and account for the signs and symptoms of decompensated HF.
- HF medications act to inhibit these neurohumoral responses.

Risk Factors

- There are a multitude of risk factors for the development and progression of HF. Common risk factors include CAD, HTN, DM, and renal dysfunction. Exposure to cardiotoxins such as chemotherapeutic drugs (e.g., anthracyclines), alcohol, and illicit drugs (e.g., cocaine) can also increase the risk of developing HF. Recent data suggest that depression, obesity, and obstructive sleep apnea may also play important roles.
- In addition, several risk factors are associated with decompensation in chronic HF. A helpful mnemonic is "Patients who are frequently hospitalized for HF eventually VANISH."
  - **V**alvular disease
  - **A**rrhythmia (AF)
  - **N**oncompliance (medications, diet)
  - **I**schemia or infection
  - **S**ubstance abuse
  - **H**ypertension

Associated Conditions

- Anemia, hypothyroidism/hyperthyroidism, DM, and renal dysfunction are common comorbidities in patients with HF. In general, they pretend a poorer prognosis, independent of the type or etiology of the cardiomyopathy. It is currently unknown whether correction of anemia and abnormal thyroid function improves outcomes. Patients with anemia should be evaluated for iron deficiency, and, if present, iron stores should be repleted.
- HF may also be associated with underlying systemic illnesses. In the case of HFpEF, examples include DM, HTN, multiple myeloma with amyloidosis, and sarcoidosis. In addition, both HFpEF and HFrEF can be seen with acromegaly, hemochromatosis, and autoimmune diseases (rheumatoid arthritis, scleroderma, antiphospholipid syndrome, and lupus). In some cases, treatment of these underlying disease processes may slow the progression of cardiomyopathy.

DIAGNOSIS

Clinical Presentation

- The clinical presentations of HF are highly variable and range from acute respiratory or circulatory compromise to gradual worsening of dyspnea on exertion. In general, patients with HF can be divided into three basic presentations:
  - Flash or acute pulmonary edema with HTN
  - Slowly progressive fluid accumulation
  - Low cardiac output state
- The most dramatic presentation is acute or flash pulmonary edema. Frequently, these patients have a rapid onset of symptoms and elevated blood pressure. The problem is usually not significant volume overload, but instead **volume redistribution secondary to increased vascular tone (increased afterload), reduced venous compliance (increased preload), and poor LV relaxation**. This can be seen in HF patients with either normal or reduced EF. The acute management of these patients should focus on the use of vasodilators rather than diuretics (see Table 10-2).

TABLE 10-2 PRESENTATION AND INITIAL MANAGEMENT OF HF

	Warm and dry	Flash pulmonary edema	Warm and wet	Cool and wet	Cool and dry
History	Exertional dyspnea Minimal orthopnea PND Minimal edema	Sudden-onset dyspnea Orthopnea PND Minimal edema	Exertional dyspnea Orthopnea PND Edema	Fatigue, dyspnea at rest Orthopnea PND Edema	Fatigue, orthostasis Minimal orthopnea PND Mild edema
Physical examination	Minimal JVD No crackles Minimal edema Normal pulses	HTN, JVD Prominent crackles Minimal edema Normal pulses	JVD/HJR Crackles Edema Normal pulses	JVD/HJR Crackles Edema Weak pulses	Hypotension Minimal JVD Minimal crackles Minimal edema Weak pulses
Laboratory	Normal/mildly increased BNP	Increased BNP	Increased BNP	Increased BNP, Cr, AST, ALT	Increased Cr, AST, ALT, acidosis
Imaging	Clear lung fields	Pulmonary edema	Pulmonary edema	Pulmonary edema	Minimal pulmonary edema
PA catheter	CI > 2 L/min Normal PCWP	CI > 2 L/min Elevated PCWP	CI > 2 L/min Elevated PCWP	CI < 2 L/min Elevated PCWP	CI < 2 L/min Normal PCWP
Management	β-Blocker, ACE-I/ARB	Vasodilator therapy (nitroglycerine, nitroprusside)	Loop diuretics, β-blocker, ACE-I/ARB/ARNI	Loop diuretics with or without thiazide diuretics with or without vasodilators with or without inotropes	Inotropes with or without IVF if PCWP <12 mm Hg

ACE-I, angiotensin-converting enzyme inhibitor; ALT, alanine aminotransferase; ARB, angiotensin II receptor blocker; ARNI, angiotensin receptor neprilysin inhibitor; AST, aspartate aminotransferase; BNP, brain natriuretic peptide; CI, cardiac index; Cr, creatinine; HF, heart failure; HJR, hepatojugular reflux; HTN, hypertension; IVF, IV fluid; JVD, jugular venous distention; PCWP, pulmonary capillary wedge pressure; PND, paroxysmal nocturnal dyspnea.

- The patient with slowly progressive fluid accumulation most commonly has chronic systolic dysfunction and is typified by normal to mildly elevated blood pressures and signs or symptoms of slowly progressive fluid accumulation. These patients have dyspnea on exertion, paroxysmal nocturnal dyspnea (PND), orthopnea, lower extremity (LE) edema, and weight gain. The use of IV diuretics combined with afterload reduction is generally very effective in the treatment of these patients.
- The third, and least common presentation, is the patient with a low cardiac output state. These patients may be either normotensive or hypotensive. They often have evidence of end-organ hypoperfusion (prerenal azotemia, cool extremities, poor energy level, and confusion). Careful questioning may reveal evidence of mesenteric ischemia and cardiac cachexia. These patients often require admission to the intensive care unit (ICU) for placement of a pulmonary artery catheter (Swan-Ganz catheter [SGC]) and/or inotropic support. In appropriate patients with refractory shock despite inotropes, mechanical circulatory support should be instituted.

History

- There are three primary objectives of the history when interviewing a patient with HF:
  - Identify etiology of HF and/or factors contributing to disease decompensation.
  - Assess progression and severity of illness.
  - Assess volume status.
- It is important to identify factors that may have contributed to etiology of the HF. For patients with a first presentation of HF, probe the likelihood of ischemic heart disease (e.g., history of MI, chest pain, atherosclerotic cardiovascular disease [ASCVD] risk factors), myocarditis or viral cardiomyopathy (e.g., recent viral illness or upper respiratory symptoms, rheumatologic disease history or symptoms), genetic cardiomyopathy (e.g., family history of HF or sudden death), toxic cardiomyopathy (e.g., alcohol or drug abuse, history of chemotherapy), and peripartum cardiomyopathy (e.g., recent pregnancy). In addition, the presence of HTN and/or diabetes should be elicited.
- For patients with a known cardiomyopathy presenting with an acute decompensation, it is important to **identify potential triggers of the exacerbation** (see Risk Factors), although no cause will be found in 50% of cases.
- The second critical area to assess in patients with new-onset or established HF is their **current functional status** and the rate of decline in their activity level. Important questions to ask include what they can currently do before becoming shortness of breath (How far can they walk? How many flights of stairs can they climb?) and how this compares with what they were able to do 6 to 12 months before. This allows categorization into an NYHA functional class and an AHA HF stage (see Chapters 11 and 12), which helps direct therapy, assess prognosis, and facilitate discussions with patients.
- The third important issue to address regards the patient's **volume status**. The inability to lie flat (**orthopnea**) and waking up at night due to shortness of breath (**PND**) **are very suggestive of volume overload in patients with chronic HF.** In addition, increases in body weight often signify fluid retention, even in the absence of other congestive symptoms. Other manifestations of increased fluid volume include abdominal bloating and/or right upper quadrant pain and LE edema.
- Additional information regarding excessive fatigue, postprandial abdominal discomfort, and orthostasis particularly after administration of HF medicines may aid in identifying patients with low cardiac output. It is important to note that many patients may report symptoms associated with low cardiac output in the absence of congestion.

Physical Examination

- The primary function of the physical examination in patients with HF is to assess volume status and characterize a patient as hypovolemic, euvolemic, or volume overloaded (see Chapter 2). This determination helps guide treatment and assess the response to therapy (Table 10-2).

- In addition, the physical examination can also provide important clues to the etiology of cardiac dysfunction. For example, the presence of a murmur or a pericardial knock may indicate a primary valvular process or pericardial constriction, respectively.
- It is important to recognize that the clinical manifestations of volume overload in HF can be highly variable and that there are several notable limitations of common physical examination findings.
  - The presence of jugular venous distention (JVD) and/or hepatojugular reflux (HJR) is the most specific and reliable physical examination indicator of volume overload (approximately 80% sensitive) and is best assessed with a penlight and the patient positioned at about 45 degrees.[5,6] The jugular venous pulse can be distinguished from carotid pulsations by the biphasic appearance of the former. Of note, elevated neck veins may also be seen with pulmonary HTN, severe tricuspid regurgitation, and pericardial diseases, such as tamponade and constriction.
  - Pulmonary crackles may be present on lung examination and indicate fluid extravasation into the alveoli due to elevated left ventricular end-diastolic pressure (LVEDP). This examination finding is often mistakenly considered mandatory for the diagnosis of decompensated HF. In reality, crackles signify either rapid increases in LVEDP or severe volume overload; they are present in only about 20-50% of chronic HF patients with elevated filling pressures.[6] In this circumstance, the gradual increase in LVEDP is compensated for by increased pulmonary lymphatic drainage; thus, crackles are often a late sign of decompensation.
  - LE edema is another marker of fluid overload when present; however, the sensitivity for predicting elevated filling pressures is relatively poor. In addition, patients can have predominantly abdominal congestive symptoms without any evidence of peripheral or pulmonary edema.
- Other examination findings suggest systolic dysfunction and volume overload: a diffuse and laterally displaced point of maximum impulse, an S_3 gallop, a mitral regurgitation murmur at the apex, diminished carotid upstrokes, ascites, and pulsatile hepatomegaly.
- Signs of low cardiac output include cool extremities, fluctuating mental status, orthostasis, resting sinus tachycardia, narrow pulse pressure, and weak pulses. Some patients may have pulsus alternans (alternating intensity of peripheral pulsus despite sinus rhythm), a sign of profoundly low cardiac output.

Diagnostic Criteria

- HF is a clinical diagnosis based on history, physical examination findings, and CXR. Although there are no universally agreed-upon diagnostic criteria for HF, the Framingham criteria are reasonable, with an HF diagnosis requiring satisfaction of two major OR one major and two minor criteria.
  - **Major criteria**: PND, JVD, crackles, cardiomegaly, pulmonary edema, S_3, HJR, weight loss with diuresis (>4.5 pounds)
  - **Minor criteria**: LE edema, nocturnal cough, dyspnea on exertion, hepatomegaly, pleural effusions, tachycardia, decrease in vital capacity
- The diagnosis of HF is further supported by laboratory values and imaging studies. These include elevated brain natriuretic peptide (BNP) or amino-terminal (NT)-proBNP and an abnormal echocardiogram (see later).

Differential Diagnosis

- It is important to consider other acute diseases that can mimic the presentation of HF with dyspnea, elevated neck veins, and LE edema (i.e., pulmonary HTN, pulmonary embolism, and pericardial diseases [constriction and tamponade]).
- Pulmonary inflammatory diseases, progressive pleural effusions, significant anemia, hypothyroidism, and some systemic neurologic disorders can also present with progressive exertional dyspnea and should remain on the differential diagnosis list if a cardiac etiology cannot be identified.

Diagnostic Testing

Laboratories

- BNP and NT-proBNP are the most useful biomarkers in diagnosing HF. These natriuretic peptides are released from the heart in response to mechanical stretch and are indicators of volume overload.
  - The normal range is <100 pg/mL for BNP and <125 pg/mL for NT-proBNP. There can be significant fluctuations in levels based on age, gender, renal dysfunction (increases level), and obesity (reduces level). In general, levels >200 pg/mL in symptomatic patients are suggestive of HF. Of note, up to 30% of patients with symptomatic HFpEF will have normal levels.
  - Renal dysfunction strongly influences BNP and NT-proBNP levels. Elevated levels over the patient's baseline (if known) may be suggestive of HF. Measuring levels in patients on dialysis is not reliable; however, elevated BNP levels are still predictive of mortality in this patient population.
  - Persistent elevations in BNP and NT-proBNP after optimization of volume status identify a population of HF patients at higher risk for morbidity and mortality.
  - The use of BNP and NT-proBNP to monitor the response to diuretic therapy may be a helpful strategy to optimize HF treatment. These biomarkers may also be useful if questions arise regarding the effectiveness of diuresis.
- The presence of hyponatremia, elevated creatinine/blood urea nitrogen, and elevated liver enzymes identify high-risk patients. These findings signify the presence of poor cardiac output and/or severe volume overload and independently portend an unfavorable prognosis.
- Persistently elevated troponin levels can be seen in a subset of both ischemic and nonischemic HF patients and are associated with a worse prognosis.
- Additional laboratory tests that may be useful include evaluations for anemia, thyroid abnormalities, dyslipidemia, diabetes, and markers of infection.

Electrocardiography

- ECG may provide diagnostic information regarding the etiology of a cardiomyopathy or point to a cause of decompensation in patients with chronic HF. Examples include Q waves characteristic of prior MI, ST-segment abnormalities suggestive of ongoing ischemia, or cardiac arrhythmias (e.g., AF/flutter).
- Both ECG and telemetry monitoring may also aid in the detection of cardiac arrhythmias that are relevant to the patient's presentation.
- QRS width and the presence of a left bundle branch block (LBBB) help identify patients who may favorably respond to cardiac resynchronization therapy.

Imaging

- CXR can help in the diagnosis of HF and in the assessment of volume status. Signs of HF decompensation include pulmonary congestion (perihilar fullness and pulmonary vascular redistribution), pulmonary edema, Kerley B lines, and pleural effusions. However, the absence of pulmonary vascular redistribution or pulmonary edema on CXR does not exclude the diagnosis of HF. The CXR can also help evaluate for other causes of dyspnea, such as emphysema, pneumonia, and pneumothorax.
- The echocardiogram is the diagnostic modality of choice for the diagnosis and characterization of HF. It is useful for the assessment of both systolic and diastolic ventricular dysfunction. Echocardiography also provides a detailed structural and functional analysis of valvular heart disease as well as assessment of congenital malformations, cardiac chamber dynamics, and pericardial diseases. Echocardiography is also useful for assessing the response to HF therapies.
- Cardiac MRI (CMR) is increasingly utilized in the assessment of new-onset cardiomyopathies. CMR may characterize structural heart disease and help define the etiology of

cardiac dysfunction. The presence and pattern of delayed gadolinium enhancement aid in the noninvasive diagnosis of specific cardiomyopathies, including ischemic, amyloid, sarcoidosis, hypertrophic, and myocarditis.

- In patients with ICM who have high-grade coronary lesions, a myocardial viability study can be useful to guide revascularization strategies. There are several types of viability imaging studies, including thallium rest/redistribution, dobutamine echocardiography, positron emission tomography, and MRI. The choice of modality should be driven by institutional expertise.

Diagnostic Procedures
- Cardiac catheterization is the gold standard for invasive assessment of CAD and cardiac hemodynamics.
  - Given the high prevalence of CAD in patients with reduced LV function, coronary angiography is recommended for the majority of patients with new-onset cardiomyopathy to evaluate the extent of CAD.
  - In patients with a high ischemic burden, revascularization can improve cardiac function and survival.
  - It is reasonable to consider noninvasive stress testing in patients at very low risk for CAD.
- Right heart catheterization (RHC) allows the measurement of intracardiac filling pressures and cardiac output, thereby providing information regarding volume status, pulmonary artery pressure, cardiac output, and the presence of an intracardiac shunt.
  - RHC is particularly beneficial for monitoring cardiac performance in patients with cardiogenic shock requiring either inotropic or mechanical support.
  - RHC is not recommended for the management of routine HF decompensation; however, it is appropriate to consider for patients not responding to medical therapy or with signs of reduced cardiac output.
- Simultaneous right and left cardiac catheterization can be considered in select patients with suspected constrictive pericarditis or valvular cardiomyopathy to aid in diagnosis and treatment options.

TREATMENT

Acute Inpatient Management

- The acute management of patients with each of these clinical presentations is unique and summarized in Table 10-2. Further details are available in Chapters 11 and 12.
- For patients with an acute exacerbation of chronic HF, management includes evaluation of outpatient medications.
  - Chronic outpatient diuretics: The inpatient initial starting dose should be $>2.5\times$ outpatient dose and should be given IV. Based on the results of the DOSE trial, there is no difference between the use of bolus or continuous IV loop diuretics in terms of symptom improvement, but patients receiving higher doses tended to do better than those receiving lower doses of diuretic.[7] A thiazide diuretic (e.g., metolazone, chlorothiazide) can be added to the IV loop diuretic for increased diuresis if response is inadequate to high-dose loop diuretics.
  - Chronic β-blocker: For patients who are not in a low cardiac output (cold) state, β-blockers can be continued at their current dose. If patients are in a low cardiac output state, the dose can be reduced by half or held until patient is compensated. For those requiring inotropic support with β-agonists (e.g., dobutamine), β-blockers should be held. Upon discharge or at first outpatient visit, β-blocker dose should be reviewed and reinstated if held in the hospital.
  - Chronic angiotensin-converting enzyme inhibitors/angiotensin receptor blockers (ACE-Is/ARBs): Most of the time, these medications can be continued during the

hospitalization, even if acute kidney injury is present as this is often due to vascular congestion. Typically, renal dysfunction will resolve with diuretics, but if it worsens despite diuresis, ACE-I/ARB discontinuation is recommended. Afterload reduction can be accomplished by switching to hydralazine and nitrates until renal function improves. For patients who are hypotensive, ACE-I/ARB should be held.

○ Initiation of sacubitril/valsartan in the hospital can be beneficial in patients with HFrEF and acute decompensation in the absence of hypotension or renal failure.

MONITORING/FOLLOW-UP

- Outpatient monitoring with the use of an implantable ambulatory pulmonary artery pressure monitoring system (CARDIOMEMS) has been shown to improve quality of life and rehospitalizations in patients with NYHA class III HF.
- Close outpatient follow-up with either primary care provider (PCP) or cardiologist within 7 to 10 days of hospital discharge is recommended.
- Outpatient medication reconciliation is important to ensure patients have resumed β-blockers, ACE-I/ARB/ARNI (angiotensin receptor neprilysin inhibitor), and aldosterone antagonists as tolerated following hospitalization.
- Initiation of sacubitril/valsartan should be strongly considered as this medication has shown a mortality benefit compared to enalapril.
- In patients with LVEF <35% and QRS >120 to 150 ms in LBBB pattern or with chronic pacing needs, cardiac resynchronization therapy pacemaker (CRT-D) implantation has been shown to improve mortality and reduce hospitalizations.
- Goals of care/overall prognosis should be discussed early in patients with HF and hospitalizations as there is significant associated mortality.

REFERENCES

1. McBride BF, White CM. Acute decompensated heart failure: a contemporary approach to pharmacotherapeutic management. *Pharmacotherapy.* 2003;23:997-1020.
2. Rosamond W, Flegal K, Friday G, et al. Heart disease and stroke statistics—2007 update: a report of the American Heart Association Statistics Committee and Stroke Statistics Committee. *Circulation.* 2007;115:e69-171.
3. Chan PS, Soto G, Jones PG, et al. Patient health status and costs in heart failure: insights from the eplerenone post-acute myocardial infarction heart failure efficacy and survival study (EPHESUS). *Circulation.* 2009;119:398-407.
4. Yancy CW, Lopatin M, Stevenson LW, et al. Clinical presentation, management, and in-hospital outcomes of patients admitted with acute decompensated heart failure with preserved systolic function: a report from the Acute Decompensated Heart Failure National Registry (ADHERE) Database. *J Am Coll Cardiol.* 2006;47:76-84.
5. Cook DJ, Simel DL. The rational clinical examination: does this patient have abnormal central venous pressure? *JAMA.* 1996;275:630-4.
6. Butman SM, Ewy GW, Standen JR, et al. Bedside cardiovascular examination in patients with severe chronic heart failure: importance of rest or inducible jugular venous distension. *J Am Coll Cardiol.* 1993;22:968-74.
7. Felker GM, Lee KL, Bull DA, et al. Diuretic strategies in patients with acute decompensated heart failure. *N Engl J Med.* 2011;364:797-805.

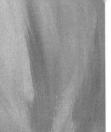

Evaluation and Management of Heart Failure with Reduced Ejection Fraction

11

Benjamin Kopecky and Justin Hartupee

GENERAL PRINCIPLES

Definition

- **Heart failure (HF)** is a complex clinical syndrome that results from any structural or functional impairment of ventricular filling or ejection of blood (cardiomyopathy [CM]) and is characterized by dyspnea, exercise intolerance, and fluid retention (CM plus symptoms = HF).
- HF is typically classified based on ejection fraction (EF): HF with reduced EF (HFrEF) (EF < 40%), HF with preserved EF (HFpEF) (EF > 50%), or midrange (EF = 40-50%). This chapter focuses on HFrEF.
- Most frequently, HF patients will present with manifestations of poor cardiac output, such as **fatigue and exercise intolerance**, or volume overload, such as **pulmonary and peripheral edema**.
- The clinical presentation of acute decompensated HF (ADHF) is described in Chapter 10.

Classification

HF may be classified by (1) etiology of CM, (2) stage, (3) symptom severity, and (4) duration/presentation.

- HF can first be divided by *etiology* as **ischemic** (a result of obstructive coronary artery disease [CAD]) or **nonischemic** (all other causes).
- The American Heart Association (AHA) *staging system* takes into account risk factors and cardiac function, ranging from those at risk for developing HF to those with the most severe consequences.[1]
- The AHA stages of HF include:
  - Stage A: patients at risk for developing HF
  - Stage B: patients with structural heart disease without symptoms of HF
  - Stage C: patients with past or current symptoms of HF
  - Stage D: patients with end-stage disease
- The New York Heart Association (NYHA) scale is frequently used to describe the severity of symptoms (see Chapter 10).[2]
- *Duration/presentation:* Patients can present with **ADHF, acute on chronic decompensated HF,** or **chronic stable HF.**

Epidemiology

- As of 2019, ~**6.2 million people** in the US had HF, with an estimated 1 million new diagnoses each year.[3]
- HF remains the primary diagnosis in >**1 million hospitalizations** in the US, with annual costs exceeding **$30 billion**.[3]
- Despite significant advances in the management of HF, mortality remains high, especially after hospitalization, where rates of death are ~22% and 42% at 1 and 5 years, respectively, with **recent trends toward worsening outcomes**.[4]

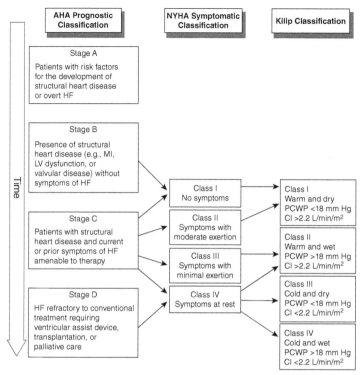

FIGURE 11-1. Classifications of heart failure. AHA, American Heart Association; CI, cardiac index; HF, heart failure; LV, left ventricular; MI, myocardial infarction; NYHA, New York Heart Association; PCWP, pulmonary capillary wedge pressure. (From McBride BF, White CM. Acute decompensated heart failure: a contemporary approach to pharmacotherapeutic management. *Pharmacotherapy.* 2003;23(8):997-1020. Reprinted by permission of John Wiley & Sons, Inc.)

Etiology

- Among patients with HF, approximately **two-thirds will have an ischemic etiology**, usually resulting from prior myocardial infarction (MI) (>1 coronary artery with >75% stenosis).[5]
- The causes of nonischemic CM in patients with HF are more varied and are shown in Table 11-1. More common etiologies include familial dilated cardiomyopathy (DCM), chemotherapy-induced DCM, infiltrative heart disease, and myocarditis/inflammation-related DCM.

Risk Factors

- There are many known factors that increase the chance of developing HF, including **advanced age, hypertension (HTN), diabetes mellitus, CAD,** and a **strong family history of CM**.
- The presence of certain risk factors will suggest a specific CM. Examples include myocarditis (recent viral illness or upper respiratory symptoms, rheumatologic disease history or symptoms), genetic CM (family history of HF or sudden cardiac death), toxic CM (alcohol or drug abuse, history of chemotherapy), and peripartum CM (recent pregnancy).

TABLE 11-1 CAUSE OF NONISCHEMIC CARDIOMYOPATHY

Primary nonischemic cardiomyopathies

Acquired	Genetic	Idiopathic
• Inflammatory (myocarditis)	• Hypertrophic CM • Arrhythmogenic right ventricular CM	
• Stress induced (Takotsubo)	• Left ventricular noncompaction	
• Peripartum	• Glycogen storage (PRKAG2, Danon)	
• Tachycardia induced	• Conduction defects	
• Infants of insulin-dependent diabetic mothers	• Mitochondrial myopathies • Congenital heart diseases	

Secondary nonischemic cardiomyopathies

• Autoimmune/ collagen-vascular:
  • Systemic lupus erythematosus
  • Dermatomyositis
  • Rheumatoid arthritis
  • Scleroderma
  • Polyarteritis nodosa
  • Churg–Strauss syndrome
	• Endomyocardial:
	  • Endomyocardial fibrosis
	  • Hypereosinophilic syndrome (Löeffler endocarditis)
	• High-output states:
	  • Arteriovenous malformation
	  • Arteriovenous fistula
		• Nutritional deficiencies:
		  • Thiamine (beriberi/B_1)
		  • Pellagra (niacin/B_3)
		  • Scurvy (vitamin C)
		  • Keshan disease (selenium)
		  • Carnitine
		  • Kwashiorkor (protein)

• Cardiofacial:
  • Noonan syndrome
  • Lentiginosis
	• Hypertensive heart disease	

• Congenital heart disease:
  • Systemic right ventricular failure (TGA)
	• Infiltrative:
	  • Amyloidosis (AL, wt-ATTR, mtATTR)
	  • Sarcoidosis
	  • Gaucher disease
	  • Hurler disease
	  • Hunter disease
		• Storage disorders:
		  • Hemochromatosis
		  • Fabry disease
		  • Glycogen storage disease (type II, Pompe)

TABLE 11-1	CAUSE OF NONISCHEMIC CARDIOMYOPATHY (*continued*)

Secondary nonischemic cardiomyopathies

- Endocrine:
  - Diabetes mellitus
  - Hyperthyroidism
  - Hypothyroidism
  - Hyperparathyroidism
  - Pheochromocytoma
  - Acromegaly

- Neuromuscular/ neurologic:
  - Friedreich ataxia
  - Duchenne, Becker, Emery– Dreifuss muscular dystrophy
  - Myotonic dystrophy
  - Neurofibromatosis
  - Tuberous sclerosis

- Toxicity:
  - Chemotherapy (anthracyclines, cyclophosphamide)
  - Radiation
  - Alcohol
  - Cocaine
  - Amphetamines
  - Heavy metals

CM, cardiomyopathy.

Pathophysiology

- Regardless of the initial insult leading to myocardial injury, there is a stereotypical **pathologic remodeling response**.
  - Over time, **negative remodeling** leads to progressive cardiac enlargement and deterioration in cardiac function, largely due to activation of compensatory **neurohormonal pathways** such as the renin–angiotensin–aldosterone system (RAAS) and the sympathetic nervous system (SNS). The initial function of these responses is to maintain cardiac output by increasing ventricular filling pressures (preload) and myocardial contractility.
  - Over time, activation of the RAAS and SNS leads to transcriptional reprogramming of cardiac myocytes, myocyte hypertrophy and cell death, extracellular matrix breakdown, left ventricular (LV) dilatation, and myocardial fibrosis. This leads to further decline in cardiac function and contributes to the increased risk of arrhythmias.[6]
- The **neurohormonal model of HF is the basis for the most effective treatments** used for HF management today.

Prevention

- Prevention, early identification, and treatment of LV dysfunction are possible by identifying and treating at-risk individuals and mitigating modifiable risk factors. The critical **modifiable risk factors** are **diabetes** (2× risk in men, 5× risk in women),[7] **HTN, dyslipidemia, CAD, tobacco/substance use**, and **alcohol abuse**; aggressive treatment of these is paramount.
  - While it is clear that diabetic control is imperative to reducing risk of HF, too intensive control may be deleterious.[8]
  - In patients with stage A HF, the optimal blood pressure should be <130/80.

Associated Conditions

Other common HF-associated conditions include **sleep-disordered breathing**, which is present in an estimated 30-40% of HF patients, and **atrial fibrillation**, which affects approximately one-third of HF patients.

DIAGNOSIS

Clinical Presentation

- Full discussion can be found in Chapter 10.
- The presentation of HFrEF is essentially the same as that of HFpEF and can be divided into two basic phenotypes:
  - Acute (or acute on chronic) systolic HF
  - Chronic systolic HF

History

- Full discussion can be found in Chapter 10.
- Four main goals to elicit from the patient's history are as follows:
  - Assess **volume status** (symptoms of pulmonary or peripheral congestion or weight change).
  - Identify **contributing factors** to the change/decline in clinical status.
  - **Assess progression and severity of illness**, particularly to classify the patient based on the AHA stage and NYHA class to aid in **risk stratification** and **need for advanced therapies**.
  - Identify opportunities for **medication clarification and optimization**.

Physical Examination

- Full discussion can be found in Chapters 2 and 10.
- The primary function of the physical examination in patients with HF is to **assess** (1) volume status and (2) cardiac output.
- It is also important to **classify** each patient as (see Figure 10.1):
  - Warm and dry
  - Warm and wet
  - Cold and dry
  - Cold and wet

Diagnostic Criteria

HF is a **clinical diagnosis** based on history and physical examination findings. Although there are no universally agreed-upon diagnostic criteria for HF, the Framingham criteria require *two major **or** one major and two minor criteria.*

- **Major criteria**: paroxysmal nocturnal dyspnea, jugular venous distention, crackles, cardiomegaly, pulmonary edema, presence of an S_3, positive hepatojugular reflux, weight loss with diuresis (>4.5 lb)
- **Minor criteria**: lower extremity edema, nocturnal cough, dyspnea on exertion, hepatomegaly, pleural effusions, tachycardia, decrease in vital capacity
- The diagnosis of HF is further supported by **laboratory values** (elevated brain natriuretic peptide [BNP] or N-terminal proBNP [NT-proBNP]), ECG, and **imaging studies** (e.g., pulmonary edema or pleural effusion on CXR; cardiac dysfunction on echocardiogram or MRI).

Diagnostic Testing

Laboratories

- Laboratory data play an important role in the detection of HF, during the assessment of ADHF, and throughout chronic HF management.
  - **BNP** is a small polypeptide released by myocytes in response to increased wall stress.
  - **NT-proBNP** is a nonactive hormone that is derived from the same precursor molecule as BNP.
    - Systemic levels of the natriuretic peptides BNP and NT-proBNP correlate with invasive intracardiac pressure measurements and are a reliable marker of volume status.
    - Both are affected by renal dysfunction, age, and obesity. The use of angiotensin receptor neprilysin inhibitors (ARNIs) will increase BNP levels, but not affect NT-proBNP.

- Screening of at-risk patients:
  - For patients at risk of developing HF (AHA stage A), natriuretic peptide (BNP, NT-proBNP) screening followed by team-based care may be useful to prevent development of LV dysfunction.[9]
  - In patients presenting with dyspnea, measurement of natriuretic peptide is useful to support or exclude HF.[9]
    - **A BNP > 400 pg/L** is consistent with HF. Levels ranging from 100 to 400 pg/mL may represent underlying LV dysfunction; however, other diseases such as acute pulmonary embolism must be considered.
    - NT-proBNP level cutoffs to help distinguish HF from other causes of dyspnea vary by patient age:
      - <50, **NT-proBNP > 450 pg/mL**
      - 50 to 75, **NT-proBNP > 900 pg/mL**
      - >75, **NT-proBNP > 1800 pg/mL**
- ADHF:
  - For hospitalized ADHF patients, laboratory data obtained should include **cardiac biomarkers**, to evaluate for myocardial stress/congestion (BNP, NT-proBNP) and ischemia (troponin), **complete metabolic panel** (CMP) for renal/liver function and electrolyte abnormalities, **hemoglobin**, and, potentially, **lactate** to assess for perfusion.
    - Measurement of **BNP or NT-proBNP** is helpful in establishing prognosis for patients admitted to the hospital with ADHF.[9,10]
    - Predischarge natriuretic peptide may be helpful to establish postdischarge prognosis.[9]
  - The presence of an elevated **troponin** may signify an acute coronary syndrome; however, mild troponin elevations can occur even in the absence of epicardial CAD. In either case, the presence of an elevated troponin signifies myocardial injury and identifies a high-risk subset of ADHF patients.
  - Additional biomarkers can be utilized if the etiology of CM is undetermined.
    - In the absence of significant CAD, additional blood work should include an **iron panel** and **ferritin level**, a test for **HIV, and hepatitis C** testing (in at-risk individuals).
    - Serum protein electrophoresis and urine protein electrophoresis should be checked if there is clinical suspicion for amyloidosis.
    - Genetic testing and counseling can be considered if there is a strong family history of CM.
    - Routine testing for viral infections is not recommended as results do not alter therapy.
    - In patients with physical findings consistent with a rheumatologic disease, additional testing such as an antinuclear antibody and/or antineutrophil cytoplasmic antibody titer can be checked.
- Chronic HF:
  - Routine labs are recommended to monitor electrolytes, especially during medication optimization.
  - NT-proBNP has prognostic value in stable patients with chronic HF.

Electrocardiography
- An ECG should be obtained in the acute setting to evaluate for ischemia, infarct, or arrhythmia.
- ECGs in HF patients may demonstrate prior infarct, left bundle branch block, conduction disease, arrhythmia, LV hypertrophy, or low voltage (infiltrative CM).

Imaging
- **CXR** can assess for evidence of pulmonary edema, pleural effusion, or cardiomegaly and rule out other causes of dyspnea (pneumonia, pneumothorax).

- A **transthoracic echocardiogram** provides information regarding systolic and diastolic function, valvular disease, LV hypertrophy, asymmetric septal hypertrophy, and pericardial disease and provides an estimation of pulmonary artery (PA) systolic pressure.
- **Cardiac MRI** has been increasingly used in the assessment of new-onset CMs, particularly for suspected infiltrative disease.
- **Positron emission tomography (PET) scan** can be useful in evaluating for cardiac sarcoidosis.

Diagnostic Procedures
- Left heart catheterization:
  - Patients with *new systolic dysfunction* should undergo an **ischemic evaluation**. For patients with multiple cardiac risk factors, chest pain, and/or segmental wall motion abnormalities on echocardiography, coronary angiography is preferred.
  - In patients with ADHF without identified cause, an ischemic evaluation is reasonable.
  - Revascularization via percutaneous intervention or coronary artery bypass grafting is indicated in patients with reduced EF if myocardium is viable.
- Right heart catheterization:
  - In some cases, placement of a **PA catheter** can help guide therapy.
  - Invasive hemodynamic data can direct the use of inotropic and vasopressor agents and can help with volume assessment (Table 11-2).
  - A PA catheter should be considered for patients who present with hypotension and evidence of cardiogenic shock.
  - The ESCAPE trial demonstrated that routine PA catheter placement does not alter mortality or length of hospital stay in ADHF. Therefore, placement of a **PA catheter** should be reserved for **hemodynamically unstable patients** or for those **not responding to therapy**.
- An endomyocardial biopsy is appropriate in select patients when the etiology for CM remains uncertain and where elucidation would change management (e.g., giant cell myocarditis, amyloidosis).

TREATMENT

Treatment must be tailored to the individual patient.

ADHF Requiring Hospitalization—Initial Management
- The treatment goals for **ADHF patients** are as follows:
  - Initiate **lifesaving** medical **therapies.**
  - Correct **hemodynamic** and **volume status**.
  - Improve patient **symptoms**.
  - **Minimize** cardiac and renal **injury**.
  - **Initiate** guideline-directed **medical therapy (GDMT)**.
- Figure 11-2 provides a guideline for the management of ADHF.
- ADHF patients can be categorized by their volume and perfusion status, which helps risk stratify and guide treatment decisions:
  - **Warm and wet:** volume overloaded but with adequate perfusion
  - **Cold and wet:** volume overloaded with poor cardiac output
  - **Cold and dry:** euvolemic with poor cardiac output
  - **Warm and dry:** appropriate cardiac output and are clinically euvolemic. Look for noncardiac etiologies of their hospital presentation.

Warm and Wet
- The immediate goal is to **stabilize respiratory status** by **lowering blood pressure** and **removing fluid**.

TABLE 11-2 INTERPRETING HEMODYNAMIC DATA IN THE HEART FAILURE PATIENT WITH A PULMONARY ARTERY CATHETER

Cardiac index (2.5–4.5 L/min/m²)	CVP (5–8 mm Hg)	Mean PAP (15–25 mm Hg)	PCWP (5–10 mm Hg)	SBP (100–120 mm Hg)	SVR (800–1200 dynes/ sec × cm⁻⁵)	Diagnosis (D) and Management (M)
↓	↓	↓ or normal	↓	↓	↑	D: Hypovolemia M: IV fluids
↓	↑	↑	↑	↑ or normal	↑↑	D: HF with high vascular tone M: Vasodilators/ afterload reduction
↓	↑	↑	↑	↓	↑↑	D: HF with poor systemic perfusion M: Inotropes, diuretics
↓	↑	↑	↑	↓↓	↑	D: HF with shock M: Inotrope, vasopressors, mechanical support
↓↑ or normal	↓ or normal	↓ or normal	↓ or normal	↓	↓	D: Distributive shock (sepsis) M: IV fluids, vasopressors, antibiotics
↓	↑	↑	↓	↓	↑	D: Pulmonary HTN, Right heart failure M: Inotropes, pulmonary vasodilators

Normal values in parentheses.
CVP, central venous pressure; HF, heart failure; HTN, hypertension; PAP, pulmonary artery pressure; PCWP, pulmonary capillary wedge pressure; SBP, systolic blood pressure; SVR, systemic vascular resistance.

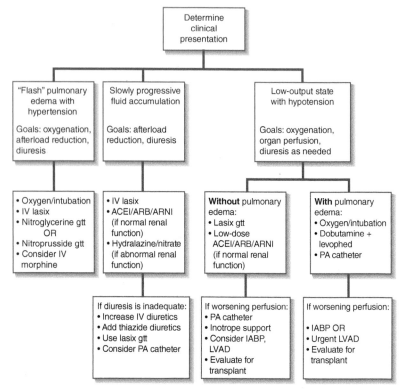

FIGURE 11-2. General approach to the management of acute decompensated heart failure (ADHF). ACEI/ARB, angiotensin-converting enzyme inhibitor/angiotensin-receptor blocker; ARNI, angiotensin receptor neprilysin inhibitor; IABP, intra-aortic balloon pump; LVAD, left ventricular assist device; PA, pulmonary artery.

- These patients should receive **oxygen, vasodilators**, and IV **diuretics**.
  - If the respiratory status is tenuous, noninvasive positive pressure ventilation or intubation may be necessary to improve oxygenation until the hemodynamic and volume status can be improved.
  - **Diuretics** are useful for reducing preload and improving patient volume status and symptoms. An initial dose of **IV diuretic** (usually **furosemide**) should be administered.
    - For patients on home oral furosemide, administer at least the same dose IV and assess response (e.g., for a patient with outpatient regimen 40 mg PO bid, use at least 40 mg IV bid).
    - As an initial strategy, IV furosemide administered as either a *bolus* or *bolus followed by continuous infusion* is reasonable (DOSE).[11] If the **diuresis is inadequate**, then the IV **dose may be increased**, the diuretic may be **changed** (furosemide, torsemide, bumetanide), or a **thiazide** diuretic (metolazone, chlorothiazide) may be added. Addition of a thiazide diuretic can cause profound potassium and magnesium depletion, so aggressive monitoring and repletion are mandatory (3T).[12]

- Poor diuresis despite these measures and/or progressive renal dysfunction may prompt **PA catheter placement** to clarify the patient's hemodynamics and/or guide the use of **inotropes** (dobutamine or milrinone).
  - Routine use of inotropes in ADHF was challenged by the OPTIME trial where milrinone infusion did not improve diuresis but did lead to an increase in adverse events.[13]
  - In addition, an association between inotrope use and worse clinical outcomes has been demonstrated.[14] Therefore, **inotropes should be reserved for patients with reduced cardiac output, resulting in end-organ dysfunction and refractory edema.** The two inotropes available in the US are the nonselective β-agonist **dobutamine** and the phosphodiesterase inhibitor **milrinone**.
    - Both increase cardiac output by increasing contractility and reducing afterload.
    - The hemodynamic effects of these agents are similar; however, dobutamine is favored when renal function is impaired and/or the systolic blood pressure (SBP) is low (85 to 90 mm Hg).
    - Milrinone may be more effective for patients with elevated PA pressures, given its potent vasodilating action.
    - Adverse events associated with inotrope infusion include hypotension (particularly in the setting of hypovolemia), atrial and ventricular arrhythmias, and accelerated decline in ventricular function. The risks and benefits must be considered very carefully before initiating inotrope therapy.
  - In **rare circumstances** when the patient has adequate cardiac output, remains volume overloaded, and is not responding to aggressive diuretics, **ultrafiltration (UF) may be considered**.
    - UF allows for fluid removal at a consistent rate without the negative consequences associated with aggressive diuretic use, such as electrolyte depletion and renal injury.
    - The UNLOAD trial was a small study that compared UF to standard therapy in patients admitted with ADHF; this showed that UF was more effective and efficient at removing fluid and reduced the risk of future hospitalizations for HF. The downside of UF is that it requires specialized peripheral venous access and the machines/equipment can be costly.
    - The larger and more recent CARRESS-HF trial found that **stepped pharmacologic therapy was superior to UF** as UF was associated with **increased adverse events**.[15]

Cold and Wet
- Patients who present with ADHF and evidence of hypoperfusion represent <5% of hospital admissions for HF.
- These patients are often in **overt cardiogenic shock**. Acute renal failure, elevated liver enzymes, metabolic acidosis, and peripheral vasoconstriction are common.
- **Patients** in early or overt cardiogenic shock **require rapid triage and admission to an intensive care unit (ICU) for stabilization**. Urgent revascularization may be required if the underlying cause of the shock state is an acute MI.
  - Empiric treatment with **dobutamine or milrinone** can often help improve end-organ perfusion and facilitate diuresis. A **continuous furosemide infusion** is often the most effective means to remove fluid from such patients without promoting further hypotension.
  - Patients with SBP <80 mm Hg will often require the addition of norepinephrine. These patients should receive a PA catheter to direct therapy (see Chapter 41).
- Many patients in cardiogenic shock may require temporary **mechanical circulatory support (MCS)**. **Short-term devices** include the percutaneously inserted pneumatic **intra-aortic balloon pump** (IABP), the axial flow **Impella**, Impella RP (for right heart support), **ProtekDuo** (for right heart support), **VA ECMO** (biventricular support), or **TandemHeart**. These devices can provide cardiac support for up to 1 to 2 months. Each device requires anticoagulation, is susceptible to hemolysis, and requires prolonged ICU care.
- See Table 11-3 for percutaneous circulatory support options.

TABLE 11-3 PERCUTANEOUS CIRCULATORY SUPPORT OPTIONS

Device	Catheters	Support	Advantages	Limitations
IABP	8-Fr arterial	Counter-pulsation 0.5 L/min	Ease of insertion Lower cost Increase in coronary perfusion	Minimal increase in CO Ineffective in tachycardia
Impella 2.5	13-Fr arterial	Microaxial impeller 2.5 L/min	Percutaneous insertion	Insufficient support for cardiogenic shock
Impella 5.0	21-Fr arterial	Microaxial impeller 5 L/min	Greater circulatory support	Large catheter size Requires surgical cutdown Vascular/bleeding complications
Impella RP	22-Fr venous	Microaxial impeller 4.0 L/min	Right ventricular support	Right ventricular support only Vascular and bleeding complications
Tandem Heart	17-Fr arterial 21-Fr venous	Centrifugal pump (extracorporeal) 4 L/min	Greater circulatory support	Large catheter size Transseptal puncture Vascular/bleeding complications

CO, cardiac output; IABP, intra-aortic balloon pump.

Cold and Dry
Patients with poor cardiac output may successfully be diuresed to euvolemia but require additional support to maintain appropriate perfusion.

Mechanical Circulatory Support
- Mechanical circulatory support (MCS) can be considered in select patients with acute or chronic end-organ hypoperfusion from cardiac dysfunction.
- Ventricular support devices are designed for short- or long-term ventricular support.
  - The **HeartMate III** is the only **long-term left ventricular assist device (LVAD)** currently being implanted (MOMENTUM).[16] Devices previously used in the US include the HeartMate II, HVAD, or pulsatile devices (Thoratec VAD and HeartMate IP, VE, and XVE and WorldHeart Novacor).
  - Compared to HeartMate II LVAD, the HeartMate III LVAD is a fully magnetically levitated centrifugal flow pump with superior survival-free time from stroke or reoperation for pump dysfunction.
  - LVADs are implanted as a bridge to transplant or are destination therapy for those who are not the transplant candidates.

- Two randomized trials of destination therapy LVADs in end-stage HF patients (REMATCH and INTrEPID studies) compared LVAD to standard medical therapy in patients with advanced HF.[17,18]
- For some patients, relieving symptoms and avoiding hospitalization may be the primary goals; therefore, **continuous inotrope infusion** and/or **hospice care** may be reasonable.
- Patients with severe HF symptoms who are **not the candidates for MCS** may benefit from **continuous home inotrope infusion**.
- In patients who are not the candidates for more aggressive HF therapy or do not want these treatments, **discussions regarding end-of-life issues are warranted**. All patients with end-stage HF should have the opportunity to interact with **palliative care**.

Acute Decompensated Heart Failure Requiring Hospitalization—Management of Stable Patient, Working Toward Discharge
- **After stabilization** of patient hemodynamics and renal function and improvement of presenting symptoms, it is important to **initiate and/or titrate medications** that have been shown to **prevent the negative remodeling** and **prolong survival** in chronic HF.
- **Patient education:** Key components to long-term success in HF management include patient education, optimal medical and device therapy, and adequate patient follow-up.
- **Posthospital follow-up**
  - An **HF team** is effective to manage the complex HF patient with randomized controlled trials (RCTs) showing improvements in death, hospitalizations, length of stay, and quality of life. Necessary infrastructure includes electronic health records, patient monitoring and engagement, care coordination, and patient education.[19]
  - Nonadherence is a common cause of HF (re-)hospitalizations.
    - **Nonadherence** is **multifactorial** (patient, medical condition, treatment side effects, socioeconomic barriers, health system).
    - Interventions to improve include discharge/clinic visit medication education, disease education, team-based care, self-management teaching, and self-monitoring.[19]
  - Before discharge, patients should be transitioned to a stable oral diuretic regimen. In general, the lowest dose of diuretic needed to maintain euvolemia should be used.
  - Several monitoring strategies have been developed in an effort to **identify subclinical volume overload**, when intervention can prevent hospitalization.
    - Blood pressure, weight, and symptoms can be monitored wirelessly and remotely via the Internet (Latitude Patient Management System, Boston Scientific), helping clinicians to direct medical therapy.
    - Thoracic impedance levels recorded from an implantable cardioverter-defibrillator/ cardiac resynchronization therapy (ICD/CRT) device can assess trends in fluid balance (OptiVol Fluid Status Monitoring, Medtronic).
    - Novel devices such as the CardioMEMS can remotely monitor PA pressures in ambulatory patients, resulting in lower rates of HF hospitalizations.[20]
  - A **basic metabolic panel** (BMP) should also be **checked regularly** to monitor electrolytes and renal function, with close attention to blood urea nitrogen (BUN) and HCO_3 levels, as they often rise with intravascular volume contraction.

Chronic, Stable Heart Failure: Outpatient Management
- Treatment goals for *chronic HF* are as follows:
  - **Initiate treatment** with **medications** and **therapies** proven to **improve survival**, **reduce** rates of **hospitalization**, increase **quality of life**, and **recover** cardiac structure and **function**.
  - Optimize **management of volume status**.
  - **Identify patients at risk** of HF exacerbation and to reduce hospitalizations.
  - **Identify patients** likely to benefit from **advanced therapies**.

- Clinic visits provide an opportunity for improved management.
  - Each visit should consist of a history, vitals, and examination and, at times, lab work.
  - The use of validated HF questionnaires should be considered, including the Minnesota Living with Heart Failure Questionnaire and the Kansas City Cardiomyopathy Questionnaire.[21]

Guideline-Directed Medical Therapy Optimization, Titration, and Monitoring

- **Four classes** of GDMT HF medication are now recognized to offer substantial benefit to patients with HFrEF and **should be prescribed** unless a contraindication exists.
  - Angiotensin-converting enzyme inhibitors (ACEIs), angiotensin-receptor blockers (ARBs), ARNIs
  - β-Blockers
  - Aldosterone antagonists
  - Sodium glucose cotransporter 2 inhibitors (SGLT2i)
- Diuretics are used as needed to control volume status.

Angiotensin-Converting Enzyme Inhibitors, Angiotensin-Receptor Blockers, Angiotensin Receptor Neprilysin Inhibitors

- Only **one drug** from among these classes should be used **at a single time**.
- The benefit of ACEIs comes from blocking the formation of angiotensin II.
  - Angiotensin II is a potent vasoconstrictor that stimulates pro-fibrotic and pro-inflammatory pathways and promotes adverse myocardial remodeling.
  - Multiple randomized trials have established the benefit of ACEIs in patients with chronic LV dysfunction (V-HEFT 2, SOLVD, CONSENSUS) and with post-MI LV dysfunction (SAVE, TRACE, AIRE).[22-26] ACEIs were consistently associated with a mortality reduction of ~20-25% at 1 to 5 years.
  - When initiating an ACEI, low doses should be used at first and then gradually titrated upward. Plasma creatinine (Cr) and potassium should be checked 1 to 2 weeks after initiation or uptitration of an ACEI. Small increases in Cr (up to 30%) are common and should not prompt discontinuation.
  - Side effects include cough (about 10% incidence), hyperkalemia, hypotension, renal insufficiency, angioedema, and teratogenicity.
- ARBs act downstream of ACEIs by inhibiting the type 1 angiotensin receptor, thereby attenuating the biologic effects of angiotensin II.
  - The largest clinical trials of ARBs in chronic HF are Val-HEFT and CHARM.[27,28] Both studies showed that **ARBs are equivalent to ACEIs with regard to HF mortality reduction**. Similar findings were seen in VALIANT for patients with LV dysfunction post-MI.[29]
  - Therefore, ARBs are an acceptable alternative for patients who are ACEI intolerant (usually secondary to cough).
  - ARBs should be initiated in a similar manner to ACEIs, with the same expected side effects with the exception of cough and angioedema.
- ARNIs are a combination of sacubitril and valsartan. Sacubitril is a prodrug that inhibits the enzyme neprilysin, which degrades natriuretic peptides (e.g., BNP).
  - ARNIs have been shown to reduce HF death and hospitalizations in NYHA classes II, III, and IV patients compared to ACEIs in both hospitalized patients stabilized from ADHF (PIONEER-HF) and stable outpatients (PARADIGM-HF).[30,31]
  - ARNIs are contraindicated with a creatinine clearance (CrCl) <30 mg/dL or a history of angioedema. ARNIs have more effect on blood pressure than ACEIs or ARBs and need to be used cautiously in those with marginal blood pressure. In euvolemic patients with lower blood pressure, reducing the diuretic dose can increase tolerability of ARNI.

○ The most recent American College of Cardiology Expert Consensus Decision Pathway states that **ARNIs are preferred from this class of medications and can be started in patients not previously treated with an ACEI or ARB.**[32] Drug affordability remains a challenge.

β-Blockers

- Therapy with a β-blocker is mandatory for all patients with HF. Once considered contraindicated in HF, β-blockers have become the most effective drugs for managing this condition.
- Carvedilol, metoprolol succinate, and bisoprolol have been shown in clinical trials to improve outcomes in HFrEF; other β-blockers should not be used to treat this condition.
  ○ **Carvedilol** has been studied in patients with mild-to-moderate HF (US carvedilol studies) or severe HF (COPERNICUS) and in the post-MI setting (CAPRICORN).[33,34] All-cause and cardiovascular mortality were consistently reduced by 25-48%.
  ○ Similar benefit was seen with **metoprolol succinate** in the MERIT-HF trial, where all-cause mortality was reduced by 34% at 1 year in NYHA classes II to III HF patients.[35]
  ○ The use of **bisoprolol** is also supported by clinical data from CIBIS I and CIBIS II.[36,37]
- β-Blockers should be started at low doses and titrated every 1 to 2 weeks until goal doses are achieved. Patients should be stable and largely euvolemic before the initiation of a β-blocker. There is strong evidence demonstrating a **dose-dependent benefit** with β-blockers. Caution should be used in patients with underlying bradycardia or conduction system disease. Fatigue is common with β-blocker treatment but generally improves after 1 to 2 weeks of treatment. If bronchospasm or low blood pressure is an issue, use of a β-selective agent (metoprolol succinate or bisoprolol) is recommended.
- The issue of how to manage β-blocker therapy during an ADHF exacerbation is a controversial and frequently discussed topic.
  ○ ADHF exacerbations are associated with high levels of systemic catecholamines, and data suggest that withdrawal of β-blockers during ADHF can worsen outcomes.
  ○ In a β-blocker–naïve patient, it is reasonable to defer β-blocker initiation until euvolemia has been achieved and the patient is on an afterload reduction regimen.
  ○ In patients already receiving β-blocker therapy, every attempt should be made to continue the medication at its current dose. If the patient is in a low-output state, the dose can be decreased.
  ○ In the event that the **patient requires inotropic therapy**, it is appropriate to **discontinue the β-blocker**.

Aldosterone Antagonists

- Aldosterone antagonists are recommended in all patients with NYHA classes II to IV HF and those with LV dysfunction post-MI. Aldosterone antagonists should be used in addition to an ACEI, ARB, or ARNI.
- Aldosterone is an adrenal hormone whose production is stimulated through angiotensin II–dependent and angiotensin II–independent pathways. In the myocardium, aldosterone leads to fibrosis and progressive pathologic remodeling.
- The effects of inhibiting aldosterone in HF were first investigated in the RALES trial, where treatment with **spironolactone** led to a 30% mortality reduction and 36% decrease in hospitalizations in patients with NYHA classes III to IV HF.[38] A beneficial effect in the setting of less severe, class II HF was seen in the EMPHASIS-HF trial using the aldosterone antagonist **eplerenone**.
- Subsequently, the EPHESUS trial demonstrated mortality benefit in patients with post-MI LV dysfunction already taking an ACEI and β-blocker.[39]
- The major side effect is hyperkalemia, especially in the setting of reduced renal function or concomitant ACEI/ARB/ARNI therapy; thus, frequent monitoring is required.

Aldosterone antagonists should be avoided in patients with a baseline potassium ≥5.0 mEq/L or with a baseline Cr >2.0 (women) or 2.5 mg/dL (men). Gynecomastia can also be seen with spironolactone, in which case eplerenone should be used.
- Monitor electrolytes (especially potassium) 2 to 3 days after titration and then after 1 week. Check every 3 months.

Sodium Glucose Transporter 2 Inhibitors
- Several recent trials have shown improved outcomes in NYHA class II, III, or IV HF patients (with or without diabetes) (e.g., DAPA-HF, EMPA-REG) already on maximally tolerated medical therapy.[40,41]
- The DAPA-HF trial demonstrated the efficacy of dapagliflozin in the treatment of HFrEF, regardless of the presence of diabetes. The primary end point of worsening HF or cardiovascular death was decreased by 26%. There was a statistically significant effect on each component of the primary end point.
- EMPEROR-Reduced demonstrated a similar effect of the SGLT2i empagliflozin on worsening HF and cardiovascular death. Again, this effect was not different based on the presence of diabetes.
- Multiple lines of evidence also suggest a renal protective effect of these medications.
- Hypoglycemia is not a concern with these medications in nondiabetics but can occur in diabetic patients on sulfonylureas or insulin. There is an increased risk of mycotic genital infections.
- These agents should not be used in patients with type 1 diabetes.

Diuretics
- Despite the lack of randomized studies to guide the optimal approach to diuretic therapy, **diuretics** are a **mainstay of medical therapy** for **volume management** in HF.
- The general consensus is to prescribe the **lowest dose of diuretic** that is necessary to maintain **euvolemia**.
- The loop diuretics **furosemide, torsemide, and bumetanide** are the primary options for volume control.
  - Torsemide or bumetanide should be considered in patients with significant right-sided HF and abdominal venous congestion, where the absorption of furosemide is frequently unpredictable.
  - The conversion ratio from furosemide to torsemide to bumetanide is ~40:20:1.
  - If high doses are required (i.e., equivalent of 120 mg furosemide bid), consider switching to a different loop diuretic or adding a thiazide diuretic.
- Given the potency of combining a thiazide with a loop diuretic, it is recommended to use only short-term dosing or a 3-day/week dosing schedule. Blood pressure, electrolytes, and renal function must be followed carefully as significant volume depletion can occur with any diuretic.
- If volume status requires treatment, adjust diuretics with clinic follow-up in 1 to 2 weeks.

Additional Options in Selected Patient Populations
- **Ivabradine** can be beneficial for NYHA classes II to III patients with EF <35% already on GDMT including maximally tolerated β-blocker who are in sinus rhythm with heart rate >70 beats per minute to reduce hospitalizations.
  - For patients >75 years of age or history of conduction defects, start with 2.5 mg bid; otherwise start with 5 mg bid.
  - Reassess heart rate in 2 to 4 weeks and increase as tolerated to a maximum of 7.5 mg bid.
- **Hydralazine/nitrate** combination can be used as an **alternative** to ACEI/ARB therapy in **patients intolerant** of these medications or **as add-on therapy** for self-identified **African American** patients.

- ○ The V-HEFT I study was the first trial to investigate hydralazine combined with nitrates (isosorbide dinitrate) in chronic HF.[42] This vasodilator combination improved patient symptoms and reduced mortality when compared to placebo and doxazosin.
  - Subgroup analysis of V-HEFT I and its counterpart V-HEFT II suggested that patients of African descent treated with this combination derived particular benefit.[42]
  - These observations led to the A-HEFT trial that demonstrated a 43% decrease in mortality and a 33% decrease in ADHF hospitalizations in African American patients with **NYHA classes III to IV HF already treated with ACEI and β-blocker.**[43] Thus, the combination of hydralazine/nitrates is **recommended in African American patients with severe HF symptoms already on aggressive medical therapy**.
  - ○ The most common side effects are headache and hypotension. Patient compliance can also be an issue, given the number of pills required per day (tid to qid dosing).
- **Digoxin can be used for symptoms of HF but does not alter survival from HF.**
  - ○ Digoxin is a cardiac glycoside that inhibits the Na–K exchange ion channel, leading to increased intracellular calcium and enhanced contractility.
  - ○ The DIG trial demonstrated that digoxin therapy, in addition to ACEIs and diuretics, decreased HF hospitalizations but did not alter mortality.[44] Of note, the best outcomes were seen in patients with **digoxin levels <1 ng/mL**. Based on these results and other studies demonstrating that digoxin can improve HF symptoms, this agent is **used for patients on optimal medical therapy who still have frequent hospitalizations for HF**.
  - ○ Caution must be used in patients with renal dysfunction as **digoxin has a narrow therapeutic index** and toxicity can occur. Adverse reactions with digoxin include cardiac arrhythmias (atrial tachycardia with atrioventricular block, bidirectional ventricular tachycardia, atrial fibrillation with regularized ventricular response), gastrointestinal symptoms, and neurologic complaints (confusion, visual disturbances).
  - ○ Digoxin toxicity usually manifests when **serum levels exceed 2 ng/mL**; however, hypokalemia and hypomagnesemia can lower this threshold.
- **Vericiguat**, an oral guanylate cyclase stimulator, reduced the incidence of death or hospitalization from HF in patients with NYHA II, III, or IV HF symptoms (VICTORIA).[45]
- **Iron supplementation:** In stabilized HF patients with iron deficiency and with a recent ADHF hospitalization, iron repletion reduced the risk for future HF hospitalizations (AFFIRM-HF).[46] However, the treatment of anemia with erythropoietin-stimulating agents is not supported (RED-HF).[47]

Device-Based Therapies

- **ICDs** are used to prevent sudden death from life-threatening ventricular arrhythmias.
  - ○ MADIT-I and MADIT-II trials established the survival benefit of ICDs in patients with ischemic HF.[48,49]
  - ○ Subsequently, the SCD-HEFT trial demonstrated a similar benefit for ICDs in patients with ischemic and nonischemic CM with EF ≤35%.[50] **ICD implantation should be considered for all HF patients with EF ≤35%.**
  - ○ The VEST trial showed that in HF patients with recent MI, the wearable cardioverter-defibrillator did not reduce the rate of arrhythmic death.[51]
- **CRT** is designed to resynchronize ventricular contraction and improve cardiac function in patients with HF and dyssynchronous electromechanical activation of the LV.
  - ○ The three largest randomized trials in CRT are COMPANION, CARE-HF, and MADIT-CRT.[52-54]
  - ○ Biventricular pacing was associated with an improvement in symptoms and a **reduction in hospitalizations** compared to patients receiving medical therapy alone. The CARE-HF trial also demonstrated a marked **decrease in mortality** associated with biventricular pacing.

- ○ CRT should be considered in patients with **dyssynchrony (QRS > 120 ms) who have NYHA classes III to IV HF symptoms despite medical therapy**. More recent indications have endorsed the use of CRT in patients with less severe HF (NYHA class I or II) but with more dyssynchrony (QRS > 150 ms).
- **MitraClip**
  - ○ Functional or secondary mitral regurgitation often develops in patients with significant LV dysfunction and remodeling and is associated with poor outcomes.
  - ○ Percutaneous transcatheter mitral valve repair using the MitraClip device was shown to decrease the primary end point of HF hospitalizations in patients with **moderate-to-severe secondary mitral regurgitation** in the COAPT trial. There was also an improvement in all-cause mortality.[55]
  - ○ In a second trial, MITRA-FR, MitraClip did not result in improved outcomes.[56] At least part of the difference in outcomes is thought to be related to differences in patient selection.
  - ○ Patients should be treated with maximally tolerated medical therapy before considering MitraClip. Based on the results of the two trials, MitraClip should be used in patients who meet entry criteria used in the COAPT trial.[56]

Lifestyle/Risk Modification

Diet
- Dietary instruction regarding sodium and fluid intake is critical in volume management in patients with HF.
- **Sodium intake** should generally be limited to **2 to 3 g per day**, though more severe restriction to <2 g per day is necessary with moderate-to-severe HF.
- **Fluid intake** must also be limited, with **1.5 to 2 L per day** recommended for those with hyponatremia or edema despite aggressive diuretic usage.

Activity
- If appropriate, exercise training can be started, preferably in a monitored setting to facilitate understanding of exercise expectations and to increase duration and intensity to a general exercise goal of 30 minutes of moderate activity/exercise, 5 days per week with warm-up and cool-down exercises.
- Outpatient exercise-based **cardiac rehabilitation** improves HF patient quality of life, functional capacity, and clinical outcomes. Unfortunately, cardiac rehabilitation is underused.[57]

REFERRAL

- Consideration of **referral to an advanced HF specialist** can be remembered with the acronym[19] "I NEED HELP":
  - **I**: IV inotropes
  - **N**: NYHA IIIb to IV
  - **E**: End-organ dysfunction
  - **E**: Ejection fraction <35%
  - **D**: Defibrillator shocks
  - **H**: Hospitalizations >1
  - **E**: Edema despite escalating diuretics
  - **L**: Low blood pressure/high heart rate
  - **P**: Progressive intolerance to GDMT
- Referral to advanced HF specialists allows for evaluation for MCS or cardiac transplantation. **Heart transplantation remains the definitive therapy for end-stage HF.**
  - ○ Successful transplantation became possible in the 1980s, when the immunosuppressant cyclosporine was used to control rejection.

- Patients considered for transplantation have severe HF symptoms despite maximally tolerated GDMT. **A VO$_{2max}$ ≤14 mL/kg per minute on cardiopulmonary exercise testing portends a significantly reduced 1-year survival, and this criterion has been used to identify patients with the greatest need for transplant.**
- Contraindications to transplant, some of which are relative, include severe, irreversible pulmonary HTN, active infection, severe chronic obstructive pulmonary disease, significant renal impairment (not thought to be reversible with improved cardiac output), severe peripheral vascular disease or carotid disease, severe psychiatric disease, primary liver disease with coagulopathy, advanced age (>70 years), diabetes with end-organ dysfunction, socioeconomic situation prohibiting follow-up care, and active malignancy.
- There are currently about 3000 heart transplants performed annually in the US.
- Survival following heart transplantation is 85%, 70%, and 50% at 1, 5, and 10 years, respectively.
- Post-transplantation:
  - During the first year after transplant, primary graft dysfunction, acute rejection, and infection (from both common and opportunistic pathogens—cytomegalovirus [CMV], *Nocardia*, and *Pneumocystis*) are the primary complications.
  - Patients typically receive two to three drug immunosuppression, infection prophylaxis, and routine endomyocardial biopsies during this time period to reduce adverse events.
  - After the first year, coronary artery vasculopathy, chronic rejection, renal insufficiency, and malignancy are the primary factors that limit survival.
  - Aggressive treatment of HTN, statin therapy, routine coronary angiography, monitored reduction of immunosuppression, and cancer screening are all important to maximize long-term survival.

OVERALL OUTCOME/PROGNOSIS FOR PATIENTS WITH HEART FAILURE

- Up to 30% of patients admitted with HF will die within 1 year.
- However, there are many factors that influence prognosis for an individual patient.
- **The Seattle HF model** is a comprehensive risk prediction tool for assessing survival probability in a given individual.[58,59] A user-friendly calculator for the Seattle Heart Failure Model is available.
- The ability to risk stratify patients with HF is useful to direct the aggressiveness of therapy and to guide discussions with patients and their families.

CONCLUSION

- HF is prevalent and associated with high morbidity and mortality.
- Early identification and intervention are essential toward improving outcomes.
- The diagnosis of HF is based on history and physical examination and is augmented by diagnostic testing.
- The goal of inpatient treatment of ADHF is to stabilize the patient's hemodynamics through aggressive medical and occasionally mechanical therapies.
- Both inpatient and outpatient initiation and optimization of GDMT are critical.
- For patients with HF despite maximally tolerated GDMT, advanced therapies may be considered and include LVAD and heart transplantation.
- For patients not wishing to pursue or who are not the candidates for advanced therapies, palliative inotropes or hospice are reasonable alternatives.

REFERENCES

1. Hunt SA, Abraham WT, Chin MH, et al. 2009 Focused update incorporated into the ACC/AHA 2005 Guidelines for the Diagnosis and Management of Heart Failure in Adults: a report of the American College of Cardiology Foundation/American Heart Association Task Force on Practice Guidelines: developed in collaboration with the International Society for Heart and Lung Transplantation. *Circulation.* 2009;119:e391-479.
2. McBride BF, White CM. Acute decompensated heart failure: a contemporary approach to pharmacotherapeutic management. *Pharmacotherapy.* 2003;23:997-1020.
3. Bozkurt B, Hershberger RE, Butler J, et al. 2021 ACC/AHA Key data elements and definitions for heart failure: a report of the American College of Cardiology/American Heart Association Task Force on Clinical Data Standards (Writing Committee to Develop Clinical Data Standards for Heart Failure). *Circ Cardiovasc Qual Outcomes.* 2021;14:e000102.
4. Ni H, Xu J. Recent trends in heart failure-related mortality: United States, 2000-2014. *NCHS Data Brief.* 2015;231:1-8.
5. Lloyd-Jones DM, Larson MG, Leip EP, et al. Lifetime risk for developing congestive heart failure: the Framingham Heart Study. *Circulation.* 2002;106:3068-72.
6. Hartupee J, Mann DL. Neurohormonal activation in heart failure with reduced ejection fraction. *Nat Rev Cardiol.* 2017;14:30-8.
7. Kannel WB, McGee DL. Diabetes and cardiovascular disease. The Framingham study. *JAMA.* 1979;241:2035-8.
8. Action to Control Cardiovascular Risk in Diabetes Study Group, Gerstein HC, Miller ME, et al. Effects of intensive glucose lowering in type 2 diabetes. *N Engl J Med.* 2008;358:2545-59.
9. Yancy CW, Jessup M, Bozkurt B, et al. 2017 ACC/AHA/HFSA Focused Update of the 2013 ACCF/AHA Guideline for the Management of Heart Failure: a report of the American College of Cardiology/American Heart Association Task Force on Clinical Practice Guidelines and the Heart Failure Society of America. *J Card Fail.* 2017;23:628-51.
10. Hartmann F, Packer M, Coats AJ, et al. Prognostic impact of plasma N-terminal pro-brain natriuretic peptide in severe chronic congestive heart failure: a substudy of the Carvedilol Prospective Randomized Cumulative Survival (COPERNICUS) trial. *Circulation.* 2004;110:1780-6.
11. Felker GM, Lee KL, Bull DA, et al. Diuretic strategies in patients with acute decompensated heart failure. *N Engl J Med.* 2011;364:797-805.
12. Cox ZL, Hung R, Lenihan DJ, et al. Diuretic strategies for loop diuretic resistance in acute heart failure: the 3T trial. *JACC Heart Fail.* 2020;8:157-68.
13. Felker GM, Benza RL, Chandler AB, et al. Heart failure etiology and response to milrinone in decompensated heart failure: results from the OPTIME-CHF study. *J Am Coll Cardiol.* 2003;41: 997-1003.
14. Abraham WT, Adams KF, Fonarow GC, et al. In-hospital mortality in patients with acute decompensated heart failure requiring intravenous vasoactive medications: an analysis from the Acute Decompensated Heart Failure National Registry (ADHERE). *J Am Coll Cardiol.* 2005;46:57-64.
15. Bart BA, Goldsmith SR, Lee KL, et al. Ultrafiltration in decompensated heart failure with cardiorenal syndrome. *N Engl J Med.* 2012;367:2296-304.
16. Mehra MR, Uriel N, Naka Y, et al. A fully magnetically levitated left ventricular assist device—final report. *N Engl J Med.* 2019;380:1618-27.
17. Rose EA, Gelijns AC, Moskowitz AJ, et al. Long-term use of a left ventricular assist device for end-stage heart failure. *N Engl J Med.* 2001;345:1435-43.
18. Rogers JG, Butler J, Lansman SL, et al. Chronic mechanical circulatory support for inotrope-dependent heart failure patients who are not transplant candidates: results of the INTrEPID Trial. *J Am Coll Cardiol.* 2007;50:741-7.
19. Yancy CW, Januzzi JL Jr, Allen LA, et al. 2017 ACC Expert Consensus Decision Pathway for Optimization of Heart Failure Treatment: answers to 10 pivotal issues about heart failure with reduced ejection fraction: a report of the American College of Cardiology Task Force on Expert Consensus Decision Pathways. *J Am Coll Cardiol.* 2018;71:201-30.
20. Shavelle DM, Desai AS, Abraham WT, et al. Lower rates of heart failure and all-cause hospitalizations during pulmonary artery pressure-guided therapy for ambulatory heart failure: one-year outcomes from the CardioMEMS Post-Approval Study. *Circ Heart Fail.* 2020;13:e006863.
21. Yee D, Novak E, Platts A, et al. Comparison of the Kansas City cardiomyopathy questionnaire and Minnesota living with heart failure questionnaire in predicting heart failure outcomes. *Am J Cardiol.* 2019;123:807-12.

22. SOLVD Investigators, Yusuf S, Pitt B, et al. Effect of enalapril on survival in patients with reduced left ventricular ejection fractions and congestive heart failure. *N Engl J Med.* 1991;325:293-302.

23. CONSENSUS Trial Study Group. Effects of enalapril on mortality in severe congestive heart failure. Results of the Cooperative North Scandinavian Enalapril Survival Study (CONSENSUS). *N Engl J Med.* 1987;316:1429-35.

24. Pfeffer MA, Braunwald E, Moye LA, et al. Effect of captopril on mortality and morbidity in patients with left ventricular dysfunction after myocardial infarction. Results of the survival and ventricular enlargement trial. The SAVE Investigators. *N Engl J Med.* 1992;327:669-77.

25. Kober L, Torp-Pedersen C, Carlsen JE, et al. A clinical trial of the angiotensin-converting-enzyme inhibitor trandolapril in patients with left ventricular dysfunction after myocardial infarction. Trandolapril Cardiac Evaluation (TRACE) Study Group. *N Engl J Med.* 1995;333:1670-6.

26. Effect of ramipril on mortality and morbidity of survivors of acute myocardial infarction with clinical evidence of heart failure. The Acute Infarction Ramipril Efficacy (AIRE) Study Investigators. *Lancet.* 1993;342:821-8.

27. Cohn JN, Tognoni G; Valsartan Heart Failure Trial Investigators. A randomized trial of the angiotensin-receptor blocker valsartan in chronic heart failure. *N Engl J Med.* 2001;345:1667-75.

28. Pfeffer MA, Swedberg K, Granger CB, et al. Effects of candesartan on mortality and morbidity in patients with chronic heart failure: the CHARM-Overall programme. *Lancet.* 2003;362:759-66.

29. Pfeffer MA, McMurray JJ, Velazquez EJ, et al. Valsartan, captopril, or both in myocardial infarction complicated by heart failure, left ventricular dysfunction, or both. *N Engl J Med.* 2003;349:1893-906.

30. Velazquez EJ, Morrow DA, DeVore AD, et al. Angiotensin-neprilysin inhibition in acute decompensated heart failure. *N Engl J Med.* 2019;380:539-48.

31. McMurray JJ, Packer M, Desai AS, et al. Angiotensin-neprilysin inhibition versus enalapril in heart failure. *N Engl J Med.* 2014;371:993-1004.

32. Writing C, Maddox TM, Januzzi JL Jr, et al. 2021 Update to the 2017 ACC Expert Consensus Decision Pathway for Optimization of Heart Failure Treatment: answers to 10 pivotal issues about heart failure with reduced ejection fraction: a report of the American College of Cardiology Solution Set Oversight Committee. *J Am Coll Cardiol.* 2021;77:772-810.

33. Packer M, Fowler MB, Roecker EB, et al. Effect of carvedilol on the morbidity of patients with severe chronic heart failure: results of the carvedilol prospective randomized cumulative survival (COPERNICUS) study. *Circulation.* 2002;106:2194-9.

34. Dargie HJ. Effect of carvedilol on outcome after myocardial infarction in patients with left-ventricular dysfunction: the CAPRICORN randomised trial. *Lancet.* 2001;357:1385-90.

35. Effect of metoprolol CR/XL in chronic heart failure: Metoprolol CR/XL Randomised Intervention Trial in Congestive Heart Failure (MERIT-HF). *Lancet.* 1999;353:2001-7.

36. A randomized trial of beta-blockade in heart failure. The Cardiac Insufficiency Bisoprolol Study (CIBIS). CIBIS Investigators and Committees. *Circulation.* 1994;90:1765-73.

37. Segev A, Mekori YA. The cardiac insufficiency bisoprolol study II. *Lancet.* 1999;353:1361.

38. Pitt B, Zannad F, Remme WJ, et al. The effect of spironolactone on morbidity and mortality in patients with severe heart failure. Randomized Aldactone Evaluation Study Investigators. *N Engl J Med.* 1999;341:709-17.

39. Pitt B, Remme W, Zannad F, et al. Eplerenone, a selective aldosterone blocker, in patients with left ventricular dysfunction after myocardial infarction. *N Engl J Med.* 2003;348:1309-21.

40. McMurray JJV, Solomon SD, Inzucchi SE, et al. Dapagliflozin in patients with heart failure and reduced ejection fraction. *N Engl J Med.* 2019;381:1995-2008.

41. Zinman B, Wanner C, Lachin JM, et al. Empagliflozin, cardiovascular outcomes, and mortality in type 2 diabetes. *N Engl J Med.* 2015;373:2117-28.

42. Cohn JN, Archibald DG, Ziesche S, et al. Effect of vasodilator therapy on mortality in chronic congestive heart failure. Results of a Veterans Administration Cooperative Study. *N Engl J Med.* 1986;314:1547-52.

43. Taylor AL, Ziesche S, Yancy C, et al. Combination of isosorbide dinitrate and hydralazine in blacks with heart failure. *N Engl J Med.* 2004;351:2049-57.

44. Digitalis Investigation Group. The effect of digoxin on mortality and morbidity in patients with heart failure. *N Engl J Med.* 1997;336:525-33.

45. Armstrong PW, Anstrom KJ, O'Connor CM, et al. Vericiguat in heart failure with reduced ejection fraction. Reply. *N Engl J Med.* 2020;383:1497-8.

46. Ponikowski P, Kirwan BA, Anker SD, et al. Ferric carboxymaltose for iron deficiency at discharge after acute heart failure: a multicentre, double-blind, randomised, controlled trial. *Lancet.* 2020;396:1895-904.

47. Swedberg K, Young JB, Anand IS, et al. Treatment of anemia with darbepoetin alfa in systolic heart failure. *N Engl J Med.* 2013;368:1210-19.
48. Moss AJ, Hall WJ, Cannom DS, et al. Improved survival with an implanted defibrillator in patients with coronary disease at high risk for ventricular arrhythmia. Multicenter Automatic Defibrillator Implantation Trial Investigators. *N Engl J Med.* 1996;335:1933-40.
49. Moss AJ, Fadl Y, Zareba W, et al. Survival benefit with an implanted defibrillator in relation to mortality risk in chronic coronary heart disease. *Am J Cardiol.* 2001;88:516-20.
50. Bardy GH, Lee KL, Mark DB, et al. Amiodarone or an implantable cardioverter-defibrillator for congestive heart failure. *N Engl J Med.* 2005;352:225-37.
51. Olgin JE, Pletcher MJ, Vittinghoff E, et al. Wearable cardioverter-defibrillator after myocardial infarction. *N Engl J Med.* 2018;379:1205-15.
52. Bristow MR, Saxon LA, Boehmer J, et al. Cardiac-resynchronization therapy with or without an implantable defibrillator in advanced chronic heart failure. *N Engl J Med.* 2004;350:2140-50.
53. Cleland JG, Daubert JC, Erdmann E, et al. The effect of cardiac resynchronization on morbidity and mortality in heart failure. *N Engl J Med.* 2005;352:1539-49.
54. Moss AJ, Hall WJ, Cannom DS, et al. Cardiac-resynchronization therapy for the prevention of heart-failure events. *N Engl J Med.* 2009;361:1329-38.
55. Stone GW, Lindenfeld J, Abraham WT, et al. Transcatheter mitral-valve repair in patients with heart failure. *N Engl J Med.* 2018;379:2307-18.
56. Obadia JF, Messika-Zeitoun D, Leurent G, et al. Percutaneous repair or medical treatment for secondary mitral regurgitation. *N Engl J Med.* 2018;379:2297-306.
57. Bozkurt B, Fonarow GC, Goldberg LR, et al. Cardiac rehabilitation for patients with heart failure: JACC Expert Panel. *J Am Coll Cardiol.* 2021;77:1454-69.
58. Levy WC, Mozaffarian D, Linker DT, et al. The Seattle Heart Failure Model: prediction of survival in heart failure. *Circulation.* 2006;113:1424-33.
59. Mozaffarian D, Anker SD, Anand I, et al. Prediction of mode of death in heart failure: the Seattle Heart Failure Model. *Circulation.* 2007;116:392-8.

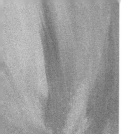

Evaluation and Management of Heart Failure with Preserved Ejection Fraction

12

Ankit K. Bhatia, Michael E. Nassif, and Justin M. Vader

GENERAL PRINCIPLES

- Heart failure (HF) incidence is increasing, given the high prevalence of diabetes and hypertension, as well as the aging population.
- Recognition and treatment of HF risk factors may curb the rise in HF incidence.
- A major contributor to an increase in HF hospitalizations has been HF with preserved ejection fraction (HFpEF), formerly known as "diastolic HF."

Definition

- Signs and symptoms of HF with left ventricular ejection fraction (LVEF) ≥50% and evidence of diastolic dysfunction:
  - HF with midrange ejection fraction (HFmrEF) LVEF 40-49%, shares many characteristics with HFpEF, with similar demographics and risk factors, but higher rates of coronary artery disease (CAD)
  - Many prior HFpEF trials have included HFmrEF patients.
- Abnormal LV diastolic function with elevated filling pressures is the hallmark of HFpEF.

Epidemiology

- Over 6 million people in the United States currently have HF, with an estimated 550,000 new diagnoses each year.[1] In the past 20 years, the incidence of HFpEF has increased relative to the incidence of HF with reduced ejection fraction (HFrEF), particularly in older patients.
- Nearly half of patients diagnosed with HF or hospitalized for acute HF have HFpEF.[2,3]
- The lifetime risk of HFpEF in the United States is >10%.[4]
- Comparison to HFrEF:
  - Common risk factors for both HFrEF and HFpEF include older age, hypertension, CAD, and diabetes.
  - Patients with HFpEF are more likely to be older, female, hypertensive, and obese.[5]
  - Markers of metabolic syndrome, obesity, and insulin resistance have a stronger association with development of HFpEF than HFrEF.[5,6]
  - Patients with HFpEF have similar rates of hospitalizations and length of hospital stay, but a slightly lower in-hospital mortality.
  - Overall mortality for patients with HFpEF is lower than mortality for patients with HFrEF.

Etiology

- Classically, hypertension was viewed as the most common cause of HFpEF, with LV hypertrophy (LVH) leading to abnormalities in myocyte relaxation.

- Increasing evidence now suggests that metabolic syndrome and excess adipose tissue play a pivotal role in the development, progression, and adverse outcomes in HFpEF.[6]
  - In the United States, >80% of HFpEF patients are overweight/obese, twice the general population rate. The population-attributable risk from overweight/obesity is similar to that of hypertension for HFpEF.
  - Excess adipose tissue promotes inflammation, hypertension, insulin resistance, and dyslipidemia, leading to impaired arterial, skeletal muscle, and myocardial function.
  - Increased body mass index (BMI) is an independent predictor of incident HFpEF. In established HFpEF, BMI is independently associated with more severe symptoms, greater exercise intolerance, cardiac dysfunction, and higher exercise pulmonary capillary wedge pressure (PCWP).
  - Large prospective cohort studies have found that obesity and insulin resistance are more strongly associated with incident HFpEF than with HFrEF.

Pathophysiology

- HFpEF symptoms result from abnormalities of cardiac structure and function, though there is increasing recognition of the roles of peripheral vascular and skeletal muscle abnormalities in HFpEF. The principal hemodynamic consequence of HFpEF is elevated left heart filling pressures.
- Mechanical abnormalities in HFpEF include:
  - Incomplete and delayed myocardial relaxation. A reduction in early passive LV filling and shift to late diastolic filling increases dependence on atrial contraction.[7]
  - Left atrial (LA) pressure rises to accommodate resistive forces in LV filling → pulmonary venous pressures rise → dyspnea ensues. Longer term structural changes due to LA hypertension include LA distension and fibrosis, altering atrial contractility and promoting atrial arrhythmias.[8]
  - HFpEF patients generally have high left heart filling pressures at rest with more pronounced pressure elevations with exercise due to impaired augmentation of LV relaxation and abnormal ventriculoarterial coupling between the LV and the aorta. This results in increased afterload.
  - Other contributing factors to HFpEF include chronotropic incompetence during exercise, reduced vasodilator reserve, and impaired right ventricular (RV)–pulmonary arterial coupling.
- The cellular mechanisms in HFpEF are not as well understood, but are thought to include abnormalities in nitric oxide/cyclic GMP signaling, disordered calcium modulation, inadequate ATP, abnormal cardiomyocyte titin content and phosphorylation and collagen deposition resulting in increased passive myocardial stiffness, microvascular endothelial dysfunction, and impaired cardiomyocyte relaxation.[9] Neurohormonal systems, including the renin–angiotensin–aldosterone system (RAAS) and the sympathetic nervous system, are activated in HFpEF, but to a lesser degree than in HFrEF.

Prevention

- Preventive measures for HFpEF include aerobic exercise, maintenance of normal weight, blood pressure control, and the use of selected antidiabetic agents in patients with diabetes.
- High-intensity exercise training is associated with reduced LV stiffness and improved cardiopulmonary fitness in middle-aged sedentary adults, but not in older (>70 years) adults. Thus, early and midlife fitness are strongly encouraged.[10]
- Antihypertensive therapy has been associated with a reduction in HF in several trials. The SPRINT trial demonstrated a 37% reduction in incident HF among nondiabetic patients at elevated cardiac risk treated to a blood pressure goal <120 mm Hg compared with a goal of <140 mm Hg.[11] Analysis of the ALLHAT trial suggests that

antihypertensive therapy with chlorthalidone is superior to lisinopril or amlodipine for HF prevention.[12]

• Sodium glucose cotransporter-2 (SGLT2) inhibitors have been shown to prevent incident HF or HF hospitalization in patients with type 2 diabetes, but the balance of HFpEF versus HFrEF prevention is unknown.[13-15]

Associated Conditions

• Due to increased LA pressure and consequent atrial remodeling, atrial arrhythmias are common in HFpEF, occurring in ~40% of patients. In HFpEF, the contribution of atrial systole to ventricular filling is more important, and atrial fibrillation (AF) can trigger HF decompensation. Consequently, AF is associated with worse outcomes in HFpEF.[16]

• More than half of HFpEF patients have chronic kidney disease (CKD) stage III or worse, and HFpEF occurs at higher rates as renal function worsens.[17]

• CAD may be present in up to two-thirds of patients with HFpEF and is associated with increased mortality and progression of ventricular dysfunction. Revascularization is associated with improved prognosis.[18]

• Iron deficiency is prevalent in patients with HFpEF and is associated with reduced cardiopulmonary fitness and quality of life.[19]

DIAGNOSIS

Clinical Presentation

Clinical history and physical examination in HF are described elsewhere (see Chapters 2 and 10).

Diagnostic Criteria

• HF is a clinical diagnosis based on history, physical examination findings, echocardiography, and CXR.

• The European Society of Cardiology defines HFpEF as satisfying three criteria:
  ○ Signs and symptoms of HF: jugular venous distention (JVD), inspiratory crackles, cardiomegaly, pulmonary edema, S3, hepatojugular reflux (HJR), weight loss with diuresis (>4.5 lb), lower extremity edema, orthopnea, nocturnal dyspnea (PND), nocturnal cough, and dyspnea on exertion (DOE)
  ○ LVEF > 50%
  ○ Elevated levels of natriuretic peptides OR at least one additional criteria:
    ▪ Relevant structural heart disease (LVH and/or left atrial enlargement [LAE])
    ▪ Diastolic dysfunction on echo

• Two scoring systems to assess the probability of HFpEF are H2FPEF[20] and HFA-PEFF.[21] These scores incorporate clinical, laboratory, and echocardiographic data (Tables 12-1 and 12-2).

Differential Diagnosis

Other diseases that can mimic symptoms of HFpEF include lung disease, thromboembolic disease, atrial arrhythmias, myocardial ischemia, obesity, pulmonary hypertension, valvular heart disease, volume overload related to renal or hepatic dysfunction, or increased afterload from hypertensive crisis (e.g., renovascular disease).

Diagnostic Testing

Because macrovascular CAD is the most common etiology of all types of HF, an ischemic evaluation is an important first step in evaluating HFpEF. This may include a combination of ECG, serum cardiac biomarkers, cardiac echocardiography (with and without stress), cardiac nuclear imaging (with and without stress), or coronary angiography.[18]

TABLE 12-1	H2FPEF SCORE		
	Clinical Variable	**Values**	**Points**
H₂	**H**eavy	Body mass index > 30 kg/m²	2
	Hypertensive	2 or more antihypertensive medicines	1
F	Atrial **F**ibrillation	Paroxysmal or Persistent	3
P	**P**ulmonary Hypertension	Doppler Echocardiographic estimated Pulmonary Artery Systolic Pressure > 35 mmHg	1
E	**E**lder	Age > 60 years	1
F	**F**illing Pressure	Doppler Echocardiographic E/e' > 9	1
	H₂FPEF score		**Sum (0-9)**

Total Points	0	1	2	3	4	5	6	7	8	9
Probability of HFpEF		0.2	0.3	0.4 0.5 0.6 0.7	0.8		0.9	0.95		

Reprinted with permission from Reddy YNV, Carter RE, Obokata M, et al. A simple, evidence-based approach to help guide diagnosis of heart failure with preserved ejection fraction. *Circulation*. 2018;138(9):861-70. Copyright ©2018 American Heart Association, Inc.

Laboratories
- Brain natriuretic peptide (BNP)
  - BNP and N-terminal ProBNP (NT-proBNP) are usually elevated in HFpEF, but not to the degree as in HFrEF.
  - Biomarker elevation may help distinguish from non-HF causes of symptoms; however, a normal BNP or NT-proBNP value **does not** exclude HFpEF as a diagnosis.[22]
  - Elevated BNP and NT-proBNP levels are associated with worse prognosis.[23]
  - BNP and NT-proBNP can be falsely low in obese patients.[24]
- Other laboratory testing:
  - Diabetes testing: blood glucose testing, hemoglobin A1C (HbA1C)
  - Iron studies to assess for iron overload states, including hemochromatosis
  - Genetic testing is indicated if rare causes of restrictive cardiomyopathy are suspected (see section Restrictive Cardiomyopathy).
  - Serum and urine protein electrophoresis with immunofixation and serum-free light-chain assay to evaluate for the presence of Ig light-chain amyloidosis in select patients
  - 5-Hydroxyindoleacetic acid (5-HIAA) testing if other features of carcinoid syndrome and tricuspid disease are present

Electrocardiogram
- ECG may provide clues to chamber enlargement and ventricular hypertrophy as well as evidence of ischemia and/or prior myocardial infarction (MI).
- Low voltages on ECG should prompt consideration of an infiltrative process.

Imaging
- Echocardiography:
  - Assessment of systolic function, chamber sizes, and hypertrophy
  - Valvular dysfunction such as aortic stenosis can lead to HFpEF.
  - Regional wall motion abnormalities may indicate ischemia and/or prior infarction.
  - Apparent LVH in the absence of a cause for pressure overload should prompt consideration of hypertrophic cardiomyopathy (HCM) or infiltrative cardiomyopathy.
  - Diastolic function is evaluated by Doppler assessment of transmitral LV filling and tissue Doppler velocities at the mitral valve annulus (see Chapter 35). Echocardiographic evidence of diastolic dysfunction supports an HFpEF diagnosis.[25]

TABLE 12-2 HFA-PEFF SCORE

	Function	Morphology	Biomarker
Major criteria (2 points)	• Mitral e' velocity < 7 cm/s (septal) or <10 cm/s (lateral) OR • Average mitral E/e' ≥ 15 OR • TR velocity > 2.8 m/s	• Left atrial volume > 34 mL/m² OR • Left ventricular mass ≥ 149 g/m² (men) or ≥122 g/m² (women) AND relative wall thickness > 0.42	• NT-proBNP > 220 pg/mL OR BNP > 80 pg/mL (normal sinus rhythm) • NT-proBNP > 660 pg/mL OR BNP > 240 pg/mL (atrial fibrillation)
Minor criteria (1 point)	• Average mitral E/e' ≥ 9–14 OR • Global longitudinal strain < 16%	• Left atrial volume > 34 mL/m² OR • Left ventricular mass ≥ 115 g/m² (men) or ≥95 g/m² (women) OR • Relative wall thickness > 0.42 OR • LV wall thickness ≥ 12 mm	• NT-proBNP > 125–220 pg/mL OR BNP 35–80 pg/mL (normal sinus) • NT-proBNP 365–660 pg/mL OR BNP 105–240 pg/mL (atrial fibrillation)

Score range 0–6 points. Score ≥ 5: HFpEF. Score 2–4: further testing.

BNP, brain natriuretic peptide; LV, left ventricular; NT-proBNP, N-terminal proBNP; TR, tricuspid regurgitation.

Adapted from Pieske B, Tschöpe C, de Boer RA, et al. How to diagnose heart failure with preserved ejection fraction: the HFA-PEFF diagnostic algorithm: a consensus recommendation from the Heart Failure Association (HFA) of the European Society of Cardiology (ESC). *Eur Heart J.* 2019;40(40):3297-317. Reproduced by permission of Oxford University Press.

- **Cardiac MRI** is useful for evaluation of infiltrative/restrictive cardiomyopathies and pericardial constriction (see Chapter 36).
- **Nuclear scintigraphy** with [99m]technetium-labeled bone scan radiotracers can be used to diagnose transthyretin cardiac amyloidosis but is inadequate for excluding light-chain cardiac amyloidosis.
- Imaging of the renal vasculature by Doppler ultrasound, magnetic resonance angiography, or renal angiography should be performed if renal artery stenosis is suspected, as in the case of recurrent hypertensive crises.

Diagnostic Procedures
- **Cardiac catheterization**:
  - Left heart catheterization can be performed for evaluation of CAD as well as to measure LV end-diastolic pressure (LVEDP).

- Right heart catheterization at rest and with exercise is the gold standard to assess the hemodynamics of patients with suspected HFpEF. PCWP and/or LVEDP >15 mm Hg at rest and >25 mm Hg with exercise are diagnostic of HFpEF.
- **Endomyocardial biopsy** can provide pathologic evidence for restrictive or infiltrative cardiomyopathies (see later).

TREATMENT

- Unlike with HFrEF, there are few clinical trials to direct optimal medical therapy in patients with HFpEF. As of December 2021, no therapies are Food and Drug Administration (FDA) approved *specifically for the treatment of HF with normal LVEF*, although sacubitril/valsartan is approved for adults with chronic HF, irrespective of LVEF. Empagliflozin has been granted "Breakthrough Therapy" designation by FDA for HFpEF and will undergo expedited review.
- Therapy is directed at control of congestive symptoms through diuretics and avoidance of excessive dietary sodium, control of blood pressure in accordance with hypertension guidelines, control of atrial arrhythmias with a preference for rhythm control when possible, control of diabetes, weight loss in obese patients, and emphasis on regular aerobic exercise.
- Antianginal therapy is indicated in patients with symptomatic CAD.
- Disease-modifying therapies are indicated in infiltrative or restrictive cardiomyopathies when such therapies exist.

Medications

- **SGLT2 inhibitors** have emerged as a promising treatment option for HFpEF.
  - SGLT2 inhibitors have been shown to reduce the composite outcome of cardiovascular (CV) death and HF hospitalizations in diabetic patients with HF and *unspecified* LVEF (dapagliflozin, empagliflozin, canagliflozin, sotagliflozin), a finding confirmed in subgroup analysis of HFpEF patients (sotagliflozin).
  - Empagliflozin reduced the composite of CV mortality and HF hospitalization in a population with HFpEF *regardless of diabetes status* in the EMPEROR-Preserved Trial.[26] Subgroup analysis revealed no heterogeneity based on LVEF or diabetes status. Dapagliflozin demonstrated improvement in HF symptoms burden, functional status, and exercise capacity in HFpEF patients with or without diabetes in the PRESERVED-HF trial.[27] A pivotal trial of dapagliflozin in HFpEF is ongoing.
  - SGLT2 inhibitors have been demonstrated to reduce the rate of decline in kidney function in patients with CKD,[28] a common comorbid condition in patients with HF.
- **Spironolactone** has been associated with improved clinical outcomes in a general HFpEF population.
  - Spironolactone decreased HF hospitalizations in patients with HFpEF in the TOPCAT trial, but did not reduce the composite outcome of CV death and hospitalization.[29]
  - Subgroup analysis demonstrated reduced HF hospitalization and CV death among patients with HFpEF and lower BNP.[30]
  - Spironolactone is not yet FDA approved specifically for HFpEF.
- **Sacubitril/Valsartan** failed to reduce mortality compared with valsartan in patients with HFpEF in the PARAGON study (mean LVEF 57%), but was associated with fewer hospitalizations.[31]
  - Secondary analysis demonstrated benefits for sacubitril/valsartan among patients recently hospitalized for HF, women, and patients with midrange LVEF (LVEF 40-50%).[32]
  - The FDA label for sacubitril/valsartan was expanded in 2021 to include all chronic HF patients, irrespective of LVEF, with an emphasis on benefit among those with LVEF

below normal. Ongoing trials will evaluate the impact of sacubitril/valsartan on hospitalizations and mortality in hospitalized HFpEF patients.

- **Diuretics:**
  - Oral thiazide diuretics (e.g., hydrochlorothiazide [HCTZ]) are indicated for antihypertensive therapy and may adequately control volume overload in mild HFpEF.
  - Loop diuretics are the most commonly used medications for maintenance of euvolemia in symptomatic HFpEF.
  - Metolazone may be added to overcome loop diuretic resistance in the setting of persistent volume overload but should be used with caution and with frequent monitoring for hypokalemia, hypomagnesemia, and renal dysfunction.
  - Loop diuretic dosage should be maximized before using metolazone.
- **Angiotensin-converting enzyme (ACE) inhibitors and angiotensin-receptor blockers** are recommended for the *prevention* of incident HFpEF in patients with a history of CAD or coronary risk factors, including diabetes.[33] These agents may be used as an antihypertensive therapy in patients with HFpEF; however, clinical trials of these agents in HFpEF have not demonstrated outcomes superior to placebo.
  - The HOPE study demonstrated a reduction in incident HFpEF with ramipril in hypertensive patients with vascular disease or multiple coronary risk factors.[34] However, no clinical trials have demonstrated reduced CV events with ACE inhibitors in patients with established HFpEF.
  - The CHARM-Preserved trial demonstrated that candesartan therapy in patients with New York Heart Association (NYHA) classes II to IV HF with LVEF >40% produced a statistically nonsignificant trend toward reduction in hospitalization and CV death, driven by reduced hospitalization.[35]
- **β-Blockers** are recommended in HFpEF patients with symptom-limiting angina or AF requiring rate control, but studies to date have not demonstrated a mortality benefit for β-blockers in HFpEF patients without another compelling indication.[36] Withdrawal of β-blockers in HFpEF patients with chronotropic incompetence may improve functional capacity.[37]
- **Calcium channel blockers** are recommended in β-blocker–intolerant HFpEF patients with symptom-limiting angina or AF requiring rate control.

Other Therapies

- Restoration and maintenance of sinus rhythm is of potential benefit in HFpEF patients with AF.
  - Loss of atrial systole compromises ventricular diastolic filling in HFpEF. Observational data suggest improved outcomes for HFpEF patients treated with a rhythm control rather than rate control strategy; however, there are no randomized clinical trials comparing rate and rhythm control strategies in AF and HFpEF.[38]
  - Rhythm control should be considered in patients with AF and HFpEF who are persistently symptomatic despite adequate rate control.
  - Antiarrhythmic drug use recommendations are similar for patients with HFrEF and HFpEF.
    - Amiodarone and dofetilide have been shown to increase conversion to and maintenance of sinus rhythm in HF patients with AF and are the first-line options in HFpEF.
    - Sotalol may be used in select HFpEF patients without significant LVH.
    - Dronedarone is generally avoided in patients with HFpEF.[39]
  - Limited data on catheter ablation of AF in HFpEF patients suggest improvement in symptoms and similar rates of effectiveness as in patients with HFrEF[40]; however, no specific guideline recommendations exist for catheter ablation of AF in the setting of HFpEF.

- Invasive pulmonary artery pressure monitoring:
  - Elevations in pulmonary artery pressure precede the development of HF symptoms and serve as a therapeutic target for diuretic and vasodilator therapies in patients with HF.
  - The CHAMPION trial demonstrated that among HFpEF patients with NYHA class III functional status and an HF hospitalization in the previous year, the use of hemodynamic pulmonary artery pressure monitoring was associated with >50% reduction in HF hospitalizations over an 18-month follow-up period.[41]
  - Pulmonary artery pressure monitoring through an implantable pulmonary artery pressure sensor (CardioMEMS) is an FDA-approved technology for the monitoring of patients with NYHA class III HF (including HFpEF) who have been hospitalized within the previous year.
- Investigational devices: interatrial shunt device (IASD):
  - Promotion of a left-to-right shunt to reduce LA pressures has been theorized as a means to mitigate the symptoms of HFpEF.
  - Use of an 8-mm IASD in a small sham-controlled study of HFpEF patients demonstrated reduction in rest and exercise PCWP as well as statistically nonsignificant improvements in HF hospitalization and NYHA functional class.[42] A larger clinical outcome trial of this technology is ongoing, and other IASD technologies are in development.

Lifestyle Modifications

- It is recommended that sodium consumption be limited to 2 to 3 g/day, similar to with HFrEF; however, supportive high-quality data are lacking. Excessive sodium restriction may be associated with adverse outcomes.
- **Regular aerobic exercise is recommended in all HFpEF patients**. Supervised exercise training can improve quality of life and exercise capacity in patients with HFpEF.[43]
- Caloric restriction and weight loss provide additive improvement in exercise capacity for obese patients with HFpEF.[44]
- Weight loss through bariatric surgery has been associated with improved HF symptoms, reduced HF admissions, and improved LV morphology and diastolic function in nonrandomized studies.[45]
- Blood pressure monitoring and measurement of daily weights are recommended to monitor for impending decompensation and/or opportunities to titrate antihypertensive medications or diuretics.
- More than half of HFpEF patients have sleep-disordered breathing, primarily obstructive sleep apnea (OSA). OSA treatment with continuous positive airway pressure (CPAP) has been associated with improved diastolic function and blood pressure control.

SPECIAL CONSIDERATIONS

Restrictive Cardiomyopathy

- Characterized by a rigid myocardium and poor ventricular filling
- Should be considered in patients presenting with HFpEF, particularly when risk factors such as hypertension, diabetes, and obesity are absent. Particular consideration should be given to genetically determined disorders in younger patients and infiltrative disorders (especially amyloidosis) in older patients.
- Pericardial diseases can present similarly but have a considerably different prognosis and treatment (see Chapter 17).
- MRI is a useful diagnostic imaging tool, with characteristic findings for certain disease states (see Chapter 36).
- When noninvasive imaging fails to differentiate between restrictive and constrictive physiology, cardiac catheterization with simultaneous hemodynamic assessment of the LV and RV is performed.

- Restrictive cardiomyopathies can be divided into noninfiltrative disease, infiltrative disease, storage disease, and endomyocardial disease.
- *Noninfiltrative disorders*:
  - Idiopathic restrictive cardiomyopathy:
    - Idiopathic restrictive cardiomyopathy is a rare and occasionally familial disorder characterized by myofilament calcium sensitivity and collagen deposition.
    - Patchy endocardial fibrosis is present and may extend into the conduction system, resulting in complete heart block.
    - Therapeutic recommendations are consistent with HFpEF therapy in general, and patients with advanced HF are considered for heart transplantation.
  - HCM (see Chapter 16):
    - HCM results from mutations in cardiomyocyte sarcomere genes, leading to cardiomyocyte hypertrophy, disordered myocardial structure, and interstitial fibrosis.
    - "Classic" hypertrophic obstructive cardiomyopathy presents as asymmetric hypertrophy of the septum at the area of the LV outflow tract and produces dynamic LV outflow tract obstruction.
    - HCM variants include nonobstructive forms with hypertrophy concentrated at other ventricular locations. This results in diastolic dysfunction and restrictive cardiomyopathy in extreme cases.
    - Cardiac myosin inhibitors have been shown to improve symptoms in patients with hypertrophic obstructive cardiomyopathy, and early-phase data suggest benefit in nonobstructive HCM with larger scale trials ongoing.
  - Systemic sclerosis (scleroderma):
    - Clinically evident cardiac involvement occurs in ~25% of cases and is more common in patients with more severe skin disease and skeletal myopathy.
    - Cardiac pathology consists of myocardial inflammation and fibrosis and coronary microvascular dysfunction, resulting in diastolic dysfunction. In more severe cases, systolic dysfunction may result.
    - Immunosuppressive therapy for systemic sclerosis is recommended.
- *Infiltrative disorders:*
  - **Cardiac amyloidosis (see Chapter 15):**
    - Deposition of misfolded protein aggregates between normal myocardial contractile elements results in decreased ventricular compliance, culminating in restrictive physiology. Aggregates may also impair normal electrical conduction and lead to arrhythmias or conduction system disease.
    - There are many types of amyloidosis, but cardiac involvement is seen most commonly in transthyretin cardiac amyloidosis (ATTR) and amyloid light-chain (AL) disease.
      - ATTR may result from mutations in the *TTR* gene (hereditary TTR) or may occur in the setting of normal *TTR* gene sequence (wild-type TTR, formerly called senile amyloidosis). Hereditary TTR generally manifests earlier in life and is more likely to be associated with neurologic symptoms.
      - AL amyloidosis is due to the overproduction of misfolded fragments of Ig light chains.
    - Amyloid deposits are demonstrated histologically as insoluble amyloid fibrils within the myocardial tissue in all chambers of the heart, classically evident with Congo red staining viewed under polarized light. Mass spectrometry may be used to determine protein type and sequence.
    - ECG classically shows low voltage with poor R-wave progression in advanced disease, **though low ECG voltage is not a sensitive marker of cardiac amyloidosis**.
    - Laboratory testing for AL amyloidosis includes serum-free light chains as well as serum and urine protein electrophoresis. Elevated NT-proBNP and troponin suggest cardiac involvement and are useful in assessing disease severity and prognosis.

- Echocardiographic findings characteristic of cardiac amyloidosis include diastolic dysfunction, increased LV wall thickness, and biatrial enlargement. Speckle tracking–derived strain mapping of the LV demonstrates preservation of apical longitudinal strain and reduction of basal segment strain ("cherry on the top" pattern).
- Cardiac MRI may be useful in identifying cardiac amyloidosis, particularly if other cardiomyopathies are in the differential.
- Increasingly, nuclear scintigraphy with bone tracers such as ^{99m}technetium-labeled pyrophosphate is used when ATTR cardiac amyloidosis is suspected, due to the high sensitivity and specificity of this test. However, AL cardiac amyloidosis cannot be excluded with a normal scan.
- Therapies for cardiac amyloidosis have evolved considerably in recent years. Transthyretin cardiac amyloidosis may be treated with disease-modifying therapies to reduce the deposition of misfolded TTR protein aggregates.
  □ Tafamidis stabilizes TTR protein tetramers and prevents monomer dissociation and misfolding.
  □ Patisiran (small interfering RNA) and inotersen (antisense oligonucleotide) are the inhibitors of TTR protein synthesis.
  □ Tafamidis is currently approved for both hereditary and wild-type TTR-CA, while patisiran and inotersen are approved for TTR amyloidosis with neurologic involvement. Other agents are in development.
- AL amyloidosis is treated in coordination with a hematologist using combined chemotherapy and immunotherapy. Autologous hematopoietic stem cell transplantation is pursued in younger patients with less severe HF and less extreme elevation in cardiac biomarkers.

○ **Cardiac sarcoidosis:**
- Cardiac involvement is likely underdiagnosed in patients with systemic sarcoidosis, having been reported in >25% of cases by autopsy study. In addition, isolated cardiac sarcoidosis may occur in the absence of systemic findings.
- Myocardial restriction results from patchy scar formation around infiltrating, noncaseating granulomas. HFpEF or HF with mild LV systolic dysfunction is a common presentation. Increasing degrees of LV diastolic dysfunction are associated with worse prognosis.
- The most common manifestation of symptomatic cardiac sarcoidosis is conduction system disease, with the most dramatic presentations being sudden cardiac death due to ventricular tachyarrhythmias or high-grade heart block.
- The diagnosis of sarcoidosis is made challenging by the patchy nature of myocardial involvement, limiting the yield of endomyocardial biopsy. Imaging with cardiac MRI or fluorodeoxyglucose-positron emission tomography (FDG-PET) is useful for demonstrating the location and extent of cardiac involvement. Active inflammatory cardiac sarcoidosis with evidence of systolic dysfunction, conduction system disease, or arrhythmia generally warrants therapy with anti-inflammatory therapy beginning with corticosteroids.

- *Storage disorders:*
  ○ **Iron overload cardiomyopathy:**
  - Excess circulating iron leads to increased intracellular iron, which forms reactive oxygen species that, in turn, mediate oxidative damage to cellular and organelle membranes and mitochondrial DNA. In addition, free iron alters calcium influx and interferes with normal excitation–contraction coupling, resulting in diastolic dysfunction.
  - Causes include hereditary hemochromatosis (characterized by an autosomal recessive mutation in the *HFE* gene) and secondary hemochromatosis, due to iron overload from exogenous sources such as blood transfusion.

- Diastolic dysfunction is the initial presentation of iron overload cardiomyopathy, evolving to dilated cardiomyopathy with systolic dysfunction in later stage disease. Extracardiac manifestations include diabetes mellitus and skin discoloration.
- Workup includes serum iron studies, with an elevated transferrin saturation being most suggestive, and cardiac MRI with T2* mapping followed by biopsy of an accessible organ (often the liver).
- Treatment of iron overload with phlebotomy or chelation therapy is required to prevent progression of disease.
- **Lysosomal storage diseases:**
  - Numerous genetic mutations may impair the function of lysosomal enzymes and result in cellular injury, including cardiomyocytes. Many of these conditions manifest clinically in childhood, but some disorders may not be diagnosed until adulthood, when they typically present as restrictive cardiomyopathy.
  - **Anderson–Fabry disease** is an X-linked recessive lysosomal storage disorder that results in reduced or absent α-galactosidase A activity, leading to an accumulation of the glycosphingolipid metabolic byproduct globotriaosylceramide in many cell types, including cardiomyocytes. The principal cardiac pathology is LVH and restrictive cardiomyopathy. Age of diagnosis ranges from the third to seventh decades. Noncardiac manifestations include peripheral neuropathy, proteinuria, cataracts, and skin lesions, such as telangiectasias and angiokeratomas. The diagnosis may be confirmed by reduced serum or leukocyte α-galactosidase A activity or by genetic sequencing. Endomyocardial biopsy is rarely necessary but demonstrates a characteristic finding of lamellar bodies in the cardiomyocyte sarcoplasm. Enzyme replacement therapy is available and can prevent disease progression.
  - **Danon disease** is an X-linked semi-dominant disease caused by deficient LAMP2. Excess glycogen storage and lysosomal dysfunction in cardiac and skeletal muscle cells results from LAMP2 deficiency. In males, cardiac hypertrophy and restrictive cardiomyopathy are the most common presentation, while females are more likely to have a dilated cardiomyopathy. Wolf–Parkinson–White syndrome is common. Intellectual disability is variable.
  - **PRKAG2 deficiency** is an autosomal dominant disease, resulting in increased cardiomyocte glucose uptake and increased glycogen storage as well as myofibril disarray and cardiac fibrosis. Clinically, this manifests as severe LVH, restrictive cardiomyopathy, and conduction system disease.
  - **Gaucher disease** is an autosomal recessive disease produced by mutations of the glucocerebrosidase gene that result in the accumulation of the lipid glucocerebroside in lysosomes, producing dysfunction in a variety of cells, including cardiomyocytes. Disease is generally evident in childhood. Restrictive cardiomyopathy may result. Enzyme replacement therapy is available.
  - The **mucopolysaccharidoses** are a family of genetic enzymatic deficiency diseases that result from the improper breakdown of glycosaminoglycans, leading to their accumulation in lysosomes, producing dysfunction in a wide variety of cell types, including cardiomyocytes. **Hurler and Hunter syndromes** are two examples of this disorder. Disease generally manifests in childhood, but attenuated forms occasionally present in early adulthood.
- *Endomyocardial disorders:*
  - **Hypereosinophilic syndromes:**
    - Prolonged hypereosinophilia and activation may lead to cardiac damage from the action of eosinophilic degranulation upon the myocardium. This condition may result from a variety of inciting factors, including malignancy, primary hematologic disorders, allergic drug reactions, parasitic infection, or idiopathic causes.

- Disease usually progresses from an acute necrotic phase to an intermediate thrombotic phase, followed by a terminal fibrotic phase characterized by restrictive cardiomyopathy.
  - Acute-phase disease is characterized clinically by elevated troponin, cardiac MRI findings of myocardial inflammation, and endomyocardial biopsy evidence of eosinophilic infiltration and cardiomyocyte damage.
  - Thrombotic-phase disease is characterized clinically by extensive mural thrombus, particularly involving the LV apex, and embolic phenomena.
  - Fibrotic-phase disease is characterized by restrictive cardiomyopathy, normal LV wall thickness, impaired valve mobility, and consequent regurgitation or stenosis.
- Corticosteroids and cytotoxic drugs in the acute phase of disease may improve symptoms and survival. Anticoagulation is recommended in the thrombotic phase when emboli have occurred. Valve repair or replacement is recommended in fibrotic-phase patients with severe valvular regurgitation or stenosis.
- **Carcinoid heart disease:**
  - Results from untreated carcinoid syndrome, where lesion formation correlates with the concentration of serotonin and 5-HIAA
  - Lesions are predominantly in the RV endocardium, where tricuspid insufficiency is prominent. Tricuspid and pulmonic stenoses can also be seen.
  - Occasionally, left-sided valvular lesions can be seen in patients with either pulmonary metastases or a patent foramen ovale (or other intracardiac shunt).
  - Therapy is focused on control of systemic carcinoid disease. Valve replacement surgery is performed in patients with severe valve disease and otherwise well-controlled systemic disease.
- **Endomyocardial fibrosis:**
  - Most commonly diagnosed in patients living in or coming from equatorial countries and rare in North America
  - Etiology is likely related to dietary (cassava-based diet, malnutrition) and infectious (helminthic parasites) factors.
  - Manifests as cardiac inflammation and eosinophilia, leading to myocardial fibrosis and restrictive cardiomyopathy with small ventricular volumes, normal LV wall thickness, and atrial dilatation
  - Surgical endocardectomy and valve repair may be considered in select cases.
- **Radiation-induced heart disease:**
  - Radiation-induced heart disease is a late consequence of mediastinal radiation.
  - Pathologically, this is characterized by early inflammation and microvascular injury, inducing ischemic changes and replacement fibrosis. Clinical presentation with diastolic dysfunction and/or valvular thickening typically occurs decades after exposure.
  - Preventive measures include limiting radiation dose, focusing radiation away from the heart, and avoiding coadministration of anthracycline chemotherapy.

OUTCOME/PROGNOSIS

- HFpEF has a fairly similar prognosis to HFrEF.[2] However, an individual patient data meta-analysis (including >10,000 patients with HFpEF) suggests that survival is better in those with HFpEF (3-year mortality about 25% vs. ~32% for those with reduced LVEF).[46]
- Many factors appear to alter prognosis for an individual patient, such as HF symptoms (NYHA class), laboratory tests (troponin, BNP, sodium, hemoglobin, creatinine), cardiac physiology (e.g., LVEF, diastolic function, pulmonary pressures, wedge pressure), HF

etiology (ischemic vs. nonischemic), associated conditions (e.g., AF, renal insufficiency), medication and device therapy, and age.[47]

- Risk prediction models for prognosis in HFrEF, such as the Seattle Heart Failure model and the MAGGIC risk score, are less accurate in patients with HFpEF, and no risk model has been developed and validated to predict prognosis in HFpEF.

REFERENCES

1. Virani SS, Alonso A, Benjamin EJ, et al. Heart disease and stroke statistics-2020 update: a report from the American Heart Association. *Circulation.* 2020;141:e139-596.

2. Steinberg BA, Zhao X, Heidenreich PA, et al. Trends in patients hospitalized with heart failure and preserved left ventricular ejection fraction: prevalence, therapies, and outcomes. *Circulation.* 2012;126:65-75.

3. Goyal P, Almarzooq ZI, Horn EM, et al. Characteristics of hospitalizations for heart failure with preserved ejection fraction. *Am J Med.* 2016;129:635.e15-26.

4. Pandey A, Omar W, Ayers C, et al. Sex and race differences in lifetime risk of heart failure with preserved ejection fraction and heart failure with reduced ejection fraction. *Circulation.* 2018;137:1814-23.

5. Dunlay SM, Roger VL, Redfield MM. Epidemiology of heart failure with preserved ejection fraction. *Nat Rev Cardiol.* 2017;14:591-602.

6. Savji N, Meijers WC, Bartz TM, et al. The association of obesity and cardiometabolic traits with incident HFpEF and HFrEF. *JACC Heart Fail.* 2018;6:701-9.

7. Freed BH, Shah SJ. Stepping out of the left ventricle's shadow: time to focus on the left atrium in heart failure with preserved ejection fraction. *Circ Cardiovasc Imaging.* 2017;10:e006267.

8. Pfeffer MA, Shah AM, Borlaug BA. Heart failure with preserved ejection fraction in perspective. *Circ Res.* 2019;124:1598-617.

9. Mishra S, Kass DA. Cellular and molecular pathobiology of heart failure with preserved ejection fraction. *Nat Rev Cardiol.* 2021;18:400-23.

10. Howden EJ, Sarma S, Lawley JS, et al. Reversing the cardiac effects of sedentary aging in middle age—a randomized controlled trial: implications for heart failure prevention. *Circulation.* 2018;137:1549-60.

11. Williamson JD, Supiano MA, Applegate WB, et al. Intensive vs standard blood pressure control and cardiovascular disease outcomes in adults aged ≥75 years: a randomized clinical trial. *JAMA.* 2016;315:2673-82.

12. The ALLHAT Officers and Coordinators for the ALLHAT Collaborative Research Group. Major outcomes in high-risk hypertensive patients randomized to angiotensin-converting enzyme inhibitor or calcium channel blocker vs diuretic: the Antihypertensive and Lipid-Lowering Treatment to Prevent Heart Attack Trial (ALLHAT). *JAMA.* 2002;288:2981-97.

13. Zinman B, Wanner C, Lachin JM, et al. Empagliflozin, cardiovascular outcomes, and mortality in type 2 diabetes. *N Engl J Med.* 2015;373:2117-28.

14. Rådholm K, Figtree G, Perkovic V, et al. Canagliflozin and heart failure in type 2 diabetes mellitus: results from the CANVAS program. *Circulation.* 2018;138:458-68.

15. Wiviott SD, Raz I, Bonaca MP, et al. Dapagliflozin and cardiovascular outcomes in type 2 diabetes. *N Engl J Med.* 2019;380:347-57.

16. Zafrir B, Lund L, Laroche C, et al. Prognostic implications of atrial fibrillation in heart failure with reduced, mid-range, and preserved ejection fraction: a report from 14964 patients in the European Society of Cardiology Heart Failure Long-Term Registry. *Eur Heart J.* 2018;39:4277-84.

17. House AA, Wanner C, Sarnak MJ, et al. Heart failure in chronic kidney disease: conclusions from a Kidney Disease: Improving Global Outcomes (KDIGO) controversies conference. *Kidney Int.* 2019;95:1304-17.

18. Hwang SJ, Melenovsky V, Borlaug BA. Implications of coronary artery disease in heart failure with preserved ejection fraction. *J Am Coll Cardiol.* 2014;63:2817-27.

19. Beale AL, Warren JL, Roberts N, et al. Iron deficiency in heart failure with preserved ejection fraction: a systematic review and meta-analysis. *Open Heart.* 2019;6:e001012.

20. Reddy YNV, Carter RE, Obokata M, et al. A simple, evidence-based approach to help guide diagnosis of heart failure with preserved ejection fraction. *Circulation.* 2018;138:861-70.

21. Pieske B, Tschöpe C, de Boer RA, et al. How to diagnose heart failure with preserved ejection fraction: the HFA-PEFF diagnostic algorithm: a consensus recommendation from the Heart Failure Association (HFA) of the European Society of Cardiology (ESC). *Eur Heart J.* 2019;40:3297-317.

22. Anjan VY, Loftus TM, Burke MA, et al. Prevalence, clinical phenotype, and outcomes associated with normal B-type natriuretic peptide levels in heart failure with preserved ejection fraction. *Am J Cardiol.* 2012;110:870-6.

23. Anand IS, Rector TS, Cleland JG, et al. Prognostic value of baseline plasma amino-terminal pro-brain natriuretic peptide and its interactions with irbesartan treatment effects in patients with heart failure and preserved ejection fraction: findings from the I-PRESERVE trial. *Circ Heart Fail.* 2011;4:569-77.

24. Mehra MR, Uber PA, Park MH, et al. Obesity and suppressed B-type natriuretic peptide levels in heart failure. *J Am Coll Cardiol.* 2004;43:1590-5.

25. Nagueh SF, Smiseth OA, Appleton CP, et al. Recommendations for the evaluation of left ventricular diastolic function by echocardiography: an update from the American Society of Echocardiography and the European Association of Cardiovascular Imaging. *J Am Soc Echocardiogr.* 2016;29:277-314.

26. Anker SD, Butler J, Filippatos G, et al. Empagliflozin in heart failure with a preserved ejection fraction. *N Engl J Med.* 2021;385:1451-61.

27. Nassif ME, Windsor SL, Borlaug BA, et al. The SGLT2 inhibitor dapagliflozin in heart failure with preserved ejection fraction: a multicenter randomized trial. *Nat Med.* 2021;27:1954-60.

28. Heerspink HJL, Stefánsson BV, Correa-Rotter R, et al. Dapagliflozin in patients with chronic kidney disease. *N Engl J Med.* 2020;383:1436-46.

29. Pitt B, Pfeffer MA, Assmann SF, et al. Spironolactone for heart failure with preserved ejection fraction. *N Engl J Med.* 2014;370:1383-92.

30. Anand IS, Claggett B, Liu J, et al. Interaction between spironolactone and natriuretic peptides in patients with heart failure and preserved ejection fraction: from the TOPCAT Trial. *JACC Heart Fail.* 2017;5:241-52.

31. Solomon SD, McMurray JJV, Anand IS, et al. Angiotensin-neprilysin inhibition in heart failure with preserved ejection fraction. *N Engl J Med.* 2019;381:1609-20.

32. Solomon SD, Vaduganathan M, Claggett B, et al. Sacubitril/valsartan across the spectrum of ejection fraction in heart failure. *Circulation.* 2020;141:352-61.

33. Yancy CW, Jessup M, Bozkurt B, et al. 2017 ACC/AHA/HFSA Focused update of the 2013 ACCF/AHA guideline for the management of heart failure: a report of the American College of Cardiology/American Heart Association Task Force on Clinical Practice Guidelines and the Heart Failure Society of America. *J Card Fail.* 2017;23:628-51.

34. Arnold JMO, Yusuf S, Young J, et al. Prevention of heart failure in patients in the heart outcomes prevention evaluation (HOPE) study. *Circulation.* 2003;107:1284-90.

35. Yusuf S, Pfeffer MA, Swedberg K, et al. Effects of candesartan in patients with chronic heart failure and preserved left-ventricular ejection fraction: the CHARM-Preserved Trial. *Lancet.* 2003;362:777-81.

36. Hernandez AF, Hammill BG, O'Connor CM, et al. Clinical effectiveness of beta-blockers in heart failure: findings from the OPTIMIZE-HF (Organized Program to Initiate Lifesaving Treatment in Hospitalized Patients with Heart Failure) Registry. *J Am Coll Cardiol.* 2009;53:184-92.

37. Palau P, Seller J, Domínguez E, et al. Effect of β-blocker withdrawal on functional capacity in heart failure and preserved ejection fraction. *J Am Coll Cardiol.* 2021;78:2042-56.

38. Kelly JP, DeVore AD, Wu JJ, et al. Rhythm control versus rate control in patients with atrial fibrillation and heart failure with preserved ejection fraction: insights from Get With The Guidelines-Heart Failure. *J Am Heart Assoc.* 2019;8:e011560.

39. January CT, Wann LS, Calkins H, et al. 2014 AHA/ACC/HRS Guideline for the management of patients with atrial fibrillation: a report of the American College of Cardiology/American Heart Association Task Force on Practice Guidelines and the Heart Rhythm Society. *J Am Coll Cardiol.* 2014;64:e1-76.

40. Black-Meier E, Ren X, Steinberg BA, et al. Catheter ablation of atrial fibrillation in patients with heart failure and preserved ejection fraction. *Heart Rhythm.* 2018;15:651-7.

41. Adamson PB, Abraham WT, Bourge RC, et al. Wireless pulmonary artery pressure monitoring guides management to reduce decompensation in heart failure with preserved ejection fraction. *Circ Heart Fail.* 2014;7:935-44.

42. Shah SJ, Feldman T, Ricciardi MJ, et al. One-year safety and clinical outcomes of a transcatheter interatrial shunt device for the treatment of heart failure with preserved ejection fraction in the Reduce Elevated Left Atrial Pressure in Patients With Heart Failure (REDUCE LAP-HF I) Trial: a randomized clinical trial. *JAMA Cardiol.* 2018;3:968-77.

43. Pandey A, Prashar A, Kumbhani D, et al. Exercise training in patients with heart failure and preserved ejection fraction: meta-analysis of randomized control trials. *Circ Heart Fail.* 2015;8:33-40.

44. Kitzman DW, Brubaker P, Morgan T, et al. Effect of caloric restriction or aerobic exercise training on peak oxygen consumption and quality of life in obese older patients with heart failure with preserved ejection fraction: a randomized clinical trial. *JAMA.* 2016;315:36-46.

45. Berger S, Meyre P, Aeschbacher S, et al. Bariatric surgery among patients with heart failure: a systematic review and meta-analysis. *Open Heart.* 2018;5:e000910.
46. Meta-Analysis Global Group in Chronic Heart Failure (MAGGIC). The survival of patients with heart failure with preserved or reduced left ventricular ejection fraction: an individual patient data meta-analysis. *Eur Heart J.* 2012;33:1750-7.
47. Yancy CW, Lopatin M, Stevenson LW, et al. Clinical presentation, management, and in-hospital outcomes of patients admitted with acute decompensated heart failure with preserved systolic function: a report from the Acute Decompensated Heart Failure National Registry (ADHERE) Database. *J Am Coll Cardiol.* 2006;47:76-84.

Heart Transplantation

13

Jonathan D. Moreno and Kory J. Lavine

GENERAL PRINCIPLES

- Heart failure remains the leading cause of morbidity and mortality in the US, affecting an estimated 5.7 million adults, and at a cost of $31 billion dollars.[1]
- Despite tremendous advancement, heart failure is a growing problem, and 5-7% of patients will progress to an end stage of disease requiring advanced therapeutic options, including durable mechanical support (e.g., left ventricular assist device [LVAD] support), or orthotopic heart transplantation.
- Orthotopic heart transplant remains the treatment of choice in carefully selected individuals, with 1-year survival ~90% and a median survival of 14 years in those patients surviving the first year.[1,2]
- LVADs can be implanted as a bridge to transplantation (BTT) or as destination therapy (DT), with 1-year survival >90%.
- This chapter discusses the care and management of heart transplantation patients as well as those with LVADs.

TRANSPLANTATION PRINCIPLES OF MANAGEMENT

Immunosuppression

- The goal of immunosuppression in orthotopic heart transplantation is to induce immune tolerance, while balancing the risk of infection with oversuppression of the immune system, the risk of graft rejection with under-immunosuppression, and the side effects of the immunosuppressive drugs.
- Immune tolerance ensures host immune tolerance to the graft while allowing the recipient to defend against pathogens and malignancy.[1]
- This careful balance of immunosuppression is key to treatment following heart transplantation and ultimately determines organ longevity.[1]
- Given the close relationship between heart transplant rejection and T-cell responses to graft antigens, effective immunosuppression is directed at the suppression of T-cell function, proliferation, and subsequent immune system activation and amplification.[1]
- Dosing, side effects, and comments regarding immunosuppressive therapy are given in Table 13-1.
- **Induction therapy**
  - In the US, approximately half of transplant institutions routinely use induction therapy, the purpose of which is to provide intense early immunosuppression when donor antigen sensitization and the risk of acute rejection are highest.
  - Those at greatest risk for early rejection include younger patients, black or African American patients, those highly sensitized, and those with previous LVAD support.[1] Induction therapy can also be used in patients with borderline renal function to delay the initiation of nephrotoxic drugs.
  - Disadvantages of induction therapy are numerous and include increased risk of infection and malignancy, development of tolerance, as well as adverse reactions (e.g., serum sickness).

TABLE 13-1 SUMMARY OF DRUGS, DOSING, AND COMMON SIDE EFFECTS

	Initial dosing	Side effects	Comments
Lymphocyte-depleting agents			
Thymoglobulin	• 2 mg/kg IV x1, 1.5 mg/kg IV x2 q24hrs	• Serum sickness (fevers, chills, tachycardia, hypotension, myalgias, rash) • Leukopenia • Thrombocytopenia • Opportunistic infections (CMV)	• Antithymocyte antibody (rabbit) • Dose adjust for leukopenia, thrombocytopenia • Reinitiate CMV and fungal PPX • Premedicate with diphenhydramine, acetaminophen, methylprednisolone
Calcineurin inhibitors			
Tacrolimus	• 1 mg bid (PO or equivalent sublingual) • Dose titrated to goal trough level (0.5–10 mg bid)	• Hypertension • Renal injury • Dyslipidemia • Tremor • Headache • Neurotoxicity (PRES, seizures) • Diabetes • Hyperkalemia	• Monitor with daily trough levels (initial trough goal 8–12 ng/mL) • 1 mg sublingual ~2 mg PO • Concurrent use with diltiazem requires empiric 50% dose reduction • Concurrent use with azole antifungals (voriconazole, itraconazole, posaconazole) requires a 66% dose reduction
Cyclosporine	• 50–100 mg PO bid • Dose titrated to goal trough level (25–200 mg bid)	• Gingival hyperplasia • Hirsutism • Hypokalemia • Nephrotoxicity • Hypertension • Hyperlipidemia • Neurotoxicity	• Monitor with daily trough levels (initial trough goal 200–300 ng/mL) • Trough levels > 400 ng/mL are considered toxic

(continued)

TABLE 13-1 SUMMARY OF DRUGS, DOSING, AND COMMON SIDE EFFECTS *(continued)*

Antimetabolites

Mycophenolate mofetil (MMF)	• 1000 mg PO bid • Dose titrated (250–1500 mg bid)	• Leukopenia • GI distress (diarrhea, abdominal bloating and cramping, nausea, vomiting) is dose dependent	• May start 500 mg bid if infection concern (open chest, ECMO, CVVHD, fever) • 1500 mg bid recommended for high-risk (black or African American, young) patients and obese patients • Teratogenic: avoid in pregnancy
Azathioprine	• 2.5 mg/kg/day PO qday • Dose titrated (50–200 mg daily)	• Leukopenia • Opportunistic infections (viral, bacterial, fungal)	• Hold for WBC < 2K/mm³; platelets < 75K/mm³ • Contraindicated with concurrent use of allopurinol or febuxostat (or dose reduce ~75%)

Steroids

Prednisone	• Initial dosing 0.7 mg/kg total daily dose PO split bid (max 35 mg bid)	• Impaired glucose tolerance • Osteopenia	• Taper according to institutional protocol
Methylprednis-olone	• 500 mg IV daily for 3 doses	• Impaired glucose tolerance	• Used for both acute cellular and antibody-mediated rejection

mTOR inhibitors

Sirolimus	• Initial 1 mg PO daily (steady state at 2 weeks) • Titrate to goal trough level (0.5–5 mg/day)	• Delayed wound healing • Hyperlipidemia/hypertriglyceridemia • Lower extremity edema • Effusions (pleural/pericardial) • Rash • Bone marrow suppression • Mucositis/stomatitis	• mTOR inhibitors not recommended with cyclosporine (switch to tacrolimus) • Goal combined mTOR inhibitor and tacrolimus troughs of ~8–10 ng/mL • Can potentiate nephrotoxic effects of cyclosporine

	Initial dosing	Side effects	Comments
Everolimus	• 0.75 mg PO bid • Titrate to goal trough level (0.5–5 mg bid) • Steady state at 6 days	• Delayed wound healing • Hyperlipidemia • Lower extremity edema • Effusions (pleural/pericardial) • Rash • Bone marrow suppression • Mucositis/stomatitis	• mTOR inhibitors not recommended with cyclosporine (switch to tacrolimus) • Goal combined mTOR inhibitor and tacrolimus troughs of ~8–10 ng/mL • Can potentiate nephrotoxic effects of cyclosporine
Prophylaxis			
Bactrim SS (PJP)	• 1 tab PO MWF	• Hyperkalemia • Agranulocytosis (rare)	• Monitor for AKI in post-op period before initiation
Dapsone (PJP)	• 100 mg PO daily	• Nausea, vomiting, dizziness, loss of appetite • Methemoglobinemia, hemolytic anemia	• Check G6PD deficiency status before initiation
Clotrimazole troche (fungal)	• 10 mg PO qid after meals and at bedtime (dissolve in mouth over 15 minutes)	• GI distress • Nausea • Pruritus	• May increase tacrolimus levels ~2-fold
Nystatin (fungal)	• 5 mL swish and swallow qid	• GI distress • Nausea, vomiting • Mouth irritation	• Should be used if patient is intubated for an extended period of time
Fluconazole (fungal)	• 100 mg daily	• GI distress • Headache • Drowsiness	

(continued)

Drug	Dosing	Side Effects	Notes
Valganciclovir (CMV)	• 450–900 mg qday (dependent on CrCl)	• Leukopenia • Tremor • Diarrhea	• HSV prophylaxis in low-risk CMV patients (not requiring valganciclovir) can be achieved with acyclovir 200 mg bid for 3 months
Aspirin (CAV)	• 81 mg daily	• GI distress	
Statins (CAV)	• 20–40 mg qday	• Muscle cramps	• Monitor LFTs post-OHTx, before initiation
Injectables			
IV immunoglobulin (IVIG)	• 100 mg/kg after each plasmapheresis session, 500 mg/kg after final session	• Few side effects	• Premedicate with acetaminophen, diphenhydramine, and methylprednisolone
Rituximab (CD20)	• 375 mg/m² IV	• Easy bruising • Bloating • Burning or stinging of skin	• Premedicate with acetaminophen, diphenhydramine, and methylprednisolone (moderate risk of cytokine-release syndrome)
Bortezomib (proteasome inhibitor)	• 1.3 mg/m² IV × 4 doses	• Numbness, paresthesia • Diarrhea, constipation • Rash • Fatigue	• Must have ANC > 1K/mm³ and platelets > 70K/mm³ before initiation
Basiliximab (IL-2)	• 20 mg IV × 2 doses (POD#0 and POD#4)	• Few side effects	• No mortality benefit proven in OHTx but some evidence of decreased early rejection
Tocilizumab (IL-6)	• 4–8 mg/kg IV	• GI side effects (diarrhea, ulcers), increased cholesterol, benign increased transaminases	• Premedicate with acetaminophen, diphenhydramine, and methylprednisolone

ACR, acute cellular rejection; AKI, acute kidney injury; AMR, antibody-mediated rejection; ANC, absolute neutrophil count; CAV, cardiac allograft vasculopathy; CMV, cytomegalovirus; CrCl, creatinine clearance; CVVHD, continuous veno-venous hemofiltration; ECMO, extracorporeal membrane oxygenation; G6PD, glucose-6-phosphate dehydrogenase; GI, gastrointestinal; HSV, herpes simplex virus; LFT, liver function test; mTOR, mammalian target of rapamycin; OHTx, orthotopic heart transplant; PJP, *Pneumocystis jirovecii* pneumonia; POD, post-op day; PPX, prophylaxis; PRES, posterior reversible encephalopathy syndrome; WBC, white blood cell.

- The induction agents used clinically include polyclonal antithymocyte antibodies ATGAM (horse) or thymoglobulin (rabbit), as well as interleukin-2 (IL-2) receptor antagonists, including basiliximab (Simulect) and daclizumab (Zenapax).[1] For both of these IL-2 receptor antagonists, there has been no mortality benefit proven, but there is some evidence of decreased early rejection.
- It is our practice that induction therapy is reserved for high-risk patients (e.g., those who are highly sensitized, have a positive crossmatch, or those with severe renal insufficiency), and the decision to use these agents is made on an individual basis.

- **Maintenance therapy**
  - Maintenance immunosuppression at most institutions is based on blocking multiple, complementary pathways of the immune system and includes a three-drug regimen that includes calcineurin inhibitor (CNI), antimetabolites, and glucocorticoids.
  - **CNIs**
    - CNIs block T-cell–receptor activation and calcineurin signaling in the T cell and inhibit the activation of NFAT (nuclear factor of the activated T cell). They also decrease the production of cytokines, which are important for T-cell proliferation, including IL-2.
    - Cyclosporine was the first CNI to be used clinically, but has since been supplanted by tacrolimus, which has a more favorable side-effect profile and has been associated with a decreased incidence of rejection episodes compared to cyclosporine.[3]
    - Side effects of tacrolimus include hypertension, nephrotoxicity, dyslipidemia, tremor, headache, posterior reversible encephalopathy syndrome (PRES), diabetes, and hyperkalemia. Cyclosporine can cause gingival hyperplasia and hypokalemia.
  - **Antimetabolites**
    - Antimetabolites interfere with the de novo synthesis of nucleic acids and inhibit the proliferation of both T and B lymphocytes.
    - The two common antimetabolites used clinically include azathioprine (Imuran) and mycophenolate mofetil (MMF) (CellCept).
    - MMF was shown to be superior in a multicenter, double-blind trial of 650 de novo heart transplant patients over azathioprine, in addition to cyclosporine (CsA) and corticosteroids.[4]
    - The most common side effects, which are dose dependent, of MMF include leukopenia and gastrointestinal (GI) upset (diarrhea, nausea, vomiting, belching, bloating, and abdominal cramping).
    - The side effects of azathioprine include nausea, vomiting, GI distress, and hair loss. Importantly, azathioprine and allopurinol coadministration should be avoided due to the toxic effects of increased 6-mercaptopurine, causing blood dyscrasias that can be fatal.
  - **Steroids**
    - Steroids are used as transcriptional regulators of many genes that affect leukocyte function. Their major effects include inhibition of gene expression that controls the production of cytokines, adhesion molecules, and inflammatory lipid modulators.[5]
    - Prednisone is gradually weaned over the course of the first year following transplant in patients considered low risk for rejection. However, high-risk patients (e.g., highly sensitized, history of prior rejection, or retransplant) should be maintained on low-dose prednisone indefinitely.
    - The benefits of steroid withdrawal include improved metabolic effects, weight loss, and improved cardiovascular risk profiles.
  - **Proliferation signal inhibitors**
    - Also known as mammalian target of rapamycin (mTOR) inhibitors, these drug block T-cell activation after stimulation by IL-2 and endothelial cell activation. Thus, their action is complementary to CNIs.

- Given their decreased incidence of nephrotoxicity, they are a useful alternative in patients with renal insufficiency.
- mTOR inhibition has also been shown to slow progression of cardiac allograft vasculopathy (CAV).
- The two common mTOR inhibitors currently in use are sirolimus (Rapamycin, Rapa, Rapamune) and everolimus (Certican).
- Major toxicities include delayed wound healing, hyperlipidemia, lower extremity edema, effusions, rash, and bone marrow suppression, leading to pancytopenia.
- **Opportunistic infection prophylaxis**
  - Following orthotopic heart transplantation, patients are at increased risk for opportunistic infections including cytomegalovirus (CMV), *Pneumocystis jirovecii* pneumonia (PJP), and oral candidiasis.
  - Depending on the patient's CMV risk status (donor status and recipient status), patients are started on valganciclovir for 3 to 6 months post-transplantation. Common side effects include leukopenia, tremor, and diarrhea.
  - All patients are started on Bactrim SS tablets tid weekly for PJP prophylaxis for the first year. If patients are allergic to Bactrim, dapsone or aerosolized pentamidine can be substituted.
  - Oral candidiasis prophylaxis includes clotrimazole troches four times daily for the first 3 months post-transplantation. Alternative therapies include nystatin or fluconazole.
  - Spontaneous bacterial endocarditis (SBE) prophylaxis is recommended during the first-year post-transplantation and includes 2 g amoxicillin 1 hour before dental procedures. Patients older than 1 year should continue to have SBE prophylaxis only if other risk factors exist (e.g., concomitant valve disease).

GRAFT SURVEILLANCE

- Because the risk of rejection is highest in the first months after transplantation, there is intensive graft surveillance immediately post-transplantation that tapers over the course of the first 2 years post-transplant.[5]
- Endomyocardial biopsy remains the gold standard for the diagnosis of acute cardiac allograft rejection.[6]
- Clinical indications for endomyocardial biopsy include routine surveillance to detect clinically silent rejection and clinical suspicion of acute rejection (e.g., onset of heart failure symptoms, hemodynamic compromise, or evidence of graft dysfunction).
- Though protocols vary, at our institution, this includes weekly biopsies and transthoracic echocardiograms (TTEs) for the first 4 weeks post-transplant, followed by biweekly for four biopsies/TTEs and then monthly until month 6 post-transplant. At that time, eligible patients are transitioned to a gene expression profiling test (AlloMAP). Additional "for-cause" biopsies are done on an individual patient basis based on the presence of rejection or after alteration of a patient's immunosuppression regimen.
- Donor-specific antibody (DSA) panels are measured at 6 months and 1 year.

EVALUATION OF SUSPECTED ALLOGRAFT REJECTION

- Rejection remains one of the most adverse outcomes to cardiac transplantation. It is often broken down into three phases: hyperacute, early cellular rejection, and antibody-mediated rejection (AMR).
- In the era of three-drug immunosuppression, the frequency of rejection is 20-40% within the first year.[2]
- Patients suspected of having an acute rejection episode should undergo a careful history and physical examination, paying particular attention to new-onset heart failure symptoms (orthopnea, shortness of breath, fluid retention) or new-onset arrhythmia.

- Physical examination findings that are abnormal may not be present or may be subtle. Evidence of heart failure including an S_3, evidence of increased jugular venous pressure (JVP), abdominal distension, and lower extremity edema should be carefully assessed.
- Hemodynamic status should be rapidly assessed, and consideration of intensive care unit (ICU)-level care should be entertained if there are signs of low-output heart failure (e.g., hypotension, oliguria, acute kidney injury, altered mentation).
- Routine blood chemistries should be obtained including complete blood count (CBC), comprehensive metabolic panel (CMP), troponin, N-terminal prohormone of brain natriuretic peptide (NT-proBNP), and coagulation profile. Other cardiac diagnostic tests including ECG, 2D echocardiogram, and CXR should be rapidly performed to assess graft function and assess for ischemia.
- Consultation with a cardiac transplantation specialist should take place early in the patient's clinical course to guide management decisions (e.g., initiation of steroids, intensified immunosuppression, or performance of an endomyocardial biopsy).
- **Cellular rejection**
  - Cellular rejection is an acute form of rejection, characterized by the histologic appearance of interstitial leukocyte infiltration with concomitant myocyte damage.[1]
  - Diagnosis is made by endomyocardial biopsy and is graded based on well-established guidelines.[6] The International Society for Heart and Lung Transplantation (ISHLT) scale goes from 0R (no abnormal histopathologic findings) to 3R (evidence of diffuse infiltrate with multifocal myocyte damage, edema, hemorrhage, and/or vasculitis).[7]
  - Cellular rejection is usually treated with a steroid burst with variable increase in baseline immunosuppression. Severe cases may require cytolytic therapies (e.g., thymoglobulin or ATGAM—thymocyte immune globulin).
  - Follow-up biopsy ~2 weeks after rejection episode is usually done to assess for resolution of rejection.
- **AMR**
  - Also known as humoral or vascular rejection, AMR results from DSA production by the recipient's immune system. Notably, up to 24% of cases of rejection demonstrate concomitant cellular and AMR processes.[1,8]
  - The criteria for diagnosis include a bland endomyocardial biopsy (minimal cellular infiltrate).
  - Immunohistochemical staining is necessary for the diagnosis including positive C3d or C4d staining, intravascular CD68+ monocytes/macrophages, and a positive DSA panel.
  - Treatment is beyond the scope of this chapter but can include a course of plasmapheresis until DSAs are no longer present, IV immunoglobulin (IVIG) infusions and a monoclonal antibody treatment (e.g., rituximab [anti-CD20], tocilizumab [IL-6R inhibitor antibody]), or bortezomib (a proteasome inhibitor that triggers plasma cell apoptosis).
- **Cardiac allograft vasculopathy (CAV)**
  - CAV represents a long-term complication and is the leading cause of mortality in orthotopic heart transplantation.
  - Risk factors include hypertension, hyperlipidemia, smoking, and diabetes, as well as transplant-related sequelae including chronic inflammation, oxidant stress, and rejection.[1]
  - CAV is characterized by both focal and diffuse intimal proliferation of the epicardial coronary arteries and microvasculature. On coronary angiography, it manifests as distal pruning of tertiary vessels with progression to secondary and primary vasculature.
  - As the transplanted heart is denervated, patients will not feel typical anginal chest pain[1,5]; thus, patients receive annual coronary angiography and left heart catheterization for the first 3 years post-transplant, followed by angiography every ~3 years,

individualized to the patient's coronary history and renal function. In the years that cardiac catheterization is not performed, patients undergo noninvasive stress testing.

○ CAV prophylaxis includes statin therapy with pravastatin 20 to 80 mg daily. If low-density lipoprotein (LDL) remains suboptimally treated (LDL > 100 mg/dL), a high-intensity statin (atorvastatin 40 to 80 mg, rosuvastatin 10 to 40 mg) is substituted. Simvastatin is avoided, given the increased risk of rhabdomyolysis, when used in combination with CNIs. Unless contraindicated, all patients should receive enteric-coated aspirin 81 mg daily.

LEFT VENTRICULAR ASSIST DEVICE PRINCIPLES OF MANAGEMENT

General Principles

• The advent of durable mechanical circulatory support devices, especially LVADs, has dramatically changed the clinical course of patients with end-stage heart failure. Between 2010 and 2019, 25,551 patients underwent continuous-flow LVAD implantation.[9]
• LVADs have become a foundational treatment strategy for patients with end-stage heart failure, both in the setting of BTT and DT. As such, more patients are implanted with LVADs and are living longer on mechanical circulatory support.
• With current-generation LVADs, the 1-year survival rate is ~90%, which is close to that seen in orthotopic heart transplant.[10,11]
• Given the intricacy of the device and the complex interplay of mechanical and physiologic mechanisms, there has been an emergence of early and late complications associated with these devices.
• Immediately following LVAD implantation, the most prevalent complications include surgical bleeding, right heart failure, and ventricular arrhythmias (early complications); whereas pump thrombosis, GI bleeding, infection, device malfunction and failure, as well as neurologic events and dysrhythmias represent the most common late complications.

COMPLICATIONS

Overview of Complications[13]

• Bleeding requiring transfusion
  ○ 50-85% complication rate
  ○ Diagnosed with hemodynamic parameters, decrease in Hb levels, etc.
• Bleeding requiring reoperation
  ○ 30% complication rate
  ○ Often diagnosed with high chest tube output (> 200 mL/hr) which requires re-exploration surgery
• Infection
  ○ 50% complication rate with up to 10% of cases fungal in etiology
  ○ Driveline infections often present with erythema, drainage, and tenderness
  ○ Deeper tissue infections often diagnosed with the assistance of imaging, demonstrating fluid collections and/or abscess
  ○ Often requires anti-microbial therapy, incision & drainage, drive-line revisions, or pump exchange
• Arrhythmia
  ○ 50% complication rate
  ○ Need to distinguish between primary (scar-related myocardium), and secondary (electrolyte imbalance, hypotension, suction events)
  ○ Manage with IV fluid challenge and electrolyte correction, adjustments to pump speed, and treatment of primary arrhythmias with pharmacologic/electric cardioversion

- Pump thrombosis
  - 2-9% complication rate
  - Symptoms of congestive heart failure associated with elevations in power and biomarker abnormalities (LDH, haptoglobin, bilirubin)
  - Manage with intensification of anticoagulation; thrombolytics; surgical correction of malpositioned inflow or outflow cannula
- Suction event
  - Should have high clinical suspicion when recurrent arrhythmias or clinical hypovolemia
  - Echocardiography demonstrating collapsed LV supportive for diagnosis.
  - Manage with IV fluids to increase preload
- Right heart failure
  - 15-25% complication rate
  - Diagnosis: Post-operative inotropes requirement >14 days, inhaled nitric oxide >48hrs; need for right-sided circulatory support; reduced cardiac index and elevated CVP in absence of tamponade
  - Management: Pulmonary vasodilators (milrinone, inhaled nitric oxide, epoprostenol); inotropes; VA-ECMO; RVAD
- Device malfunction
  - <5% complication rate
  - Diagnosis: Alterations in pump speed, flows, power, or pulsatility index; clinical evidence of heart failure or hemolysis; absence of pump "hum" and MAP <40 mm Hg
  - Management: Ensuring adequate hydration; surgical correction of malpositioning or device malfunction; replacement of device. ACLS protocol if clinically indicated
- Stroke
  - 10-15% complication rate
  - Should obtain urgent non-contrast head CT when patient presents with acute neurological symptoms
  - If evidence of intracranial hemorrhage, strongly consider reversal of anticoagulation and expert consultation with neurosurgery or interventional radiology
- Cardiac arrest
  - ACLS treatment protocols should be followed
  - Chest compressions are appropriate and improve RV circulation
  - Defibrillation pads should be placed away from device

Bleeding

- Bleeding complications are unfortunately relatively common, with contemporary estimates being 20-30% for continuous flow (CF) LVADs.[12]
- With systemic anticoagulation and open sternotomy, early surgical site bleeding is prevalent, and treatment is left to the discretion of the surgical service but often includes delayed sternal closure and thoracic washout. Further treatment of surgical bleeding is beyond the scope of this chapter, but the reader is referred to Kilic et al.[13]
- Common etiologies in late nonsurgical site bleeding include systemic anticoagulation, acquired von Willebrand syndrome (similar pathophysiology to Heyde syndrome for aortic stenosis), and GI bleeding due to arteriovenous malformations (AVMs).
- Treatment includes medical management and endoscopic intervention; endoscopy remains the mainstay of intervention, and the diagnostic yield of conventional endoscopy is ~60-80%.
- Lesions identified with high-risk bleeding stigmata can achieve successful initial hemostasis in 80-90% of patients, although rebleeding commonly occurs in up to 50%.[12]
- Medical stabilization and management of GI bleeding remains the same, regardless of the presence of LVAD support (large-bore IV access, red blood cell [RBC] transfusion, acid suppression for melena, and hemodynamic support); however, fluid resuscitation must be done cautiously in this patient population.[12]

- Additional strategies with moderate data include the use of octreotide,[14-16] a somatostatin analog, which decreases acid secretion, splanchnic blood flow, and inhibition of angiogenesis and platelet aggregation, as well as thalidomide to treat AVMs and angiodysplasia.[17] Its mechanism is thought to be related to suppression of vascular endothelial growth factor (VEGF).
- Except for profound, hemodynamically significant bleeding, and drastically deranged international normalized ratio (INR), reversal of anticoagulation is generally deferred, in lieu of supportive management. Given the substantial risk of systemic thrombosis, reversal of anticoagulation needs to be made on a case-by-case basis, with the expertise of a multidisciplinary team.

Right Ventricular Failure

- Right ventricular failure (RVF) is a well-known and poorly understood postoperative complication of LVAD implantation and is associated with increased morbidity and mortality.[18,19]
- The diagnosis is typically made in patients who fail to wean from inotropes for >14 days or require mechanical right ventricular assist device (RVAD) support. Other hemodynamic variables that are suggestive include a cardiac index of <2.0 L/min/m^2, mixed venous O_2 saturation <55%, central venous pressure (CVP) >16 mm Hg, and a mean arterial pressure (MAP) <55 mm Hg.[13]
- The estimated prevalence of RVF is between 9 and 44% following LVAD implantation.[18,20]
- After LVAD implant, the altered hemodynamics of increased RV preload, increased RV diameter due to interventricular septal shift, and an increased demand for RV output to match the LV predispose to RVF.[21,22]
- Prevention of RVF is supported by pre-LVAD hemodynamic optimization, with aggressive diuresis to maintain a CVP < 15 mm Hg. Minimization of surgical site bleeding and the need for blood products reduces the risk of volume overload.[13]
- When RVF does occur, management strategies remain suboptimal and include optimization of LVAD flow to minimize septal shift and pharmacologic therapy for RV afterload reduction and pulmonary vasodilation (e.g., epoprostenol, inhaled nitric oxide).
- Inotropic support is sometimes necessary, with milrinone having the synergistic benefit of pulmonary vasodilation and improved cardiac contractility. Early biventricular support may be suitable for patients deemed to be at high risk.
- Given the increased morbidity and mortality of RVF, BTT patients with RVF should strongly be considered for expedited cardiac transplantation.[20]

Pump Thrombosis

- Patients with CF LVADs are at increased risk for pump thrombosis and hemolysis, which can place the patient at risk for device malfunction, peripheral emboli, stroke, hemodynamic instability, and death.[23]
- Pump thrombosis should be suspected in patients with hemolysis, unexplained heart failure, and abnormal pump parameters. Confirmed thrombosis is established by visual inspection or radiographic evidence.[24]
- Risk factors for pump thrombosis fall into three categories: (1) patient-related, (2) device-related, and (3) management-related factors.
  - Patient-related factors include infection, malignancy, hypercoagulable states (e.g., factor V Leiden mutation, antiphospholipid syndrome, protein C or S deficiency), atrial fibrillation, preexisting LV thrombus, and medical noncompliance.
  - Device-related factors include heat generated by the pump, blood/surface interactions, sheer stress–induced platelet interactions, areas of flow stasis, and inflow/outflow graft malposition (kinking or compression).

- ○ Management-related factors include inadequate anticoagulation, inadequate antiplatelet agents, and low pump speeds (which may have to be balanced in patients with GI bleeding and aortic insufficiency).[13]
- Key physical examination findings suggestive of pump thrombosis include an easily palpable pulse, a "grinding" LVAD sound, and an accentuated S_2 (increased aortic component). Patients may endorse hemoglobinuria (dark cola-colored urine).
- LVAD interrogations that suggest thrombosis include transient or sustained LVAD power elevations, decreased pump flows, or a change in the pulsatility index.
- Laboratory markers that are suggestive of hemolysis include anemia, elevated bilirubin and increased lactate dehydrogenase (LDH) (often defined as 2.5× the upper limit of normal), increased plasma-free hemoglobin (>20 mg/dL), decreased haptoglobin, and increased creatinine.[20]
- Initial diagnostic approach includes imaging such as CT angiography to confirm the position of inflow and outflow cannulas and to assess for the presence of thrombus.
- Echocardiography can be used to assess LV dilatation, presence of thrombus, mitral regurgitation, aortic valve opening, and pressure gradients at the inflow cannula. A ramp study can also be used to assess the severity of thrombus.[25,26]
- Initial management includes intensification of systemic anticoagulation with IV heparin and discontinuation of long-acting anticoagulants. IV fluid hydration should be used as clinically able to limit kidney injury from ongoing hemolysis and the nephrotoxic effects of sediment. Adjunct antiplatelet agents such as glycoprotein IIb/IIIa inhibitors and dipyridamole have also been used.
- With worsening heart failure symptoms, admission to an ICU for inotropic support, diuresis, and heparin may become necessary. A failure to improve clinically necessitates urgent consideration of candidacy for transplantation or pump exchange.
- Thrombolytics should be reserved for those patients deemed not to be surgical candidates.[13] After resolution of the acute event, our practice is to intensify oral anticoagulation with an INR goal of 2.5 to 3.5.
- Notably, the incidence of pump thrombosis has dramatically decreased with improvements in LVAD technology.[27]

Infection

- LVAD implantation is associated with a unique risk of infection, given combined internal and external components to the LVAD.
- In general, infection can manifest in the hardware, the body surfaces that are in contact with the hardware, the pump pocket, anastomoses, the percutaneous driveline, or the tunnel.[28]
- Driveline infection is the most common and is often caused by driveline trauma at the skin interface.[23,29] The most common pathogens associated with driveline and pump pocket infections tend to be *Staphylococcus aureus*, *Staphylococcus epidermidis*, and *Enterococcus*. These infections can track up into the pump pocket and subsequently lead to pump pocket infection and bloodstream infection.
- In general, most infections manifest with common local and systemic symptoms, including localized pain, erythema, induration or tenderness, and drainage, as well as fever, malaise, leukocytosis, and systemic response symptoms, though these "classic" signs were only present in 50% of patients in a retrospective review of 247 LVAD patients.[29]
- An initial treatment approach includes obtaining basic blood chemistries (e.g., leukocyte count, C-reactive protein [CRP], erythrocyte sedimentation rate [ESR]), multiple sets of blood cultures, aspirate for Gram stain and culture, tissue culture, and initiation of broad-spectrum antibiotics until culture sensitivities return.
- CT or ultrasound is useful for assessing for fluid collection or abscess and delineating the extent of the infection.[13]
- Treatment varies based on the extent of the infection, and consultation from infectious disease specialists to tailor antibiotic choice and duration of treatment is recommended.

If conservative management is not successful, or the extent of the infection is substantial, surgical management including incision and drainage and debridement may be necessary.
- In addition to driveline infection, pump-related infection should be considered with bacteremia in the absence of any other source of infection.[30] If LVAD-associated endocarditis is suspected, a transesophageal echocardiogram (TEE) should be obtained, but the diagnosis remains challenging, given suboptimal visualization with the metal surfaces of the LVAD.
- Explantation of the device may be required if the infection is associated with sepsis, septic emboli, or end-organ dysfunction.[13]

Device Malfunction and Failure

- Device malfunction and mechanical failure is a rare but potentially deadly complication of LVAD therapy. There are two common alarms on most LVADs, hazard and advisory alarms, which can be activated as a result of a change in the patient's circulatory physiology (e.g., low blood volume, hypertension, or thrombosis) or device-related such as battery failure or lead disconnection.[23,31,32]
- Hazard alarms indicate low-flow, pump turnoff or disconnection, low-voltage requiring immediate battery replacement or alternative power source, or complete loss of power.[33] Low-flow alarms indicate either an obstruction to the inflow pathway or device malfunction.
- In order of importance:
  ○ Ensure that the percutaneous driveline is properly connected to the controller, as well as a stable power source.
  ○ Auscultate the chest to determine whether the pump is actually running. Signs of pump failure include inability to auscultate the motor, undetectable blood pressure via Doppler, or the absence of the power light on the controller.[23,34] If the pump is not working, the pump should be restarted as soon as possible, given increasing risk of blood stasis and thrombus formation.
  ○ If the pump has ceased to function and cannot be restarted, immediate consultation with CT surgery, the on-call LVAD engineer, and the LVAD support team should be undertaken, while concurrently supporting the patient hemodynamically.
- Driveline fracture also tends to be a relatively common issue[35]; this is also known as short-to-shield. A majority of these fractures were isolated to the external portion of the driveline, with successful nonoperative reinforcement in most instances.[20,35] However, it is possible for driveline fracture and fault to happen to the internal, tunneled portion of the driveline, which may require surgical intervention. For short-to-shield events, ensure that the patient is either connected to batteries or on an **ungrounded** power cable.
- A full review of all of the device malfunction and alarms for each type of LVAD is beyond the scope of this chapter. The reader is urged to consult with the operating manual of the respective manufacturer, as well as the local LVAD support team, including the on-call LVAD engineer, CT surgeon, and LVAD nurse coordinator.
- Lastly, it is important to note that the basic and advanced cardiac life support (ACLS) pathways are always indicated in the right clinical context. As such, in the absence of a perfusing rhythm, chest compressions, external defibrillation, and pharmacologic support are never contraindicated and should be performed, regardless of the presence of the LVAD.[36]

Stroke and Intracranial Hemorrhage

- Stroke and intracranial hemorrhage remain among the most feared complications of LVAD use. In a study of the INTERMACS registry, the 1-month, 3-month, and 1-year stroke rates were 3, 5, and 11%, respectively.[37]
- Importantly, rates of stroke seem to be pump dependent, with rates of postimplant stroke being higher with the HeartWare device compared to the HeartMate 3. The ENDURANCE supplemental trial found an association between tighter blood pressure control

and decreased risk of adverse neurologic events. It is recommended that patients with the HeartWare HVAD aim for an MAP < 70 mm Hg.[38]

- Regarding management of an acute neurologic event, an emergent workup should include assessment of anticoagulation status (current anticoagulants, antiplatelets, INR, and basic laboratories) and imaging with a noncontrast head CT to differentiate ischemic and hemorrhagic stroke.
- In the setting of a hemorrhagic stroke, reversal agents must be weighed against the potential risk of pump thrombosis, and decisions should be made within a team-based approach. For large intracranial hemorrhages, reversal agents include prothrombin complex concentrate (PCC), fresh-frozen plasma, vitamin K, and desmopressin acetate. The decision of which agent(s) to use is generally institution specific.

Dysrhythmias

- The incidence of arrhythmias in end-stage heart failure is relatively high, with both LVAD-independent (primary) and LVAD-dependent (secondary to LVAD implantation) mechanisms contributing to their high prevalence.
- While the incidence of arrhythmia is highest in the first 30 days postimplant, ventricular arrhythmia can also manifest as a late complication.[39]
- With LVAD support, many (but not all) patients can maintain a perfusing cardiac output despite tachyarrhythmia. This has allowed liberalization of tachy therapy parameters, with increasing detection limits and additional antitachycardia pacing (ATP) before ultimately requiring defibrillation. It is important to note, however, that extended periods of ventricular arrhythmia can predispose to suck-down events, thrombus formation, RV dysfunction, and poor perfusion.[23,40,41]
- The emergency management of tachyarrhythmia follows the same ACLS algorithm, regardless of the presence of an LVAD.[23,36] As mentioned however, patients are often able to tolerate tachyarrhythmias for extended periods of time before becoming hemodynamically unstable. As such, expanded maneuvers to stabilize the heart rhythm before defibrillation can and should be attempted. These include chemical cardioversion (e.g., amiodarone bolus) as well as manual ATP therapy if a patient has an implanted device.
- In parallel, evaluation for the underlying etiology should commence; principal causes for arrhythmia include suck-down events caused by inadequate preload and hypovolemia. A fluid bolus and emergent echo to assess volume status can help rule in this diagnosis. Electrolyte abnormalities should be corrected.
- If the clinical presentation is consistent with acute coronary syndrome, coronary angiography should be considered.[23]
- Lastly, ambulatory implantable cardioverter-defibrillator (ICD) firing should be evaluated for potential inappropriate shocks secondary to lead issues, oversensing, or electromagnetic interference.[39]

REFERENCES

1. Furiasse N, Kobashigawa JA. Immunosuppression and adult heart transplantation: emerging therapies and opportunities. *Expert Rev Cardiovasc Ther.* 2017;15:59-69.
2. Lund LH, Edwards LB, Kucheryavaya AY, et al. The registry of the International Society for Heart and Lung Transplantation: thirty-second official adult heart transplantation report—2015; focus theme: early graft failure. *J Heart Lung Transplant.* 2015;34:1244-54.
3. Kobashigawa JA, Miller LW, Russell SD, et al. Tacrolimus with mycophenolate mofetil (MMF) or sirolimus vs. cyclosporine with MMF in cardiac transplant patients: 1-year report. *Am J Transplant.* 2006;6:1377-86.
4. Kobashigawa J, Miller L, Renlund D, et al. A randomized active-controlled trial of mycophenolate mofetil in heart transplant recipients. Mycophenolate Mofetil Investigators. *Transplantation.* 1998;66:507-15.

5. Edwards NM, Chen JM, Mazzeo PA, eds. *Cardiac Transplantation: The Columbia University Medical Center/New York-Presbyterian Hospital Manual.* Humana Press; 2014.

6. Costanzo MR, Dipchand A, Starling R, et al. The international society of heart and lung transplantation guidelines for the care of heart transplant recipients. *J Heart Lung Transplant.* 2010;29:914-56.

7. Stewart S, Winters GL, Fishbein MC, et al. Revision of the 1990 working formulation for the standardization of nomenclature in the diagnosis of heart rejection. *J Heart Lung Transplant.* 2005;24:1710-20.

8. Kfoury AG, Hammond ME, Snow GL, et al. Cardiovascular mortality among heart transplant recipients with asymptomatic antibody-mediated or stable mixed cellular and antibody-mediated rejection. *J Heart Lung Transplant.* 2009;28:781-4.

9. Molina EJ, Shah P, Kiernan MS, et al. The Society of Thoracic Surgeons Intermacs 2020 annual report. *Ann Thorac Surg.* 2021;111:778-792.

10. Strueber M, Larbalestier R, Jansz P, et al. Results of the post-market Registry to Evaluate the Heart-Ware Left Ventricular Assist System (ReVOLVE). *J Heart Lung Transplant.* 2014;33:486-91.

11. Netuka I, Sood P, Pya Y, et al. Fully magnetically levitated left ventricular assist system for treating advanced HF: a multicenter study. *J Am Coll Cardiol.* 2015;66:2579-89.

12. Cushing K, Kushnir V. Gastrointestinal bleeding following LVAD placement from top to bottom. *Dig Dis Sci.* 2016;61:1440-7.

13. Kilic A, Acker MA, Atluri P. Dealing with surgical left ventricular assist device complications. *J Thorac Dis.* 2015;7:2158-64.

14. Rennyson SL, Shah KB, Tang DG, et al. Octreotide for left ventricular assist device-related gastrointestinal hemorrhage: can we stop the bleeding? *ASAIO J.* 2013;59:450-1.

15. Coutance G, Saplacan V, Belin A, et al. Octreotide for recurrent intestinal bleeding due to ventricular assist device. *Asian Cardiovasc Thorac Ann.* 2014;22:350-2.

16. Dang G, Grayburn R, Lamb G, et al. Octreotide for the management of gastrointestinal bleeding in a patient with a heartware left ventricular assist device. *Case Rep Cardiol.* 2014;2014:826453.

17. Chan LL, Lim CP, Lim CH, et al. Novel use of thalidomide in recurrent gastrointestinal tract bleeding in patients with left ventricular assist devices: a case series. *Heart Lung Circ.* 2017;26:1101-04.

18. Morine KJ, Kiernan MS, Pham DT, et al. Pulmonary artery pulsatility index is associated with right ventricular failure after left ventricular assist device surgery. *J Card Fail.* 2016;22:110-16.

19. Kang G, Ha R, Banerjee D. Pulmonary artery pulsatility index predicts right ventricular failure after left ventricular assist device implantation. *J Heart Lung Transplant.* 2016;35:67-73.

20. Grimm JC, Magruder JT, Kemp CD, Shah AS. Late complications following continuous-flow left ventricular assist device implantation. *Front Surg.* 2015;2:42.

21. Matthews JC, Koelling TM, Pagani FD, Aaronson KD. The right ventricular failure risk score a pre-operative tool for assessing the risk of right ventricular failure in left ventricular assist device candidates. *J Am Coll Cardiol.* 2008;51:2163-72.

22. Topilsky Y, Hasin T, Oh JK, et al. Echocardiographic variables after left ventricular assist device implantation associated with adverse outcome. *Circ Cardiovasc Imaging.* 2011;4:648-61.

23. Robertson J, Long B, Koyfman A. The emergency management of ventricular assist devices. *Am J Emerg Med.* 2016;34:1294-301.

24. Rosenthal JL, Starling RC. Coagulopathy in mechanical circulatory support: a fine balance. *Curr Cardiol Rep.* 2015;17:114.

25. Goldstein DJ, John R, Salerno C, et al. Algorithm for the diagnosis and management of suspected pump thrombus. *J Heart Lung Transplant.* 2013;32:667-70.

26. Uriel N, Morrison KA, Garan AR, et al. Development of a novel echocardiography ramp test for speed optimization and diagnosis of device thrombosis in continuous-flow left ventricular assist devices: the Columbia ramp study. *J Am Coll Cardiol.* 2012;60:1764-75.

27. Mehra MR, Naka Y, Uriel N, et al. A fully magnetically levitated circulatory pump for advanced heart failure. *N Engl J Med.* 2017;376:440-50.

28. Hannan MM, Husain S, Mattner F, et al. Working formulation for the standardization of definitions of infections in patients using ventricular assist devices. *J Heart Lung Transplant.* 2011;30:375-84.

29. Nienaber JJ, Kusne S, Riaz T, et al. Clinical manifestations and management of left ventricular assist device-associated infections. *Clin Infect Dis.* 2013;57:1438-48.

30. Nienaber J, Wilhelm MP, Sohail MR. Current concepts in the diagnosis and management of left ventricular assist device infections. *Expert Rev Anti Infect Ther.* 2013;11:201-10.

31. Fukamachi K, Shiose A, Massiello AL, et al. Implantable continuous-flow right ventricular assist device: lessons learned in the development of a Cleveland Clinic device. *Ann Thorac Surg.* 2012;93:1746-52.

32. Sayer G, Naka Y, Jorde UP. Ventricular assist device therapy. *Cardiovasc Ther.* 2009;27:140-50.
33. Federal Drug Administration. HeartMate II® LVAS—left ventricular assist system: instructions for use. 2009. https://www.accessdata.fda.gov/cdrh_docs/pdf6/P060040S005c.pdf
34. Greenwood JC, Herr DL. Mechanical circulatory support. *Emerg Med Clin North Am.* 2014;32:851-69.
35. Puehler T, Ensminger S, Schoenbrodt M, et al. Mechanical circulatory support devices as destination therapy-current evidence. *Ann Cardiothorac Surg.* 2014;3:513-24.
36. Wilson SR, Givertz MM, Stewart GC, Mudge GH Jr. Ventricular assist devices the challenges of outpatient management. *J Am Coll Cardiol.* 2009;54:1647-59.
37. Kirklin JK, Naftel DC, Kormos RL, et al. Fifth INTERMACS annual report: risk factor analysis from more than 6,000 mechanical circulatory support patients. *J Heart Lung Transplant.* 2013;32:141-56.
38. Milano CA, Rogers JG, Tatooles AJ, et al. HVAD: the ENDURANCE supplemental trial. *JACC Heart Fail.* 2018;6:792-802.
39. Nakahara S, Chien C, Gelow J, et al. Ventricular arrhythmias after left ventricular assist device. *Circ Arrhythm Electrophysiol.* 2013;6:648-54.
40. Ziv O, Dizon J, Thosani A, et al. Effects of left ventricular assist device therapy on ventricular arrhythmias. *J Am Coll Cardiol.* 2005;45:1428-34.
41. Klein T, Jacob MS. Management of implantable assisted circulation devices: emergency issues. *Cardiol Clin.* 2012;30:673-82.

Cardio-Oncology: Essentials for Effective Consultation

14

Joshua D. Mitchell and Daniel J. Lenihan

GENERAL PRINCIPLES

- Cancer therapy, including radiation, chemotherapy, and targeted agents, can have substantial effects on the vasculature, myocardium, electrical system, and pericardium.
- Patients seen within the realm of Cardio-Oncology (CO) are often complex with significant comorbidities that can directly affect their cardiovascular (CV) care. Thrombocytopenia, for instance, often influences treatment decisions.
- **A collaborative multidisciplinary team, including cardiologists and oncologists, is essential to optimizing patient management.** The team should work together to select the best cancer therapy for a given patient's overall survival, limiting and mitigating cardiotoxicity, if possible, and minimizing treatment interruptions.
- **Cardiac risk factors** should be assessed and treated in all patients.
- **Screening programs** help identify patients with early CV toxicity. Early treatment of left ventricular (LV) dysfunction has been shown to limit long-term sequelae.
- Patients at highest risk for cardiotoxicity may benefit from prophylactic **cardioprotective medications** that can include dexrazoxane, β-blockers, angiotensin-converting enzyme inhibitors (ACE-Is) and angiotensin-receptor blockers (ARBs), aldosterone antagonists, aspirin, anticoagulants, and statins.

Definition

- **CO** broadly addresses the CV care of a patient with cancer or a history of cancer and **includes the prevention of, screening for, and treatment of cardiotoxicity secondary to the short- or long-term effects of their cancer therapy**. The importance of having CO specialists has grown as a direct result of the explosion of new cancer therapies with varying mechanisms of action and adverse effects on the CV system.
- Cardiotoxicity/CV toxicity refers to damage to the heart and/or vasculature. For patients undergoing cancer treatment, or for those with a history of exposure, clinicians should have a high index of suspicion that the cancer therapy could be a contributing factor.
- **CV toxicity can be clinically apparent immediately, years, or even decades after anticancer therapy**.

Classification

- Cardiotoxicity can be classified using the **Common Terminology Criteria for Adverse Events (CTCAE)** developed by the National Cancer Institute for codification of adverse events during oncology trials[1] (https://ctep.cancer.gov/protocolDevelopment/adverse_effects.htm). In the classification scheme, adverse events are graded from 1 (mild) to 5 (death).
- Due to discrepancies in definitions and reporting with CTCAE, **events are often underreported in oncology trials**.[2] Real-world patients also have a higher incidence of CV comorbidities, placing them at higher risk for CV events.[3] Postmarketing analysis, therefore, often reveals higher incidence/prevalence of cardiac events than anticipated during the oncology trials. Some adverse effects, such as myocarditis with checkpoint inhibitors, may go unrecognized until after the drug hits the market.

- While anticancer therapies can have wide-ranging cardiotoxic effects, most classification schemes have focused more narrowly on LV dysfunction. Various cutoffs for evaluating LV dysfunction have been defined in addition to the CTCAE (Table 14-1), which can complicate comparative reporting of events.

Epidemiology

- As of January 2019, there were 16.9 million cancer survivors, a number expected to grow to by 31% to 22.2 million by 2029.[4]
- **CV events are second only to malignancy in their impact on morbidity and mortality among cancer survivors in general**.[5]
- In older patients diagnosed with breast cancer, CV death has been found to be even more prevalent than death due to the cancer itself.[6]
- The cumulative incidence of heart failure (HF) continues to steadily increase yearly following anthracycline and trastuzumab therapy, measuring 20.1% at 5 years.[7]
- The incidence and prevalence of CV disease is higher in real-world patients outside clinical trials.[3]

Etiology

- **CV events** are prevalent in patients with cancer due to **common risk factors** (age, tobacco use, etc.) as well as on-target and off-target **effects of anticancer therapies**. The **cancer type** may also play a role. HF, for instance, has been noted much more frequently in patients with multiple myeloma, irrespective of treatment.[8]
- Documented CV toxicities include, but are not limited to, arrhythmias and QTc prolongation, fulminant myocarditis or HF from checkpoint inhibitors, hemorrhagic pericarditis from cyclophosphamide, constrictive pericarditis from radiation, hypertension and associated LV dysfunction from vascular endothelial growth factor (VEGF) signaling pathway (VSP) inhibitors, arterial and thromboembolism from VSP inhibitors and immunomodulatory agents, and LV dysfunction from anthracyclines, HER2 antagonists, proteasome inhibitors, and MEK inhibitors.

Risk Factors

- **Cardiotoxicity from anthracyclines and radiation is directly related to the total dose or exposure**. Mediastinal radiation $\geq$ 30 Gray (with the heart in the treatment field), doxorubicin $\geq$ 250 mg/m^2 (or epirubicin $\geq$ 600 mg/m^2), and the combination of anthracyclines or radiation at any dose have been identified as particularly significant risk factors for LV dysfunction and HF.[9]
- In addition to the increased relative risk for the development of cardiac dysfunction related to specific anticancer therapies, traditional cardiac risk factors increase the likelihood of CV toxicity from any anticancer treatment.
- Risk factors for the development of HF include older age, smoking, hypertension, hyperlipidemia, diabetes mellitus, obesity, baseline LV dysfunction or prior HF, history of atherosclerotic CV disease, valvular heart disease, frailty, and poor cardiorespiratory fitness.
- Presence of hypertension, specifically, leads to a relative risk of coronary artery disease (CAD) requiring treatment 24-fold over radiation alone and also to a relative risk of HF 44-fold over anthracycline alone in childhood survivors of cancer.[10]
- For **childhood survivors of cancer within 5 years of their cancer diagnosis, a CV risk calculator** can be found at https://ccss.stjude.org/tools-documents/calculators-other-tools/ccss-cardiovascular-risk-calculator.html.[11]
- A risk score for incident HF within 3 years of receiving trastuzumab has also been developed and includes adjuvant chemotherapy, age, and the presence of CAD, atrial fibrillation/flutter, diabetes mellitus, hypertension, and renal failure.[12]

TABLE 14-1 CARDIOTOXICITY CLASSIFICATION CRITERIA FOR HEART FAILURE AND LV DYSFUNCTION

	Severity		
	Mild	Moderate	Severe
Cardiac review and evaluation committee, definition of chemotherapy-induced cardiotoxicity	Any one of the following: 1) Reduction of LVEF, either global or specific in the interventricular septum 2) Symptoms of congestive HF 3) Signs associated with HF, such as S_3 gallop, tachycardia, or both 4) Reduction in LVEF from baseline ≥5% to <55% in the presence of signs or symptoms of HF, or a reduction in LVEF ≥10% to <55% without signs or symptoms of HF		
NYHA classification	Class I No symptoms.	Class II Mild symptoms and slight limitation during ordinary activity	Class III Marked limitation due to symptoms, even with less than ordinary activity.	Class IV Symptoms at rest.
ACCF/AHA stages of HF	Stage A At high risk for HF but without structural disease or symptoms of HF.	Stage B Structural heart disease but without signs or symptoms of HF.	Stage C Structural heart disease with prior or current symptoms of HF.	Stage D Refractory HF requiring specialized interventions.
CTCAE v5.0 Ejection fraction decreased[a]		Grade 2 Resting EF 50-40%; 10-19% drop from baseline	Grade 3 Resting EF 39-20%; ≥20% drop from baseline	Grade 4 Resting EF < 20%
CTCAE v5.0 LV systolic dysfunction[a]		Grade 3 Symptomatic due to drop in EF responsive to intervention	Grade 4 Symptomatic due to drop in EF due to drop in EF responsive to intervention	Grade 4 Refractory or poorly controlled HF due to drop in EF; intervention such as ventricular assist device, IV vasopressor support, or heart transplant indicated

	Grade 1	Grade 2	Grade 3	Grade 4
CTCAE v5 Heart failure[a]	Asymptomatic with laboratory (e.g., BNP) or cardiac imaging abnormalities	Symptoms with moderate activity or exertion	Symptoms at rest or with minimal activity or exertion; hospitalization; new onset of symptoms	Life-threatening consequences; urgent intervention indicated (e.g., continuous IV therapy or mechanical hemodynamic support)
Package insert guidelines to hold cancer therapy due to LV dysfunction	**Trastuzumab** ≥16% absolute decrease in LVEF or ≥10% drop to below institutional limits of normal		**Pertuzumab** ≥10% drop in LVEF to <50% for early breast cancer, ≥10% drop in LVEF to 40–45% for metastatic breast cancer, or drop to < 40%	
2014 Echo guidelines for subclinical LV dysfunction	**Subclinical LV dysfunction** > 15% relative drop in GLS from baseline		**CTRCD** Drop in LVEF of > 10 percentage points to a level < 53%. Should be confirmed by repeat testing.	
2016 ESC position statement	**Mild (asymptomatic)** LVEF < 50% or LVEF reduction > 10% from baseline, should be repeated within 3–4 weeks		**Moderate (symptomatic from HF)** LVEF <50%	
2017 ASCO guideline		**All cancer therapy** Cardiotoxicity not specifically defined		
2020 ESMO guideline	**Mild (asymptomatic)** LVEF > 15% from baseline if LVEF >50%	**Anthracycline or trastuzumab related**	**Moderate** Symptomatic HF regardless of LVEF **Moderate** LVEF ≥10% from baseline, or Any drop of LVEF to <50% but ≥40%	**Severe** LVEF < 40%

	Severity		
	Mild	Moderate	Severe
2021 ICOS definition asymptomatic CTRCD (with or without additional biomarkers)	**Mild** New LVEF reduction to ≥50% AND new fall in GLS by >15% With or without new rise in cardiac biomarkers[b]	**Moderate** New LVEF reduction to >10% and to 40-49% New LVEF reduction by <10% and to 40-49% AND new fall in GLS by >15% With or without new rise in cardiac biomarkers[b]	**Severe** New LVEF reduction to <40%
2021 ICOS definition symptomatic CTRCD (with LVEF and supportive diagnostic biomarkers)	**Mild** Mild HF symptoms, no intensification of therapy required	**Moderate** Need for outpatient intensification of diuretic and HF therapy	**Severe** HF hospitalization
			Very Severe Requiring inotropic support, mechanical circulatory support, or consideration for transplantation

ACCF, American College of Cardiology Foundation; AHA, American Heart Association; ASE, American Society of Echocardiography; BNP, brain natriuretic peptide; CTCAE, Common Terminology Criteria for Adverse Events; CTRCD, cancer therapeutics-related cardiac dysfunction; ESC, European Society of Cardiology; ESMO, European Society for Medical Oncology; GLS, global longitudinal strain; HF, heart failure; ICOS, International Cardio-Oncology Society; LVEF, Left ventricular ejection fraction; NYHA: New York Heart Association.

[a] Oncology trial investigators can choose to classify a given event under "ejection fraction decreased," "LV systolic dysfunction," or "Heart Failure" with associated grades if they decide the adverse effect is related to the intervention. This contributes to difficulty in comparing results of trials and effects of cancer therapies. Grade 1 – Grade 4 (mild to severe). Death = Grade 5. No grade 5 for "ejection fraction decreased."

[b] Cardiac troponin I/T >99th percentile, BNP ≥ 35 pg/mL, NT-proBNP ≥125 pg/mL

PATHOPHYSIOLOGY AND SPECIFIC TOXICITIES

- While comprehensive, this should not be considered a complete list of toxicities (Table 14-2). Adverse effects may only be noted with postmarketing surveillance, and actual risk may be higher in patients outside clinical trials due to higher incidence of comorbidities.
- Clinicians treating patients with cancer should always maintain an index of suspicion that the underlying therapy can contribute to the patient's CV presentation.

Alkylating Agents

- **Examples**: cyclophosphamide, ifosfamide, cisplatin, melphalan
- **Mechanism of action**: adds methyl, alkyl, or other side groups to DNA leading to DNA fragments, cross-linking, and/or nucleotide mispairing, ultimately leading to cell death
- **Main CV adverse effects**:
  - ○ Hemorrhagic myopericarditis (7-25% with high-dose cyclophosphamide >150 mg/kg)[13]
  - ○ Symptomatic cardiomyopathy (22% with cyclophosphamide)
  - ○ Venous and arterial thromboembolism: 12.9% with cisplatin in patients with urothelial transitional cell carcinoma[14]
  - ○ Hypertension (9.4%), hyperlipidemia (7.9%), and Raynaud phenomenon (33.4%) with cisplatin in patients with testicular cancer[15]

Androgen Deprivation Therapy and Antiandrogens

- **Examples**:
  - ○ Gonadotropin-releasing hormone (GnRH) agonists: goserelin, histrelin, leuprolide, triptorelin
  - ○ GnRH antagonists: degarelix
  - ○ Androgen synthesis inhibitor: abiraterone
  - ○ Antiandrogens: bicalutamide, enzalutamide, flutamide, nilutamide
- **Mechanism of action**: modulates the gonadotropin–testosterone axis to reduce testosterone levels to castrate levels. Can result in overproduction of other adrenal hormones, such as aldosterone
- **Main CV adverse effects**: metabolic syndrome, coronary heart disease, myocardial infarction, hypertension. The exact CV impact of androgen deprivation therapy remains controversial. Androgen deprivation therapy consistently results in an unfavorable metabolic profile; however, studies have been conflicted regarding the degree it increases CV events above that of baseline risk factors.[16]
- Due to the mechanism of action, an aldosterone antagonist would be uniquely suited to treat associated hypertension, though this has not been directly studied.

Anthracyclines

- **Examples**: daunorubicin, doxorubicin, epirubicin, idarubicin, mitoxantrone
- **Mechanism of action**: inhibits topoisomerase II, inducing DNA strand breaks and apoptosis
- **Main adverse CV effects**:
  - ○ LV dysfunction—7% at dose of 150 mg/m^2 of doxorubicin[17]
  - ○ HF—26% at dose of 550 mg/m^2 of doxorubicin[17]
- Inhibition of topoisomerase IIb in cardiac tissue has been implicated in causing LV dysfunction.
- Anthracyclines also lead to generation of free radicals and reactive oxidant species with resultant oxidative damage.
- Toxicity is dose dependent, with ≥250 mg/m^2 of doxorubicin equivalent (≥600 mg/m^2 of epirubicin) found to be a threshold for increased risk for toxicity. Conversion rates and thresholds for toxicity are specific to the anthracycline used.

TABLE 14-2 TOXICITIES ASSOCIATED WITH CANCER THERAPIES

Anticancer agents	Type of cardiotoxicity	Reported frequency
Alkylating agent (cyclophosphamide, ifosfamide, cisplatin)	Hemorrhagic myopericarditis (with high dose)	7–25%
	Symptomatic cardiomyopathy	22%
	Venous and arterial thromboembolism	12.9%
	Hypertension	9.4%
	Hyperlipidemia	7.9%
	Raynaud phenomenon	33.4%
Androgen deprivation therapy/antiandrogen	Metabolic syndrome	[a]
	Aldosterone-associated hypertension	
Anthracyclines (doxorubicin, daunorubicin, epirubicin, idarubicin, mitoxantrone)	LV dysfunction (dose dependent)	7% at 150 mg/m^{2b}
	Heart failure (dose dependent)	26% at 550 mg/m^{2b}
Checkpoint inhibitors (ipilimumab, nivolumab, pembrolizumab)	Myocarditis (rare but potentially fatal)	1%
	Heart failure	[a]
	Arrhythmia	[a]
Chimeric antigen receptor (CAR) T-cell therapy	Tachycardia	26–57%
	Grade 3 or higher	2–4%
	Arrhythmia	23%
	Grade 3 or higher	7%
	Cardiac arrest	4%
	Cardiac failure	6–7%
Fluoropyrimidine (5-FU, capecitabine)	Coronary vasospasm	0–19%
	Myocardial infarction	0–2%
HER2-targeted therapy (trastuzumab, pertuzumab)	LV dysfunction	9.4%
	with anthracyclines	18.6%
	Heart failure	0.4–12%
	with anthracyclines	2–20%

Immunomodulatory agent
(thalidomide, lenalidomide, pomalidomide)

Venous thromboembolism	0–75%
Arterial thromboembolism	~5%
Sinus bradycardia (thalidomide)	26%
severe or life-threatening	3%

MEK/BRAF inhibitors
(binimetinib, cobimetinib, trametinib; dabrafenib, encorafenib, vemurafenib)

LV dysfunction	7–26%
QTc prolongation (especially vemurafenib—concentration dependent)	

PI3K/AKT/mTOR inhibitors
(everolimus, idelalisib, temsirolimus)

Hyperglycemia, hypercholesterolemia, hypertriglyceridemia	>50%

Proteasome inhibitors
(bortezomib, carfilzomib)

Hypertension	8–23%
Heart failure (carfilzomib)	4%

Radiation (mediastinal/thoracic)

Arrhythmia	16%
Autonomic dysfunction	30–45%
Coronary heart disease	19–20%
Heart failure	11–12%
Pacemaker/ICD malfunction	3%
Pericardial disease	5%
Valvular heart disease	11–31%

Tyrosine kinase inhibitors
(see also VSP inhibitors, HER2 antagonists, and mTOR inhibitors)
Incidence of adverse effects varies with specific drugs.

Arterial thromboembolic event (ponatinib)
Atrial fibrillation (ibrutinib)
Atherosclerosis (nilotinib)
Bleeding (ibrutinib)
Bradyarrhythmia (trametinib)
Edema (imatinib)
Hypertension (ibrutinib, trametinib, nilotinib)
LV dysfunction (ponatinib, trametinib)
QT prolongation (trametinib, dabrafenib, nilotinib)
Venous thromboembolic event (ponatinib, erlotinib, trametinib, nilotinib)

(continued)

TABLE 14-2 TOXICITIES ASSOCIATED WITH CANCER THERAPIES (continued)

Anticancer agents	Type of cardiotoxicity	Reported frequency
VSP inhibitors (bevacizumab, pazopanib, sunitinib, sorafenib, axitinib)	Arterial thromboembolic event	0–5.4%
	Hypertension	20–91%
	LV dysfunction	10–15%
	Venous thromboembolic event	2–11.9%
	QT prolongation > 500 ms (vandetanib)	2.7%
Other cancer therapies		
Arsenic trioxide	QT prolongation	38%
	Heart failure, myocardial infarction, supraventricular tachycardia	<5% [a]
Decitabine	Autonomic dysfunction	3%
Docetaxel/paclitaxel	QT prolongation	23%
Ribociclib	Arrhythmias	6%
Tretinoin	Heart failure	3.2%
Vorinostat	QT prolongation	

LV, left ventricle; CAR, chimeric antigen receptor; FU, fluorouracil; HER2, human epithelial growth factor; ICD, implantable cardioverter-defibrillator; mTOR, mammalian target of rapamycin; VSP, vascular endothelial growth factor signaling pathway.

[a] Exact incidence unknown and/or studies conflicting.

[b] Doxorubicin equivalent dose.

- As a general rule of thumb, patients receive 50 mg/m^2 of doxorubicin per cycle of chemotherapy in breast cancer and lymphoma.
- Dexrazoxane is US Food and Drug Administration (FDA) approved to prevent cardiotoxicity from anthracyclines. Evidence suggests that dexrazoxane may achieve its cardioprotective benefit from its antioxidant properties and interfering with the effect of anthracyclines on topoisomerase IIb in the heart.
- Carvedilol may achieve part of its cardioprotective benefit due to its antioxidant properties, a characteristic not shared by metoprolol.

Checkpoint Inhibitors (PD-1/PDL-1 and CTLA-4 Inhibitors)

- **Examples**: atezolizumab, avelumab, cemiplimab, durvalumab, ipilimumab, nivolumab, pembrolizumab
- **Mechanism of action**: PD-1/PDL-1 and CTLA-4 serve as checkpoints on the immune system. Some cancers are able to activate these receptors to turn the immune system off. By inhibiting these checkpoints, the immune system is activated and attacks the cancer.
- **Main adverse CV effects**:
  - Myocarditis is rare (1%) but can be fatal.[18-20]
  - HF can occur with or without signs of myocarditis (case studies, no systematic reports).[19]
  - Accelerated atherosclerosis[21]
  - Arrhythmia (case studies)
- Due to the activated immune system, immune-mediated side effects can occur throughout the body, including the heart.
- Expert opinion currently favors corticosteroids for treatment and higher intensity immunosuppression in severe cases if not steroid responsive. Higher intensity immunosuppression therapy, however, has been associated with severe infection and death.[22]

Chimeric Antigen Receptor T-Cell Therapy

- **Examples**: axicabtagene ciloleucel, tisagenlecleucel
- **Mechanism of action**: T cells are genetically engineered to produce chimeric antigen receptors (CARs) that target tumor cells.
- **Main adverse CV effects**:
  - Tachycardia: 26-57%; grade 3 or higher: 2-4% (package inserts)
  - Arrhythmia (axicabtagene ciloleucel): 23%; grade 3 or higher: 7% (package insert)
  - Cardiac arrest: 4%; package inserts
  - Cardiac failure: 6-7%; package inserts
- Up to 94% of patients will have symptoms of the cytokine-release syndrome (CRS), which can be fatal in ~4%.

Fluoropyrimidine

- **Examples**: 5-fluorouracil (5-FU), capecitabine
- **Mechanism of action**: inhibits the synthesis of thymidine, a nucleoside (pyrimidine) required for the construction of DNA
- **Main CV adverse effects**:
  - Coronary vasospasm (0-19%; systematic review)[23]
  - Myocardial infarction (0-2%)

HER2-Targeted Therapies

- **Examples**: trastuzumab, pertuzumab, lapatinib
- **Mechanism of action**: recombinant humanized monoclonal antibodies against human epidermal growth factor 2 (HER2, aka ErbB2). HER2 promotes cell proliferation through growth signaling pathways.

- **Main adverse CV effect** (trastuzumab, pertuzumab):
  ○ LV dysfunction: trial data: 9.4% at 65 months; 18.6% in combination with anthracycline[24]
  ○ HF
    ▪ Trial data: 0.4% at 65 months, 2.0% in combination with anthracyclines[24]
    ▪ Retrospective cohort (real world): 12% at 5 years; 20% at 5 years with trastuzumab plus anthracycline[7]
- HER2 is also present in cardiac tissue and likely is important in the stress response in the heart.[25] Knockout mice without HER2 develop dilated cardiomyopathy.[26]
- Lapatinib is a tyrosine kinase inhibitor (TKI) that affects the HER2 signaling pathway. It is uncommonly associated with LV dysfunction or HF. Pertuzumab has similar CV risk to trastuzumab but does not appear to have significant additive risk when used in conjunction with trastuzumab.

Immunomodulatory Agents

- **Examples**: thalidomide, lenalidomide, pomalidomide
- **Mechanism of action**: The drugs have antiangiogenic and immunomodulatory properties that include T-cell activation and reduced production of pro-inflammatory cytokines.[25] Drugs in this class are synthetically derived from thalidomide.
- **Main adverse CV effects**:
  ○ Venous thromboembolism (VTE)[26,27]
    ▪ 0-33% incidence for lenalidomide
    ▪ 8-75% when lenalidomide given with dexamethasone
    ▪ Reduced with prophylaxis
  ○ Arterial thromboembolism 1.98% (myocardial infarction) and 3.4% (cerebrovascular events) with lenalidomide and dexamethasone[28,29]
  ○ Sinus bradycardia with thalidomide (not seen with newer metabolites)
    ▪ 26% including asymptomatic patients
    ▪ 3% with severe or life-threatening bradycardia (phase II trial)[30]
- Consider prophylactic anticoagulation for VTE prevention in patients with multiple myeloma on lenalidomide.

PI3K/AKT/mTOR Inhibitor

- **Examples**: everolimus, idelalisib, temsirolimus
- **Mechanism of action**: inhibits the PI3K/AKT/mTOR signaling cascade, resulting in reduced cell growth, proliferation, and angiogenesis
- **Main CV adverse effects**: The PI3K/AKT/mTOR signaling cascade is important in a number of cellular processes, including tissue metabolism and glucose homeostasis. There was over a 50% incidence of hyperglycemia, hypercholesterolemia, and hypertriglyceridemia in clinical trials, though new onset of diabetes mellitus was <1% and hyperglycemia in patients being treated for cancer is common in general. As the drugs were approved by the FDA in 2017, the true incidence of CV effects is currently unknown. Hypertension (4%) and HF (1%) are reported in the package insert.

Proteasome Inhibitors

- **Examples**: bortezomib, carfilzomib, ixazomib
- **Mechanism of action**: The proteasome is responsible for degradation of proteins within the cell. Inhibiting the proteasome subsequently leads to apoptosis.
- **Main adverse CV effects**:
  ○ HF
    ▪ Few reports with bortezomib
    ▪ 4% in systematic review of clinic trials of carfilzomib[31]

○ Hypertension
  ▪ 18% in systematic review of carfilzomib[31]
  ▪ Bortezomib: 8-23% based on package insert
• Carfilzomib is associated with increased incidence of HF compared to bortezomib.

Radiation (Mediastinal)

• **Mechanism of action**: damages DNA directly and through free radical production, leading to cell death
• **Main CV adverse effects**:
  ○ Arrhythmia: 16% (9-year median follow-up)
  ○ Autonomic dysfunction: 30-45% (19-year median follow-up)[32]
  ○ Coronary heart disease: 19-20% (9- to 20-year median follow-up)[33,34]
  ○ HF: 11-12% (9- to 20-year median follow-up)[33,34]
  ○ Pericardial disease: 5% (9-year median follow-up)[34]
  ○ Pacemaker/implantable cardioverter-defibrillator (ICD) malfunction: 3%[35]
  ○ Valvular heart disease: 11-31% (9- to 20-year median follow-up)[33,34]
• Mediastinal radiation: ≥30 Gray (with the heart in the treatment field), and the combination of anthracyclines or radiation at any dose has been identified as especially high-risk factors for LV dysfunction.[9]
• Radiation, whether to the mediastinum or peripherally, also increases risk of vascular disease within the treated field (Figure 14-1).
• More recent radiation protocols have incorporated a number of different measures to reduce toxicity. It is expected that the cardiac impact will be lower in the future, though the degree of which it will be lower is unknown.

Tyrosine Kinase Inhibitors

• See also Vascular Endothelial Growth Factor Signaling Pathway inhibitors, HER2 antagonists, and mTOR inhibitors.
• **Examples**:
  ○ MEK inhibitors: trametinib, binimetinib, cobimetinib
  ○ BRAF inhibitors: vemurafenib, dabrafenib, encorafenib
  ○ ABL kinase inhibitors: imatinib, dasatinib, ponatinib, nilotinib
  ○ BTK inhibitor: ibrutinib
  ○ EGFR inhibitor: erlotinib, cetuximab, lapatinib
  ○ ALK inhibitor: ceritinib, crizotinib
  ○ MET inhibitor: capmatinib

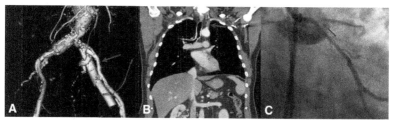

FIGURE 14-1. Radiation-induced vascular disease. **(A)** Peripheral atherosclerosis and left iliac vein occlusion with stent placement due to pelvic radiation (arrow). **(B)** CXR-induced left subclavian stenosis (arrow). **(C)** Subtotal occlusion of the left anterior descending artery in a young patient due to prior CXR and chronic graft-versus-host disease (arrow).

- **Mechanism of Action**: inhibit tyrosine kinases directly or by inhibiting the kinase receptor, blocking downstream cell signaling. There are several tyrosine kinase targets to date, and some drugs can affect multiple targets.
- **Main adverse CV effects** (not consistent across class, relatively more toxic drugs listed as examples):
  - Arterial thromboembolic event (ponatinib)
  - Atrial fibrillation (ibrutinib)
  - Atherosclerosis (nilotinib)
  - Bleeding (ibrutinib)
  - Bradyarrhythmia (trametinib)
  - Edema (imatinib, capmatinib)
  - Hypertension (ibrutinib, trametinib, nilotinib)
  - LV dysfunction (ponatinib, MEK inhibitors)
  - QT prolongation (nilotinib, vemurafenib)
  - VTE event (ponatinib, erlotinib, trametinib, nilotinib)

Vascular Endothelial Growth Factor Signaling Pathway Inhibitors

- Includes VEGF-receptor inhibitors and antiangiogenic TKIs
- **Examples**: bevacizumab, pazopanib, sunitinib, sorafenib, axitinib, vandetanib, regorafenib, cabozantinib, ziv-aflibercept, ramucirumab, lenvatinib
- **Mechanism of action**: inhibit angiogenesis through the VEGF pathway. Bevacizumab directly binds the VEGF receptor, while drugs such as sunitinib are TKIs that block downstream signaling.
- **Main adverse CV effects**: Side effects are generally a class effect, though hypertension and LV dysfunction are lower with some medications such as bevacizumab than with the antiangiogenic TKIs such as sunitinib. QT prolongation is specific to the medication, with vandetanib reporting the highest incidence of significant QT prolongation, though the incidence is still low (<3%).
  - Hypertension (20-91%; clinical trials)[36]
  - LV dysfunction (14% with sunitinib; cohort study)[37]
  - Arterial thromboembolic event (0-5.4%; clinical trials)[36]
  - VTE event (2-11.9%; clinical trials)[36]
  - QT prolongation (vandetanib −2.7% with QTc > 500 ms)

Select Other Medications and Cardiovascular Adverse Effects

- Arsenic trioxide: QT prolongation (38%; retrospective analysis)[38]
- Decitabine (hypomethylating agent): <5% incidence of cardiac failure, myocardial infarction, atrial fibrillation, supraventricular tachycardia
- Docetaxel/paclitaxel (antimicrotubules): autonomic dysfunction (incidence not well defined)
- Ribociclib (CDK4/CDK6 inhibitor): QT prolongation (3%); package insert
- Rituximab (anti-CD20 antibody): hypotension in 10% (infusion reaction), grade 3 or 4 in 1%
- Tretinoin: arrhythmias (23%), HF (6%); package insert
- Vorinostat (histone deacetylase inhibitor): QT prolongation > 500 ms (3.2%)[39]

PREVENTION

- **Preventive measures should always include baseline and ongoing assessment for cardiac risk factors accompanied by guideline-directed treatment.**
- Patients with cancer also often have CT scans of the chest done for screening or staging that can be reviewed for presence of **coronary artery calcifications**, a marker of CAD. Identification of coronary artery calcifications can help trigger appropriate preventive therapy for coronary events (Figure 14-2).

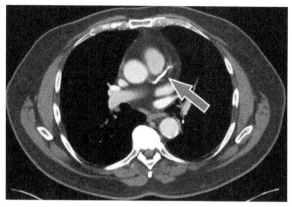

FIGURE 14-2. Coronary artery calcifications noted on staging CT scan. Extensive coronary artery calcium is noted in the left anterior descending artery on a staging CT scan in a patient with newly diagnosed prostate cancer. The patient eventually underwent three-vessel coronary artery bypass surgery after subsequently developing unstable angina 1 year later.

ABCDEs

The **ABCDEs** have had modifications for use in screening to prevent CV disease in patients with breast[40] and prostate cancer. It can be a useful screening tool.

- **A:** Awareness of risks of heart disease, Aspirin
- **B:** Blood pressure, Biomarkers
- **C:** Cholesterol, Cigarette/tobacco Cessation
- **D:** Diet and weight management, Dose of chemotherapy or radiation, Diabetes mellitus prevention/treatment
- **E:** Exercise, Echocardiogram

Coronary Vasospasm

- Secondary prevention of vasospasm associated with fluoropyrimidines (5-FU, capecitabine) can be achieved with bolus as opposed to continuous infusion of 5-FU as well as use of calcium channel blockers (nifedipine, diltiazem) and nitrates.[41]
- While **diltiazem** may be the most effective at preventing vasospasm, any use of diltiazem should be carefully considered due to its **interactions with the cytochrome P450 system** and associated risk of adverse drug interactions as well as its association with worsening LV function in patients with systolic dysfunction.
- Given their underlying endothelial dysfunction, all patients should be considered for treatment for CAD, specifically aspirin and a statin.

Left Ventricular Dysfunction

- LV dysfunction is most classically associated with anthracyclines, HER2-targeted agents, and mediastinal radiation. Other cancer therapies with established links to cardiomyopathy include MEK inhibitors/BRAF inhibitors, proteasome inhibitors, VEGF/VSP inhibitors, and immune checkpoint inhibitors.
- In patients receiving VEGF/VSP inhibitors, treatment of associated hypertension may help prevent subsequent LV dysfunction, although more study is needed.

- In high-risk patients for LV dysfunction receiving doxorubicin, cardiotoxicity can be limited through continuous infusion instead of bolus dosing and the use of the liposomal formulation.[42]
- **Dexrazoxane** is the only agent with specific FDA approval for the prevention of anthracycline cardiotoxicity and is generally considered for patients receiving over 300 mg/m² of doxorubicin or equivalent. A Cochrane meta-analysis found it successfully reduced incident HF without affecting progression free or overall survival.[43]
- Studies have also found potential benefit for the use of some ACE-Is, ARBs, and β-blockers including carvedilol, enalapril, and candesartan for the prevention of LV dysfunction.[44-46] Metoprolol has not shown benefit.[45]
- More limited direct evidence supports possible use of statins and aldosterone antagonists.[47-50] It is unknown if the hormonal, antiandrogen effects of spironolactone have a clinical impact in tumors tied to the hormonal axis (prostate, breast, etc.).
- Patients at the highest risk for LV dysfunction, based on patient characteristics or treatment regimen, are likely to derive the most benefit from protective medications. Patients with elevated troponin receiving anthracyclines, for instance, showed benefit from enalapril and carvedilol versus placebo in reducing LV dysfunction.[44]
- Cardioprotective medication also reduced the prevalence of subsequent drop in LVEF when initiated after a relative reduction of 12% in global longitudinal strain (GLS) in patients receiving anthracycline chemotherapy.[51]

Thrombosis

Patients with multiple myeloma on lenalidomide should be considered for thromboembolism prophylaxis with anticoagulation.[28,29]

Torsades de Pointes

- Several chemotherapy drugs have the potential to prolong the QTc interval, notably arsenic trioxide as well as certain TKIs (dabrafenib, nilotinib, trametinib, vandetanib), the histone deacetylase inhibitor vorinostat, and the CDK4/CDK6 inhibitor ribociclib.
- Ribociclib specifically requires an FDA-mandated ECG on C1D1 (Cycle 1 Day 1), C1D14, and C2D1 (package insert).
- Patients with cancer are routinely exposed to other QT-prolonging medicines such as antiemetics, which could place them at higher risk for arrhythmia.
- ECGs and possibly telemetry should be considered for patients initiated on new QT-prolonging medications or with clinical status changes such as electrolyte abnormalities. Electrolytes should be monitored and replaced as needed to reduce risk for arrhythmia.

SCREENING AND DIAGNOSIS

General Principles

- Clinical signs and symptoms of CV toxicity can develop immediately or be delayed for up to decades later.
- Cardiologists may be consulted before treatment for preoperative assessment, during chemotherapy initiation due to immediate adverse effects, or in survivorship clinic for monitoring or treatment of long-term sequelae.
- Screening **protocols** are optimally **individualized** to the patient based on the **incidence of cardiotoxicity** of the patient's cancer therapy, the patient's **known and estimated CV risk**, and collaboration between the oncologist and the cardiologist.[52,53] Recommended guidelines for echocardiography screening based on specific cancer therapies can be found in Table 14-3, although complete cancer screening protocols can and should include the use of interval CV history and examination as well as the use of biomarkers.

TABLE 14-3 TRANSTHORACIC ECHOCARDIOGRAPHIC SURVEILLANCE STRATEGIES IN THE CANCER PATIENT

Cancer therapy	Baseline evaluation[a]	During treatment[a]	Following treatment[a]
Anthracyclines	Recommended	• After >240 mg/m^2 doxorubicin equivalent • Every additional 100–150 mg/m^2 doxorubicin equivalent or every 2 cycles	6–12 months after final cycle Consider annually for 2–3 years in high-risk patients, otherwise 5 yearly review
HER2 receptor antagonists	Recommended	• Every 3 months until treatment conclusion	6–12 months after treatment in patients who received anthracyclines or are at otherwise high CV risk
Alkylating agents	Consider	If change in clinical status	[b]
Antimetabolites	Consider	If change in clinical status	[b]
Proteasome inhibitors	Consider, especially with carfilzomib and to evaluate for AL in patients with MM	If change in clinical status	[b]
ICIs	Consider	Consider in patients at high risk (combination ICI, other cardiotoxic treatments, high baseline CV risk)	[b]
Anti-VEGF TKIs	Recommended	• Consider every 4 months during the first year of treatment • Consider 6–12 monthly TTE thereafter	[b]

(continued)

203

TABLE 14-3 TRANSTHORACIC ECHOCARDIOGRAPHIC SURVEILLANCE STRATEGIES IN THE CANCER PATIENT (*continued*)

Cancer therapy	Baseline evaluation[a]	During treatment[a]	Following treatment[a]
BCR-ABL TKIs (second and third generation)	Consider	• Consider 6–12 monthly TTE	[b]
MEK/BRAF inhibitors	Recommended	• After 1 month and then every 3 months until treatment conclusion	[b]
Dasatinib	Recommended to assess for baseline pulmonary HTN	• Low threshold if cardiac symptoms develop	[b]
Radiation therapy	Consider, especially if high CV risk or in combination with other cardiotoxic treatments	Monitoring during XRT itself generally not required due to brief treatment times	In patients with anthracycline chemotherapy, 6–12 months after treatment. Further TTE based on CV risk: High: every 5 years Moderate/low: 10 years after treatment conclusion, then every 5 years

Suggested transthoracic echocardiographic surveillance strategies derived from expert consensus statements and from known incidence of cardiovascular events associated with treatment.

AL, light-chain amyloidosis; CV, cardiovascular; HER2, human epithelial growth factor; HTN, hypertension; ICIs, immune checkpoint inhibitors; MM, multiple myeloma; TKIs, tyrosine kinase inhibitors; TTE, transthoracic echo; XRT, radiation therapy; VEGF, vascular endothelial growth factor.

[a] Consider the summative patient risk based on existing CV disease and cancer therapy, both planned and delivered.

[b] Not required if asymptomatic and normal LV function during treatment.

- The **goal of screening is to identify any cardiotoxicity early in its course to help direct management and mitigate more severe progression.** Ultimately, the objective is to **maximize delivery of cancer therapy** while limiting associated toxicity.
- Importantly, **the diagnosis of cardiotoxicity should not automatically prompt cessation of therapy.** Cancer treatment can often be continued with the support of cardioprotective medications and close monitoring (Figure 14-3). The decision to withhold or discontinue a particular form of cancer therapy should always include **multidisciplinary discussion** regarding CV risk, cancer prognosis, availability of alternative treatments, and patient goals of care.

Clinical Presentation

History
- All patients should receive a comprehensive screening for traditional CV risk factors (hypertension, smoking, diabetes mellitus, dyslipidemia, physical activity, diet, obesity) and receive guideline-directed treatment as indicated.
- The CO history should be tailored to the specific CV concern but always include:
  ○ Underlying cancer prognosis
  ○ Previous treatments received
  ○ Ongoing and planned therapy

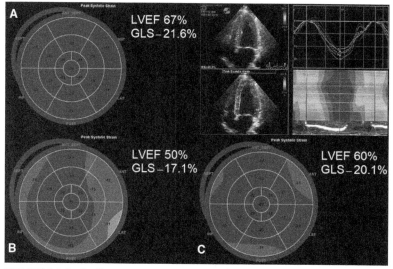

FIGURE 14-3. Facilitating cancer treatment with cardioprotective medications. A 41-year-old undergoing treatment for breast cancer stage IIB invasive ductal carcinoma. **(A)** Baseline transthoracic echocardiogram shows normal LV systolic function (LVEF 67%, GLS −21.6%). **(B)** On screening echocardiogram after five cycles of paclitaxel, carboplatin, and trastuzumab, the patient has an asymptomatic drop in her LVEF to 50% with a GLS reduction to −17.1%. Trastuzumab is held, and she is referred to cardio-oncology. She is started on carvedilol and lisinopril, and her cancer therapy with trastuzumab is resumed. **(C)** Three months later, her LVEF has normalized to 60% with GLS of −20.1%. LVEF, left ventricular ejection fraction; GLS, global longitudinal strain.

- Information on past/present treatment regimen should include cumulative dose of anthracycline and mediastinal radiation.
- All patients should be screened for history of:
  ○ Cardiomyopathy, HF, or LV dysfunction
  ○ CAD
  ○ Arrhythmia or QT prolongation including symptoms of presyncope/syncope
  ○ Arterial thromboembolism or VTE
- During cancer treatment, patients are at high risk for orthostatic hypotension and should be monitored for symptoms of presyncope/syncope.

Physical Examination
- A few noteworthy comments relevant to the differential diagnosis in patients with cancer:
  ○ Isolated elevated jugular venous pressure (JVP) can occur after administration of IV fluids even in a patient without documented LV dysfunction.
  ○ Graft-versus-host disease (GVHD) and radiation pneumonitis can mimic pulmonary edema on lung auscultation and plain radiography, though other signs of HF would be absent.
- Importantly, cardiac tamponade remains a clinical diagnosis, and physical examination should assess for patient distress, tachycardia, elevated JVP, and pulsus paradoxus.

Diagnostic Criteria
- Diagnostic criteria for cardiotoxicity are generally consistent with the diagnostic criteria for CV events in patients without cancer. In addition to cardiotoxicity, all common etiologies should still be considered (e.g., ischemic cardiomyopathy).
- The diagnosis of subclinical LV dysfunction and cardiotoxicity in patients with cancer often incorporates GLS (Table 14-1) and/or use of biomarkers. Patients with subclinical LV dysfunction should be considered for cardioprotective medications. As mentioned earlier, in a trial of 331 patients receiving anthracyclines, cardioprotective medication reduced the prevalence of subsequent drop in LVEF when initiated after a relative reduction of 12% in GLS.[51]

Screening and Diagnostic Testing
- In addition to the standard evaluation for any patient for HF, acute coronary syndrome, or other CV disease, screening and diagnostic testing specific to patients with cancer are presented herein.
- Patients receiving cancer treatment should receive appropriate monitoring during and after treatment. CV disease can become evident years after therapy is completed.
- Patients on VSP inhibitors should check their blood pressure regularly.

Laboratories
- Both troponin and brain natriuretic peptide (BNP) have shown some promise in detecting subclinical cardiotoxicity and predicting future events.[54-56] The optimal timing for testing in all cancers and with specific anticancer therapy has not been fully defined.
- Baseline biomarkers can be helpful before initiation of cancer therapy with a significant incidence of LV dysfunction to identify patients at highest risk.[57-60]

Imaging
- Echocardiogram (or potentially MRI) should be considered:
  ○ At baseline for patients scheduled to undergo cancer therapy associated with high risk of HF or LV dysfunction
  ○ For patients with signs (elevated JVP, edema) or symptoms (orthopnea, paroxysmal nocturnal dyspnea, dyspnea on exertion) of HF

- ○ Routine surveillance in patients at moderate-to-high risk of LV dysfunction (high baseline CV risk, regimen with HER2 antagonist and/or anthracycline, mediastinal radiation)
- ○ 6 to 12 months after completion of cancer therapy at moderate-to-high risk of LV dysfunction, even in asymptomatic patients
- Echocardiogram is generally the test of choice due to lower cost and better availability. The advantages of MRI include reproducibility and obtaining diagnostic images in patients with poor acoustic windows.
- In patients undergoing echocardiogram evaluation, the addition of GLS may be helpful in detecting subclinical dysfunction and patients at higher risk for developing future HF.[61]
- Strain can also be used as an additional data point when determining the presence of true cardiotoxicity and has reduced variability and increased reliability relative to LVEF measurements alone (Figure 14-4.).

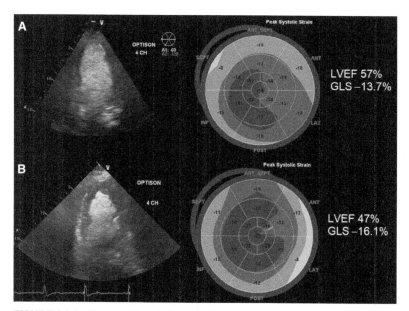

FIGURE 14-4. Myocardial strain is a useful tool in diagnosing cardiotoxicity. A 71-year-old female with metastatic leiomyosarcoma receiving doxorubicin with concurrent dexrazoxane on trial is on the 16th cycle of anthracycline-based therapy (cumulative doxorubicin dose 1200 mg/m²). **(A)** Her most recent TTE 6 weeks ago showed LVEF of 57% with GLS of −13.7%. **(B)** Her TTE performed today is read in a standard clinical fashion with an LVEF of 47%, and she is subsequently removed from study due to concern for cardiotoxicity. However, her LV strain, a measure with reduced variability, is stable, if not improved, compared to previous measures (GLS −16.1%). Subsequent blinded analysis of her echocardiograms from the research central core lab showed that her LVEF had actually remained unchanged (prior LVEF 60.7% with current LVEF 57.4%). Thus, the patient was erroneously removed from the clinical trial, and her cancer therapy was altered as a result of an incomplete interpretation of her LV function. LVEF, left ventricular ejection fraction; GLS, global longitudinal strain; TTE, transthoracic echocardiogram.

Electrocardiography

- A baseline ECG should be obtained in all patients to screen for conduction disorders (including QT prolongation) as well as signs of prior myocardial infarction or other significant cardiac disease.
- ECGs and possibly telemetry should be used to monitor patients initiated on new QT-prolonging medications or with clinical status changes, such as electrolyte abnormalities.

TREATMENT

- Treatment for CV events (HF, acute coronary syndrome) in the cancer population mirrors treatment in the noncancer population, but comorbidities (such as thrombocytopenia, orthostatic hypotension) often limit management options.
- In patients with active cancer, **treatment goals should always include minimizing stoppages or cessation of cancer therapy**. In patients with planned or current treatment for cancer and indication for coronary evaluation, the expected treatment course and platelet trend should be considered when making management decisions.
- Radial approach for invasive coronary evaluation can be considered to minimize bleeding in patients with thrombocytopenia.

Medications

- Patients with **HF with reduced ejection fraction** (HFrEF) should receive guideline-directed medical therapy as with all other patients.
- **LV dysfunction** not meeting criteria for HFrEF (EF > 40% and lower than institutional normal) is treated more aggressively to reduce ongoing decline in function and potentially allow for continued cancer treatment, if needed.
- **In patients with thrombocytopenia requiring antiplatelets or anticoagulation**, the following practice recommendations[62,63] are based on expert opinion and review of the available literature. Decisions, though, should be individualized based on patient specific risk factors and goals of care.
  - Platelets > 10,000 = aspirin in patients with CAD
  - Platelets > 30,000 = dual antiplatelet therapy in indicated patients after percutaneous coronary intervention (PCI)
  - Platelets > 50,000 = acute VTE, full dose low-molecular-weight heparin (LMWH) anticoagulation for platelets
    - If 30 to 50,000, then 50% dose reduction
    - If <30,000, then hold anticoagulation
  - Platelets 50 to 100,000 = nonacute VTE, 75% LMWH anticoagulation dose. If 30 to 50,000, then 50% or more dose reduction
- For treatment of **hypertension**, cardioprotective medications (ACE-I/ARB or carvedilol) should be considered as a first line for antihypertensives in all patients undergoing treatment with potential for LV dysfunction. Per the HF guidelines, these patients are considered stage A HF.
- Given increased arterial stiffness and resistive load seen during treatment with sunitinib[64] and potentially other antiangiogenic TKIs, patients may also benefit from vasodilator therapy such as dihydropyridine calcium channel blockers as well as combined α- and β-blockade (e.g., carvedilol) for the treatment of associated hypertension.
- Nondihydropyridines (e.g., diltiazem, verapamil) inhibit the cytochrome P450 system and affect the metabolism of TKIs and other cancer therapies. They should thus be avoided or used with caution in patients with cancer after checking all drug–drug interactions.

Lifestyle/Risk Modification

Diet

- In addition to diet's role in CV disease, diet has also been linked to the development of cancer.
- Saturated fats may reduce survival from cancer in addition to increasing risk for CV disease.
- Eating sufficient fruits and vegetables as well as foods high in fiber has been linked to a lower risk of certain cancers, while certain processed and red meat, as well as high levels of smoked food, has been linked to an increased risk of colorectal and stomach cancer, respectively.
- Patients with cancer can frequently have poor nutrition due to anorexia or adverse effects of cancer treatment on the gastrointestinal mucosa. In these patients, maximizing calories often becomes the priority.
- Certain diets, such as lower fiber, may also be recommended to counteract symptoms of diarrhea or trouble digesting food.

Activity

- Peak exercise capacity, as measured by peak oxygen consumption, is often substantially reduced in patients with cancer, and patients can benefit from interventions improving their exercise capacity.
- In women with nonmetastatic breast cancer, the incidence of CV events is reduced proportionately with increasing amounts of exercise.[65]
- Exercise has also been shown to reduce breast cancer–related death and all-cause mortality.[66]
- Given the wide range in capabilities and comorbidities of individual patients, experts have recommend tailoring the exercise plan to the individual patient and giving specific recommendations (number of times per week, duration), when able.

SPECIAL CONSIDERATIONS

- Care should be individualized to the patient's goals of care and quality of life. Some patients may simply be focused on relieving or reducing symptoms, while others may want more aggressive care.
- Delay in recognition of cardiotoxicity can significantly worsen prognosis and recovery.

REFERRAL

- Referral to a CO specialist is preferred in any patient with significant baseline CV risk or with plans for therapy with intermediate-to-high risk for cardiotoxicity.
- These CV specialists will have the most experience working with the oncologist in selecting the optimal treatment regimen and mitigating any potential cardiotoxicity.

PATIENT EDUCATION

- All patients should be educated on their cancer regimen, potential toxicities, and recommended follow-up.
- Patients should be counseled on important factors in maintaining overall CV health. The American Heart Association Life's Simple 7 is a useful guide that advocates for a healthy weight, tobacco cessation, a healthy diet, regular physical activity as well as blood pressure, cholesterol, and glucose management. Patients can be directed to their website.[67]
- The American College of Cardiology (ACC) is also developing a number of patient resources through CardioSmart at https://www.cardiosmart.org/Heart-Conditions/Cardio-Oncology.[68]

MONITORING/FOLLOW-UP

- Close follow-up, ideally within 2 weeks, is recommended after discharge from the hospital in patients being treated for cancer. In such patients, delays in care can contribute to increased or more prolonged stoppages of cancer therapy. Such stoppages can have a significant impact on mortality.
- Patients on cardiotoxic regimens should have ongoing evaluation of their risk factors and for signs of toxicity.
- Patients with prior mediastinal radiation should undergo evaluation for CAD/ischemia and valvular disease starting 5 years after completion of therapy at regular intervals thereafter. While there are little data to recommend any particular screening test, a history and physical examination should be completed with consideration for other stress testing as clinically appropriate.
- Patients who have received cancer therapy associated with moderate-to-high risk of LV dysfunction should receive an echocardiogram 6 to 12 months after completion of therapy, even if asymptomatic.

OUTCOME/PROGNOSIS

- Prognosis varies significantly depending on cancer type and stage, as well as whether the cancer is refractory to initial treatment options. The patient's prognosis should be considered in management decisions by the multidisciplinary team.
- It is important to note that new treatment options can allow for much longer survival even in the setting of metastatic disease. Patients with metastatic renal cell cancer can be controlled for years on VSP inhibitor therapy as can metastatic breast cancer patients on hormonal therapy. Immunotherapy with checkpoint inhibitors has also led to significantly prolonged survival in patients with metastatic cancers. These patients can often continue to benefit from appropriate primary and secondary prevention for CV disease.

REFERENCES

1. National Institutes of Health. Cancer therapy evaluation program. Last accessed 08/19/21. https://ctep.cancer.gov/protocolDevelopment/adverse_effects.htm
2. Groarke JD, Cheng S, Moslehi J. Cancer-drug discovery and cardiovascular surveillance. *N Engl J Med.* 2013;369:1779-81.
3. Karanis YB, Canta FAB, Mitrofan L, et al. "Research" vs "real world" patients: the representativeness of clinical trial participants. *Ann Oncol.* 2016;27(suppl 6):vi526-44.
4. National Cancer Institute. Cancer statistics. Last accessed 05/19/21. https://www.cancer.gov/about-cancer/understanding/statistics
5. Armstrong GT, Kawashima T, Leisenring W, et al. Aging and risk of severe, disabling, life-threatening, and fatal events in the childhood cancer survivor study. *J Clin Oncol.* 2014;32:1218-27.
6. Patnaik JL, Byers T, DiGuiseppi C, et al. Cardiovascular disease competes with breast cancer as the leading cause of death for older females diagnosed with breast cancer: a retrospective cohort study. *Breast Cancer Res.* 2011;13:R64.
7. Bowles EJ, Wellman R, Feigelson HS, et al. Risk of heart failure in breast cancer patients after anthracycline and trastuzumab treatment: a retrospective cohort study. *J Natl Cancer Inst.* 2012;104:1293-1305.
8. Strongman H, Gadd S, Matthews A, et al. Medium and long-term risks of specific cardiovascular diseases in survivors of 20 adult cancers: a population-based cohort study using multiple linked UK electronic health records databases. *Lancet.* 2019;394:1041-54.
9. Armenian SH, Lacchetti C, Barac A, et al. Prevention and monitoring of cardiac dysfunction in survivors of adult cancers: American Society of Clinical Oncology Clinical Practice Guideline. *J Clin Oncol.* 2017;35:893-911.
10. Armstrong GT, Oeffinger KC, Chen Y, et al. Modifiable risk factors and major cardiac events among adult survivors of childhood cancer. *J Clin Oncol.* 2013;31:3673-80.

11. St. Jude Children's Research Hospital. CCSS cardiovascular risk calculator. Last accessed 06/05/22. https://ccss.stjude.org/tools-documents/calculators-other-tools/ccss-cardiovascular-risk-calculator. html

12. Ezaz G, Long JB, Gross CP, Chen J. Risk prediction model for heart failure and cardiomyopathy after adjuvant trastuzumab therapy for breast cancer. *J Am Heart Assoc.* 2014;3:e000472.

13. Pai VB, Nahata MC. Cardiotoxicity of chemotherapeutic agents: incidence, treatment and prevention. *Drug Saf.* 2000;22:263-302.

14. Czaykowski PM, Moore MJ, Tannock IF. High risk of vascular events in patients with urothelial transitional cell carcinoma treated with cisplatin based chemotherapy. *J Urol.* 1998;160:2021-4.

15. Kerns SL, Fung C, Monahan PO, et al. Cumulative burden of morbidity among testicular cancer survivors after standard cisplatin-based chemotherapy: a multi-institutional study. *J Clin Oncol.* 2018;36:1505-12.

16. Nguyen PL, Alibhai SMH, Basaria S, et al. Adverse effects of androgen deprivation therapy and strategies to mitigate them. *Eur Urol.* 2015;67:825-36.

17. Swain SM, Whaley FS, Ewer MS. Congestive heart failure in patients treated with doxorubicin: a retrospective analysis of three trials. *Cancer.* 2003;97:2869-79.

18. Johnson DB, Balko JM, Compton ML, et al. Fulminant myocarditis with combination immune checkpoint blockade. *N Engl J Med.* 2016;375:1749-55.

19. Heinzerling L, Ott PA, Hodi FS, et al. Cardiotoxicity associated with CTLA4 and PD1 blocking immunotherapy. *J Immunother Cancer.* 2016;4:50.

20. Mahmood SS, Fradley MG, Cohen JV, et al. Myocarditis in patients treated with immune checkpoint inhibitors. *J Am Coll Cardiol.* 2018;71:1755-64.

21. Drobni ZD, Alvi RM, Taron J, et al. Association between immune checkpoint inhibitors with cardiovascular events and atherosclerotic plaque. *Circulation.* 2020;142:2299-2311.

22. Naidoo J, Wang X, Woo KM, et al. Pneumonitis in patients treated with anti-programmed death-1/programmed death ligand 1 therapy. *J Clin Oncol.* 2017;35:709-17.

23. Polk A, Vaage-Nilsen M, Vistisen K, Nielsen DL. Cardiotoxicity in cancer patients treated with 5-fluorouracil or capecitabine: a systematic review of incidence, manifestations and predisposing factors. *Cancer Treat Rev.* 2013;39:974-84.

24. Slamon D, Eiermann W, Robert N, et al. Adjuvant trastuzumab in HER2-positive breast cancer. *N Engl J Med.* 2011;365:1273-83.

25. Odiete O, Hill MF, Sawyer DB. Neuregulin in cardiovascular development and disease. *Circ Res.* 2012;111:1376-85.

26. Crone SA, Zhao YY, Fan L, et al. ErbB2 is essential in the prevention of dilated cardiomyopathy. *Nat Med.* 2002;8:459-65.

27. Kotla V, Goel S, Nischal S, et al. Mechanism of action of lenalidomide in hematological malignancies. *J Hematol Oncol.* 2009;2:36.

28. Palumbo A, Rajkumar SV, Dimopoulos MA, et al. Prevention of thalidomide-and lenalidomide-associated thrombosis in myeloma. *Leukemia.* 2008;22:414-23.

29. Musallam KM, Dahdaleh FS, Shamseddine AI, Taher AT. Incidence and prophylaxis of venous thromboembolic events in multiple myeloma patients receiving immunomodulatory therapy. *Thromb Res.* 2009;123:679-86.

30. Rajkumar SV, Gertz MA, Lacy MQ, et al. Thalidomide as initial therapy for early-stage myeloma. *Leukemia.* 2003;17:775-9.

31. Waxman AJ, Clasen S, Hwang W, et al. Carfilzomib-associated cardiovascular adverse events: a systematic review and meta-analysis. *JAMA Oncol.* 2018;4:e174519.

32. Groarke JD, Tanguturi VK, Hainer J, et al. Abnormal exercise response in long-term survivors of Hodgkin lymphoma treated with thoracic irradiation: evidence of cardiac autonomic dysfunction and impact on outcomes. *J Am Coll Cardiol.* 2015;65:573-83.

33. van Nimwegen FA, Schaapveld M, Janus CP, et al. Cardiovascular disease after Hodgkin lymphoma treatment: 40-year disease risk. *JAMA Intern Med.* 2015;175:1007-17.

34. Maraldo MV, Giusti F, Vogelius IR, et al. Cardiovascular disease after treatment for Hodgkin's lymphoma: an analysis of nine collaborative EORTC-LYSA trials. *Lancet Haematol.* 2015;2:e492-502.

35. Zaremba T, Jakobsen AR, Sogaard M, et al. Radiotherapy in patients with pacemakers and implantable cardioverter defibrillators: a literature review. *Europace.* 2016;18:479-91.

36. Li W, Croce K, Steensma DP, et al. Vascular and metabolic implications of novel targeted cancer therapies: focus on kinase inhibitors. *J Am Coll Cardiol.* 2015;66:1160-78.

37. Narayan V, Wang L, Putt M, et al. Risk of left ventricular systolic dysfunction with sunitinib therapy in patients with metastatic renal cell carcinoma: a prospective cohort study. *J Clin Oncol.* 2016;34(15 suppl):e16104.

38. Barbey JT, Pezzullo JC, Soignet SL. Effect of arsenic trioxide on QT interval in patients with advanced malignancies. *J Clin Oncol*. 2003;21(19):3609-15.

39. Porta-Sánchez A, Gilbert C, Spears D, et al. Incidence, diagnosis, and management of qt prolongation induced by cancer therapies: a systematic review. *J Am Heart Assoc*. 2017;6:e007724.

40. Montazeri K, Unitt C, Foody JM, et al. ABCDE steps to prevent heart disease in breast cancer survivors. *Circulation*. 2014;130:e157-9.

41. Clasen SC, Ky B, O'Quinn R, et al. Fluoropyrimidine-induced cardiac toxicity: challenging the current paradigm. *J Gastrointest Oncol*. 2017;8:970-9.

42. Smith LA, Cornelius VR, Plummer CJ, et al. Cardiotoxicity of anthracycline agents for the treatment of cancer: systematic review and meta-analysis of randomised controlled trials. *BMC Cancer*. 2010;10:337.

43. van Dalen EC, Caron HN, Dickinson HO, Kremer LC. Cardioprotective interventions for cancer patients receiving anthracyclines. *Cochrane Database Syst Rev*. 2011(6):Cd003917.

44. Cardinale D, Colombo A, Sandri MT, et al. Prevention of high-dose chemotherapy-induced cardiotoxicity in high-risk patients by angiotensin-converting enzyme inhibition. *Circulation*. 2006;114:2474-81.

45. Gulati G, Heck SL, Ree AH, et al. Prevention of cardiac dysfunction during adjuvant breast cancer therapy (PRADA): a 2 x 2 factorial, randomized, placebo-controlled, double-blind clinical trial of candesartan and metoprolol. *Eur Heart J*. 2016;37:1671-80.

46. Bosch X, Rovira M, Sitges M, et al. Enalapril and carvedilol for preventing chemotherapy-induced left ventricular systolic dysfunction in patients with malignant hemopathies: the OVERCOME trial (preventiOn of left Ventricular dysfunction with Enalapril and caRvedilol in patients submitted to intensive ChemOtherapy for the treatment of Malignant hEmopathies). *J Am Coll Cardiol*. 2013;61:2355-62.

47. Akpek M, Ozdogru I, Sahin O, et al. Protective effects of spironolactone against anthracycline-induced cardiomyopathy. *Eur J Heart Fail*. 2015;17:81-9.

48. Seicean S, Seicean A, Plana JC, et al. Effect of statin therapy on the risk for incident heart failure in patients with breast cancer receiving anthracycline chemotherapy: an observational clinical cohort study. *J Am Coll Cardiol*. 2012;60:2384-90.

49. Acar Z, Kale A, Turgut M, et al. Efficiency of atorvastatin in the protection of anthracycline-induced cardiomyopathy. *J Am Coll Cardiol*. 2011;58:988-9.

50. McKay RR, Lin X, Albiges L, et al. Statins and survival outcomes in patients with metastatic renal cell carcinoma. *Eur J Cancer*. 2016;52:155-62.

51. Thavendiranathan P, Negishi T, Somerset E, et al. Strain-guided management of potentially cardiotoxic cancer therapy. *J Am Coll Cardiol*. 2021;77:392-401.

52. Celutkiene J, Pudil R, Lopez-Fernandez T, et al. Role of cardiovascular imaging in cancer patients receiving cardiotoxic therapies: a position statement on behalf of the Heart Failure Association (HFA), the European Association of Cardiovascular Imaging (EACVI) and the Cardio-Oncology Council of the European Society of Cardiology (ESC). *Eur J Heart Fail*. 2020;22:1504-24.

53. Rao VU, Reeves DJ, Chugh AR, et al. Clinical approach to cardiovascular toxicity of oral antineoplastic agents: JACC state-of-the-art review. *J Am Coll Cardiol*. 2021;77:2693-716.

54. Cardinale D, Sandri MT, Colombo A, et al. Prognostic value of troponin I in cardiac risk stratification of cancer patients undergoing high-dose chemotherapy. *Circulation*. 2004;109:2749-54.

55. Ky B, Putt M, Sawaya H, et al. Early increases in multiple biomarkers predict subsequent cardiotoxicity in patients with breast cancer treated with doxorubicin, taxanes, and trastuzumab. *J Am Coll Cardiol*. 2014;63:809-16.

56. Lenihan DJ, Stevens PL, Massey M, et al. The utility of point-of-care biomarkers to detect cardiotoxicity during anthracycline chemotherapy: a feasibility study. *J Card Fail*. 2016;22:433-8.

57. Curigliano G, Cardinale D, Dent S, et al. Cardiotoxicity of anticancer treatments: epidemiology, detection, and management. *CA Cancer J Clin*. 2016;66:309-25.

58. Lipshultz SE, Rifai N, Sallan SE, et al. Predictive value of cardiac troponin T in pediatric patients at risk for myocardial injury. *Circulation*. 1997;96:2641-8.

59. Cardinale D, Sandri MT, Martinoni A, et al. Myocardial injury revealed by plasma troponin I in breast cancer treated with high-dose chemotherapy. *Ann Oncol*. 2002;13:710-15.

60. Kilickap S, Barista I, Akgul E, et al. cTnT can be a useful marker for early detection of anthracycline cardiotoxicity. *Ann Oncol*. 2005;16:798-804.

61. Plana JC, Galderisi M, Barac A, et al. Expert consensus for multimodality imaging evaluation of adult patients during and after cancer therapy: a report from the American Society of Echocardiography and the European Association of Cardiovascular Imaging. *J Am Soc Echocardiogr*. 2014;27:911-39.

62. Chang HM, Moudgil R, Scarabelli T, et al. Cardiovascular complications of cancer therapy: best practices in diagnosis, prevention, and management: part 1. *J Am Coll Cardiol.* 2017;70:2536-51.
63. Saccullo G, Marietta M, Carpenedo M, et al. Platelet cut-off for anticoagulant therapy in cancer patients with venous thromboembolism and thrombocytopenia: an expert opinion based on RAND/ UCLA Appropriateness Method (RAM). *Blood.* 2013;122:581.
64. Narayan V, Keefe S, Haas N, et al. Prospective evaluation of sunitinib-induced cardiotoxicity in patients with metastatic renal cell carcinoma. *Clin Cancer Res.* 2017;23:3601-9.
65. Jones LW, Habel LA, Weltzien E, et al. Exercise and risk of cardiovascular events in women with nonmetastatic breast cancer. *J Clin Oncol.* 2016;34:2743-9.
66. Lahart IM, Metsios GS, Nevill AM, Carmichael AR. Physical activity, risk of death and recurrence in breast cancer survivors: a systematic review and meta-analysis of epidemiological studies. *Acta Oncol.* 2015;54:635-54.
67. American Heart Association. Life's simple 7®. Last accessed 8/19/21. https://www.heart.org/en/ professional/workplace-health/lifes-simple-7
68. American College of Cardiology. Cancer treatment and your heart. Last accessed 8/19/21. https:// www.cardiosmart.org/topics/cancer-treatment-and-your-heart

Cardiac Amyloidosis

Kathleen W. Zhang and Daniel J. Lenihan

GENERAL PRINCIPLES

Definition

- Amyloidosis is a systemic disease that results from the deposition of misfolded protein aggregates as amyloid fibrils in extracellular tissue.
- Cardiac amyloidosis results when amyloid fibrils deposit in myocardium, typically producing a restrictive cardiomyopathy with signs and symptoms of heart failure.

Classification

- Over 30 precursor proteins have been associated with amyloidosis. However, >95% of cardiac amyloidosis cases are due to light-chain amyloidosis (AL) or transthyretin amyloidosis (ATTR).
- AL results from overproduction of clonal Igs by a plasma cell neoplasm, leading to misfolding and deposition of light-chain fragments as amyloid fibrils. Only 10-15% of AL occurs in association with multiple myeloma.[1]
- ATTR results from misfolding of transthyretin, a serum transport protein for thyroxine and retinol. Transthyretin misfolding may occur as an acquired wild-type variant or due to a point mutation in the transthyretin gene.
- Less common types of cardiac amyloidosis include secondary amyloidosis (AA) and apolipoprotein A1 amyloidosis (AApoA1).

Epidemiology

- AL is an uncommon condition with an annual incidence of >4000 in the US, of which at least 30-50% have symptomatic cardiac involvement. Median age at diagnosis is 63.[2]
- Wild-type ATTR is a disease of the elderly (median age at diagnosis is 76) that predominantly affects Caucasian men.[3]
  - Wild-type transthyretin cardiac amyloidosis (ATTR-CM) has been identified in 13% of patients hospitalized for heart failure with preserved ejection fraction and in 13% of patients with severe aortic stenosis referred for transcatheter aortic valve replacement.[4,5]
  - Carpal tunnel syndrome is common among patients with wild-type ATTR-CM (25% prevalence).[6]
- Hereditary ATTR is a rare, autosomal dominant disease with incomplete penetrance that leads to a familial cardiomyopathy, polyneuropathy, or both.
  - Age of onset varies by the mutation involved, but generally precedes onset of wild-type ATTR by several decades.
  - Val122Ile is the most common genetic variant found in the US and presents in individuals of African descent as a restrictive cardiomyopathy and/or polyneuropathy. In all, 3-4% of African Americans are carriers for the Val122Ile mutation.[7]
  - Thr60Ala is the second most common genetic variant in the US and presents as a mixed cardiomyopathy and polyneuropathy in patients typically of Irish descent.

DIAGNOSIS

- The diagnosis of cardiac amyloidosis is frequently missed and requires a high index of clinical suspicion.
- "Red flag" findings on history, physical examination, and diagnostic testing can raise clinical suspicion for cardiac amyloidosis.

Clinical Presentation

History

- Heart failure is the most prominent manifestation of AL cardiac amyloidosis (AL-CM) and ATTR-CM. Atrial arrhythmias are common with both types.
- Proteinuria is common with AL and may lead to diffuse anasarca.
- Sensorimotor peripheral neuropathy (numbness and tingling), orthostatic hypotension, and gastrointestinal symptoms (unintentional weight loss, early satiety, nausea, constipation, and diarrhea) are commonly seen in AL and hereditary ATTR.
- Wild-type ATTR-CM is associated with aortic stenosis, especially paradoxical low-flow, low-gradient aortic stenosis.
- Carpal tunnel syndrome (especially bilateral disease), lumbar spinal stenosis, and biceps tendon rupture are associated with amyloidosis, particularly ATTR.

Physical Examination

- Cardiac examination findings of cardiac amyloidosis are consistent with restrictive cardiomyopathy and include pulmonary rales, elevated jugular venous pressure, and peripheral edema.
- Findings of right heart failure (ascites, lower extremity edema) are particularly prominent in patients with AL-CM, especially those with significant proteinuria.
- Autonomic dysfunction may manifest with low blood pressure and/or significant postural hypotension.
- Symmetric sensorimotor polyneuropathy, carpal tunnel syndrome, or spinal stenosis may be seen on neurologic examination.
- Macroglossia and periorbital purpura ("raccoon eyes") are uncommon, but virtually pathognomonic for AL-CM in the presence of a cardiomyopathy.

Initial Diagnostic Testing

Laboratories

- Mild elevation in serum troponin on multiple occasions is common in patients with cardiac amyloidosis.
- Brain natriuretic peptide (BNP) or N-terminal proBNP (NT-proBNP) levels are often markedly elevated. In patients with AL, NT-proBNP is highly sensitive for cardiac involvement and is part of the staging system for diagnosis and prognosis.[8]

Electrocardiography

- Individual ECG findings have limited diagnostic accuracy for cardiac amyloidosis.
- Hallmark ECG findings of cardiac amyloidosis include low-voltage QRS amplitude in the limb leads, pseudoinfarct pattern, and relative low-voltage QRS amplitude in the setting of increased left ventricular wall thickness on echocardiography (Figure 15-1).
- Other ECG findings include intraventricular conduction delay, atrioventricular block, and atrial fibrillation/atrial flutter.

Imaging

Transthoracic echocardiography:

- Hallmark echocardiography findings of cardiac amyloidosis include increased left and right ventricular wall thickness (Figure 15-1B,C), diastolic dysfunction, biatrial enlargement, and a small pericardial effusion (Figure 15-1C).

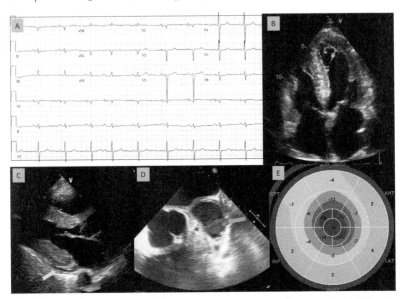

FIGURE 15-1. ECG and echocardiographic findings in cardiac amyloidosis. **(A)** Pseudoinfarct pattern and low QRS voltage in the limb leads on ECG. **(B)** Increased left and right ventricular wall thickness on transthoracic echocardiography. **(C)** Increased left ventricular wall thickness and a small pericardial effusion (arrow). **(D)** Left atrial appendage thrombus on transesophageal echocardiography (arrow). **(E)** Relative apical sparing of left ventricular longitudinal strain on echocardiography.

- Left ventricular ejection fraction (LVEF) is typically preserved ($\geq 50\%$), though reduced LVEF may be seen with advanced disease.
- Intracardiac thrombus (i.e., left atrial appendage thrombus) is more common in patients with cardiac amyloidosis, including those on systemic anticoagulation (Figure 15-1D).
- Relative apical sparing of left ventricular longitudinal strain is suggestive of cardiac amyloidosis and is thought to reflect preferential deposition of amyloid fibrils in the mid and basal segments of the heart (Figure 15-1E).
- Global longitudinal strain is usually severely abnormal in patients with cardiac amyloidosis. Abnormalities in atrial strain may also be early indicators of cardiac involvement.[9]

Differential Diagnosis

Hypertensive cardiomyopathy, hypertrophic cardiomyopathy, and other infiltrative cardiomyopathies are other causes of heart failure associated with left ventricular hypertrophy. A multimodality approach is usually necessary.[10]

Establishing the Diagnosis of Cardiac Amyloidosis

Once cardiac amyloidosis is suspected, definitive diagnostic testing should be pursued using technetium-labeled bone scintigraphy, endomyocardial biopsy, or cardiac MR imaging (CMR) with a noncardiac biopsy (Figure 15-2).

Diagnostic Criteria
- Endomyocardial biopsy with mass spectrometry is the gold standard for the diagnosis of cardiac amyloidosis.

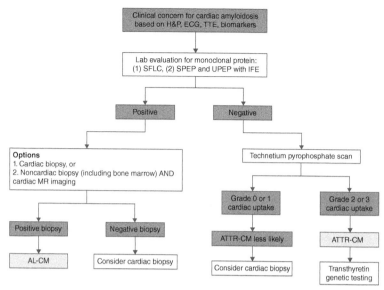

FIGURE 15-2. Establishing the diagnosis of cardiac amyloidosis. A suggested diagnostic algorithm for light-chain and transthyretin cardiac amyloidosis. AL-CM, light-chain cardiac amyloidosis; ATTR-CM, transthyretin cardiac amyloidosis; H&P, history and physical examination; IFE, immunofixation; SFLC, serum-free light-chain assay; SPEP, serum protein electrophoresis; TTE, transthoracic echocardiography; UPEP, urine protein electrophoresis.

- Technetium-labeled bone scintigraphy has been validated for noninvasive diagnosis of ATTR-CM with 91% sensitivity and 100% specificity in the absence of a monoclonal protein.[11]
- Noncardiac biopsy with mass spectrometry in combination with characteristic findings on CMR can be used for diagnosis of AL-CM in most cases.
- Transthyretin genotyping is necessary for all patients with ATTR to identify potential hereditary variants.

Endomyocardial Biopsy
- Endomyocardial biopsy is the diagnostic gold standard for cardiac amyloidosis and is safely performed at experienced centers.
- Histopathologic examination reveals apple-green birefringence with Congo red staining under polarized light microscopy.
- Confirmation of the fibril type with mass spectrometry is essential for accurate diagnosis.

Technetium-Labeled Bone Scintigraphy
- Technetium (^{99m}Tc)-labeled bisphosphonates localize to cardiac transthyretin amyloid deposits and may be used for noninvasive diagnosis of ATTR-CM. ^{99m}Tc-labeled pyrophosphate (PYP) is the most commonly used tracer in the US. Other tracers used in Europe include ^{99m}Tc-labeled 3,3-diphosphono-1,2-propanodicarboxylic acid (DPD) and ^{99m}Tc-labeled hydroxymethylene diphosphonate (HMDP).
- Scans are scored on a semi-quantitative grading scale (Figure 15-3A-C):
  ○ Grade 3 = cardiac uptake greater than bone

- ○ Grade 2 = cardiac uptake equal to bone
- ○ Grade 1 = cardiac uptake less than bone
- ○ Grade 0 = no cardiac uptake
- A study is considered positive for ATTR-CM in the setting of grade 2 or 3 uptake. Single-photon emission CT (SPECT) imaging should be used to confirm intramyocardial tracer uptake and not blood pool uptake (Figure 15-3D).
- As a quantitative measure, a heart-to-contralateral lung ratio of tracer uptake >1.5 is consistent with the diagnosis of ATTR-CM.
- Because the majority of false-positive scans are due to AL-CM, AL must be excluded before interpreting the technetium scan. This is typically done by checking serum-free light-chain assay along with serum and urine protein electrophoresis with immunofixation (Figure 15-2).

Cardiac Magnetic Resonance Imaging
- Diffuse, subendocardial late gadolinium enhancement (LGE) is highly specific for cardiac amyloidosis, though other nonvascular patterns of LGE can also be seen.
- Increased extracellular volume is also characteristic of cardiac amyloidosis.
- Prolonged native T1 relaxation times identify cardiac amyloidosis without need for gadolinium contrast.

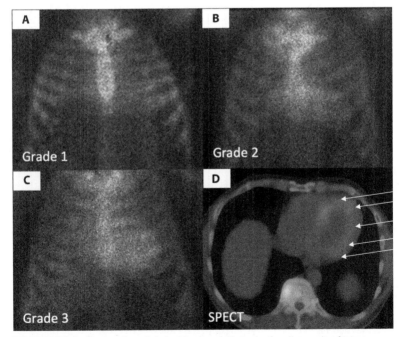

FIGURE 15-3. Technetium-labeled bone scintigraphy for diagnosis of transthyretin cardiac amyloidosis. Planar images demonstrate grade 1 **(A)**, grade 2 **(B)**, and grade 3 **(C)** uptake in patients with transthyretin cardiac amyloidosis. Single-photon emission CT (SPECT) imaging is critical to ensure tracer uptake within the myocardium (**D**, noted by arrows).

Noncardiac Biopsy

- To maximize diagnostic yield, biopsy of the clinically most affected organ should be performed.
- Diagnostic sensitivity of fat pad biopsy is higher for AL (80%) than hereditary ATTR (55%) or wild-type ATTR (15%).[12,13]

TREATMENT

- Inhibition of amyloid fibril production is the mainstay of therapy for AL-CM and ATTR-CM. This is accomplished using chemotherapy and/or autologous stem cell transplantation (ASCT) for AL-CM, and transthyretin stabilizers or transthyretin synthesis inhibitors for ATTR-CM (Table 15-1).
- Management of heart failure, arrhythmias, and orthostatic hypotension are additional components of cardiac amyloidosis management.

Targeted Therapy for Light-Chain Amyloidosis

- High-dose melphalan chemotherapy with ASCT imparts the highest chance of complete hematologic response and overall survival benefit for patients with AL.
- Increased risk for ASCT-related mortality include age, more than two organs involved with AL, advanced cardiac disease (symptomatic heart failure, arrhythmias, baseline hypotension), and renal dysfunction.
- Only about 20% of AL patients are eligible for ASCT at diagnosis; therefore, the majority are treated with bortezomib-based combination chemotherapy.
- Cyclophosphamide, bortezomib, and dexamethasone (CyBorD) is the most commonly used frontline regimen. Hematologic response is seen in 60-70% of patients, and cardiac response in about 33% of patients at 12 months. Overall survival among responders is comparable to that seen after ASCT.[14]
- Daratumumab plus CyBorD is a novel combination with superior hematologic response rates as compared to CyBorD alone in clinical trials and will likely represent a new standard of care.[15]
- Doxycycline inhibits the formation of light-chain amyloid fibrils in vivo and may improve survival in patients with AL-CM when used in conjunction with chemotherapy.[16]
- Management should be guided by a multidisciplinary team with expertise in the complexities of AL.

Targeted Therapy for Transthyretin Amyloidosis

Transthyretin Stabilizers

- Formation of transthyretin amyloid fibrils requires dissociation of the transthyretin homotetramer into monomers, which misfold and aggregate into insoluble fibrils.
- Transthyretin stabilizers prevent dissociation of the homotetrameric structure.[17]
- Tafamidis is approved by the US Food and Drug Administration (FDA) for the treatment of wild-type and hereditary ATTR-CM.
  - In the ATTR-ACT trial, tafamidis reduced all-cause mortality and cardiovascular hospitalization as compared to placebo and was also associated with lower rates of decline in 6-minute walk distance and quality of life.[18]
  - Patients with New York Heart Association (NYHA) class IV heart failure and/or advanced renal dysfunction (estimated glomerular filtration rate [eGFR] <25 mL/min) were excluded.
- Diflunisal is an NSAID that reduced rate of disease progression for ATTR with polyneuropathy in clinical trials.[19]
  - Renal dysfunction, worsening of heart failure, and bleeding are potential adverse effects.
  - Diflunisal may be considered in carefully selected patients with normal renal function and stable volume status when tafamidis is not available.

| TABLE 15-1 | TARGETED DRUG THERAPY FOR LIGHT-CHAIN AND TRANSTHYRETIN AMYLOIDOSIS | | |

Therapy	Amyloidosis FDA approval	Route and frequency	Notable toxicities
Transthyretin amyloidosis			
Transthyretin stabilizers			
Tafamidis	ATTR cardiomyopathy	PO, daily	GI symptoms
Diflunisal	—	PO, bid	Renal dysfunction, bleeding
Transthyretin synthesis inhibitors			
Patisiran	Hereditary ATTR with polyneuropathy	IV, every 3 weeks	Vitamin A deficiency, infusion reaction
Inotersen	Hereditary ATTR with polyneuropathy	SC, weekly	Thrombocytopenia, glomerulone- phritis, vitamin A deficiency, infusion reaction
Light-chain amyloidosis			
Bortezomib	—	IV, twice weekly for 2 weeks per 28-day cycle	Peripheral neurop- athy, diarrhea, thrombocytopenia
Cyclophosphamide	—	PO, once weekly per 28-day cycle	GI symptoms, pancytopenia
Daratumumab	Newly diagnosed AL	IV, once weekly (then once) per 28-day cycle	Respiratory infec- tions, diarrhea
Doxycycline	—	PO, bid	GI symptoms, photo- sensitive rash

AL, light-chain amyloidosis; ATTR, transthyretin amyloidosis; FDA, US Food and Drug Administration; GI, gastrointestinal.

Transthyretin Synthesis Inhibitors
- Patisiran and inotersen are small interfering RNA therapeutics approved by the FDA for the treatment of hereditary ATTR with polyneuropathy. Phase III studies of therapeutic efficacy in patients with ATTR-CM are ongoing (NCT03997383, NCT04136171).
- In the APOLLO trial, patisiran improved neuropathy impairment scores and quality of life. In addition, patisiran reduced NT-proBNP levels and left ventricular wall thickness and mitigated worsening of global longitudinal strain, suggesting cardiac benefit.[20] Pa- tients with NYHA classes III and IV heart failure were excluded.

- In the NEURO-TTR trial, inotersen improved neuropathy impairment scores and quality of life, without change in echocardiographic parameters.[21]
  ○ Thrombocytopenia and glomerulonephritis are important safety concerns.
  ○ Patients with NYHA classes III and IV heart failure were excluded.

Cardiac-Specific Therapy

- Diuretic agents and sodium restriction are the mainstays for symptom management in patients with cardiac amyloidosis. A combination of loop diuretics and potassium-sparing agents (i.e., spironolactone or eplerenone) is most effective to maintain adequate volume and potassium balance. Torsemide is preferred to furosemide due to its higher bioavailability and longer duration of action, as many patients have significant gut wall edema.
- Traditional neurohormonal antagonists are generally poorly tolerated due to a dependency on heart rate for cardiac output and tendency toward orthostatic hypotension.
- β-Blockers may be cautiously used in the setting of rapid atrial arrhythmias, although amiodarone will likely be better tolerated.[22]
- Anticoagulation is mandatory for all patients with atrial fibrillation.
- Pacemaker therapy is indicated according to established guidelines. There is no proven benefit to prophylactic pacemaker or implantable defibrillator placement.[23,24]
- Postural hypotension may be due to over-diuresis or autonomic neuropathy. Midodrine and droxidopa can be effective to alleviate symptoms related to autonomic dysfunction.
- Orthotopic heart transplantation (OHT) is reasonable for patients with end-stage ATTR-CM who are otherwise acceptable transplant candidates.[25] OHT may be considered in patients with AL-CM in whom disease is limited to the heart and systemic chemotherapy is deemed to be too toxic to be tolerated due to cardiac disease.

OUTCOME/PROGNOSIS

Light-Chain Cardiac Amyloidosis

- Cardiac involvement is highly prognostic of worse outcomes in patients with AL. Untreated, median survival from the onset of heart failure in AL-CM is ~6 months.
- The revised Mayo classification system utilizes troponin-T, NT-proBNP, and difference between involved and uninvolved free light-chain levels (dFLC) to designate three stages of disease with progressively worsening mortality. Patients receive 1 point each for troponin-T ≥ 0.025 ng/mL, NT-proBNP ≥ 1800 pg/mL, and dFLC ≥ 18 mg/dL.[8]
- Median overall survival after ASCT is ~5 years for patients with cardiac involvement.[26]

Transthyretin Cardiac Amyloidosis

- Untreated, median survival for ATTR-CM is 4.8 years.[27] This is expected to improve with targeted transthyretin therapy.
- Troponin-T, NT-proBNP, and eGFR can be used to stratify patients into prognostic categories, with worse clinical outcomes with troponin-T ≥ 0.05 ng/mL, NT-proBNP ≥ 3000 pg/mL, and eGFR < 45 mL/min.[27,28]

REFERENCES

1. Falk RH, Alexander KM, Liao R, Dorbala S. AL (light-chain) cardiac amyloidosis: a review of diagnosis and therapy. *J Am Coll Cardiol.* 2016;68:1323-41.
2. Quock TP, Yan T, Chang E, Guthrie S, Broder MS. Epidemiology of AL amyloidosis: a real-world study using US claims data. *Blood Adv.* 2018;2:1046-53.
3. Maurer MS, Hanna M, Grogan M, et al. Genotype and phenotype of transthyretin cardiac amyloidosis: THAOS (Transthyretin Amyloid Outcome Survey). *J Am Coll Cardiol.* 2016;68:161-72.
4. González-López E, Gallego-Delgado M, Guzzo-Merello G, et al. Wild-type transthyretin amyloidosis as a cause of heart failure with preserved ejection fraction. *Eur Heart J.* 2015;36:2585-94.

5. Scully PR, Patel KP, Treibel TA, et al. Prevalence and outcome of dual aortic stenosis and cardiac amyloid pathology in patients referred for transcatheter aortic valve implantation. *Eur Heart J.* 2020;41:2759-67.

6. Milandri A, Farioli A, Gagliardi C, et al. Carpal tunnel syndrome in cardiac amyloidosis: implications for early diagnosis and prognostic role across the spectrum of aetiologies. *Eur J Heart Fail.* 2020;22:507-15.

7. Quarta CC, Buxbaum JN, Shah AM, et al. The amyloidogenic V122I transthyretin variant in elderly black Americans. *N Engl J Med.* 2015;372(1):21-9.

8. Kumar S, Dispenzieri A, Lacy MQ, et al. Revised prognostic staging system for light chain amyloidosis incorporating cardiac biomarkers and serum free light chain measurements. *J Clin Oncol.* 2012;30:989-95.

9. Huntjens PR, Zhang KW, Soyama Y, et al. Prognostic utility of echocardiographic atrial and ventricular strain imaging in patients with cardiac amyloidosis. *JACC Cardiovasc Imaging.* 2021;14(8):1508-19.

10. Zhang KW, Zhang R, Deych E, et al. A multi-modal diagnostic model improves detection of cardiac amyloidosis among patients with diagnostic confirmation by cardiac biopsy. *Am Heart J.* 2021;232:137-45.

11. Gillmore JD, Maurer MS, Falk RH, et al. Nonbiopsy diagnosis of cardiac transthyretin amyloidosis. *Circulation.* 2016;133(24):2404-12.

12. Quarta CC, Gonzalez-Lopez E, Gilbertson JA, et al. Diagnostic sensitivity of abdominal fat aspiration in cardiac amyloidosis. *Eur Heart J.* 2017;38(24):1905-8.

13. Fine NM, Arruda-Olson AM, Dispenzieri A, et al. Yield of noncardiac biopsy for the diagnosis of transthyretin cardiac amyloidosis. *Am J Cardiol.* 2014;113:1723-27.

14. Manwani R, Cohen O, Sharpley F, et al. A prospective observational study of 915 patients with systemic AL amyloidosis treated with upfront bortezomib. *Blood.* 2019;134:2271-80.

15. Schwotzer R, Manz MG, Pederiva S, et al. Daratumumab for relapsed or refractory AL amyloidosis with high plasma cell burden. *Hematol Oncol.* 2019;37:595-600.

16. Wechalekar AD, Whelan C. Encouraging impact of doxycycline on early mortality in cardiac light chain (AL) amyloidosis. *Blood Cancer J.* 2017;7:89-91.

17. Zhang KW, Stockerl-Goldstein KE, Lenihan DJ. Emerging therapeutics for the treatment of light chain and transthyretin amyloidosis. *JACC Basic Transl Sci.* 2019;4:1-11.

18. Maurer MS, Schwartz JH, Gundapaneni B, et al. Tafamidis treatment for patients with transthyretin amyloid cardiomyopathy. *N Engl J Med.* 2018;379:1007-16.

19. Berk JL, Suhr OB, Obici L, et al. Repurposing diflunisal for familial amyloid polyneuropathy. *JAMA.* 2013;310:2658.

20. Adams D, Gonzalez-Duarte A, O'Riordan WD, et al. Patisiran, an RNAi therapeutic, for hereditary transthyretin amyloidosis. *N Engl J Med.* 2018;379:11-21.

21. Benson MD, Waddington-Cruz M, Berk JL, et al. Inotersen treatment for patients with hereditary transthyretin amyloidosis. *N Engl J Med.* 2018;379:22-31.

22. Giancaterino S, Urey MA, Darden D, Hsu JC. Management of arrhythmias in cardiac amyloidosis. *JACC Clin Electrophysiol.* 2020;6:351-61.

23. Sayed RH, Rogers D, Khan F, et al. A study of implanted cardiac rhythm recorders in advanced cardiac AL amyloidosis. *Eur Heart J.* 2015;36:1098-1105.

24. Lin G, Dispenzieri A, Kyle R, Grogan M, Brady PA. Implantable cardioverter defibrillators in patients with cardiac amyloidosis. *J Cardiovasc Electrophysiol.* 2013;24:793-98.

25. Barrett CD, Alexander KM, Zhao H, et al. Outcomes in patients with cardiac amyloidosis undergoing heart transplantation. *JACC Heart Fail.* 2020;8:461 LP-468.

26. Madan S, Kumar SK, Dispenzieri A, et al. High-dose melphalan and peripheral blood stem cell transplantation for light-chain amyloidosis with cardiac involvement. *Blood.* 2012;119:1117-22.

27. Gillmore JD, Damy T, Fontana M, et al. A new staging system for cardiac transthyretin amyloidosis. *Eur Heart J.* 2017;39:2799-806.

28. Grogan M, Scott CG, Kyle RA, et al. Natural History of Wild-Type Transthyretin Cardiac Amyloidosis and Risk Stratification Using a Novel Staging System. *J Am Coll Cardiol.* 2016;68(10):1014-1020.

Hypertrophic Cardiomyopathy

16

Natasha K. Wolfe and Sharon Cresci

GENERAL PRINCIPLES

- Hypertrophic cardiomyopathy (HCM) is **the most common heritable cardiac disease**; HCM is transmitted in an autosomal dominant manner but has incomplete penetrance and variable expression.[1-4]
- The prevalence of HCM is estimated to be ~1 in 200 to 1 in 500 and is caused by one of >1500 **mutations in genes encoding cardiac sarcomeric proteins.**[2,5]
- Mutations of β-myosin heavy-chain and myosin-binding protein C are the most common, accounting for nearly 80% of the identifiable pathologic variants. The mutations result in **inappropriate myocardial hypertrophy, myocyte disarray, and fibrosis.**[1,3,6,7]
- The clinical picture of HCM varies considerably and can be associated with chest pain, shortness of breath, syncope, or no symptoms at all. It is the most common cause of **sudden death among young athletes in the US.**[8,9]
- Summary of management of HCM:
  - Control symptoms.
  - Avoid strenuous exertion.
  - Screen for risk factors for sudden cardiac death (SCD) and consider a primary prevention implantable cardioverter-defibrillator (ICD) in high-risk patients.
  - Screen first-degree relatives.

Definition

- A characteristic feature of HCM is **left ventricular (LV) wall thickening in the absence of a cardiac or systemic cause** (e.g., aortic stenosis or hypertension). The usual clinical diagnostic criterion for HCM is **maximal LV wall thickness >15 mm** with wall thickness of 13 or 14 mm considered borderline.[4]
- The most common location of LV wall thickness is the interventricular septum, resulting in **asymmetric septal hypertrophy (ASH**; Figure 16-1). The increased thickening of the interventricular septum may geometrically narrow the LV outflow tract (LVOT). Elongation of the anterior mitral valve (MV) leaflet is also common in patients with HCM (etiology is currently not known). **Systolic anterior motion (SAM)** of the anterior MV leaflet further decreases the LVOT area, and **dynamic LVOT obstruction** of blood exiting the heart can occur. This dynamic process of **LVOT obstruction is present in approximately one-third of patients at rest and another third with provocation.**[10,11]

Classification

- It is important to distinguish between the **obstructive and nonobstructive forms** of HCM via 2D echocardiography. An outflow tract **gradient ≥50 mm Hg** at rest or after provocation represents severe LVOT obstruction.
- In patients with no obstruction at rest, provocative maneuvers such as exercise or the Valsalva maneuver should be performed to identify latent obstruction.
- The pattern of hypertrophy in HCM is asymmetric and can involve any portion of the ventricular septum or LV free wall. Thickening confined to the most distal portion of LV chamber, apical HCM (Figure 16-2), is a morphologic form often associated with a "spade" deformity of the LV and marked deep T waves on the ECG.[12]

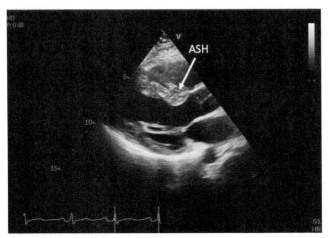

FIGURE 16-1. Parasternal long-axis view on echocardiogram showing asymmetric septal hypertrophy (ASH; arrow) in a patient with hypertrophic cardiomyopathy.

Epidemiology

- The prevalence of HCM is estimated to be from 1 in 200 to 1 in 500[5]; it is thought that up to 80% of individuals do not know they have the diagnosis. It is the most common genetic cardiovascular disease.[4]
- >1500 mutations, predominantly in the genes encoding sarcomeric proteins, have been associated with HCM.[3,13]
- HCM is inherited in an **autosomal dominant** manner but has **variable or incomplete penetrance** (not all individuals who inherit the mutation will develop the disease) and **variable expression** (location and extent of disease differs, even in individuals with the same causative mutation).[11]

Etiology

- HCM is a primary disorder of the sarcomere.
- Phenotypic expression of HCM is variable and depends on a complex interplay of genetic, environmental, and molecular factors.[3] Myocytes of involved cardiac tissue in HCM show bizarre shapes and disorganized patterns (myocardial disarray). There is often replacement fibrosis in the interstitium of the myocardium.
- Intramyocardial coronary microvessels in patients with HCM can have thickened walls with abnormal function.[4]
- MV leaflets are elongated [even in genotype (+)/phenotype (−) family members].[14]

Pathophysiology

- LVOT obstruction may result from the geometric narrowing of the LVOT due to ASH and/or SAM of the MV.
- SAM is felt to be a result of a combination of the Venturi phenomenon (high-velocity LV ejection jet pulls the mitral leaflet toward the septum), drag effect (a pushing force of flow directly on the leaflets), and intrinsic abnormalities of the MV (e.g., elongated anterior MV leaflet).[15,16] These factors cause the MV leaflets to be drawn toward the interventricular septum, resulting in leaflet–septal contact and LVOT obstruction.

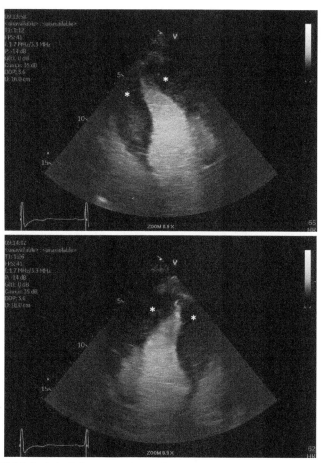

FIGURE 16-2. Apical views on echocardiogram with image enhancement showing apical hypertrophy (marked by asterisks) and spade-shaped left ventricle in patient with apical hypertrophic cardiomyopathy.

- The pathophysiology of **SAM-related mitral regurgitation (MR)** is distinct from, and should be differentiated from, intrinsic MR.[17] During LV ejection, the MR resulting from SAM is predominantly caused by the preferential motion of the anterior MV leaflet that results in an interleaflet gap and a posteriorly directed regurgitant jet into the left atrium.[18] As opposed to intrinsic MR that tends to be holosystolic, the MR associated with obstructive HCM (oHCM) may occur only in late systole and, as a result, may appear late peaking.[19]
- **LVOT obstruction is dynamic** and reduced by maneuvers that decrease myocardial contractility and increase ventricular volume. It is increased by maneuvers that reduce ventricular volume or increase myocardial contractility.
  - The pharmacologic agent phenylephrine increases systemic vascular resistance (afterload) and thus decreases the murmur of HCM.

○ The pharmacologic agent amyl nitrite decreases systemic vascular resistance (afterload) and preload, which increases LVOT obstruction and the murmur of HCM.
• Diastolic dysfunction arises from multiple factors that ultimately affect both ventricular relaxation and chamber stiffness.
• Myocardial ischemia and even infarction may occur in HCM. Ischemia is frequently unrelated to obstructive epicardial coronary artery disease but is caused by supply–demand mismatch.[4]
• Midcavity obstruction can also occur; usually due to hypertrophied papillary muscles and small LV cavity size. The profile of midcavitary obstruction is different than that of LVOT obstruction (Figure 16-3).

Prevention

All individuals with a first-degree family member with HCM are at risk and should undergo surveillance screening (see later).

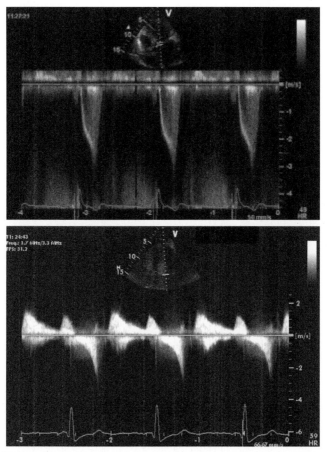

FIGURE 16-3. Typical late-peaking dagger-shaped profile of left ventricular outflow tract obstruction in a patient with hypertrophic cardiomyopathy **(A)**. Typical scythe-shaped profile of midcavitary obstruction **(B)**.

DIAGNOSIS

Clinical Presentation

History
- Many patients with HCM are **asymptomatic**.
- The most commonly reported symptom is **dyspnea**, often secondary to elevated LV diastolic filling pressures and diastolic dysfunction.[20,21]
- Other symptoms include **angina** (from myocardial oxygen mismatch due to increased myocardial mass, small vessel disease, or wall stress), **syncope** (due to LVOT obstruction or arrhythmias), and **arrhythmia** (manifesting as palpitations, syncope, or sudden death).

Family History
- A complete family history, including at least three generations, is recommended as part of the initial evaluation.[4]
- Compared with classic HCM, patients with apical variant HCM are less likely to have a positive family history of disease.[12]

Physical Examination
- A classic finding on auscultation is a **crescendo–decrescendo systolic murmur**, audible in at least two-thirds of patients with HCM, best heard along the left sternal border but may be heard throughout the precordium.
- The **murmur is dynamic** (changes in intensity with changes in loading conditions).
  - **The murmur increases** with maneuvers that decrease preload, like standing after squatting and the Valsalva maneuver, or with maneuvers or agents that decrease afterload.
  - Conversely, the **murmur decreases** in intensity with squatting (which increases preload and afterload) and handgrip (which increases afterload).
- The carotid pulse typically rises briskly and then declines in mid-systole as the gradient develops, followed by a secondary rise.
- The jugular venous pulse may demonstrate a prominent a wave secondary to diminished ventricular compliance.

Diagnostic Criteria

HCM can be diagnosed by a combination of physical examination, ECG, and imaging techniques; appropriate diagnostic testing can include echocardiography and MRI, cardiac catheterization, and/or genetic testing.

Diagnostic Testing

Laboratories
- Genetic testing can be performed, starting with the index case (proband) to allow for **cascade screening of all first-degree family members**.
- Genetic variants identified on genetic tests are categorized as pathogenic (P), likely pathogenic (LP), variant of uncertain significance (VUS), likely benign, or benign.
- ~60% of HCM patients will be found to have a P or LP variant on genetic testing, but the yield is higher in those with a family history of HCM. The yield is even higher if an individual has multiple specific clinical and phenotypic features (yield increases to ~80% if aged 45 years or older, maximal wall thickness of ≥ 20 mm, family history of HCM and SCD, and reverse curve type of septal morphology is present).[16]
- An individual's HCM phenotype, prognosis, clinical course, or response to medications cannot be predicted based on a particular genetic variant (with the possible exception that prognosis may be worse among those with multiple P/LP variants and/or P/LP variant with a VUS).[22]

- The decision to undergo genetic testing should be a shared decision between the patient and the physician. It should include a comprehensive discussion of the yield of genetic testing, the implications for cascade testing of relatives, and benefits and risks for the patient and their family.[4]

Electrocardiography
- ECG is usually abnormal in HCM patients; however, at least 10% of patients with HCM may have a normal ECG.
- **No particular ECG pattern is classic for HCM.** ST-segment and T-wave abnormalities are the most common, followed by evidence of LV hypertrophy.
- Prominent Q waves in the inferior leads, precordial leads, or both can occur in up to 50% of patients.
- Deep negative T waves in the mid-precordial leads are characteristic of apical HCM (Figure 16-4).[12]

Imaging
- Echocardiography is diagnostic for HCM. Wall thickness, MV abnormalities including elongated leaflets, MR, and LVOT obstruction can be accurately assessed.
- **MRI** has similar diagnostic capabilities as echocardiography and is particularly useful when echo images are suboptimal. It can also assess the presence and extent of myocardial fibrosis by assessment of late gadolinium enhancement.[23]

Diagnostic Procedures
- **Cardiac catheterization** can be useful to quantify the LVOT obstruction and LV pressures, along with evaluating coronary artery anatomy.
- Most symptomatic patients with HCM complain of angina or chest pain. Left heart catheterization can evaluate epicardial coronary artery abnormalities as a cause for angina, such as the presence of coronary artery disease or myocardial bridging.

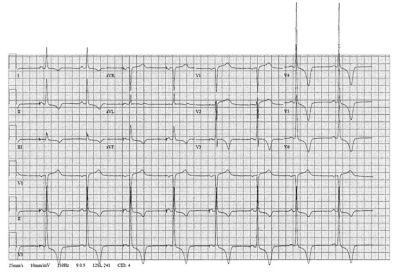

FIGURE 16-4. ECG with deep negative T waves (arrows) in the mid-precordial leads characteristic of apical hypertrophic cardiomyopathy.

TREATMENT

Many patients with HCM have no or mild symptoms and do not require treatment. For symptomatic patients, the majority can be managed medically without the need for invasive procedures.

Medications

* **β-Blockers are usually the first-line drugs** and are useful to treat angina, palpitations, and shortness of breath due to dynamic LVOT obstruction (gradients also respond well to β-blockade).[4,24]
* **Calcium channel blockers, especially verapamil,** can also be useful in relieving symptoms among patients who do not respond to or who do not tolerate a β-blocker.[4,25]
* **Disopyramide,** a class I antiarrhythmic drug, is a potent negative inotrope that can reduce LVOT obstruction and relieve symptoms. Disopyramide should be initiated in hospital with telemetry monitoring. Disopyramide is usually combined with a β-blocker.[4,26]
* New agents, such as **myosin inhibitors,** have recently been tested in clinical trials and found to be beneficial.[27,28]

Septal Reduction Therapy

* **Septal reduction therapy** can be considered in patients with severe symptoms (New York Heart Association [NYHA] class III or IV) **refractory to medications** and an LVOT gradient of at least 50 mm Hg at rest or with provocation.[4]
* Septal reduction can be achieved by septal myectomy or alcohol septal ablation. Both should be performed by experienced operators.[4]
* **Septal myectomy** is the gold standard for septal reduction treatment. There is over 50 years of experience, a low operative mortality (<1-2%), and studies show substantial reduction in heart failure symptoms.
* **Alcohol septal ablation** is an effective percutaneous catheter–based method for septal reduction that is also associated with substantial symptomatic benefit and may be preferred among patients at increased surgical risk or who prefer a nonsurgical approach. Recovery time is less than surgical myectomy.[4,29]
* Alcohol ablation is associated with an increased risk of conduction abnormalities, including complete heart block requiring pacemaker implantation among about 10% of patients.[29]
* The choice of treatment strategy should be a shared decision between the patient and the physician and include a comprehensive discussion of the success rates, benefits, and risks of each option.[4]

Lifestyle/Risk Modification

* Syncope in patients with HCM should be reported promptly, as it may represent aborted sudden cardiac arrest.
* Given autosomal dominant inheritance, the risk of transmitting the causative genetic mutation from affected parents to their children is 50%.
* First-degree relatives should be screened with an ECG, echocardiogram, and physical examination; genetic testing can also be considered if the proband has a causative mutation.
* Activity:
  ○ HCM is the **most common cause of sudden death in athletes aged <35 years**.[8,9]
  ○ All patients with HCM should be advised to **avoid strenuous exertion, including competitive sports**.
  ○ Patients can walk, jog, or ride a bike as long as they do so at a low-to-moderate (less than strenuous) workload.

MONITORING/FOLLOW-UP

- Patients with HCM should be seen at least every 6 to 12 months. Baseline evaluation should include echocardiogram, stress testing if symptomatic and/or to determine baseline functional capacity, Holter monitoring, and risk assessment for SCD (which may include MRI).[4]
- Every 1 to 2 years, or with change in symptoms, patients should have an evaluation including clinical assessment, echocardiogram, and Holter monitoring. A reassessment for SCD risk (unless an ICD has already been placed) should also be completed.[4]
- Exercise stress testing should be performed in symptomatic patients to reassess functional status every 2 to 3 years.[4]
- Reassessment with MRI to help with SCD risk assessment may be considered every 3 to 5 years.[4]
- Cardiopulmonary exercise testing should be performed if considering advanced heart failure therapies.[4]
- Family screening of first-degree relatives is indicated and should be discussed at every visit (if not yet completed).

SPECIAL CONSIDERATIONS

- All individuals with a first-degree family member with HCM should be screened for HCM with a history and physical examination, 12-lead ECG, and 2D echocardiogram with provocative maneuvers.[4]
  - Children and adolescents with a family member with a known P or LP variant should be screened at the time of diagnosis of their family member and every 1 to 2 years thereafter.
  - All other children and adolescents should be screened at any time after the diagnosis of their family member but no later than puberty and every 2 to 3 years thereafter.
  - Adults (aged >18 to 21 years) should be screened at the time of diagnosis of their family member and every 3 to 5 years thereafter.
- Patients may experience different emotions on receiving the diagnosis of HCM, both negative (anxiety, denial, upset) and positive (acceptance, increased mindfulness toward healthy habits).[30]

OUTCOME/PROGNOSIS

- HCM mortality rates have improved with the advent of current treatment strategies, including ICDs for at-risk individuals and cardiac transplantation. Some studies suggest annual mortality among HCM patients is equal to that of the general US population.[20,31]
- In referral cohorts, ~30-40% of patients with HCM have adverse clinical outcomes, including heart failure, atrial fibrillation, and SCD events.[21]
- A multicenter registry report has suggested that the lifelong risk of adverse events caused by HCM may be greater among patients with pathogenic sarcomeric gene variants or those diagnosed early in life.[32]
- Patients with HCM may be at **increased risk of SCD** due to abnormal myocardial substrate (ischemia, fibrosis, necrosis, and abnormal myocytes). Risk for SCD should be assessed at initial presentation and repeated every 1 to 2 years. One risk factor may be sufficient to recommend an ICD.[4]
  - **Risk factors for sudden death include:**
    - Prior cardiac arrest or sustained ventricular arrhythmia
    - Family history of sudden death in first-degree relative
    - Unexplained syncope particularly in young patients or when exertional and recurrent
    - LV thickness ≥30 mm
    - LV ejection fraction (LVEF) of ≤50%
    - LV apical aneurysm
    - Frequent runs of nonsustained ventricular tachycardia
    - Extensive late gadolinium enhancement on MRI

○ The American Heart Association (AHA) has developed a risk calculator to help estimate the 5-year risk of SCD in patients with HCM who are 16 years or older and have at least one major risk factor for SCD (https://professional.heart.org/en/guidelines-and-statements/hcm-risk-calculator).[33] It should not be used in elite athletes, HCM phenocopies, or in patients with HCM who have had SCD or sustained ventricular arrhythmias (who should receive ICD for secondary prevention). The risk calculator may help patients understand the magnitude of their individual risk for SCD and can be used in shared decision-making discussions between the patient and their physician.

• ~5% of patients with HCM develop LV dilatation and LV systolic dysfunction.
  ○ In patients with HCM, an LVEF <50% is considered significant LV systolic dysfunction.
  ○ These patients have a poor prognosis and should be treated similarly to other patients who have systolic dysfunction, including medications such as angiotensin-converting enzyme (ACE) inhibitors and consideration of advanced therapies.[4]

REFERRAL

• HCM patients should be managed by a cardiologist familiar with the disease.[4]
• HCM Centers of Excellence can help confirm the diagnosis of HCM, provide genetic counseling and testing, and provide advanced therapies, including septal reduction and heart failure therapies.[4]

PATIENT EDUCATION

• Time should be spent explaining HCM to patients and their families.
• There are several available resources for patients and their families.
  ○ The AHA provides professionals (https://professional.heart.org/en/education/hypertrophic-cardiomyopathy-for-professionals)[34] and patients (https://www.heart.org/en/health-topics/cardiomyopathy/what-is-cardiomyopathy-in-adults/hypertrophic-cardiomyopathy)[35] educational resources, webinars, podcasts, and patient stories.
  ○ The Hypertrophic Cardiomyopathy Association (HCMA) (https://4hcm.org/) started one of the first patient **advocacy** websites and can provide further education, support, and advocacy to patients and families with HCM.[36]

REFERENCES

1. Arad M, Seidman JG, Seidman CE. Phenotypic diversity in hypertrophic cardiomyopathy. *Hum Mol Genet.* 2002;11:2499-506.
2. Sabater-Molina M, Pérez-Sánchez I, Hernández Del Rincón JP, Gimeno JR. Genetics of hypertrophic cardiomyopathy: a review of current state. *Clin Genet.* 2018;93:3-14.
3. Marian AJ, Braunwald E. Hypertrophic cardiomyopathy: genetics, pathogenesis, clinical manifestations, diagnosis, and therapy. *Circ Res.* 2017;121(7):749-70.
4. Ommen SR, Mital S, Burke MA, et al. 2020 AHA/ACC guideline for the diagnosis and treatment of patients with hypertrophic cardiomyopathy: a report of the American College of Cardiology/American Heart Association Joint Committee on Clinical Practice Guidelines. *Circulation.* 2020;142:e558-e631.
5. Semsarian C, Ingles J, Maron MS, Maron BJ. New perspectives on the prevalence of hypertrophic cardiomyopathy. *J Am Coll Cardiol.* 2015;65:1249-54.
6. Maron BJ, Maron MS. Hypertrophic cardiomyopathy. *Lancet.* 2013;381:242-55.
7. Cui H, Schaff HV, Lentz Carvalho J, et al. Myocardial histopathology in patients with obstructive hypertrophic cardiomyopathy. *J Am Coll Cardiol.* 2021;77:2159-70.
8. Maron BJ, Doerer JJ, Haas TS, et al. Sudden deaths in young competitive athletes: analysis of 1866 deaths in the United States, 1980-2006. *Circulation.* 2009;119:1085-92.
9. Wasfy MM, Hutter AM, Weiner RB. Sudden cardiac death in athletes. *Methodist Debakey Cardiovasc J.* 2016;12:76-80.
10. Maron MS, Olivotto I, Zenovich AG, et al. Hypertrophic cardiomyopathy is predominantly a disease of left ventricular outflow tract obstruction. *Circulation.* 2006;114:2232-9.
11. Rowin EJ, Maron BJ, Maron MS. The hypertrophic cardiomyopathy phenotype viewed through the prism of multimodality imaging: clinical and etiologic implications. *JACC Cardiovasc Imaging.* 2020;13:2002-16.

12. Hughes RK, Knott KD, Malcolmson J, et al. Apical hypertrophic cardiomyopathy: the variant less known. *J Am Heart Assoc.* 2020;9:e015294.
13. Cirino AL, Seidman CE, Ho CY. Genetic testing and counseling for hypertrophic cardiomyopathy. *Cardiol Clin.* 2019;37:35-43.
14. Maron MS, Olivotto I, Harrigan C, et al. Mitral valve abnormalities identified by cardiovascular magnetic resonance represent a primary phenotypic expression of hypertrophic cardiomyopathy. *Circulation.* 2011;124:40-7.
15. Sherrid MV, Gunsburg DZ, Moldenhauer S, Pearle G. Systolic anterior motion begins at low left ventricular outflow tract velocity in obstructive hypertrophic cardiomyopathy. *J Am Coll Cardiol.* 2000;36:1344-54.
16. Geske JB, Ommen SR, Gersh BJ. Hypertrophic cardiomyopathy: clinical update. *JACC Heart Fail.* 2018;6:364-75.
17. Moreno JD, Bach RG, Damiano RJ, et al. Phenylephrine provocation to evaluate the cause of mitral regurgitation in patients with obstructive hypertrophic cardiomyopathy. *Circ Cardiovasc Imaging.* 2021;14(5):e012656.
18. Yu EH, Omran AS, Wigle ED, et al. Mitral regurgitation in hypertrophic obstructive cardiomyopathy: relationship to obstruction and relief with myectomy. *J Am Coll Cardiol.* 2000;36:2219-25.
19. Grigg LE, Wigle ED, Williams WG, et al. Transesophageal Doppler echocardiography in obstructive hypertrophic cardiomyopathy: clarification of pathophysiology and importance in intraoperative decision making. *J Am Coll Cardiol.* 1992;20:42-52.
20. Maron BJ. Clinical course and management of hypertrophic cardiomyopathy. *N Engl J Med.* 2018;379(7):655-68.
21. Rowin EJ, Maron MS, Chan RH, et al. Interaction of adverse disease related pathways in hypertrophic cardiomyopathy. *Am J Cardiol.* 2017;120:2256-64.
22. Burns C, Bagnall RD, Lam L, et al. Multiple gene variants in hypertrophic cardiomyopathy in the era of next-generation sequencing. *Circ Cardiovasc Genet.* 2017;10:e001666.
23. Maron MS. Clinical utility of cardiovascular magnetic resonance in hypertrophic cardiomyopathy. *J Cardiovasc Magn Reson.* 2012;14:13.
24. Nistri S, Olivotto I, Maron MS, et al. β blockers for prevention of exercise-induced left ventricular outflow tract obstruction in patients with hypertrophic cardiomyopathy. *Am J Cardiol.* 2012;110:715-19.
25. Bonow RO, Dilsizian V, Rosing DR, et al. Verapamil-induced improvement in left ventricular diastolic filling and increased exercise tolerance in patients with hypertrophic cardiomyopathy: short-and long-term effects. *Circulation.* 1985;72:853-64.
26. Sherrid MV, Barac I, McKenna WJ, et al. Multicenter study of the efficacy and safety of disopyramide in obstructive hypertrophic cardiomyopathy. *J Am Coll Cardiol.* 2005;45:1251-8.
27. Olivotto I, Oreziak A, Barriales-Villa R, et al. Mavacamten for treatment of symptomatic obstructive hypertrophic cardiomyopathy (EXPLORER-HCM): a randomised, double-blind, placebo-controlled, phase 3 trial. *Lancet.* 2020;396:759-69.
28. Spertus JA, Fine JT, Elliott P, et al. Mavacamten for treatment of symptomatic obstructive hypertrophic cardiomyopathy (EXPLORER-HCM): health status analysis of a randomised, double-blind, placebo-controlled, phase 3 trial. *Lancet.* 2021;397:2467-75.
29. Batzner A, Pfeiffer B, Neugebauer A, et al. Survival after alcohol septal ablation in patients with hypertrophic obstructive cardiomyopathy. *J Am Coll Cardiol.* 2018;72:3087-94.
30. Zytnick D, Heard D, Ahmad F, et al. Exploring experiences of hypertrophic cardiomyopathy diagnosis, treatment, and impacts on quality of life among middle-aged and older adults: an interview study. *Heart Lung.* 2021;50:788-93.
31. Maron BJ, Rowin EJ, Casey SA, et al. Hypertrophic cardiomyopathy in adulthood associated with low cardiovascular mortality with contemporary management strategies. *J Am Coll Cardiol.* 2015;65:1915-28.
32. Ho CY, Day SM, Ashley EA, et al. Genotype and lifetime burden of disease in hypertrophic cardiomyopathy: insights from the Sarcomeric Human Cardiomyopathy Registry (SHaRe). *Circulation.* 2018;138:1387-98.
33. American Heart Association. HCM risk calculator. Last accessed 08/20/21. https://professional.heart.org/en/guidelines-and-statements/hcm-risk-calculator
34. American Heart Association. Hypertrophic cardiomyopathy for professionals. Last accessed 08/20/21. https://professional.heart.org/en/education/hypertrophic-cardiomyopathy-for-professionals
35. American Heart Association. Hypertrophic cardiomyopathy (HCM). Last accessed 08/20/21. https://www.heart.org/en/health-topics/cardiomyopathy/what-is-cardiomyopathy-in-adults/hypertrophic-cardiomyopathy
36. Hypertrophic Cardiomyopathy Association. Last accessed 08/20/21. https://4hcm.org/

Diseases of the Pericardium

17

Natasha K. Wolfe and Sharon Cresci

Introduction

- The pericardium is a fibrous sac surrounding the heart and consisting of two layers:
  - Visceral pericardium is a thin inner layer of mesothelial cells and collagen and elastin fibers attached to the epicardium.
  - Parietal pericardium is a 2-mm fibrous outer layer.
- The layers are separated by the pericardial space, which normally contains 15 to 50 mL of fluid.
- Pericardial fluid consists of an ultrafiltrate continuously produced from the mesothelial cells of the visceral pericardium and is resorbed via lymphatics and venules.
- Although it is not absolutely essential for cardiac performance, several functions have been attributed to the pericardium, including:
  - Tethering of the heart within the mediastinum
  - Lubrication of the movements of the heart
  - Augmentation of diastolic function
  - Serving as a barrier to infection and inflammation
  - Participation in autonomic reflexes and paracrine signaling

Acute Pericarditis

GENERAL PRINCIPLES

- Acute pericarditis is the most common pericardial syndrome, caused by inflammation of the pericardium, resulting in characteristic clinical features.
- Usually affects young and middle-aged individuals and frequently recurs[1]
- Can occur from a variety of diseases, but most cases are considered idiopathic

Classification

- Pericarditis can be classified as acute or recurrent.
- Recurrent pericarditis can occur after the resolution of the inciting cause of an acute attack. Approximately 15-30% with idiopathic acute pericarditis will suffer a relapse. Women and those who initially fail treatment with NSAIDs are at increased risk.[2]

Epidemiology

- The exact incidence and prevalence are unknown, as undoubtedly many cases are undiagnosed.
- It is diagnosed in 1 out of every 1000 hospital admissions.[3]
- Pericarditis accounts for 0.2% of all hospital cardiovascular admissions and is diagnosed in 5% of patients presenting with nonischemic chest pain in emergency departments.[1]

Etiology

- See Table 17-1 for common causes of acute pericarditis.

TABLE 17-1	ETIOLOGIES OF ACUTE PERICARDITIS

- Idiopathic
- Infectious
  - Viral (echovirus, coxsackievirus, Epstein–Barr virus, adenovirus, cytomegalo-virus, HIV)
  - Bacterial (*Pneumococcus, Staphylococcus, Streptococcus, Mycoplasma,* Lyme disease, *Haemophilus influenzae, Neisseria meningitides*)
  - Mycobacteria
- Inflammatory
  - Connective tissue disease (SLE, RA, scleroderma, dermatomyositis)
  - Drug induced
  - Postcardiac surgery
- Postmyocardical infarction
  - Early
  - Late (Dressler)
- Malignancy, chemotherapy, and radiation
- Uremia
- Thyroid disease

RA, rheumatoid arthritis; SLE, systemic lupus erythematosus.

- **Most cases of pericarditis are idiopathic. (highlight the work "idiopathic").** Diagnostic workup for the cause of acute pericarditis rarely establishes a specific diagnosis.
- **Viral infections** represent the second most common cause of acute pericarditis.
  - Patients typically will have upper respiratory tract infection symptoms before presentation.
  - Coxsackie and echoviruses are the most common viral agents.
- **Autoimmune** phenomena collectively represent a major cause of acute pericarditis, including connective tissue disease, drug induced, postpericardiotomy, and Dressler syndrome.
- **Uremic** pericarditis occurs in up to one-third of patients with chronic uremia.
  - It is typically associated with a pericardial effusion.
  - It is associated with higher levels of azotemia (blood urea nitrogen [BUN] > 60 mg/dL).
- **Tuberculous** or **HIV**-associated pericarditis should be suspected in high-risk patients (history of exposure, immunocompromised state).
- Pericarditis **after acute myocardial infarction** (AMI) is declining in incidence in the reperfusion era, and Dressler syndrome is now rare.
  - Post-MI pericarditis presents in the first few days up to a week after an infarct, due to transmural necrosis with inflammation affecting the adjacent pericardium.
  - Dressler syndrome is a type of postinfarction pericarditis that occurs 1 to 8 weeks after the infarct. It occurs in 1% of patients after AMI and is thought to be immune mediated.

DIAGNOSIS

Clinical Presentation

History
- Typically, patients will present with recent-onset chest pain.
- The chest pain can be quite severe and often described as:
  - Pleuritic, sharp

○ Substernal or left sided
○ Radiation to the back, neck, and/or shoulders
○ Pain along the trapezius ridge is classic for pericarditis and uncommon in ischemic disease.
○ May be worsened with swallowing
- Classically, the pain will improve when the patient leans forward and worsen when the patient is supine.
- Associated symptoms can include dyspnea, cough, and, occasionally, hiccups.
- It is important to ask the patient about any fevers, chills, shaking, lethargy, myalgias, or upper respiratory symptoms, which raise suspicion for an infectious etiology.
- In patients with suspected autoimmune disorders, it is key to also ask about arthralgias, including morning stiffness, skin changes, Raynaud phenomenon, abdominal pain, and neuropathy.

Physical Examination
- Patients may have a low-grade fever and sinus tachycardia.
- Otherwise, the only abnormal physical finding is the pericardial friction rub, which is present in approximately one-third of patients presenting with acute pericarditis.
- A **pericardial friction rub** is:
  ○ Caused by friction between the inflamed visceral and parietal pericardia
  ○ Described as high pitched, grating, or scratching
  ○ Classically has three components per cardiac cycle (i.e., ventricular systole, early diastole, and atrial systole), but in many patients, only one or two components may be present
  ○ Often fleeting and dynamic
  ○ Best heard by placing the diaphragm of the stethoscope at the left lower sternal border while the patient is leaning forward

Diagnostic Criteria

To diagnose acute pericarditis, at least two of the following four symptoms should be present:
- Typical chest pain
- Pericardial friction rub
- Suggestive ECG changes
- New or worsening pericardial effusion

Differential Diagnosis

- Acute pericarditis–type chest discomfort can mimic several diseases, including:
  ○ Acute coronary syndrome (ACS)
  ○ Aortic dissection
  ○ Pulmonary embolism
  ○ Pneumonia
  ○ Pneumothorax
- It can be difficult to differentiate pericarditis from ACS.

Diagnostic Testing

Laboratories
- Laboratory tests may reveal nonspecific markers of inflammation, such as an elevated erythrocyte sedimentation rate (ESR), C-reactive protein (CRP), or leukocytosis.
- Serum cardiac enzymes (troponin or creatine kinase-MB [CK-MB]) are often slightly elevated due to inflammation of the adjacent myocardium.
- More specific tests, such as antinuclear antibody (ANA), rheumatoid factor, thyroid function, tuberculin testing, blood or viral cultures, and cytology, should be ordered based on the clinical scenario.

Electrocardiography

- ECG changes are present in most cases, but their absence does not exclude pericarditis (Figure 17-1).
- Serial ECGs during the initial hours to days of acute pericarditis reveal a characteristic evolution present in about 60% of patients:
  ○ Stage 1: diffuse concave ST-segment elevation and PR depression in all leads, except aVR. Also, helpful is concomitant ST depression and PR elevation in lead aVR
  ○ Stage 2: normalized ST segments with decreasing or flattened T waves
  ○ Stage 3: T-wave inversion
  ○ Stage 4: ECG normalization
- Stage 1 is highly specific and diagnostic for acute pericarditis.
- **The crucial distinction between stage 1 ECG changes in acute pericarditis and acute ST-segment elevation MI lies in the noncoronary distribution of the ST changes** (e.g., leads I, II, and III), as well as the presence of PR depression in acute pericarditis.

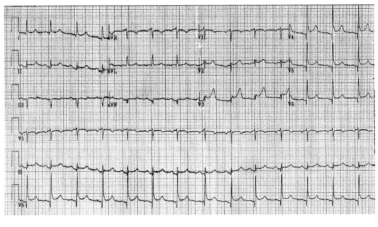

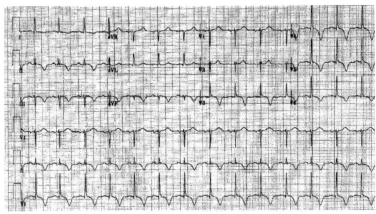

FIGURE 17-1. ECG in pericarditis. **(A)** Stage 1 pericarditis, exhibiting diffuse concave ST-segment elevations and PR depression, except in aVR, where the abnormalities are reversed. **(B)** Stage 3 pericarditis, 1 day later in the same patient, showing diffuse T-wave inversion after ST segments had normalized.

- An equally important distinction is that in acute pericarditis, **T-wave inversion only occurs after the ST-segment elevation has resolved**, whereas in ST-segment elevation MI, both T-wave inversion and ST-segment elevation are found concurrently.
- However, due to significant overlap in the ECG findings in these two entities, urgent echocardiography can be useful to rule out segmental wall motion abnormalities, which would be expected with ongoing myocardial ischemia.

Imaging
- Transthoracic echocardiography (TTE) is obtained at diagnosis and usually 1 to 2 weeks after initiation of treatment to rule out a significant pericardial effusion.
- Large effusions are not typical in uncomplicated viral or idiopathic pericarditis.
- The presence of larger effusion alerts the physician to a broader differential diagnosis, such as chronic inflammation, constriction, tamponade, or malignancy.
- Cardiac CT or MRI may be used as second-line imaging techniques to evaluate for evidence of pericardial inflammation and assess for constrictive and/or effusive-constrictive physiology in cases where the diagnosis is uncertain.[1]

TREATMENT

- Typically, acute pericarditis is self-limited.
- Treatment generally consists of a short course of an NSAID with or without the addition of colchicine.

Medications
- **NSAIDs**:
  - NSAIDS that are commonly used include aspirin (ASA), ibuprofen, naproxen, or indomethacin
  - All patients should be treated for at least 2 weeks to minimize the risk for scarring.
    - Ibuprofen: 600 to 800 mg every 8 hours
    - ASA: 650 to 1000 mg every 8 hours for 2 to 4 weeks
  - ASA is suggested in patients with post-MI pericarditis or Dressler syndrome as other NSAIDs are contraindicated in the setting of an AMI. Glucocorticoids should be avoided early after an AMI due to a risk for impaired ventricular healing, which can increase the risk for ventricular rupture.
- **Colchicine**:
  - There is considerable evidence that supports the use of colchicine as an adjunct to NSAIDs.
  - In a meta-analysis including seven studies of medical therapy for pericarditis, colchicine was associated with a reduced risk of treatment failure (odds ratio 0.23) and recurrent pericarditis (odds ratio 0.39).[4]
  - The Colchicine for acute Pericarditis (COPE) trial found that adding colchicine to an ASA regimen significantly reduced the recurrence of acute pericarditis compared with placebo with a number needed to treat of 5.[5]
    - Colchicine was given as 1 to 2 mg for 1 day, then 0.5 to 1.0 mg per day for 3 months.
    - The ASA regimen for the study was 800 mg every 6 to 8 hours for 7 to 10 days with a gradual taper over 3 to 4 weeks.
  - Some patients may not be able to tolerate the gastrointestinal side effects.
  - Less frequent but important side effects include hepatoxicity, myotoxicity, and bone marrow suppression; thus, the patient's serum creatinine, CK, transaminases, and blood cell count should be followed.
  - To avoid toxicity, it must be used with caution in elderly patients and in those with renal insufficiency.

- **Glucocorticoids**:
  - Treatment with high-dose corticosteroid with a rapid taper is an independent risk factor for recurrence of pericarditis.[5] Therefore, corticosteroids are not typically used as a first-line therapy, except in specific cases, such as autoimmune pericarditis (especially if secondary to connective tissue disease), or for refractory symptoms despite NSAID therapy and/or colchicine.
  - If steroids are necessary, lower initial doses (0.2 to 0.5 mg/kg/day) with a slow taper every 2 to 4 weeks is preferred. Tapering should be guided by symptoms and potentially by serial measurement of serial high-sensitivity CRP.
  - Some clinicians will add NSAIDs with or without colchicine during the steroid taper.
- **Interleukin-1 (IL-1) blockers and additional immunosuppressive agents:**
  - IL-1 blockade with anakinra has been demonstrated in a small randomized controlled trial to be beneficial for the treatment of recurrent pericarditis in patients resistant to colchicine and dependent on corticosteroids.[6]
  - Additional small studies have demonstrated efficacy of azathioprine in the treatment of long-term recurrent pericarditis requiring high doses of steroids.[7]
  - Other studies have demonstrated some benefit of methotrexate and mycophenolate mofetil in patients with idiopathic recurrent pericarditis who are not responsive to steroids, are steroid dependent, or had unacceptable steroid-related side effects.[7]

Nonpharmacologic Therapies

- Pericardiocentesis (diagnostic and/or therapeutic) may be considered in patients with moderate or large pericardial effusion with:
  - Symptoms attributable to the effusion
  - Cardiac tamponade (see later)
  - Concern for a purulent, tuberculous, or malignant effusion
- Any patient with a high fever, bacteremia, or signs of sepsis should undergo urgent pericardiocentesis for diagnosis as there is increased risk for the development of tamponade, sepsis, and death in patients with purulent pericarditis.

Surgical Management

Pericardiectomy may be considered in patients with severe recurrent disease despite intensive medical therapy.

COMPLICATIONS

- Complications include:
  - Recurrent or chronic pericarditis which occurs in 15-30% of patients with idiopathic acute pericarditis.
  - Pericardial constriction (usually resulting from chronic pericarditis). Studies suggest this can occur in 1.5% of patients with acute pericarditis. It is more likely in those who have an identified cause of acute pericarditis. It is rare in viral/idiopathic cases.[8]
  - Pericardial effusion and tamponade (including hemopericardium). Large pericardial effusions are uncommon among patients with acute pericarditis, especially those with idiopathic or viral etiology.
  - Development of atrial fibrillation
- **Anticoagulants should be avoided** to decrease the risk of hemopericardium, an uncommon complication that can lead to cardiac tamponade.

MONITORING/FOLLOW-UP

- Patients should be seen within 2 to 4 weeks of initiating medical therapy for acute pericarditis.

- Patients with pericardial effusions should be followed up with serial TTEs.
- Strenuous activity should be avoided for at least 4 weeks in case of concomitant myocardial involvement.
- Serial high-sensitivity CRP can be used to monitor response to treatment.

Pericardial Effusion and Tamponade

GENERAL PRINCIPLES

- A pericardial effusion represents an increased amount of fluid in the pericardial space.
- The significance of a pericardial effusion is determined by its size, rate of accumulation, and cause.
- Effusions become clinically detectable around 50 mL and can reach up to 2 L or more.
- Cardiac tamponade is a complication of pericardial effusion, which can be life-threatening. It is a condition that exists when the pericardial space contains fluid under sufficient pressure to interfere with cardiac filling, resulting in decreased cardiac output. It is considered a medical emergency, as cardiogenic shock and death can rapidly ensue.

Classification

- Effusions are often classified based on their etiology.
- Another distinction is based on the chronicity of the effusion.
  - Acute effusions may develop hemodynamic compromise (i.e., tamponade) with small amounts of fluid (<200 mL).
  - With chronic effusions, large amounts of fluid may accumulate without cardiac tamponade due to pericardial stretching over time.

Etiology

- Typically, a patient has an established underlying diagnosis before the development of the pericardial effusion.
- Any cause of pericarditis (Table 17-1) can lead to a pericardial effusion.
- In one U.S. study, malignancy was the most common cause (23%), followed by radiation (14%), viral infection (14%), collagen-vascular disease (14%), and uremia (12%).[9]
- Tamponade is more common in pericardial effusions due to infection (bacterial, fungal, and HIV-associated), bleeding, and malignancy.
- Purulent pericarditis should be suspected in any patient with high fevers or signs of sepsis.

Pathophysiology

- The etiology of an effusion can be categorized by the mechanisms leading to the effusion:
  - Increased fluid production (e.g., chronic inflammation)
  - Decreased resorption due to disruption of lymphatics and veins
  - Altered oncotic balance (e.g., congestive heart failure, renal failure, or hypoalbuminemia)
  - Foreign substance (e.g., blood, pus, lymph, or tumor infiltration)
- Cardiac tamponade is the result of an effusion that causes circulatory compromise from reduced cardiac output. As fluid accumulates in the pericardial space, intrapericardial pressure increases and impairs diastolic filling.
- Cardiac tamponade results in increased ventricular interdependence and reduced stroke volume.
  - Normal physiology
    - During inspiration, decreased intrathoracic pressure facilitates increased venous return to the right side of the heart.

- With increased right ventricular (RV) filling, the intraventricular septum slightly blows into the left ventricular (LV) cavity; this mildly reduces LV filling.
- This leads to a small physiologic decline in the systolic blood pressure (<10 mm Hg) during inspiration.
  ○ Tamponade physiology
    - During inspiration, there continues to be increased venous return to the right side of the heart.
    - Due to increased intrapericardial pressures, the RV can only expand at the intraventricular septum, resulting in exaggerated bowing of the septum and decreased diastolic filling of the LV.
    - Thus, the normal ventricular interdependence is exaggerated and results in reduced LV preload.
- Adrenergic compensation with increased heart rate, contractility, and vasoconstriction occur in response to reduced cardiac output. However, if the pericardial pressure continues to rise, the compensatory mechanisms eventually fail and the patient develops shock.

DIAGNOSIS

Clinical Presentation

Pericardial effusions have marked variability in their clinical presentation, ranging from asymptomatic to life-threatening.

History
- Symptoms of pericardial effusion, when present, are often vague and nonspecific.
- Fatigue, decreased exercise capacity, and dyspnea are common.
- Patients may complain of a dull ache or chest pressure.
- Large effusions may compress extrinsic structures and lead to complaints of dysphagia, nausea, hiccups, hoarseness (due to recurrent laryngeal nerve impingement), or cough.
- Symptoms of tamponade include restlessness, dyspnea, cough, chest discomfort, extreme fatigue, presyncope, anxiety, or agitation.
- With progression, shock may occur, resulting in decreased urine output, mental status changes, obtundation, and eventual cardiac arrest.

Physical Examination
- Physical examination often yields no unique findings for pericardial effusion.
- Despite a substantial effusion, a pericardial rub may still be present in the setting of pericarditis.
- The three classic signs of cardiac tamponade are known as Beck's triad, which include **hypotension, jugular venous distention (JVD), and decreased heart sounds**.
- Physical examination findings of tamponade include the following:
  ○ JVD: The neck veins may also show a prominent x descent and lack of y descent (Figure 17-2),[10] characteristic of tamponade.
  ○ Tachycardia
  ○ Decreased heart sounds
  ○ Hypotension with decreased pulse pressure
  ○ Tachypnea
  ○ Signs of cardiogenic shock
  ○ Pulsus paradoxus:
    - **Pulsus paradoxus is an exaggerated drop in systolic pressure on inspiration**. It should be assessed in all patients with suspected cardiac tamponade. It is due to the interventricular dependence that occurs in tamponade.

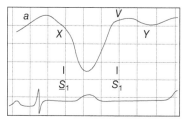

FIGURE 17-2. Right atrial pressure tracing in pericardial tamponade. Note the prominent *x* descent and absent *y* descent. (Reprinted with permission from Murphy JG. *Mayo Clinic Cardiology Review.* 2nd ed. Lippincott Williams & Wilkins; 2000:854.)

- Pulsus paradoxus can be checked by inflating the blood pressure cuff above the systolic pressure and deflating until Korotkoff sounds are heard only during expiration.
- Then, the cuff is further deflated until Korotkoff sounds are heard with both inspiration and expiration.
- Pulsus paradoxus is the difference between these pressures.
- The sensitivity is 98% if >10 mm Hg, and the specificity is 70% if >10 mm Hg and 83% if >12 mm Hg.[11]
- Other disorders that may be associated with an abnormal pulsus paradoxus include chronic obstructive pulmonary disease, constrictive pericarditis, and RV failure from infarction or pulmonary embolism.

Diagnostic Testing

Laboratories
If the clinical evaluation is suspicious for a certain etiology, lab studies may be indicated to support the clinical diagnosis.

Electrocardiography
- ECG may reveal low voltage of the QRS complex and/or electrical alternans.
- Amplitude of the entire QRS complex (R + S):
  - Limb leads <5 mm
  - Precordial leads <10 mm

Imaging
- **TTE**:
  - TTE is **the study of choice** for diagnosis and follow-up of pericardial effusions. **As soon as tamponade is suspected, TTE should be performed urgently to confirm the diagnosis**.
  - TTE can detect size and location of the effusion. It can also detect other features, such as pericardial thickness, fibrinous stranding, and fluid loculations or masses.
  - TTE can also detect loculated effusions that occur more often in patients after recent cardiac surgery.
  - In tamponade, TTE will typically reveal a large effusion and may show swinging of the heart within the effusion. The size of the effusion will depend on its chronicity.
  - Some TTE findings that suggest cardiac tamponade are as follows:
    - Right atrial notching in late diastole
    - RV collapse in early diastole
    - Abnormal ventricular septal motion

- Dilated, noncompressible inferior vena cava with blunted respiratory changes
- Respiratory variation of tricuspid valve inflow velocities of >40% or mitral valve inflow velocities of >25%
  - Of note, tamponade is a clinical diagnosis, and echocardiography has a confirmatory role. Thus, the decision of how and when to best perform drainage is best determined by the patient's clinical status and not the specific echo findings.
  - If tamponade is suspected in postcardiotomy cases or following cardiac trauma, TTE provides inadequate assessment because of the possibility of localized or loculated effusions and usually poor echocardiographic windows.
    - The most common location of hemorrhage postcardiotomy is posterior to the left atrium, which is virtually invisible by TTE.
    - Transesophageal echocardiography (TEE) should be used instead to confirm the diagnosis.
- **Ancillary imaging**:
  - Chest radiography (CXR) may reveal enlargement of the cardiac silhouette if the effusion is >250 mL.
  - A globular or water bottle–shaped heart may also be seen.
  - CT and MRI can determine the size of an effusion and estimate pericardial thickness and have the added advantage of imaging surrounding structures.

Diagnostic Procedures
- **Pericardiocentesis**:
  - Diagnostic pericardiocentesis should be considered if an effusion is large and readily accessible and if further diagnostic information would affect management decisions.
  - **The diagnostic yield of a diagnostic pericardiocentesis is fairly low but variable**.[3,9,12]
  - Pericardial effusion analysis should be considered in patients:
    - Undergoing drainage for tamponade
    - With a high suspicion for neoplastic, purulent, or tuberculous pericarditis
    - With a moderate-to-large effusion of unknown etiology
  - Pericardial fluid is typically sent for:
    - Cell count and differential (though rarely helpful in establishing a cause)
    - Gram stain
    - Culture
    - Cytology
    - Possibly polymerase chain reaction testing for certain organisms
  - Further specific testing (e.g., adenosine deaminase level in suspected tuberculous effusion) is based on the clinical scenario.
  - In patients with an established malignancy and a new pericardial effusion, it is important to perform a fluid analysis as up to 50% of patients will not have a malignant pericardial effusion (i.e., positive pathologic evidence of tumor).
- **Pericardial biopsy**:
  - Pericardial biopsy can be performed percutaneously at experienced centers but is typically performed surgically.
  - Biopsy is done in patients with an effusion of unknown etiology or in patients with recurrent effusions despite drainage.
  - Patients with malignant effusions may undergo biopsy to help establish the primary cancer.

TREATMENT

- Therapy for pericardial effusion is directed at the underlying cause.
- Drainage is indicated for symptomatic or refractory cases or when an infectious cause is present.

- Drainage may be considered in large effusions with echocardiographic features of tamponade.
- All patients with clinical tamponade need to be drained expediently. Options for drainage include percutaneous needle pericardiocentesis or surgical drainage.
- Malignant effusions frequently recur and may require an indwelling catheter.
- Anticoagulation is generally avoided until the effusion resolves to minimize the risk of hemopericardium.
- Pericardiectomy or "pericardial window" is warranted in certain patients undergoing biopsy or in patients with:
  ○ Recurrent effusions
  ○ Loculated effusion, especially posterior effusions that cannot be approached percutaneously

Medication

- Patients with tamponade **must be resuscitated aggressively** with intravenous fluids to reduce chamber collapse. Pressor support (e.g., norepinephrine) may be added for blood pressure support if necessary.
- In addition, endotracheal intubation when indicated must be undertaken with caution owing to the decrease in preload both with sedative agents and with positive pressure ventilation, which could precipitate complete circulatory collapse.

MONITORING/FOLLOW-UP

- Patients should be followed up closely depending on the size of the pericardial effusions.
- All large pericardial effusions should be followed up with serial TTE.

OUTCOMES/PROGNOSIS

Prognosis depends on the underlying cause for the pericardial effusion.

Constrictive Pericarditis

GENERAL PRINCIPLES

- Constrictive pericarditis occurs when chronic inflammation renders the pericardium thickened and scarred.
- The pericardial space is obliterated, resulting in a **loss of normal pericardial compliance**.
- This exerts an **external volume constraint** on the heart, thus interfering with normal cardiac filling.

Etiology

- Any chronic insult to the pericardium, including host immune response, can result in constriction.
- The **most common causes** include:
  ○ Idiopathic or viral pericarditis accounts for roughly half of the cases.
  ○ Postcardiac surgery constrictive pericarditis occurs as a late complication and is more common in surgeries complicated by postoperative pericarditis or hemorrhage into the pericardial space.
  ○ Constrictive pericarditis post-chest radiation is a late complication, occurring years after radiation therapy.
  ○ Connective tissues disorders

○ Postinfectious, with tuberculosis being the most common cause in developing countries
○ End-stage renal disease
○ Malignancy, typical associated cancers include breast, lung, and lymphoma
- **Effusive-constrictive pericarditis** is a unique and rare variant of constrictive pericarditis caused by **constriction of the visceral layer of pericardium**.
  ○ Its hallmark feature is constrictive physiology (see later) in the presence of a pericardial effusion.
  ○ Typically, patients will present with suspected tamponade and undergo pericardiocentesis. However, right atrial pressures will remain elevated after drainage.
  ○ Specifically, the diagnosis should be suspected in patients who fail to reduce right atrial pressure by >50% or <10 mm Hg following adequate drainage (i.e., intrapericardial pressure = 0 mm Hg),[13] though this can also occur in patients with RV failure or severe tricuspid regurgitation.
  ○ Treatment and clinical course depend on the cause for pericarditis, and some patients may require pericardiectomy.

Pathophysiology

- Thickening and fibrosis of the pericardium decrease pericardial compliance.
- The pericardium often becomes calcified and adherent to the epicardium of the heart.
- This results in **decreased ventricular compliance** as the ventricle cannot expand during diastolic filling. As the ventricle fills, **diastolic pressures rapidly increase and filling ceases** due to the elevated pressures in both ventricles.
  ○ Rapid ventricular filling occurs in early diastole only.
  ○ Atrial systole does not contribute to ventricular filling due to the elevated ventricular pressures.
- The increased end-diastolic pressures become equal in all four chambers of the heart, and the elevated pressures in both ventricles lead to **elevated systemic and pulmonary venous pressures**.

DIAGNOSIS

Clinical Presentation

History
- The signs and symptoms of constrictive pericarditis are due to elevated filling pressures causing left- and right-sided heart failure.
- In early stages, patients may complain of fatigue, weakness, and decreased exercise tolerance.
- As filling pressures continue to rise, patients complain of right-sided heart failure symptoms, such as lower extremity edema, increased abdominal girth and ascites, and, eventually, left-sided heart failure symptoms, such as dyspnea on exertion, orthopnea, and paroxysmal nocturnal dyspnea.

Physical Examination
- Physical examination in constriction typically reveals impressive **findings of right-sided heart failure**, including markedly elevated jugular venous pulse (JVP), hepatomegaly, ascites, and lower extremity edema.
- Findings of left-sided heart failure, such as frank pulmonary edema, are less common.
- Physical examination findings that are more specific for constriction include:
  ○ Increased JVP with prominent *y* descent due to rapid early diastolic filling (Figure 17-3)[10]
  ○ **Kussmaul sign**: lack of expected decrease or an obvious increase of JVP on inspiration
  ○ **Pericardial knock**: early, loud, high-pitched S3 derived from rapid pressure equalization after initial ventricular filling, best heart at left sternal border or apex

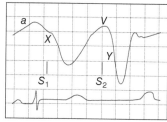

FIGURE 17-3. Right atrial pressure tracing in constrictive pericarditis. Note the prominent *y* descent. (Reprinted with permission from Murphy JG. *Mayo Clinic Cardiology Review.* 2nd ed. Lippincott Williams & Wilkins; 2000.)

Diagnostic Testing

No single study provides definitive evidence of constrictive pericarditis; thus, several different studies are often necessary in the evaluation of suspected constriction.

Electrocardiography
- ECG findings commonly include low QRS voltage, generalized T-wave flattening, or left atrial enlargement.
- Atrial fibrillation is fairly common in patients with constrictive pericarditis.

Imaging
- CXR may reveal:
  - Calcified pericardium (best seen in the lateral views)
  - Pleural effusions
  - Evidence of biatrial enlargement
- TTE can reveal several indirect features suggestive of constriction:
  - Thickened, echogenic pericardium
  - Tram-tracking: adherence to and movement of the pericardium with the myocardium during contraction
  - Dilated, noncompressible inferior vena cava
  - Septal bounce due to rapid early diastolic filling
  - **Ventricular interdependence** on Doppler examination. No echo findings are pathognomonic of constriction, although ventricular interdependence is the closest physiologic correlate. Because of the external volume constraint, RV and LV fill at the expense of each other. Mitral inflow velocities decrease with inspiration and increase with expiration, and tricuspid velocities conversely increase with inspiration and decrease with expiration.
  - **Mitral annular tissue Doppler assessment** demonstrates normal or paradoxically increased medial early diastolic mitral annular velocity (e') despite elevated filling pressures ("annulus paradoxus") or medial greater than lateral e' ("annulus reversus").[14]
- CT and MRI are useful for detecting pericardial thickening, dilated hepatic veins, dilated right atrium, and other findings that support constrictive pericarditis. These studies are not diagnostic and should be used only to support a diagnosis of pericardial constriction.

Diagnostic Procedures
- **Right and left heart catheterizations** are done simultaneously to assess right- and left-sided pressures, determine cardiac output, and help differentiate constrictive from restrictive physiology.[15]

- Hemodynamic measurements reveal **elevated and equal pressure in all four chambers in diastole** before the *a* wave.
- Right atrial measurements reveal a preserved *x* descent and a **steep *y* descent** from the increased flow during early diastole (Figure 17-3)[10] and Kussmaul sign.
- Ventricular hemodynamic measurements reveal the **dip and plateau ("square root" sign) during diastole** due to rapid early diastolic filling, which is abruptly halted once the constricted volume is reached (Figure 17-4).[16]
- A common diagnostic dilemma is the **distinction between pericardial constriction and restrictive cardiomyopathy**.
  - Decreased compliance of either the pericardium or the myocardium leads to similar defects in ventricular filling, and substantial overlap exists in signs, symptoms, and hemodynamic measurements.
  - The distinction is critical, however, as patients with restrictive cardiomyopathy carry an exceptionally high mortality risk with cardiac surgery.
  - Restrictive cardiomyopathy and constriction can be present in the same patient (e.g., after chest radiation).
  - The most sensitive (97%) and specific (100%) catheterization criterion for constrictive pericarditis is a **systolic area index** >1.1 (the ratio of RV to LV systolic pressure–time area in inspiration vs. expiration).[17]

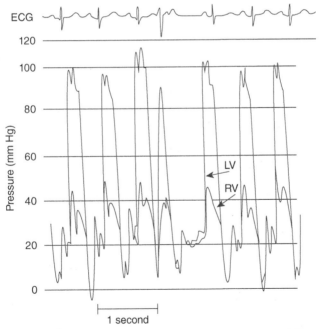

FIGURE 17-4. Simultaneous RV and LV pressure tracings in constrictive pericarditis. Note the prominent dip and plateau (square root sign), particularly post-PVC. LV, left ventricular; PVC premature ventricular complex; RV, right ventricular. (Reprinted with permission from Marso SP, Griffin BP, Topol EJ, eds. *Manual of Cardiovascular Medicine.* Lippincott Williams & Wilkins; 2000.)

○ Endomyocardial biopsy may occasionally be required to rule out a myocardial process before surgery.

○ Figure 17-5 highlights some the major differences between constriction and restriction.[14]

TREATMENT

• Constrictive pericarditis is a difficult disease to manage medically. For most, surgical pericardiectomy is the definitive treatment.

• If possible, it is desirable to treat the underlying cause.

• A small subset of patients will have spontaneous resolution or respond to medical therapy.

Medication

• Medical therapy is dictated by the underlying cause for constriction.

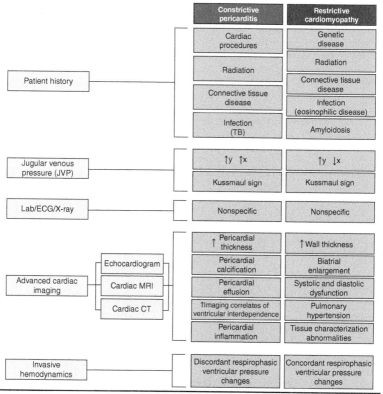

Differentiation of constriction and restriction requires a multifaceted approach inclusive of history, physical examination, laboratory testing, and multimodality imaging. Even with this toolset, hemodynamic catheterization remains necessary to provide definitive hemodynamic assessment for a subset of patients. CP = constrictive pericarditis; CT = computed tomography; ECG = electrocardiogram; JVP = jugular venous pressure; MRI = magnetic resonance imaging; RCM = restrictive cardiomyopathy; TB = tuberculosis.

FIGURE 17-5. Diagnostic approach to constrictive pericarditis and restrictive cardiomyopathy. (Reprinted from Geske JB, Anavekar NS, Nishimura RA, et al. Differentiation of constriction and restriction: complex cardiovascular hemodynamics. *J Am Coll Cardiol.* 2016;68(21):2329-47. Copyright © 2016 by the American College of Cardiology Foundation. With permission.)

- For patients with heart failure symptoms, diuretics, angiotensin-converting enzyme (ACE) inhibitors, and a low-salt diet form the cornerstone of therapy but often meet with limited success.
- Because sinus tachycardia is a compensatory mechanism, β-blockers and calcium channel blockers that slow the heart rate should be avoided.

Surgical Management
- **Surgical pericardiectomy (stripping) is the definitive therapy of choice**.
- The operative mortality rate can be as high as 20%.
- The majority of patients report symptomatic improvement with pericardiectomy.
- Surgery should be performed early, as constrictive pericarditis is a progressive disease, and patients with poor functional class are at higher risk of perioperative death.

Pericardial Tumors

GENERAL PRINCIPLES
- Patients may present with a mass (or multiple masses) within the pericardium.
- Tumors can be categorized as primary (i.e., derived initially from pericardial tissue) or metastatic.

Etiology
- **Primary pericardial tumors are very rare**. Five entities make up the bulk of tumors in this category.
  - Pericardial cyst:
    - Pericardial cysts are fluid-filled fibrous sacs lined with mesothelial cells and represent **the most common primary pericardial tumor**.
    - They are usually <3 cm in size and are often located at the right heart border.
    - Surgery is curative but is often not necessary, as there is no malignant potential.
  - Teratoma:
    - Teratomas occur more often in young women.
    - **Although benign, they are quite aggressive** and are likely to cause compressive symptoms.
  - Mesothelioma:
    - Mesotheliomas are malignant, with features similar to the better-known pleural mesothelioma.
    - Association with asbestos exposure is still controversial.
  - Angiosarcoma: Angiosarcomas are aggressive malignancies that can be derived from pericardial or myocardial tissue.
  - Lipoma: Pericardial lipomas are similar to lipomas in other locations.
- **Pericardial metastases are 100- to 1000-fold more common than primary tumors**.
  - They typically represent a late-stage process; thus, identification of the primary tumor is usually well established at the time of presentation.
  - The most common malignancies (accounting for two-thirds of cases) found to metastasize to the pericardium include:
    - Lung cancer (most common)
    - Breast cancer
    - Hematologic malignancies
  - Although less common overall, **melanoma has the highest propensity to spread to the pericardium**.

○ There are three routes of metastasis to the pericardium:
- Lymphatic spread (lung and breast cancer), associated with significant pericardial effusion
- Hematogenous spread (leukemia, lymphoma, melanoma), which tends to result in hemorrhagic effusion
- Direct extension (lung and esophageal cancer)

DIAGNOSIS

Clinical Presentation

Common presentations include:
- Symptoms from compression of the cardiac chambers (usually dyspnea or syncope)
- Pericarditis
- Effusion/tamponade
- Arrhythmias

Diagnostic Testing

Diagnosis typically involves:
- Imaging with multiple modalities (CXR, TTE, CT, or MRI)
- Pericardial fluid analysis
- Tissue biopsy (if needed)

TREATMENT

In addition to systemic chemotherapy, treatment includes local control with drainage procedures, radiation, and, occasionally, instillation of chemotherapeutic drugs into the pericardial space.

REFERENCES

1. Imazio M, Gaita F, LeWinter M. Evaluation and treatment of pericarditis: a systematic review. *JAMA.* 2015;314(14):1498-506.
2. Imazio M, Bobbio M, Cecchi E, et al. Colchicine as first-choice therapy for recurrent pericarditis: results of the CORE (Colchicine for Recurrent pericarditis) trial. *Arch Intern Med.* 2005;165:1987-91.
3. Imazio M, Trinchero R. Triage and management of acute pericarditis. *Int J Cardiol.* 2007;118:286-94.
4. Lotrionte M, Biondi-Zoccai G, Imazio M, et al. International collaborative systematic review of controlled clinical trials on pharmacologic treatments for acute pericarditis and its recurrences. *Am Heart J.* 2010;160(4):662-70.
5. Imazio M, Bobbio M, Cecchi E, et al. Colchicine in addition to conventional therapy for acute pericarditis: results of the Colchicine for Acute Pericarditis (COPE) trial. *Circulation.* 2005;112:2012-6.
6. Brucato A, Imazio M, Gattorno M, et al. Effect of Anakinra on recurrent pericarditis among patients with colchicine resistance and corticosteroid dependence: the AIRTRIP Randomized Clinical Trial. *JAMA.* 2016;316(18):1906-12.
7. Chiabrando JG, Bonaventura A, Vecchié A, et al. Management of acute and recurrent pericarditis: JACC State-of-the-Art review. *J Am Coll Cardiol.* 2020;75(1):76-92.
8. Imazio M, Cecchi E, Demichelis B, et al. Indicators of poor prognosis of acute pericarditis. *Circulation.* 2007;115:2739-44.
9. Corey GR, Campbell PT, Van Trigt P, et al. Etiology of large pericardial effusions. *Am J Med.* 1993;95:209-13.
10. Murphy JG. *Mayo Clinic Cardiology Review.* 2nd ed. Lippincott Williams & Wilkins; 2000.
11. Roy CL, Minor MA, Brookhart MA, et al. Does this patient with a pericardial effusion have cardiac tamponade? *JAMA.* 2007;297:1810-18.
12. Permanyer-Miralda G, Sagristá-Sauleda J, Soler-Soler J. Primary acute pericardial disease: a prospective series of 231 consecutive patients. *Am J Cardiol.* 1985;56:623-30.

13. Miranda WR, Oh JK. Effusive-constrictive pericarditis. *Cardiol Clin.* 2017;35(4):551-8.
14. Geske JB, Anavekar NS, Nishimura RA, et al. Differentiation of constriction and restriction: complex cardiovascular hemodynamics. *J Am Coll Cardiol.* 2016;68(21):2329-47.
15. Welch TD. Constrictive pericarditis: diagnosis, management and clinical outcomes. *Heart.* 2018;104(9):725-31.
16. Marso SP, Griffin BP, Topol EJ, eds. *Manual of Cardiovascular Medicine.* Lippincott Williams & Wilkins; 2000.
17. Talreja DR, Nishimura RA, Oh JK, et al. Constrictive pericarditis in the modern era: novel criteria for diagnosis in the cardiac catheterization laboratory. *J Am Coll Cardiol.* 2008;51:315-9.

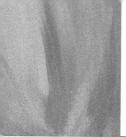

Pulmonary Hypertension, Pulmonary Arterial Hypertension, and Right Heart Failure

18

Suraj Sunder and Murali M. Chakinala

GENERAL PRINCIPLES

Definition

- *Pulmonary hypertension* (PH) is a broad term denoting increased blood pressure within the pulmonary vasculature.
- The Sixth World Symposium on Pulmonary Hypertension (WSPH) **defines PH as mean pulmonary artery pressure (PAP) > 20 mm Hg**. PAPs rise modestly with age.[1]

    Based on the pulmonary vascular resistance (PVR), PH can be classified as **precapillary** (PVR ≥ 3 Wood units), **isolated postcapillary** (PVR < 3 Wood units), or **combined precapillary and postcapillary** (PVR ≥ 3 Wood units + increased left-sided filling pressures).

Classification

Five major categories of PH are based upon the underlying pathophysiology and are presented in Table 18-1.[1]

Etiology

- **Pulmonary arterial hypertension (PAH)**, group 1, has a prevalence of 15 to 26 cases per million.[2]
  - Idiopathic PAH (IPAH) is a rare sporadic disease with prevalence of five cases per million people but is still the largest fraction of PAH cohorts.
  - Heritable forms of PAH (HPAH) are often due to mutations in the bone morphogenetic protein receptor 2 (*BMPR2*) gene, but many other genes have been identified. Incomplete penetrance is notable with BMPR2 mutations.[3]
  - Toxin- and drug-induced PAH are linked to many exposures, including anorexigens (e.g., fenfluramine, dexfenfluramine) and toxic rapeseed oil; **most frequent contemporary risk exposure is methamphetamines**.[1]
  - Associated PAH (APAH) is the second largest group of PAH patients and represents a diverse group of disorders with extrapulmonary origins that also lead to PAH.
    - PAH develops in ~12% of patients with systemic sclerosis (or scleroderma).
    - Portopulmonary PH occurs in 5-7% of cirrhotic patients with portal hypertension referred for liver transplantation.
    - Prevalence of PAH in congenital heart disease varies by the type of systemic-to-pulmonary shunt, with ventricular septal defects (VSDs) and patent ductus arteriosus having the highest rate of developing PAH and Eisenmenger syndrome. PH may occur in patients with atrial septal defects (ASDs), but only 6% develop pulmonary vascular remodeling and PAH.
  - PAH with overt features of venous/capillary involvement designates a very rare subgroup of patients with "pan-vasculopathy" and replaces the older diagnoses of pulmonary veno-occlusive disease and pulmonary capillary hemangiomatosis.[1]

TABLE 18-1	CLINICAL CLASSIFICATION OF PULMONARY HYPERTENSION

Group 1—Pulmonary arterial hypertension
- Idiopathic pulmonary arterial hypertension
- Heritable pulmonary arterial hypertension
- Drug-/toxin-induced pulmonary arterial hypertension
- Associated pulmonary arterial hypertension
  - Connective tissue disorders
  - HIV infection
  - Portal hypertension
  - Congenital heart disease (systemic-to-pulmonary shunt)
  - Schistosomiasis
- PAH long-term responders to calcium channel blockers
- PAH with overt features of venous/capillaries (PVOD/PCH) involvement

Group 2—Pulmonary hypertension due to left heart disease
- PH due to heart failure with preserved ejection fraction
- PH due to heart failure with reduced ejection fraction
- Valvular disease

Group 3—Pulmonary hypertension due to lung disease and/or hypoxia
- Obstructive lung diseases
- Restrictive lung diseases
- Other pulmonary diseases with mixed restrictive and obstructive pattern
- Hypoxia without lung disease
- Development lung disorders

Group 4—Pulmonary hypertension due to pulmonary artery obstructions
- Chronic thromboembolic pulmonary hypertension
- Other pulmonary artery obstructions

Group 5—Pulmonary hypertension with unclear and/or multifactorial mechanisms
- Hematologic disorders
  - Myeloproliferative disorders
  - Hemoglobinopathies
- Systemic and metabolic disorders
  - Sarcoidosis, pulmonary Langerhans cell histiocytosis, lymphangioleiomyomatosis, neurofibromatosis
  - Glycogen storage disease, Gaucher disease
- Other disorders: tumoral obstruction, fibrosing mediastinitis, chronic renal failure on dialysis
- Complex congenital heart defects

- Most common cause of PH is **group 2 or PH due to left heart disease**. Diastolic dysfunction and **sustained elevated left ventricular (LV) filling pressures** are instrumental for developing PH. This is commonly seen in the setting of heart failure with preserved ejection fraction (HFpEF), heart failure with reduced ejection fraction (HFrEF), or severe mitral regurgitation and in obstructive left-sided heart disease, such as aortic valve stenosis, subaortic stenosis, and hypertrophic obstructive cardiomyopathy. A subset of group 2 patients will develop combined precapillary and postcapillary PH (CpcPH).

- Second most common cause of PH is **group 3 or PH due to lung diseases and/or hypoxia**.
  - Typically mild (mean PAP 20 to 30 mm Hg) and correlates with the severity of underlying lung disease and/or hypoxemia, but can be more severe in susceptible individuals due to other mechanisms of hypoxia[4]
  - PH can be severe in mixed lung disorders, such as chronic obstructive pulmonary disease (COPD) plus obstructive sleep apnea (OSA) or combined pulmonary fibrosis and emphysema.
    - Mean PAP > 35 mm Hg warrants workup for additional conditions (e.g., OSA, chronic thromboembolic disease, LV dysfunction).
    - Hypoventilation leading to chronic hypercarbia is often associated with more significant PH.
- **Group 4** represents **PH due to pulmonary artery obstructions**, with **chronic thromboembolic pulmonary hypertension (CTEPH)** comprising the dominant form.[5]
  - 1-2% of pulmonary embolism (PE) survivors develop CTEPH. Features of PE linked to CTEPH include recurrent events, unprovoked PE, younger age of onset, and larger acute clot burden.
  - ~40% have no history of acute veno-thromboembolism.
  - Associated with chronic endovascular devices (e.g., pacemaker/defibrillator leads, ventriculoatrial shunts, vascular access catheters), postsplenectomy state, inflammatory bowel disease, and chronic inflammatory states
- **Group 5** encompasses a broad group of disorders that develop **PH from unclear and/or multiple mechanisms**, depending on the underlying disorders and their respective pathophysiology.
  - Notable entities include sarcoidosis, hemoglobinopathies (e.g., sickle cell disease), myeloproliferative disorders, end-stage renal disease (ESRD), and fibrosing mediastinitis.
  - Some cases present like group 1 conditions and may be treated similarly, but only after thorough evaluation of the underlying mechanisms for PH.
- Patients with multiple conditions associated with PH ("mixed PH") can have more severe hemodynamic abnormalities and symptoms.

Pathophysiology

- PAH involves a complex interplay of factors, resulting in **vascular remodeling** at the arteriolar level, including endothelial cell and smooth muscle cell proliferation, vasoconstriction, and in situ thrombosis. Vessel wall thickening and luminal narrowing restrict blood flow and lead to higher-than-normal pressures, which are quantifiable by an elevated PVR.
  - Elevated PVR leads to increased right ventricular (RV) afterload, causing an increase in RV wall tension and stroke work while reducing contractility; ultimately, cardiac output declines, and progressive exercise intolerance ensues.
  - The RV has limited ability to hypertrophy and tolerate high afterload, leading to vascular–ventricular uncoupling, chamber dilation, and encroachment on the LV. **Leading cause of death in PAH is right-sided heart failure (RHF)**.
- Group 2 PH involves the persistent elevation in left-sided filling pressures that secondarily cause pulmonary venous hypertension and "passive" elevation of PAPs without the proliferative vasculopathy encountered in group 1 conditions.
  - Sustained reduction of left-sided filling pressures rapidly corrects PH in most patients.
  - Pulmonary vascular remodeling may occur in a subset of patients and requires a longer interval after corrective action (e.g., mitral valve surgery for mitral stenosis) to resolve PH, or it may not resolve at all.
- Multiple mechanisms contribute to group 3 PH, including vasoconstriction due to alveolar hypoxia and/or hypercarbia, interstitial fibrosis, vascular bed compression and destruction, inflammation, and direct effect of noxious gases.

- CTEPH, the main disorder in group 4 PH, reflects the combination of proximal vessel obstruction from organized thromboembolic material and vascular remodeling of arterioles, similar to group 1 conditions.
- Group 5 PH can result from a myriad of mechanisms, including any of the processes delineated earlier in groups 1 to 4 PH, with more than one mechanism having relevance in a particular disorder or individual.[6]

DIAGNOSIS

Clinical Presentation

- Symptoms of PH are progressive dyspnea, palpitations, and reduced exercise tolerance. Symptoms in groups 2 and 3 PH are also tied to the underlying heart or lung disorder.
- As RHF develops, additional complaints include fatigue, swelling, weight gain, exertional dizziness, and syncope.
- The average delay in the diagnosis of PAH remains very lengthy (~2.5 years).

History
- Explore underlying risk factors and comorbid conditions that could lead to PH (Table 18-1).
- Inquire about symptoms that could indicate heart failure.

Physical Examination
- Cardiac auscultation reveals accentuated S_2 with a loud P_2 component.
- RV dysfunction results in systolic tricuspid regurgitant murmur (early), diastolic pulmonary insufficiency murmur (late), and RV S_3.
- Peripheral manifestations of RHF include distended jugular venous pulsation, lower extremity edema, hepatojugular reflux, hepatomegaly, pulsatile liver, and ascites.
- Findings of underlying conditions linked to PAH should be sought out (e.g., skin changes of scleroderma, stigmata of liver disease, clubbing in congenital heart disease, abnormal breath sounds in parenchymal lung disease).
- Bruits in the chest are a clue for CTEPH.

Diagnostic Testing

- A multistep strategy is necessary to translate the detection of PH ultimately to one of the diagnostic categories indicates in Table 18-1.
- Findings on basic investigations are helpful when abnormalities are present, but insensitive in milder cases of PH.
  - CXR: PA enlargement and prominence of right atrium or RV
  - ECG: RV hypertrophy and right-axis deviation
- A series of investigations (Figure 18-1) is necessary to clarify the clinical group of PH and the specific etiology within the PAH group (Table 18-1) and evaluate the severity through functional and hemodynamics measures.

Laboratories
- Investigate causative conditions: hepatic function panel, HIV, antinuclear antibody (ANA), extractable nuclear antigens (ENAs), anticentromere and anti-topoisomerase antibodies (systemic sclerosis), and hematological disorders. Contingent testing may include hepatitis B and C serologies, hemoglobin electrophoresis, antiphospholipid antibody, and lupus anticoagulant.

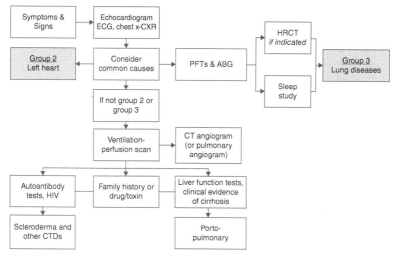

FIGURE 18-1. Diagnostic flowchart for the evaluation of pulmonary hypertension. ABG, arterial blood gas; CTEPH, chronic thromboembolic pulmonary hypertension; ECG, electrocardiogram; HRCT, high-resolution CT; HTN; hypertension; PFT, pulmonary function test.

- Assess the severity of cardiac impairment: creatinine and blood urea nitrogen (BUN), and NT-pro brain natriuretic peptide (NT-proBNP).
- Arterial blood gas can demonstrate hypercarbia and a hypoventilation.

Imaging
- **Transthoracic echocardiography** (TTE) with Doppler and agitated saline injection is the preferred initial test to identify PH.
  - Doppler interrogation of tricuspid valve regurgitation estimates the pulmonary artery systolic pressure (PASP).
    - Sensitivity for PH is 80-100%, and the correlation coefficient with invasive measurement is 0.6 to 0.9.
    - Generally, PASP > 35 mm Hg is noteworthy, but the presence of right-sided cardiac abnormalities should heighten suspicion, regardless of PASP estimate.
  - TTE can identify left-sided cardiac causes of PH. Clues for diastolic dysfunction and elevated left-sided filling pressures (grade II or III diastolic dysfunction) include left atrial enlargement, decreased mitral valve tissue Doppler velocities, and an elevated average ratio between early mitral inflow velocity and mitral annular early diastolic velocity (E/e′ > 14).
  - Several TTE measures provide important functional and morphologic information about the RV, including the degree of hypertrophy and/or dilatation, tricuspid annular plane systolic excursion (TAPSE <1.8 portends poorer prognosis), tricuspid valve tissue Doppler, wall strain, and fractional area change.
  - Agitated saline or "bubble study" can identify congenital systemic-to-pulmonary shunts (e.g., ASDs, VSDs) or a patent foramen ovale (PFO).
- **Transesophageal echocardiography** (TEE) may be necessary to evaluate atrial septal anatomy (for an ASD) and mitral valve disease, if indicated.
- **Cardiac MRI** demonstrates cardiac anomalies, especially if TEE is contraindicated, and provides functional RV data, such as RV ejection fraction and stroke volume.

- **Ventilation–perfusion (V/Q) lung scan is the preferred screening test to exclude chronic thromboembolic disease but can also be abnormal in pulmonary veno-occlusive disease and fibrosing mediastinitis.**
  - **CT angiography** may miss subtle findings of chronic thromboembolic disease, particularly when read by inexperienced radiologists.
  - **Pulmonary angiography** can confirm chronic thromboembolic disease and determine surgical accessibility of organized thrombotic material.
- **High-resolution chest CT** can reveal relevant parenchymal and mediastinal findings when suspected.

Diagnostic Procedures
- **Pulmonary function testing** (PFT) to assess for obstructive (e.g., COPD) or restrictive (e.g., interstitial lung diseases [ILDs]) ventilatory abnormalities.
- **Polysomnography** should be done if symptoms of sleep-disordered breathing are present.
- **Nocturnal oximetry** can disclose nocturnal desaturations, which are common in PH even in the absence of daytime hypoxemia and should be treated with supplemental oxygen.
- **Six-minute walk** is a critical test for establishing the severity of impairment and predicting short- and intermediate-term survivals in PAH. A 6-minute distance <300 mm is associated with a poor prognosis.[2]
- **Right heart catheterization (RHC)** is the gold standard for diagnosing PH.
  - Based on clinical presentation and noninvasive evaluation, a clinical impression for the type of PH should be formulated and catheterization should be designed to solidify that clinical impression.
  - **RHC should be performed on any patient suspected to have PAH and before the initiation of therapy**.
  - Critical measurements include PAP, right atrial pressure, pulmonary artery wedge pressure (PAWP), mixed venous saturation, cardiac output (thermodilution or Fick methods), and PVR.
    - If PAWP is unreliable, LV end-diastolic pressure (LVEDP) should be measured.
  - Significant "step-up" in saturation measurements (>5-7%) anywhere from the vena cava, right atrium, RV, and PA suggests a left-to-right shunt. Right (Qp) and left (Qs) flow measures should be performed if a shunt is detected, in order to calculate flow (Qp/Qs) and resistance ratios.
  - **Acute vasodilator testing** is recommended for patients with IPAH, HPAH, and drug-/toxin-induced PAH.[2]
    - Short-acting vasodilators (e.g., intravenous adenosine, epoprostenol, or inhaled nitric oxide) should be administered.
    - Should not be done when severe RHF present (RAP > 20 mm Hg or cardiac index <1.5 L/min/m[2])
    - **Response to vasodilator testing is defined by a decline in mean PAP ≥ 10 mm Hg and concluding mean PAP < 40 mm Hg without a decline in cardiac output.**[2]
    - Sodium nitroprusside should be considered in cases of CpcPH to determine reversibility of PH if LV filling pressures can be acutely lowered.
  - **Provocative testing**, such as rapid fluid challenge or exercise, can be performed if resting hemodynamics are inconsistent with the clinical impression of PH or if uncertainty about the type of PH (precapillary versus postcapillary PH) persists.[7]
    - If PAWP > 18 mm Hg with 500-mL fluid challenge over 5 minutes, postcapillary contribution to PH should be suspected.
    - While exercise protocols vary significantly, a total pulmonary resistance (TPR = mean PAP/cardiac output) > 3 is considered abnormal.

TREATMENT

Management of PH heavily depends on the specific category determined by comprehensive evaluation.

Medications

First Line
- See Table 18-2 for approved therapies for PH.
- Group 2 PH is managed by optimizing the underlying left heart conditions with a hemodynamic goal of lowering the PAWP as much as possible.
  - **HFpEF** should be managed with **afterload-reducing agents** (to minimize LV afterload) and **diuretics** (to avoid excess volume). Chronic anemia and nonsteroidal anti-inflammatory drugs (NSAIDs) use can aggravate heart failure and should be avoided.
  - A subset of patients with HFrEF **and associated PH** may benefit from **sildenafil** (a phosphodiesterase-5 inhibitor [PDE5-I]), in terms of exertional capacity, exercise hemodynamics, and quality of life, after being optimized on goal-directed medical therapy.[8]
  - Pulmonary vasodilators have not benefitted and may even cause harm when used in HFpEF or left-sided valvular disease.[9]
- **Group 3** should be managed with appropriate **therapies for the underlying pulmonary condition**, whether it is obstructive lung disease, ILD, or OSA.
  - Supplemental oxygen to maintain $SpO_2 > 89\%$ and avoid hypoxic vasoconstriction and remodeling
  - Subset of patients with PH associated with ILD can benefit from the inhaled pulmonary vasodilator, treprostinil.[10] See Table 18-2.
- **CTEPH (group 4)** is primarily managed with surgical **pulmonary thromboendarterectomy** at specialized centers and requires careful evaluation to determine resectability. **Balloon pulmonary angioplasty** has quickly become an option for more distal disease and offers durable hemodynamic benefits.[5]
  - Pulmonary vasodilators, primarily riociguat, are an option for patients considered inoperable due to distal disease or persistent PH after aforementioned interventions.[11] See Table 18-2.
- **Mainstay of group 1 management is pulmonary vasodilator therapy**, which improves hemodynamics, exercise capacity, functional class, and quality of life, while reducing hospitalization and "time to clinical worsening." Long-term survival benefit is inferred by observational data and large-scale contemporary registries. See Table 18-2.
  - **Calcium channel blockers (CCBs) should only be used in vasoresponders** identified by acute vasodilator challenge (as noted earlier).[2]
    - **Indiscriminate CCB use can induce hemodynamic collapse and syncope** in non-vasoresponders.
    - Chronic CCB therapy (e.g., amlodipine, nifedipine, or diltiazem) should start at a low dose and titrated over several weeks, while monitoring systemic pressures and avoiding RHF.
    - Patients who do not have near-normalization of PAPs within a few months of CCB therapy should be considered for additional vasodilator therapy.
  - **Vast majority of group 1 patients will require careful risk assessment**, utilizing validated instruments such as **the REVEAL 2.0 risk calculator or the French PH Registry method**, to determine an initial treatment regimen. Risk assessment tools apply multiple pieces of data collected during the initial evaluation to estimate short- and intermediate-term survival.[12-14] See Figure 18-2.
    - Low- and intermediate-risk patients can generally be initiated on dual oral pulmonary vasodilator therapy.

TABLE 18-2 APPROVED PULMONARY VASODILATORS FOR GROUP 1 PH

Drug	Therapeutic class	Route of delivery	Dosing range	Adverse effects	Cautions
Nifedipine, amlodipine, diltiazem	Calcium channel blocker	PO	Varies by patient tolerance	Peripheral edema, hypotension, fatigue	**Use only in patients who are vasoresponders.** Avoid in low cardiac output state or decompensated right heart failure
Sildenafil Tadalafil	Phosphodiesterase-5 inhibitor	PO	20 mg tid 40 mg/day	Headache, hypotension, dyspepsia, myalgias, visual disturbances	Avoid using with **nitrates** or **protease inhibitors**
Riociguat	Soluble guanylate cyclase stimulator	PO	2.5 mg tid	Hypotension	Avoid using with **nitrates. Approved for PAH and CTEPH that is inoperable or** persistent after endarterectomy
Bosentan	Endothelin-receptor antagonist	PO	125 mg bid	Hepatotoxic, teratogen, peripheral edema	**Monthly liver function monitoring;** avoid using with glyburide and glipizide
Ambrisentan	Endothelin-receptor antagonist	PO	5–10 mg/day	Teratogen, peripheral edema	Fluid retention, particularly in older patients
Macitentan	Endothelin-receptor antagonist	PO	10 mg/day	Teratogen, peripheral edema	Monitor for anemia

Drug	Class	Route	Dose	Side effects	Notes
Iloprost Treprostinil	Prostacyclin analog	IH	2.5–5 µg 6–8/day ≥9 breaths qid	Cough, flushing, headache, trismus	**Suboptimal adherence due to dosing frequency** Treprostinil has been shown beneficial in PH-ILD
Selexipag	Prostacyclin-receptor agonist	PO	200–1600 µg bid	Headache, jaw pain, diarrhea, extremity pain	Hyperthyroidism
Treprostinil	Prostacyclin analog	SC, IV, or PO	Varies by patient tolerance	Headache, jaw pain, diarrhea, extremity pain	**With continuous parenteral use,** catheter-related complications (IV). **Site pain/ reaction (SC).** GI distress with PO use.
Epoprostenol	Prostacyclin analog	IV	Varies by patient tolerance	Headache, jaw pain, diarrhea, extremity pain	**Continuous parenteral agent with very short half-life Catheter-related complications (IV);** high output state at higher doses

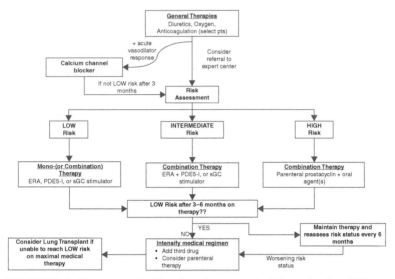

FIGURE 18-2. Treatment algorithm for pulmonary arterial hypertension. ERA, endothelin-receptor antagonist; PDE5-I, phosphodiesterase-5 inhibitor; sGC, soluble guanylate cyclase.

- High-risk patients should receive advanced therapy with a parenteral prostacyclin analog in conjunction with oral pulmonary vasodilator.
- Risk should be reassessed within 3 to 6 months of initiating therapy with the goal of achieving low risk. Patients not improving to a low-risk category should be considered for additional vasodilator therapy.
  ○ **Endothelin-receptor antagonists** (ERAs) block the binding of endothelin-1 to its receptors on PA smooth muscle cells and endothelial cells, thus mitigating vasoconstriction and cellular hypertrophy/growth. ERAs are teratogenic and require monthly monitoring.
  ○ **PDE5-Is** increase nitric oxide signaling by enhancing intracellular cGMP levels, thereby inducing vasodilation and inhibiting cellular growth. Must avoid using concomitantly with nitrates.
  ○ Riociguat is the lone **soluble guanylate cyclase stimulator** that also enhances cGMP signaling but cannot be used in conjunction with nitrates or PDE5-Is.
  ○ **Prostacyclin pathway activators** (PPAs) are potent pulmonary vasodilators that also inhibit cellular growth and platelet aggregation. PPAs are available in oral, inhaled, and parenteral forms with their respective complexities, side effects, and challenges to administration.
    - Parenteral administration is considered the most potent route of administration and used in the most high-risk cases. Inhaled agents are less likely to lower systemic blood pressure and worsen V/Q mismatching.
    - Adverse effects include drug-related side effects (e.g., jaw pain, flushing, headache, gastrointestinal side effects, leg/foot pain) and delivery system complications (e.g., bloodstream infections, catheter-related thrombosis, inadvertent interruptions of drug administration with very short-acting continuous infusions).
    - **Optimal dosing is vital to maximizing therapeutic effect and minimizing side effects.**

Second Line

- **Diuretics** to optimize RV preload and RV–LV interaction
  - May require combination of a loop diuretic, aldosterone antagonist, and thiazide
  - Potential to aggravate chronic renal dysfunction, particularly in an individual with long-standing RHF or intrinsic renal disease; inotropic support may be needed.
- **Anticoagulation with warfarin is now generally reserved for IPAH and HPAH patients with a target INR < 2.5**. CTEPH patients require therapeutic anticoagulation to avoid recurrent acute thromboembolism.
- **Management of acute decompensated RHF** requires a multi-pronged approach geared to optimize RV preload, afterload, and contractility, often in an intensive care setting.[15] See Figure 18-3.
  - **Potential precipitating factors:** interruption of chronic PAH therapy, dietary/fluid indiscretion, infection (particularly bloodstream infection if indwelling central venous catheter present), atrial tachyarrhythmias, PE, thyrotoxicosis, pregnancy, and induction for general anesthesia
  - **Early use of vasopressors to combat hypotension and optimize RV preload.** Low systemic diastolic pressure coupled with elevated RV end-diastolic pressure narrow the myocardial perfusion gradient during diastole and induce RV ischemia. Norepinephrine, vasopressin, and phenylephrine are available options.

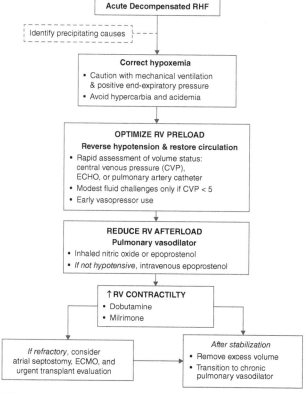

FIGURE 18-3. Approach to the management of acute decompensated right heart failure. RHF, right heart failure.

○ **Afterload reduction** with selective PA dilation is critical to breaking the spiral of RV decompensation and hypotension.

- Intravenous epoprostenol and treprostinil are potent pulmonary vasodilators but can also aggravate hypotension.

- Inhaled agents preferentially lower PVR with minimal decreases in systemic vascular resistance while minimizing V/Q mismatching and hypoxemia. Continuous nebulized options are nitric oxide and epoprostenol.

- Nonselective vasodilators (e.g., nitroprusside, nitroglycerin, hydralazine, calcium channel antagonists) should strictly be avoided in isolated RHF.

○ **Inotropic support enhances RV contractility** and can resolve a low-flow state and unmet peripheral metabolic needs (i.e., lactic acidosis or renal hypoperfusion). Options include dobutamine, epinephrine, and milrinone but must guard against hypotension and tachyarrhythmias.

Nonpharmacologic Therapies

- **Supplemental oxygen** to maintain normoxemia and avoid hypoxic vasoconstriction if possible, as anatomic shunts, including a PFO, may preclude normoxemia

- **In line IV filters** to prevent paradoxical air emboli in patients with significant intracardiac right-to-left shunts

- **Fluid and sodium restriction** is appropriate for individuals with RHF.

- **Pulmonary rehabilitation** and exercise training for select individuals to overcome physical deconditioning.

Surgical Management

- **Lung or heart-lung transplantation** is reserved for suitable PAH patients who remain in advanced functional classes (III to IV) with ominous hemodynamics (RAP >15 mm Hg and cardiac index < 2.0 L/min/m^2) despite maximal medical therapy, including a parenteral prostanoids.[16]

  ○ RV recovery after isolated lung transplantation can reserve heart-lung transplantation for cases with irreparable complex congenital defects.

  ○ Median survival after lung transplantation is ~6 years.

- **Atrial septostomy** percutaneously creates a right-to-left interatrial shunt that increases blood flow to the systemic circulation and oxygen to peripheral tissues. Indicated in refractory RHF (e.g., recurrent syncope, severe ascites, or poor systemic end-organ perfusion).

- ASDs can be closed in carefully selected cases in order to prevent or minimize progression of PAH.

  ○ Prerequisite criteria include significant net left-to-right shunting (Qp/Qs ≥ 2.0) and low PVR < 5 Wood units and pulmonary/systemic resistance ratio ≤ 0.3.

  ○ Ostium secundum defects can be closed percutaneously.

SPECIAL CONSIDERATIONS

- Comorbidities, social support, and a patient's overall health care literacy are important to consider due to the nature and complexity of certain PAH therapies.

- Vaccination against *Streptococcus pneumoniae* and *Influenza* should be offered.

- Patients in RHF should **avoid high-risk situations** that can acutely decrease RV preload and/or increase RV afterload, such as:

  ○ Strong **Valsalva maneuvers** (e.g., severe coughing paroxysms, straining during defecation or micturition, vigorous exercise including resistance training, or lifting heavy items)

  ○ **High altitudes** (>5000 feet) may be dangerous due to low inspired concentration of oxygen.

- **Avoid pregnancy** due to the marked hemodynamic alterations that can further strain a compromised RV. Choice of contraception should be based on effectiveness without increasing risk of thromboembolism.
- **Systemic sympathomimetic agents** with vasoactive properties (e.g., over-the-counter decongestants, nicotine, cocaine) should be avoided.

MONITORING/FOLLOW-UP

- PAH remains incurable in spite of current therapies. Patients require close follow-up (i.e., every 3 to 6 months) and frequent monitoring to detect declining RV function and clinical progression.[14]
- Utilizing the same risk assessment tools that determine initial treatment, long-term treatment goals should be to achieve and maintain low-risk status.
  - Because some patients will never meet low-risk criteria due to comorbidities, hemodynamic monitoring and RV imaging should be relied upon.

REFERENCES

1. Simonneau G, Montani D, Celermajer DS, et al. Haemodynamic definitions and updated clinical classification of pulmonary hypertension. *Eur Respir J.* 2019;53;1801913.
2. McLaughlin VV, Archer SL, Badesch DB, et al. ACCF/AHA 2009 expert consensus document on pulmonary hypertension a report of the American College of Cardiology Foundation Task Force on expert consensus documents and the American Heart Association developed in collaboration with the American College of Chest Physicians; American Thoracic Society, Inc.; and the Pulmonary Hypertension Association. *J Am Coll Cardiol.* 2009;53:1573-19.
3. Morrell NW, Aldred MA, Chung WK, et al. Genetics and genomics of pulmonary arterial hypertension. *Eur Respir J.* 2019;53:1801899.
4. Nathan SD, Barbera JA, Gaine SP, et al. Pulmonary hypertension in chronic lung disease and hypoxia. *Eur Respir J.* 2019;53:1801914.
5. Kim NH, Delcroix M, Jais X, et al. Chronic thromboembolic pulmonary hypertension. *Eur Respir J.* 2019;53:1801915.
6. Lahm T, Chakinala MM. World Health Organization group 5 pulmonary hypertension. *Clin Chest Med.* 2013;34:753-78.
7. Vachiery JL, Tedford RJ, Rosenkranz S, et al. Pulmonary hypertension due to left heart disease. *Eur Respir J.* 2019;53:1801897.
8. Lewis GD, Shah R, Shahzad K, et al. Sildenafil improves exercise capacity and quality of life in patients with systolic heart failure and secondary pulmonary hypertension. *Circulation.* 2007;116:1555-62.
9. Bermejo J, Yotti R, Garcia-Orta R, et al. Sildenafil for improving outcomes in patients with corrected valvular heart disease and persistent pulmonary hypertension: a multicenter, double-blind, randomized clinical trial. *Eur Heart J.* 2018;39:1255-64.
10. Waxman A, Restrepo-Jaramillo R, Thenappan T, et al. Inhaled treprostinil in pulmonary hypertension due to interstitial lung disease. *N Engl J Med.* 2021;384:325-34.
11. Ghofrani HA, D'Armini AM, Grimminger F, et al. Riociguat for the treatment of chronic thromboembolic pulmonary hypertension. *N Engl J Med.* 2013;369:319-29.
12. Benza RL, Gomberg-Maitland M, Elliott CG, et al. Predicting survival in patients with pulmonary arterial hypertension: the reveal risk score calculator 2.0 and comparison with esc/ers-based risk assessment strategies. *Chest.* 2019;156:323-37.
13. Boucly A, Weatherald J, Savale L, et al. Risk assessment, prognosis and guideline implementation in pulmonary arterial hypertension. *Eur Respir J.* 2017;50.
14. Galie N, Channick RN, Frantz RP, et al. Risk stratification and medical therapy of pulmonary arterial hypertension. *Eur Respir J.* 2019;53:1801889.
15. Lahm T, McCaslin CA, Wozniak TC, et al. Medical and surgical treatment of acute right ventricular failure. *J Am Coll Cardiol.* 2010;56:1435-46.
16. Hoeper MM, Benza RL, Corris P, et al. Intensive care, right ventricular support and lung transplantation in patients with pulmonary hypertension. *Eur Respir J.* 2019;53:1801906.

Peripheral Arterial Disease 19

Prashanth D. Thakker, Nathan L. Frogge,
and Jasvindar Singh

Introduction

- Peripheral arterial disease (PAD) consists of a group of disorders that lead to progressive stenosis, occlusion, or aneurysmal dilation of the aorta and its noncoronary artery branches, such as the carotid artery, upper extremity, visceral, and lower extremity arterial branches.
- The importance of PAD has been increasingly recognized, with lower extremity PAD affecting >200 million people worldwide and 8.5 million Americans above the age of 40 years.[1]
- PAD is also associated with increased prevalence of concomitant coronary artery disease (CAD) and an increased risk of myocardial infarction (MI), cerebrovascular accident (CVA), and death.[1,2]
- This chapter primarily focuses on vascular disease processes that lead to ischemia of the lower extremity, kidney, and carotid artery territories.

Lower Extremity Peripheral Arterial Disease

GENERAL PRINCIPLES

Classification

- Patients with lower extremity PAD range from those who are asymptomatic to those with acute limb-threatening emergencies. The clinician must differentiate between the severity of symptoms in deciding on further workup and the urgency of a treatment plan.
- Lower extremity PAD is commonly defined by presentation:
  - Asymptomatic
  - Claudication
  - Critical limb ischemia (CLI)
  - Acute limb ischemia (ALI)

Epidemiology

- The prevalence increases with age, with ~15-20% of patients over the age 70 having an abnormal ankle–brachial index (ABI).[2]
- In a high-risk patient population older than 50 to 69 years with a history of cigarette smoking or diabetes, the prevalence of PAD is estimated at 29%.[3]

Etiology

The most common cause of PAD is atherosclerosis (Table 19-1). Other etiologies include vasculitis and connective tissue disorders.

TABLE 19-1   ETIOLOGY OF PERIPHERAL ARTERIAL DISEASE

- Atherosclerosis
- Connective tissue diseases
  - Marfan syndrome
  - Ehlers–Danlos syndrome
- Dysplastic disease: Fibromuscular dysplasia
- Vasculitic diseases
  - **Large vessels:** Giant cell (temporal) arteritis, Takayasu arteritis
  - **Medium-sized vessels:** Kawasaki disease, polyarteritis nodosa
  - **Small-vessel disease (arterioles and microvessels):** Wegener granulomatosis, microscopic polyangiitis, Churg–Strauss syndrome, Henoch–Schönlein purpura, cryoglobulinemic vasculitis
  - Thromboangiitis obliterans (Buerger disease)
- Prothrombotic diseases
- Vasospastic diseases

Risk Factors

- **The major cause of lower extremity PAD is atherosclerosis.** Identified risk factors include smoking, diabetes, hypertension, hyperlipidemia, hyperhomocysteinemia, and family history of CAD.
- **Cigarette smoking** is associated with a dose-dependent increase in the prevalence of PAD.[3]

Associated Conditions

- Although PAD can cause significant morbidity, the shared pathophysiology and risk factors between PAD and CAD mean that the **majority of these patients will die from cardiovascular diseases, such as MI or ischemic stroke.**
- Patients with lower extremity PAD have an increased risk of the following[1]:
  - Developing a stroke or transient ischemic attack (TIA)
  - Dying due to coronary heart disease events

DIAGNOSIS

Clinical Presentation

- **Asymptomatic** lower extremity PAD:
  - Limb function is not necessarily normal.
  - Patients may not have classic exertional limb discomfort but may have less typical symptoms, such as decreased walking speed or poor balance.
- **Claudication:**
  - Claudication symptoms are due to exercise-induced ischemia.
  - Symptoms of chronic lower extremity atherosclerotic occlusion are variable but are frequently described as **reproducible cramping or fatigue with walking,** with resolution shortly after rest.
  - Symptoms may occur anywhere in the lower extremity, including buttocks, thighs, or calves.
- **CLI:**
  - CLI is limb pain that occurs at rest (**rest pain**) or **impending limb loss** that is caused by severe compromise of blood flow to the affected extremity.
  - This term should be used to describe all patients **with chronic pain at rest, ulcers, or gangrene attributable to objectively proven arterial occlusive disease.**

- **ALI:**
  - ○ ALI is caused by a sudden decrease in limb perfusion that threatens tissue viability. Symptoms occur as a result of thrombosis of an atherosclerotic plaque or an embolism, frequently of cardiac or aortic origin.

History
- Asymptomatic patients aged 50 years or older with cardiovascular risk factors and all patients aged 70 years or older should be asked about walking impairment, rest pain, and nonhealing wounds. If positive, further testing should be initiated.
- Claudication can be confused with pseudoclaudication from spinal stenosis. Classically, limb discomfort associated with spinal stenosis is not reliably reproduced with exertion; it is exacerbated by standing and relieved only by sitting.
- **CLI usually presents with rest pain that is worse while lying in a supine position**. Patients with CLI will often maintain limbs in a dependent position and are frequently unable to walk.
- The typical symptoms and signs of ALI include "the six P's": **pain, paralysis, paresthesias, pulselessness, pallor**, and **polar (cold).**

Physical Examination
- Visualization:
  - ○ Capillary refill
  - ○ Nonhealing wounds or ulcers
  - ○ Livedo reticularis (in the case of atheroembolization)
  - ○ Calf atrophy
  - ○ Alopecia over the dorsum of the foot
  - ○ Auscultation and palpation: bruits over major vascular beds as well as palpation of peripheral pulses over the femoral, popliteal, posterior tibial, and dorsalis pedis arteries (Figure 19-1). The presence of a bruit or a thrill only describes turbulent flow but does not confirm arterial stenosis. In addition, both the volume and quality of the peripheral pulses should be noted.
- **Elevation-dependency test:**
  - ○ This is a screening maneuver. While the patient is supine, elevate the lower extremities to 60 degrees above the horizontal. Development of pallor in the sole of the foot indicates arterial disease in that extremity.
  - ○ Have the patient sit upright and swing their legs so that they are hanging off the examination table. Delayed return of color and venous engorgement in either lower extremity may confirm inadequate circulation.
  - ○ With more advanced disease, a deep red color develops along with dependent edema, the so-called **dependent rubor**.

Diagnostic Testing
- All patients with symptomatic claudication should undergo measurement of the ABI to confirm the diagnosis and to establish a baseline result (Figure 19-2).
  - ○ Calculate the ABI for each leg by comparing the higher pressure in the posterior tibialis or dorsalis pedis arteries to the higher pressure in the right or left arm
  - ○ right ABI = (higher right ankle pressure, mm Hg) / (higher arm pressure, mm Hg)
  - ○ left ABI = (higher left ankle pressure, mm Hg) / (higher arm pressure, mm Hg)
  - ○ The calculation of the interpreted index is based on this ratio
    > 0.90 = normal
    0.71-0.90 = mild obstruction
    0.41-0.70 = moderate obstruction
    0.00- 0.40 = severe obstruction
  - ○ Advanced age and diabetes mellitus contribute to vessel rigidity and make the ABI test less reliable. When this occurs and the ABI is >1.40, a toe–brachial index (TBI) can be used instead.[1]
    - ■ Toe pressure <30 mm Hg indicates ischemia, impaired wound healing, and increased risk of amputation.
    - ■ An ABI <0.9 and a TBI of <0.7 are considered diagnostic of lower extremity PAD.

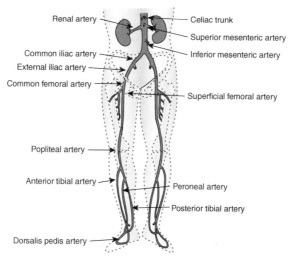

FIGURE 19-1. Diagram of major branches of lower extremity peripheral arterial anatomy.

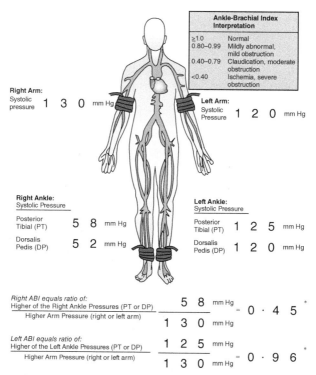

FIGURE 19-2. Ankle-Brachial Index Interpretation. Adapted with permission from Diepenbrock NH. *Quick Reference to Critical Care.* 5th ed. Wolters Kluwer; 2016.

- ○ If the resting ABI is normal and clinical suspicion is high, ABI can be repeated after exercise or **plantar flexion test**.
    - ■ For the plantar flexion test, the patient raises their heels off the ground, standing on the tips of their toes, and then returns to the normal position.
    - ■ When symptoms develop or after 50 repetitions, the ABI is repeated.
    - ■ The test is a reasonable alternative if a treadmill is not available.[1]
- ○ **Segmental limb pressure examination** may be helpful to further identify the location and extent of lower extremity PAD. Cuffs are placed on the upper thigh, lower thigh, and upper calf. A drop of 20 mm Hg in the systolic pressure between segments is consistent with arterial stenosis.
- ○ **Pulse volume recordings** use plethysmographic waveforms to identify changes in pulse contour and amplitude. In the presence of arterial disease, the slope flattens, the pulse width widens, and the dicrotic notch is lost.
- **Duplex ultrasonography**
    - ○ Duplex ultrasonography combines Doppler velocity and waveform analysis with gray-scale visualization of the arterial wall.
    - ○ A normal waveform is triphasic, with forward flow in cardiac systole followed by a brief flow reversal in early diastole followed by forward flow in late diastole.
    - ○ With arterial stenosis, distal blood flow velocities increase. In severe stenosis, the flow reversal component is absent as well (Figure 19-3).[4] The degree of stenosis is determined by combining waveform analysis and measurement of the peak-systolic velocity.
- For specific anatomic delineation to guide revascularization, additional imaging with **computed tomography (CT)**, **magnetic resonance angiography (MRA)**, or **digital subtraction angiography** can be used.
    - ○ **Digital subtraction angiography** (Figure 19-4) remains the gold-standard test, but it is invasive and carries risks related to the use of contrast and radiation exposure.
    - ○ **CT angiography** is rapid and noninvasive but carries similar contrast and radiation risks. Calcium found in atherosclerotic lesions can create so-called blooming artifacts, rendering images less accurate.
    - ○ **MRA** carries fewer risks and gives detailed information, although prior stent placement can affect image quality.

TREATMENT

- The primary goal should be prevention of the development and progression of PAD through **risk factor modification**, especially smoking cessation.
- When prevention fails, early detection and lifestyle modification, along with medical and, in some cases, mechanical reperfusion therapy, should be combined to maintain and improve quality of life and to avoid progression to limb- and life-threatening disease.

Medications

- Antiplatelet therapy **aspirin** (75 to 325 mg daily) or **clopidogrel** (75 mg daily)
    - ○ The use of antiplatelet therapy in patients with PAD carries a class I indication in symptomatic PAD due to the benefit in reducing cardiovascular events, including MI, stroke, or vascular death.[1]
    - ○ It is reasonable to treat patients with antiplatelet therapy in the setting of asymptomatic PAD.
- **Rivaroxaban** (2.5 mg twice daily), a Xa inhibitor, with aspirin (100 mg daily) has shown to be beneficial in patients with lower extremity PAD by reducing vascular and cardiovascular events; this occurs at the expense of increased bleeding.[5] In patients who have undergone lower limb revascularization, rivaroxaban and aspirin significantly lowered the risk of ALI, major amputations, MI, stroke, or death.[6]
- **Cilostazol**, a phosphodiesterase type 3 inhibitor, has both vasodilatory and platelet-inhibitory properties and has been shown to improve walking distance. As other phosphodiesterase

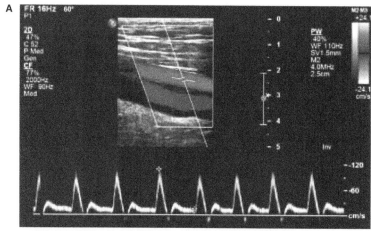

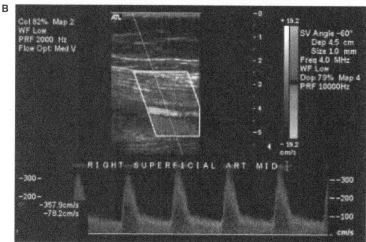

FIGURE 19-3. Doppler arterial waveforms from patients without **(A)** and with **(B)** peripheral arterial disease (PAD). In the setting of PAD, the peak-systolic velocity increases and the diastolic flow reversal is lost. (Reprinted with permission from Begelman SM, Jaff MR. Noninvasive diagnostic strategies for peripheral arterial disease. *Cleve Clin J Med.* 2006;73(suppl 4):S22-29. Copyright © 2006 Cleveland Clinic Foundation. All rights reserved.)

inhibitors are associated with an increased mortality in patients with heart failure, care should be taken to avoid cilostazol in patients with left ventricular dysfunction.[1]

- **Lipid-lowering therapy**, such as with high-intensity statin therapy, should be employed with a goal low-density lipoprotein (LDL) <70 mg/dL.[1]
- **Antihypertensive therapy** should be pursued with a goal blood pressure <130/80 mm Hg.[1]
- **Glucose control** with goal hemoglobin A1C <6.5% has been shown to have better limb-related outcomes and decreased amputations compared to those with more loosely controlled A1C.[1]

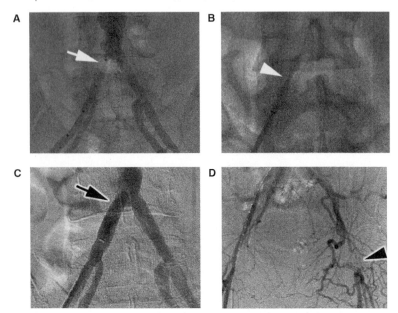

FIGURE 19-4. Lower extremity peripheral arterial disease angiography and percutaneous intervention. **(A)** Severe hazy lesion in the ostial right common iliac artery (white arrow). A marker pigtail has been used to perform angiography to allow assessment of lesion length. **(B)** Deployment of a 7.0- × 16-mm Racer bare metal stent (Medtronic, Minneapolis) in the right common iliac lesion (white arrowhead). **(C)** Post–stent digital subtraction angiography demonstrates brisk flow through the stent (black arrow) and patency of the right common iliac artery. **(D)** Digital subtraction angiography demonstrating a chronic total occlusion of the left common femoral artery (black arrowhead) with well-developed collaterals in the same patient.

Nonpharmacologic Therapies

- Smoking cessation[1]:
  - Patients with PAD should be advised to quit at every visit.
  - They should be assisted in developing a plan for quitting that includes pharmacotherapy and/or referral to a smoking cessation program.
- Daily foot inspection and proper foot care
- **Supervised exercise program**: Improvements in functional capacity occur over several months, with long-term data suggesting persistent benefit of supervised exercise in patients with claudication.[1]

Percutaneous and Surgical Management

- For symptomatic patients with **claudication** that causes limitations in quality of life or vocational ability and who do not respond adequately to a supervised exercise program and medical management, a **revascularization procedure** may be considered.[1]
- **Endovascular treatments** such as percutaneous transluminal angioplasty (PTA), lithotripsy, and atherectomy, with or without stenting (Figure 19-4); catheter-based thrombolysis; mechanical thrombectomy; and open surgical procedures are reasonable treatment options based on comorbidities and vascular anatomy.[1]
- In patients presenting with **CLI**, revascularization should be considered and performed to minimize tissue loss with either endovascular or open surgical approach.[1]

REFERRAL

- For rapid disease progression, urgent referral to a vascular specialist is warranted to limit the extent of tissues necrosis and increase the chance of limb salvage.
- **If signs of ALI are present (the six P's), the vascular consult is emergent**, and immediate concerns should address anticoagulation to prevent the propagation of thrombus material and initiate plans for urgent or emergent revascularization.

MONITORING/FOLLOW-UP

- Clinically stable patients should be regularly evaluated with history and physical examination as well as noninvasive studies such as ABI.
- Patients with progressive symptoms may require more intense evaluation, including imaging or invasive angiography.
- All patients with PAD require regular follow-up for continued medical management of both PAD and other cardiovascular disease.

Renal Artery Stenosis

GENERAL PRINCIPLES

Epidemiology

- Renovascular hypertension resulting from renal artery stenosis (RAS) is the **most common correctable cause of secondary hypertension**.
- The prevalence of RAS in patients with refractory hypertension, multivessel CAD, and newly initiated hemodialysis has been noted to be as high as 20-40%.[7]

Etiology

- **Atherosclerotic disease is the cause of most RAS**. Less common causes of RAS are listed in Table 19-2.
- Fibromuscular dysplasia (FMD) is the second most common cause of RAS. Although occurring in both genders, the typical presentation of FMD is that of hypertension in a young female.

Pathophysiology

- Renal hypoperfusion leads to **activation of the renin–angiotensin system**. The vasoactive properties of aldosterone and angiotensin II lead to volume expansion and elevated systemic blood pressures.

TABLE 19-2	CAUSES OF RENAL ARTERY STENOSIS

- Atherosclerosis
- Fibromuscular dysplasia
- Renal artery aneurysms
- Aortic or renal artery dissection
- Vasculitis
- Thrombotic or cholesterol embolization
- Collagen vascular disease
- Retroperitoneal fibrosis
- Trauma
- Post-transplantation stenosis
- Postradiation

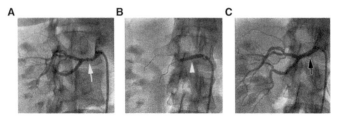

FIGURE 19-5. Fibromuscular dysplasia of the renal artery in a patient with severe refractory hypertension. **(A)** Invasive angiography of the right renal artery with classic "beads-on-a-string" stenotic appearance (white arrow) of the right renal artery. **(B)** Inflation of a 4.0- × 20-mm Angiosculpt (Angioscore, Fremont) scoring angioplasty balloon (white arrowhead) to treat the stenotic lesion. **(C)** Final postintervention angiography reveals brisk flow through the right renal artery lesion (black arrow) following further dilatation with a noncompliant angioplasty balloon.

- Progression of high-grade RAS can result in loss of renal function/mass and ultimately, ischemic nephropathy.
- Atherosclerotic RAS tends to involve the ostium of the renal arteries and the aorta.
- FMD involves the mid- and distal renal artery and may extend into the side branches. The characteristic "string-of-beads" appearance (Figure 19-5) and location within the renal artery help differentiate FMD from atherosclerotic RAS. FMD can also affect other arterial beds, especially the carotid and vertebral arteries.

DIAGNOSIS

Clinical Presentation
- RAS may be clinically silent in many individuals.
- **Severe hypertension** and **fluid retention** are the hallmark findings of RAS. Clinical features that should prompt evaluation for RAS include[8]:
  - Onset of hypertension before the age of 30 years
  - Onset of severe hypertension after the age of 55 years
  - Accelerated hypertension (sudden and persistent worsening of previously controlled hypertension)
  - Resistant hypertension (refractory despite three drugs, one of which must be a diuretic)
  - Malignant hypertension (coexistent evidence of acute end-organ damage)
  - Worsening renal function after the administration of an angiotensin-converting enzyme (ACE) inhibitor or angiotensin-receptor blocker (ARB)
  - An unexplained atrophic kidney or >1.5-cm size discrepancy between the two kidneys
  - Sudden unexplained pulmonary edema or refractory angina

Diagnostic Testing
- **Duplex ultrasonography with Doppler** is recommended as an initial test for the detection of RAS and has a high sensitivity and specificity in identifying stenosis >60%.[8]
- **CT or MRA** can define lesion characteristics and is helpful in imaging patients in whom ultrasonography proves difficult.

○ CT uses iodinated contrast, which can lead to further renal ischemic injury and subsequent worsening hypertension within this RAS population.

○ MRA uses gadolinium contrast, traditionally thought to be less nephrotoxic than CT contrast. When the glomerular filtration rate is <30 mL/min, however, there is an association between gadolinium use and nephrogenic systemic fibrosis.

• If initial tests are inconclusive or considered too risky, **catheter angiography** could be considered for definitive diagnosis and is considered the gold standard for diagnosing RAS.

• Owing to the **high prevalence of atherosclerotic RAS in patients with lower extremity PAD and CAD**, a renal angiogram should be considered in patients with CAD and clinical suspicion for RAS who are already undergoing invasive angiography.[8]

• Because of the association with cerebral aneurysms, all patients with renal FMD should undergo MRA screening or CT angiography of the head.

TREATMENT

Medications

Medical treatment for atherosclerotic RAS focuses mainly on **controlling renovascular hypertension**.[9]

Surgical Management

• A revascularization strategy may be considered for **hemodynamically significant RAS**, which is defined as follows[7]: (1) any stenosis ≥70% diameter stenosis by angiography or intravascular ultrasound; or (2) ≥50% to 70% diameter stenosis with a renal P_d/P_a ≤0.8, hyperemic pressure gradient >20 mm Hg, or a mean resting gradient ≥10 mm Hg.

• In particular, intervention in the following scenarios is considered appropriate[7]:
  ○ Accelerated, refractory, or malignant hypertension
  ○ Hypertension with an unexplained unilateral small kidney
  ○ Hypertension with intolerance to medication
  ○ Chronic kidney disease with bilateral RAS or with RAS affecting a solitary functioning kidney
  ○ Recurrent, sudden unexplained pulmonary edema
  ○ Recurrent angina in the setting of severe hypertension

• Percutaneous intervention (Figure 19-5) with stenting has resulted in a higher clinical success rate and lower restenosis rate, especially for ostial lesions, especially with the use of intravascular imaging.

• Patients with FMD are an exception; in such individuals, balloon angioplasty alone is the therapy of choice.

• In some situations, specifically macroaneurysmal disease and small, multiple renal arteries, the anatomy is unfavorable for percutaneous therapy and vascular surgical reconstruction may be the treatment of choice.

Lifestyle/Risk Modification

Cardiovascular risk factor reduction may aid in the treatment of RAS and reduce the risk of other cardiovascular disease:
• Smoking cessation
• Blood pressure control (<130/80)
• Goal serum lipid levels
• Goal serum glucose control

Carotid Artery Stenosis

GENERAL PRINCIPLES

- Stroke is the third leading cause of death in the United States and represents a major cause of long-term disability.
- The detection of carotid artery stenosis presents an opportunity to identify patients at high risk for stroke and prevent cerebrovascular events and other adverse cardiovascular events.
- **Nearly half of patients with atherosclerotic carotid artery disease have severe CAD.** As a result, although recent trials have focused on the role of percutaneous carotid intervention versus carotid endarterectomy in the prevention of stroke, the management of carotid artery disease must be multimodal and include the treatment of modifiable risk factors, such as hypertension, dyslipidemia, diabetes, and tobacco abuse.

Classification

- *Asymptomatic carotid stenosis* is defined as identifiable carotid artery plaque in the absence of neurologic symptoms, such as amaurosis fugax, TIA, or stroke.
- Symptomatic carotid stenosis, in contrast, is the presence of neurologic symptoms suggestive of embolic or ischemic disease.
- Transcranial Doppler studies have demonstrated that embolic events may be present in asymptomatic carotid stenosis and are associated with a higher rate of symptomatic events.

Epidemiology

- Carotid stenosis >50% is present in 7% of men older than and 5% of women older than 65 years.[10]
- Although strokes and TIAs have multiple etiologies, ~80% are ischemic in origin. About 7% of all first ischemic strokes were associated with an extracranial carotid stenosis >60% or more.[10]
- Modifiable risk factors for stroke include hypertension, tobacco use, dyslipidemia, and diabetes.
- In general, relative risk of stroke increases as the degree of stenosis progresses.

Pathophysiology

- Carotid artery stenosis is most commonly the result of atherosclerotic plaque formation, although, less commonly, FMD, cystic medial necrosis, or arteritis may play a role.
- Atherosclerotic carotid artery disease may result in cerebrovascular ischemic events via two mechanisms:
  - **Flow limitation:** Although collateral circulation via the circle of Willis may compensate, severe stenosis or acute plaque rupture of the internal carotid artery can lead to potential ischemia and/or infarction of the affected hemisphere.
  - **Cerebral embolic event:** Embolization of thrombus or atheromatous debris from the carotid plaque can result in a TIA or stroke.

DIAGNOSIS

Clinical Presentation

History

- Atherosclerotic carotid artery stenosis can present as an asymptomatic carotid bruit, TIA, or stroke.
- Focal neurologic symptoms suggestive of cerebrovascular ischemia or infarction include, but are not limited to, unilateral weakness, paresthesia, or sensory loss, neglect, abnormal visual–spatial ability, monocular blindness, hemianopsia, aphasia, ataxia, cranial nerve deficits, visual field loss, dizziness, imbalance, and incoordination.

Physical Examination
- Auscultation: Patients presenting to a cardiovascular specialist should undergo auscultation of the carotid arteries. Most bruits detected will be during systole; if the bruit extends into diastole, this indicates a significant gradient in the carotid artery with stenosis of about 80%.
- Neurologic evaluation: Patients with a carotid bruit should be evaluated for neurologic signs via a brief neurologic examination for strength, sensation, and orientation. Pre-existing neurologic deficits should be examined and documented in patients who have previously had a stroke.

Diagnostic Testing

Laboratories
Routine evaluation of patients with asymptomatic and symptomatic carotid stenosis should include factors important for the medical management of systemic atherosclerosis:
- Fasting lipid profile
- Renal function studies
- Fasting glucose and hemoglobin A1C

Imaging
- **Ultrasound with Doppler:**
  - Ultrasound has been reported to have a sensitivity of 87-99% and specificity of 69-96% in the identification of >50% stenosis.[10]
  - All symptomatic patients with ischemic focal neurologic symptoms should undergo carotid ultrasound.
  - Although most recent recommendations from the US Preventive Services Task Force (USPSTF) recommend against screening for asymptomatic carotid artery disease for the general population, society-specific guidelines note that screening in selective patients with known vascular disease or in patients aged 65 years or older with risk factors can be considered. In addition, screening for patients undergoing coronary artery bypass grafting surgery should also be performed to understand their perioperative stroke risk.[11,12]
- **MRA:**
  - MRA allows high-resolution imaging of the carotid anatomy as well as the aortic arch vessels up to the circle of Willis.
  - Contrast MRA improves imaging of high-grade stenosis and slow-flowing blood.
  - Sensitivity of MRA has been reported as 97-100% and sensitivity of 82-96%; a weakness of MRA is the overestimation of the degree of stenosis.[9]
- **CT angiography:**
  - CT angiography allows imaging of the carotid as well as the arch vessels and cerebral vessels.
  - Multidetector imaging with three-dimensional reconstruction has improved the quality of imaging significantly and now may be near comparable to the resolution of invasive angiography with a sensitivity of 100% and specificity of 63%.[10]
  - Heavily calcified lesions as well as metallic dental or cranial implants can cause significant imaging artifacts.
  - Iodinated contrast is required, which can be nephrotoxic to individuals with preexisting renal insufficiency.
- **Invasive angiography:**
  - Angiography offers excellent resolution of vascular anatomy, though the invasive nature of this technique incurs significant risk, in part dependent on variations in carotid and aortic arch anatomy and potential stroke risk.
  - Outside a planned catheter-based intervention, the use of routine diagnostic angiography has generally fallen out of favor, except for resolving conflicting noninvasive test results.

TREATMENT

Medications

- Medical treatment should focus on control of the modifiable risk factors of cerebrovascular events.
- Antiplatelet medications[10]:
  - If not contraindicated, antiplatelet therapy with **aspirin** (75 to 325 mg daily) should be administered.
  - **Clopidogrel** (75 mg daily) may be considered instead of aspirin.
  - **Dipyridamole** may be considered in conjunction with aspirin in select patients.
- For patients with a history of TIA or stroke, control of risk factors including hypertension, diabetes, and cholesterol is paramount.

Surgical Management

- **Asymptomatic carotid artery stenosis**[10]:
  - Carotid endarterectomy or carotid artery stenting may be considered in select asymptomatic patients, if the risk of perioperative stroke, MI, and death is low, with >70% stenosis (Doppler ultrasound) or 60% by angiography.
- **Symptomatic carotid artery stenosis**[10]:
  - For patients with a recent (<6 months) TIA or ischemic stroke with ipsilateral severe (>70% by noninvasive or >50% by invasive imaging) carotid stenosis, endarterectomy by a surgeon can be undertaken if at average or low surgical risk.
  - Carotid artery stenting may be an alternative in patients with an average or low risk of complications associated with endovascular intervention.
  - The decision for stenting versus endarterectomy should be undertaken on a case-by-case basis factoring in operator experience, patient clinical scenario, vessel anatomy, and lesion complexity.

REFERENCES

1. Gerhard-Herman MD, Gornik HL, Barrett C, et al. 2016 AHA/ACC guideline on the management of patients with lower extremity peripheral artery disease: a report of the American College of Cardiology/American Heart Association Task Force on Clinical Practice Guidelines. *Circulation.* 2017;135:e726-79.
2. Lee JY, Lee SW, Lee WS, et al. Prevalence and clinical implications of newly revealed, asymptomatic abnormal ankle–brachial index in patients with significant coronary artery disease. *JACC Cardiovasc Interv.* 2013;6:1303-13.
3. Hirsch AT, Criqui MH, Treat-Jacobson D, et al. Peripheral arterial disease detection, awareness, and treatment in primary care. *JAMA.* 2001;286:1317-24.
4. Begelman SM, Jaff MR. Noninvasive diagnostic strategies for peripheral arterial disease. *Cleve Clin J Med.* 2006;73:S22-9.
5. Anand SS, Bosch J, Eikelboom JW, et al. Rivaroxaban with or without aspirin in patients with stable peripheral or carotid artery disease: an international, randomised, double-blind, placebo-controlled trial. *Lancet.* 2018;391:219-29.
6. Bonaca MP, Bauersachs RM, Anand SS, et al. Rivaroxaban in peripheral artery disease after revascularization. *N Engl J Med.* 2020;382:1994-2004.
7. Li J, Parikh SA. Management of renal arterial disease. *Interv Cardiol Clin.* 2014;3(4):501-16.
8. Parikh SA, Shishehbor MH, Gray BH, et al. SCAI expert consensus statement for renal artery stenting appropriate use. *Catheter Cardiovasc Interv.* 2014;84:1163-71.
9. Bailey SR, Beckman JA, Dao TD, et al. ACC/AHA/SCAI/SIR/SVM 2018 appropriate use criteria for peripheral artery intervention: a report of the American College of Cardiology Appropriate Use Criteria Task Force, American Heart Association, Society for Cardiovascular Angiography and Interventions, Society of Interventional Radiology, and Society for Vascular Medicine. *J Am Coll Cardiol.* 2019;73:214-37.

10. Brott TG, Halperin JL, Abbara S, et al. 2011 ASA/ACCF/AHA/AANN/AANS/ACR/ASNR/CNS/SAIP/SCAI/SIR/SNIS/SVM/SVS guideline on the management of patients with extracranial carotid and vertebral artery disease: executive summary. A report of the American College of Cardiology Foundation/American Heart Association Task Force on Practice Guidelines, and the American Stroke Association, American Association of Neuroscience Nurses, American Association of Neurological Surgeons, American College of Radiology, American Society of Neuroradiology, Congress of Neurological Surgeons, Society of Atherosclerosis Imaging and Prevention, Society for Cardiovascular Angiography and Interventions, Society of Interventional Radiology, Society of Neuro Interventional Surgery, Society for Vascular Medicine, and Society for Vascular Surgery. *Circulation.* 2011;124:489-532.
11. U.S. Preventive Services Task Force., & United States. *U.S. Preventive Services Task Force (USPSTF).* U.S. Dept. of Health & Human Services, Agency for Healthcare Research and Quality; 2021.
12. Ricotta JJ, Aburahma A, Ascher E, et al. Updated Society for Vascular Surgery guidelines for management of extracranial carotid disease: executive summary. *J Vasc Surg.* 2011;54:832-6.

Diseases of the Aorta

20

Tarun Ramayya and Alan C. Braverman

Introduction

- The aorta is divided into two anatomic components.
  - The **thoracic aorta** is divided into the ascending, arch, and descending segments. The ligamentum arteriosum marks the point at which the arch joins the descending segment and denotes the aortic isthmus, which is an area most vulnerable to deceleration trauma.
  - The **abdominal aorta** is divided into the suprarenal and infrarenal segments.
- The aorta is composed of three separate histologic layers:
  - The **intima** is the thin innermost lining, comprising primarily endothelium.
  - The **media** is the muscular middle layer, comprising smooth muscle cells and elastin.
  - The **adventitia** is the fibrous outer layer.
- The nutrient supply to the vessel wall is a combination of passive diffusion from the lumen and the vasa vasorum, which supplies most of the aorta, with the exception of the infrarenal abdominal aorta.
- Aortopathies, or diseases of the aorta, are a spectrum of diseases that usually involve the intima or media of the aorta, and the pathophysiology will depend upon the underlying disease state.
- Some basic principles of physiology, however, are pertinent to the understanding of all aortopathies.
  - The smooth intimal layer and elastic media allow the aorta to have low vascular resistance and a natural distensibility.
  - The elasticity of the aorta is directly related to blood pressure (BP); the higher the pressure, the stiffer the walls of the aorta become, as the load is borne less by elastin and more by collagen.
  - With age, there is an increase in the collagen-to-elastin ratio in the aortic wall, resulting in a less compliant structure.
  - Atherosclerosis also serves to lessen the elasticity of involved aortic segments and may disrupt the intimal layer as well.
  - Genetically triggered aortic diseases usually lead to abnormalities of the aortic media, with decreased distensibility, cystic medial degeneration (CMD), progressive wall weakness, and subsequent aneurysmal enlargement and risk of aortic dissection (AD).
  - Though the underlying pathophysiologic processes that cause aortic diseases vary, the clinical consequences may be severe.

Aortic Aneurysms

- Aortic aneurysms are a pathologic segment of aortic dilation that can expand and rupture or dissect; there are true aneurysms and pseudoaneurysms ("false" aneurysms).
  - **True aneurysms** involve dilation of all three layers of the vessel wall but leave the vessel wall intact; they are either saccular or fusiform.

- Fusiform aneurysms are the most common and are symmetrically dilated with involvement of the entire aortic circumference.
- Saccular aneurysms are less common and are a focal outpouching.
  - **Pseudoaneurysms** occur when there is rupture of the wall typically from trauma resulting in a contained periaortic hematoma in continuity with the aortic lumen.
- Aortic aneurysms are further divided by location as either abdominal or thoracic aneurysms.

Abdominal Aortic Aneurysms

GENERAL PRINCIPLES

- An *abdominal aortic aneurysm* (AAA) is defined as an **abdominal aortic diameter >3.0 cm**.
- It is the most common type of aortic aneurysm.
- About 4-7% of men older than 50 years have AAA, and AAA is fivefold more common in men than women.[1]
- It is thought to be related to a chronic inflammatory state in the aortic wall, which, over time, degrades the elastin and smooth muscle cells, weakens the vessel wall, and leads to dilation.
- Risk factors include age, male gender, Caucasian race, smoking (fivefold increased risk), atherosclerosis, emphysema, hypertension (HTN), hyperlipidemia, the presence of other large artery aneurysms, and family history.
- Up to 20% of patients with AAAs report a family history of AAA.[2,3]

DIAGNOSIS

Clinical Presentation

- Most commonly (80%) located in the infrarenal aorta
- AAAs have an insidious course over years, with relative paucity of symptoms.
  - The vast majority of AAAs are small.
  - Enlargement may cause abdominal or back pain.
  - Complications include mural thrombus formation, distal thromboembolism, rapid expansion, or rupture and, less commonly, dissection.
- **Size of the aneurysm predicts 1-year risk of rupture**.[3]
  - 9% for AAA 5.5 to 5.9 cm in diameter
  - 10% for AAA 6.0 to 6.9 cm in diameter
  - 33% for AAA ≥7.0 cm in diameter
- Enlargement of the aneurysm is also nonlinear; the larger the diameter, the faster the growth rate.
- Aneurysm rupture:
  - 30-50% of patients with ruptured AAA die before reaching hospital.
  - Symptoms include abdominal or back pain; hypotension with rupture into the peritoneal cavity.
  - Rupture is associated with >40-50% operative mortality.
  - Although aneurysm diameter is most important in predicting rupture, the aneurysm's rate of expansion, wall tension, wall stiffness, and peak wall stress all contribute to risk of rupture.[2,3]

Diagnostic Testing

- **Ultrasound:**
  - It is widely available, relatively accurate, inexpensive, and involves no radiation.
  - Limited by body habitus, overlying bowel and gas, and operator expertise

○ The United States Preventive Services Task Force (USPSTF) recommends a one-time screening for AAA in men aged 65 to 75 years with a history of smoking and selective screening for women aged 65 to 75 years who have ever smoked.[4]

○ The Society of Vascular Surgery recommends a one-time AAA ultrasound screening for men and women aged 65 to 75 years who have a history of tobacco use.[2]

○ Ultrasound screening for AAA in first-degree relatives of patients with AAA is recommend (to begin at age 65 years).[2]

- **Computed tomography (CT):**
  ○ CT angiography (CTA) is highly accurate and allows for visualization of the proximal and distal aorta and branch vessels.
  ○ It provides valuable information such as the presence of mural thrombus, calcification, and coexisting anatomic abnormalities and is used for staging of endovascular repair.
  ○ It has replaced angiography for the routine imaging of AAA.
  ○ Limited by the need for IV contrast and radiation

- **Magnetic resonance imaging (MRI):**
  ○ MRI and MR angiography (MRA) are highly accurate for diagnosing and sizing AAA.
  ○ It does not utilize IV iodinated contrast.
  ○ No radiation exposure
  ○ Limited by availability

TREATMENT

Medications

- The following modifications and therapy are important in AAA disease:
  ○ Treatment of HTN
  ○ Treatment of hyperlipidemia with statin therapy to lower atherosclerotic cardiovascular risk
  ○ Angiotensin-converting enzyme inhibitors, angiotensin-receptor blockers (ARBs), β-blockers (BBs), and doxycycline have beneficial effects in animal models of AAA; however, they have not been proven to modify the disease course in humans.[5,6]

Nonpharmacologic Therapies

- Smoking cessation
- Moderate exercise

Surgical Management

- For AAA <5.0 to 5.5 cm, surgery is not indicated unless a complication occurs.[2,6]
- For AAA >5.0 to 5.5 cm, or those with complications, surgical or endovascular **treatment is indicated**.[2]
  ○ Open surgical repair (OSR) involves directly visualizing the AAA and excision of the aneurysm, followed by a Dacron graft sewn end to end to the proximal and distal aorta. Complications of OSR are related to abdominal incision (hernia, bowel obstruction), perianastomotic aneurysm, graft infection, graft-enteric fistula, and graft limb occlusions with lower extremity edema.
  ○ Endovascular aortic repair (EVAR) involves a catheter-based approach, through which a stent graft is placed across the aneurysmal portion of the aorta, excluding it from exposure to arterial blood flow and pressures.
    ■ Stent grafts are fabric (woven polyester, similar to material used in open repair) that is suspended on a metal (usually stainless steel) frame.
    ■ The proximal and distal ends of the stent graft lie outside the aneurysm, and therefore, it excludes the aneurysm from the lumen of the aorta, without resection of the aneurysm itself.
    ■ The anatomy must allow enough space for deployment, with appropriate "landing zones" proximally and distally to anchor the stent graft.

- Complications of EVAR include leaks through or around the fabric ("endoleak"), stent migration or fracture, and infection.
  - For asymptomatic infrarenal AAA, there is a lower 30-day mortality rate with EVAR than with OSR, but EVAR has a significantly higher incidence of repeat interventions. Long-term (8-year) follow-up shows no difference in AAA-related or all-cause mortality for EVAR or OSR.[7]
  - In the setting of ruptured AAA, endovascular repair is preferred to surgical repair (if anatomically feasible).[2]

MONITORING/FOLLOW-UP

- For aortic diameters of 2.5 to 2.9 cm, repeat screening in 10 years is suggested.
- For aortic diameters of 3.0 to 3.9 cm, repeat imaging at 3 years is suggested.
- For aortic diameters of 4.0 to 4.9 cm, repeat imaging at 12 months is suggested.
- For aortic diameters of 5.0 to 5.4 cm, repeat imaging at 6 months is suggested.[2]

Thoracic Aortic Aneurysm

GENERAL PRINCIPLES

Definition

- Generally, an **aortic size >4.0 cm in the thorax** is considered abnormal. Age, body surface area (BSA), and sex must be considered when diagnosing a thoracic aortic aneurysm (TAA).
- Nomograms relating BSA, age, and aortic root and ascending aortic diameter are readily available.

Epidemiology

- TAAs are less common than AAAs, with an incidence of about 5 to 10 in 100,000 person-years.[6]
- Most commonly involve the ascending aorta (60%), followed by the descending aorta (35%) and the aortic arch (<10%)

Etiology

- TAAs are caused by a variety of pathogenic mechanisms, including degenerative (atherosclerotic), infectious, inflammatory, and genetic diseases (Table 20-1).[6,8,9]
- **CMD** is a histologic finding of bland, mucoid-appearing, basophilic-staining cysts in the media that represents degeneration of the elastin and collagen fibers, and smooth muscle cell loss.
  - CMD appears in the elderly, to varying degrees, and is exacerbated by chronic HTN.
  - It is also seen in genetic diseases, such as Marfan syndrome (MFS), Loeys–Dietz syndrome (LDS), hereditary thoracic aortic aneurysm disease (H-TAD), Turner syndrome (TS), and bicuspid aortic valve (BAV) disease.
  - The loss of the main components that provide the load-bearing support for the aortic wall leads to progressive dilation and aneurysm formation.
- **Atherosclerosis** involves the descending aorta more commonly than the ascending aorta. Risk factors for degenerative (atherosclerotic) aneurysms are the same as those for coronary artery disease (CAD).
- **MFS** is an autosomal dominant heritable connective tissue disorder that affects 1 in 5000 to 10,000 individuals.
  - Caused by a mutation in *FBN1* on chromosome 15, which encodes fibrillin-1, a structural protein that is the major component of the microfibrils and controls the activation and signaling of transforming growth factor-β (TGF-β) and ERK signaling pathways

TABLE 20-1	ETIOLOGY OF THORACIC AORTIC ANEURYSMS

- Cystic medial degeneration (CMD)
  - Aging and hypertension accelerate CMD
- Genetic disorders[a]
  - Marfan syndrome
  - Loeys–Dietz syndrome
  - Hereditary thoracic aortic aneurysm disease
  - Vascular Ehlers–Danlos syndrome
- Congenital conditions
  - Bicuspid aortic valve[a]
  - Turner syndrome
  - Aortic coarctation
  - Congenital heart disease

- Atherosclerosis
- Aortic dissection
- Inflammatory/infectious conditions
  - Giant cell arteritis
  - Takayasu arteritis
  - HLA-B27 spondyloarthropathies
  - Rheumatoid arthritis
  - Systemic lupus erythematosus
  - ANCA-associated vasculitis
  - IgG subclass 4 disease
  - Behçet disease
  - Syphilitic aortitis
  - Bacterial aortitis

ANCA, antineutrophil cytoplasmic antibody; CMD, cystic medial degeneration.
[a]First-degree relatives of patients with these conditions should be screened for aortic disease.

- ○ Aortic root aneurysms in MFS typically involve the aortic root and are largest at the sinuses of Valsalva.
- ○ MFS is a phenotypically variable disease, affecting the skeleton, eyes (ectopia lentis), skin, dura (dural ectasia), and lung (spontaneous pneumothorax).
- ○ Overactivation of TGF-β is observed in tissues affected in MFS, and drugs that block TGF-β, such as ARBs, are known to attenuate aneurysm formation in Marfan mice. Prospective trials of these agents in people with MFS have shown no difference in aortic growth in patients treated with BBs or ARBs.[10,11]
- **LDS** is an autosomal dominant aortic aneurysm syndrome due to mutations in *TGFBR1* and *TGFBR2* and is characterized by the triad of hypertelorism (wide-set eyes), bifid or broad uvula, and generalized arterial tortuosity. Patients may have cleft palate, velvety, translucent skin, pectus deformities, clubfeet, and arachnodactyly.[8,12,13]
  - ○ Patients have a high risk of AD or rupture at an earlier age and with smaller aortic sizes than in MFS.
  - ○ LDS leads to aneurysms in the aortic root (most commonly) but may also affect the aorta from the root to the pelvis and may cause cerebral or aortic branch vessel aneurysms.
  - ○ Mutations in *SMAD3* (aneurysm-osteoarthritis syndrome), *TGFB2*, and *TGFB3* are sometimes included within the LDS family of disorders due to shared phenotype. Other experts include these disorders in the H-TAD category.
- **H-TAD** is a group of disorders characterized by an autosomal dominant inheritance pattern of aneurysm and AD, which have variable phenotypic expression and age of onset. BAV and/or cerebral aneurysms may be present in some individuals. Some also have mild skeletal features.
  - ○ Mutations in multiple genes lead to H-TAD, including genes involved in extracellular matrix proteins, TGF-β signaling, and vascular smooth muscle contraction (Table 20-2).[11]
  - ○ Livedo reticularis, moyamoya, and premature CAD/stroke complicate *ACTA2* mutations; patent ductus arteriosus may be present in *MYH11*.
  - ○ Mutations in the vascular smooth muscle genes *MYH11* and *ACTA2* occur in 1% and 14% of H-TAD, respectively.[8,11]
- Approximately 20% of first-degree relatives of the individual with unexplained TAA or dissection will also have thoracic aortic disease. Thus, it is imperative to screen all first-degree relatives of the proband with a TAA or dissection for familial disease. If a

TABLE 20-2	GENES ASSOCIATED WITH HEREDITARY THORACIC AORTIC ANEURYSM DISEASE (H-TAD)
Extracellular matrix genes	• *FBN1* (Marfan syndrome) • *COL3A1* (vascular Ehlers–Danlos syndrome) • *EFEMP2* (cutis laxa) • *MFAP5*
TGF-β signaling genes	• *TGFBR1, TGFBR2, SMAD3, TGFB2, TGFB3* (Loeys–Dietz syndrome disorders) • *SKI* (Shprintzen–Goldberg syndrome) • *SLC2A10* (arterial tortuosity syndrome)
Vascular smooth muscle contraction genes	*ACTA2, MYH11, MYLK, PRKG1, MAT2A, FLNA* (H-TAD)

H-TAD, hereditary thoracic aortic aneurysm disease; TGF-β, transforming growth factor-β.

mutation in a gene leading to TAA is found, other family members may be tested for the same mutation. If mutation analysis is not performed or is negative, each first-degree relative should have imaging screening at baseline and periodically thereafter.

- **Vascular Ehlers–Danlos syndrome (vEDS)** is a rare disorder caused by a mutation in the *COL3A1* gene.[11]
  - Inherited in an autosomal dominant pattern, vEDS is characterized by spontaneous rupture or dissection of medium–large arteries and the aorta, often in the absence of significant aneurysm formation, spontaneous colonic rupture, pneumothorax, easy bruising, varicose veins, and atrophic scars.
  - BB therapy with celiprolol showed improved outcomes in vEDS in one randomized controlled trial (RCT).[14]
  - Surgical repair of the vessel is very difficult due to poor vascular connective tissue and the lack of appropriate collagen to provide support for sutures.
- **BAV** occurs in ~1-2% of the population and is associated with increased risk of aortic root and/or ascending aortic aneurysm, AD, and coarctation of the aorta.[15,16]
  - Over half of patients with BAV have aortic dilatation, generally of the ascending aorta and/or aortic root, independent of valvular stenosis or regurgitation. Aneurysms in BAV most commonly affect the mid-ascending aorta.
  - The risk of AD is four to eight times higher in BAV than in the normal population because of abnormalities of elastic tissue in the aortic media.[16]
  - BAV may be familial in about 9% of cases and may be inherited as an autosomal dominant trait with reduced penetrance; patients with BAV and aneurysm should have their first-degree relatives screened for BAV and/or TAA.
  - Hemodynamic stress on the aortic wall due to abnormal flow patterns accompanying the BAV may underlie the pathophysiology of medial changes, leading to TAA in this disorder.
- **TS** is a genetic disorder caused by complete or partial loss of the second sex chromosome (XO or Xp), and 50-75% of patients with TS have several cardiovascular defects, including BAV (30%), aortic coarctation (12%), and ascending aortic dilation (33%).
  - CMD can occur in TS, which may lead to ascending TAA.
  - Because TS is associated with short stature, aortic size must be corrected for BSA. An aortic size index >2.5 cm/m^2 is associated with an increased risk for AD in TS.
- **Inflammatory aortitis** includes a broad spectrum of diseases divided into noninfectious and infectious causes.
- **Noninfectious:** giant cell arteritis (temporal arteritis), Takayasu arteritis, the HLA-B27 spondyloarthropathies (ankylosing spondylitis, reactive arthritis), rheumatoid arthritis,

systemic lupus erythematosus, antineutrophil cytoplasmic antibodies (ANCAs)-associated vasculitis (granulomatosis with polyangiitis, polyarteritis nodosa, microscopic polyangiitis), Behçet disease, Cogan syndrome, relapsing polychondritis, sarcoidosis, idiopathic aortitis, and IgG subclass 4 disease
- **Infectious (or mycotic aneurysms):** can be caused by acute infections involving *Staphylococcus, Streptococcus,* or *Salmonella* species.
  - Patients present with fever, pain, and bacteremia.
  - Infected aneurysms tend to be saccular, may progress rapidly, and have high risk for rupture.
  - Syphilitic aortitis is very rare and involves the ascending aorta. Pathologic features include lymphocytic and plasma cell inflammation in aortic adventitia and classic appearance of "tree bark" or wrinkled appearance of aortic intima.

DIAGNOSIS
Clinical Presentation
- **Most TAAs are asymptomatic and incidentally found** on radiologic studies or echocardiograms done for other reasons.
- When they occur, symptoms are related to enlarging aneurysms, which may cause chest or back pain, or due to rupture, impending rupture, or dissection.
  - Aortic root dilation may lead to significant aortic regurgitation (AR).
  - Mural thrombus formation may lead to thromboembolism.
- The most serious complications are aortic rupture and dissection.
- The natural history and progression of TAA depends upon the etiology.
  - While age-related CMD or atherosclerosis may cause an aneurysm to slowly grow over years, a TAA related to LDS, vEDS, aortitis, or infection may grow more rapidly or lead to acute dissection in the setting of a relatively small aneurysm.
  - The rate of dilation and risk of rupture are also dependent on the size of the aorta.
    - Similar to AAA, the relationship between size and risk of rupture is nonlinear.
    - The yearly risk of rupture, dissection, or death for descending TAAs of 5 cm is ~5%; for TAAs of 5.5 cm is ~7%; for TAAs of 6 cm is ~9%; and for TAAs of 7 cm is ~15%.
    - The risk of rupture, dissection, or death for ascending TAA ≥6 cm is 15.6%.[17,18]

Diagnostic Testing
- **Chest radiography** (CXR) may show a widened mediastinum or prominent aortic knob. Small aneurysms may not be appreciable on CXR, and CXR is not a useful test to exclude the presence of TAA.
- **Transthoracic echocardiogram** (TTE) is useful for defining the dimensions of the aortic root, the proximal ascending aorta, and the structure and function of the aortic valve. The ascending and proximal descending aorta may be seen but with less accuracy than with TEE, CT, or MRI.
- **Transesophageal echocardiogram** (TEE) is an excellent modality to image the aortic root, arch, and descending aorta.
  - There is a small blind spot at the level of the mid-high ascending aorta that may be missed by TEE.
  - It also provides useful information about cardiac and valve function.
- **CTA** and **MRI/MRA** are excellent tests to image the entire thoracic aorta.
  - Measurement of aneurysms needs to be carefully done, especially if the aorta is tortuous, because the axial slices may image the aorta at an oblique angle that may provide inaccurate measurements of the true transverse dimension of the aorta. A double oblique technique for measuring the aortic diameter is recommended.
  - MRI/MRA may be preferred as the imaging modality of choice for chronic surveillance, due to the lack of radiation and iodinated contrast.

TREATMENT

Medications

- Patients with degenerative TAAs should receive cholesterol-lowering therapy, such as a statin.
- In the absence of genetically triggered TAA or HTN, there are no clinical data showing a benefit for prophylactic BBs and ARBs.
- Adequate BP control (goal <120/60 mm Hg) is recommended, however, to minimize the risk of progressive dilation, rupture, and dissection by lowering the shear forces on the aorta.
- BBs lower BP and lessen the rate of change in pressure with each systole (dP/dt) and thus are indicated in TAA patients with HTN. In the absence of H-TAD, there are no data demonstrating benefit of BBs for sporadic, non–H-TAD patients.
- ARBs, by antagonizing TGF-β, have been demonstrated to be noninferior to BBs for slowing the aortic growth rate in MFS. While used in other H-TADs, there are no clinical trials available to inform their use in management.[10]

Nonpharmacologic Therapies

- Smoking cessation is imperative.
- Patients must be educated and made aware of the condition and the risk of AD and rupture.
- Avoidance of strenuous physical activity such as isometric exercise, heavy weightlifting, and sports that involve body collisions is important and may impact participation in certain jobs and sports.[19]
- Pregnancy in the setting of genetically triggered aneurysm syndromes increases the risk of rupture or dissection, so contraception and timing of pregnancy must be discussed with patients.[12,19,20]

Surgical Treatment

- Ascending TAA:
  - Surgical resection and repair of the aorta is the treatment of choice.
  - Surgery is recommended for ascending aortic aneurysms at the following size thresholds (but must consider age, sex, BSA, family history, aortic growth rate, and surgical risk):
    - **Degenerative aneurysm ≥5.5 cm**
    - **BAV ≥5.5 cm** (≥5.0 cm if family history of dissection, rapid growth, aortic coarctation, or low surgical risk)
    - **MFS ≥5.0 cm** (≥4.5 cm if family history of dissection or rapid growth)
    - **H-TAD ≥4.5 to 5.0 cm** (depending upon gene, aortic growth, family history)
    - **LDS ≥4.5 cm** (≥4.0 if rapid growth, marked craniofacial features, female, *TGFBR2* mutation, young age, patient/surgeon preference)
  - Involvement of the aortic root and presence of AR are two factors that impact the surgical procedure.
  - When there is significant AR from an abnormal aortic valve and aortic root involvement, the modified Bentall procedure (or a valve-sparing root replacement in selected patients) is performed.
    - After resection of the aortic valve, root and proximal ascending aorta, a prosthetic valve is suspended in a tube made of woven Dacron polyester, which is sutured in an end-to-end manner.
    - The coronary arteries are preserved with "buttons" of native aortic wall and are reimplanted into the aortic graft.
  - If the aortic valve itself is normal, it may be possible to resuspend the patient's native aortic valve in the graft; this is termed a *valve-sparing surgery.*

- Descending TAA:
  - Surgical resection of the aneurysm is followed by an end-to-end anastomosis of a graft.
    - Small branches of the descending aorta are ligated.
    - Cardiopulmonary bypass is necessary.
    - The operative morbidity and mortality may be very significant, depending upon comorbidities.
  - Thoracic endovascular aortic aneurysm repair (TEVAR) is often possible and is performed in patients with the appropriate anatomy.
    - There is a significantly lower procedure-related mortality with TEVAR compared to traditional open repair.[12,21]
    - Stent grafts are fabric (woven polyester, similar to material used in open repair) that is suspended on a metal (usually stainless steel) frame.
    - The proximal and distal ends of the stent graft lie outside the aneurysm, and therefore, it excludes the aneurysm from the lumen of the aorta, without resection of the aneurysm itself.
    - The anatomy must allow enough space for deployment, with appropriate landing zones proximally and distally to anchor the stent graft.
    - Complications of TEVAR include leaks through or around the fabric ("endoleak"), stent migration or fracture, and infections.
    - TEVAR is not recommended for general use in genetic aortopathy disorders.
  - The surgical threshold for descending aortic aneurysm is ≥5.5 to 6 cm depending upon the cause of aneurysm, underlying disease, and whether TEVAR is a suitable option (≥5.5 cm) or OSR is required (≥6 cm). OSR may be appropriate at lower size thresholds for genetic aortopathies.

MONITORING/FOLLOW-UP

- Long-term surveillance must be performed even after definitive repair, and the imaging modality (TTE, CTA, or MRI) and timing depend upon the location, size, and underlying etiology of the TAA.
- In general, after the initial diagnosis, imaging should be performed at more frequent intervals (every 6 months), until the TAA is deemed to be stable. Thereafter, imaging should be performed every year, with intervals depending upon the aortic size, growth rate, and underlying condition.

Acute Aortic Syndromes: Aortic Dissection and Variants

GENERAL PRINCIPLES

Definition
- **See** Figure 20-1.[6]
- **Classic AD** is a tear in the intima, which allows blood to enter the aortic wall creating a false lumen or channel, which propagates in an anterograde or retrograde manner (Figure 20-2A).[6]

Aortic dissection

Aortic intramural hematoma

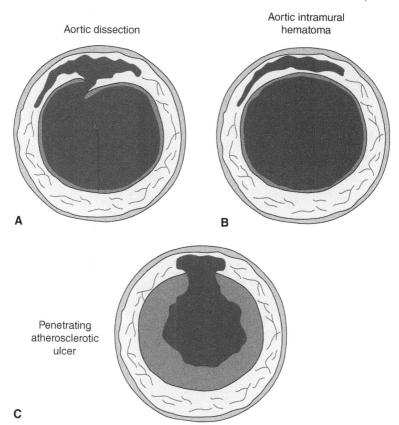

A

B

Penetrating atherosclerotic ulcer

C

FIGURE 20-1. Schematics of acute aortic syndromes with cross section of the aorta demonstrating each pathophysiologic subtype. **(A)** Classic aortic dissection. **(B)** Aortic intramural hematoma. **(C)** Penetrating atherosclerotic ulcer. (Reprinted from Braverman AC, Schermerhorn M. Diseases of the aorta. In: Zipes DP, Libby P, Bonow RO, et al, eds. *Braunwald's Heart Disease: A Textbook of Cardiovascular Medicine.* 11th ed. Elsevier; 2018:1295-327. Copyright © 2019 Elsevier. With permission.)

- **Aortic intramural hematoma** (IMH) is a hemorrhage in the aortic media without a visible flap, which may result from a microscopic intimal defect or from a spontaneous rupture of the vasa vasorum (Figure 20-2B).[6]
- **Penetrating aortic ulcer** (PAU) results from an atherosclerotic lesion that penetrates through the media and may lead to aortic rupture, dissection, pseudoaneurysm, or late aneurysm formation (Figure 20-2C).[6]

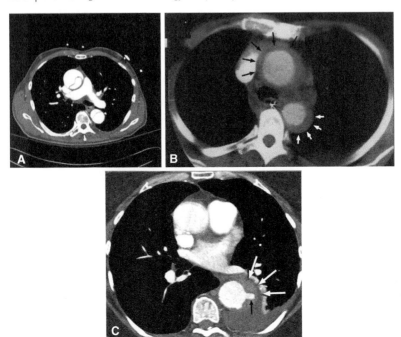

FIGURE 20-2. Acute aortic syndromes. **(A)** Classic aortic dissection. Black arrows point to the intimal flap (TL, true lumen). **(B)** Intramural hematoma (IMH) of the aorta. Black arrows indicate IMH in ascending aorta; white arrows denote crescentic IMH in descending aorta. **(C)** Penetrating atherosclerotic ulcer (PAU) of the aorta (black arrow). White arrows point to associated contained hematoma. (Modified from Braverman AC, Thompson RW, Sanchez LA. Diseases of the aorta. In: Bonow RO, Mann DL, Zipes DP, et al, eds. *Braunwald's Heart Disease: A Textbook of Cardiovascular Medicine*. 9th ed. Elsevier; 2012:1309-37. Copyright © 2012 Elsevier. With permission.)

Classification

- There are several classification systems for ADs, and involvement of the ascending aorta is the defining characteristic.[12,13,22] See Figure 20-3 for classification.[23]
- Stanford type A or DeBakey types I and II dissections involve the ascending aorta.
- Stanford type B or DeBakey type III dissections do not involve the ascending aorta.
- Classification of the anatomy is important because the decision regarding surgical or medical management is dependent on the location of the dissection. Dissections of the ascending aorta (type A, I, or II) require immediate surgical repair, while those involving the descending aorta (type B or III) are initially treated medically.
- AD may be classified as hyperacute (<24 hours), acute (2 to 7 days), subacute (8 to 30 days), and chronic (>30 days) based upon time from symptom onset. A type A dissection has a 20% mortality rate in the first 24 hours and then 30% by 48 hours.[22]

Epidemiology

AD is a rare, but life-threatening condition, with an incidence of 2 to 6 cases per 100,000 person-years. It occurs at least twice as often in males than females and presents most often in individuals aged 50 to 60 years (type A dissection) and 60 to 70 years (type B dissection).[13]

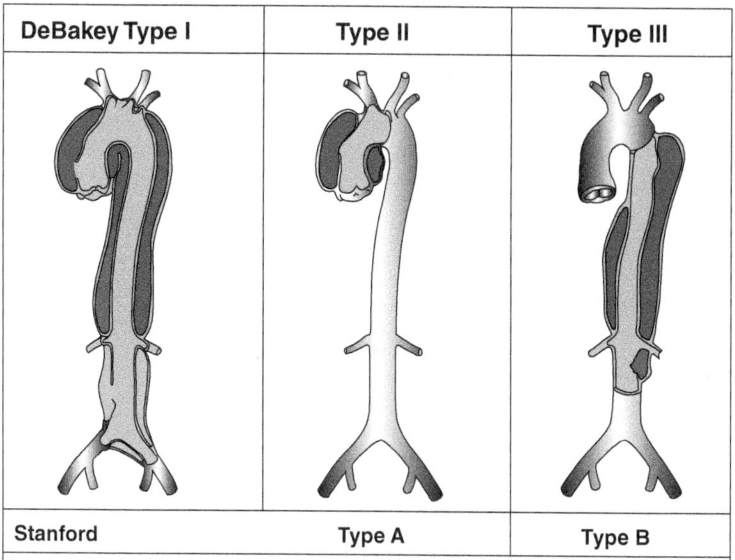

DeBakey Type I	Type II	Type III
Stanford	Type A	Type B

DeBakey

Type I   Originates in the ascending aorta, propagates at least to the aortic arch and often beyond it distally.

Type II   Originates in and is confined to the ascending aorta.

Type III   Originates in the descending aorta and extends distally down the aorta or, rarely, retrograde into the aortic arch and ascending aorta.

Stanford

Type A   All dissections involving the ascending aorta, regardless of the site of origin

Type B   All dissections not involving the ascending aorta

FIGURE 20-3. Classification systems for aortic dissection: Stanford and DeBakey. (Reprinted with permission from Nienaber CA, Eagle KA. Aortic dissection: new frontiers in diagnosis and management. Part I: from etiology to diagnostic strategies. *Circulation.* 2003;108(5):628-35.)

Etiology

- Several conditions predispose the aorta to dissection, most as a result of abnormalities in the arterial wall composition or hemodynamic stress on the aortic wall (Table 20-3).
- Approximately 75% of patients with AD have HTN.[24]
- Patients with genetic disorders such as the MFS, LDS, vEDS, BAV, or H-TAD are particularly prone to aortic dilation and dissection.[25]
- Cocaine or methamphetamine-induced HTN, inflammatory conditions such as giant cell arteritis, or direct trauma from catheterization or aortic surgery can disrupt the aortic intima and lead to dissection.

TABLE 20-3	RISK FACTORS FOR AORTIC DISSECTION

Hypertension
- Genetic disorders[a]
  - Marfan syndrome
  - Loeys–Dietz syndrome
  - Hereditary thoracic aortic aneurysm diseases
  - Vascular Ehlers–Danlos syndrome
- Congenital conditions
  - Bicuspid aortic valve[a]
  - Turner syndrome
  - Aortic coarctation
  - Supravalvular aortic stenosis
- Cocaine/methamphetamine use
- Atherosclerosis/penetrating aortic ulcer

- Trauma—iatrogenic or blunt
  - Catheter induced
  - Intra-aortic balloon pump
  - Aortic valve surgery/TAVR
  - Coronary artery bypass grafting
  - Deceleration injury (e.g., motor vehicle accident)
- Inflammatory/infectious conditions
  - Giant cell arteritis
  - Takayasu arteritis
  - Behçet disease
  - Aortitis
  - Syphilitic aortitis
- Pregnancy[b]
- Weightlifting[b]

TAVR, transcatheter aortic valve replacement.
[a]First-degree relatives of patients with these conditions should be screened for aortic disease.
[b]In the setting of aortopathy.

DIAGNOSIS

Clinical Presentation

- The clinical presentation of AD may be quite variable, and one must maintain a high index of suspicion for the diagnosis.
- The American College of Cardiology/American Heart Association (ACC/AHA) TAD guidelines emphasize considering AD in all patients presenting with chest pain with special attention to the patient with following features: (1) **high-risk conditions** (TAA, Marfan and related disorders, BAV, H-TAD, positive family history, or instrumentation), (2) **high-risk symptoms** (abrupt-onset severe pain, ripping/tearing, syncope), and (3) **high-risk examination** (AR, pulse deficits). If at least one such feature is present and another diagnosis is not obvious, evaluation for AD is recommended.[26]
- Significant morbidity and mortality from dissection are attributed to end-organ damage and aortic rupture (Table 20-4).
- Organ systems may be compromised by compression of branch vessels by an expanding false lumen (dynamic malperfusion) or direct extension of a dissection into the vessel with thrombosis (static malperfusion).
- Cardiovascular and neurologic manifestations are two particularly devastating complications of AD.
  - When the ascending aorta is involved, **acute AR** may lead to heart failure; AR is a key diagnostic feature of type A dissections, occurring in 41-76% of patients.[13]
  - **Cardiac tamponade**, **aortic rupture**, or **myocardial infarction** from coronary artery involvement may lead rapidly to hemodynamic shock and death.
    - Dissection complicated by acute hemopericardium may lead to cardiac tamponade.
    - Poor outcomes have been reported from pericardiocentesis secondary to recurrent bleeding and acute decompensation. Therefore, pericardiocentesis should generally be avoided in favor of emergent surgery unless required for refractory shock.
  - Neurologic sequelae may result from acute dissection involving the carotid or vertebral arteries, and cerebral hypoperfusion may lead to syncope, altered mental status, and

TABLE 20-4	COMPLICATIONS OF AORTIC DISSECTION
Cardiovascular	Aortic rupture, cardiac arrest, syncope, aortic regurgitation, congestive heart failure, coronary ischemia, myocardial infarction, cardiac tamponade, pericarditis
Pulmonary	Pleural effusion, hemothorax, hemoptysis (from aortotracheal or bronchial fistula)
Renal	Acute renal failure, renovascular hypertension, renal ischemia or infarction
Neurologic	Stroke, transient ischemic attack, paraparesis or paraplegia, encephalopathy, coma, spinal cord syndrome, ischemic neuropathy
Gastrointestinal	Mesenteric ischemia or infarction, pancreatitis, hemorrhage (from aortoenteric fistula)
Peripheral vascular	Upper or lower limb ischemia
Systemic	Fever, shock

stroke. Transverse myelitis, myelopathy, paraplegia, or quadriplegia may result from spinal malperfusion.
○ Mesenteric ischemia due to dissection may be difficult to diagnose and can be fatal.

History
• In contrast to the crescendo discomfort of angina pectoris, the pain of acute dissection is typically sudden and is maximal at its onset; it often characterized as a severe, sharp, or stabbing pain in the chest, neck, or interscapular areas. However, in some patients, the pain is not severe and may mimic other more common conditions.
• In addition to the dissection itself, presenting symptoms may also be related to malperfusion or complications involving various organ systems.

Physical Examination
• Physical examination should include a complete pulse examination and BP in both arms and legs, as there may be pulse or pressure deficits.
• Cardiac auscultation may reveal an AR murmur.
• Pulse differentials and an AR murmur are present in the minority of patients, and physical examination alone is not sufficient to rule out AD.

Diagnostic Testing
Laboratories
• D-Dimer may be of assistance in the evaluation; it is usually elevated in acute AD and has a high negative predictive value (95%) when it is <500 ng/mL.
• In IMH or PAU, the D-dimer may not be elevated. Thus, in the setting of a high-risk subset or a high clinical index of suspicion, a negative D-dimer does not rule out an acute AD.[13]
• After dissection is diagnosed, laboratory evaluation includes comprehensive metabolic panel (CMP), complete blood count (CBC), lactate, troponin, creatine kinase (CK), amylase, and lipase levels.

Imaging
• CXR
○ It may demonstrate a widened mediastinum or abnormal aortic contour.

○ Pleural effusion may represent hemothorax, and displaced calcium at the aortic knob may occasionally be present.

○ Up to 20% of ADs are associated with a normal CXR. Therefore, **a normal CXR does not rule out an AD.**[6,24]

• Given the critical nature of ADs, immediate diagnostic confirmation and definition of the extent of the dissection are imperative. The choice of imaging should be made on the basis of sensitivity, specificity, clinical stability, and operator availability and experience (Table 20-5).[24]

○ **If the patient presents with hemodynamic instability or hypotension, rapid evaluation by CT or TEE (or TTE) should be performed** to assess for complications of dissection, including pericardial effusion, AR, or aortic rupture.

○ CT is widely and rapidly available and is the test most commonly used. IV contrast is required to evaluate for dissection and offers outstanding imaging of the entire aorta, branch vessels, and heart (Figure 20-2A).

○ TEE requires an experienced operator and esophageal intubation to perform the procedure; however, it can be performed at the bedside and visualizes the aortic valve, aortic root, and pericardium well.

○ Because of the time delay and difficulties with hemodynamic monitoring, MRI is usually not the first test of choice.

○ While TTE may be rapidly performed and may diagnose an AD, the sensitivity and specificity of this approach are far less than other diagnostic modalities. Thus, lack of diagnostic findings on TTE cannot exclude an AD.

TABLE 20-5	COMPARISON OF DIAGNOSTIC IMAGING MODALITIES FOR AORTIC DISSECTION			
Test	Sensitivity (%)	Specificity (%)	Advantages	Disadvantages
TEE	95	95	Excellent evaluation of aortic root and descending thoracic aorta, aortic valve, and pericardium	Requires esophageal intubation; limited to thoracic aorta, little information about branch vessels
CT	95–100	95–100	Widely and rapidly available; superior imaging of entire aorta, heart, branch vessels, and complications such as rupture, hemopericardium, and malperfusion	Nephrotoxic iodinated contrast required
MRI	98	98	High accuracy, sensitivity, and specificity for all types of dissection	Limited availability, time-consuming procedure, less monitoring during scan

TEE, transesophageal echocardiogram.

TREATMENT

Medications

- **When AD is suspected, immediate initiation of BB therapy** (even when normotensive) to reduce shear forces is recommended while pursuing confirmation of the diagnosis (Table 20-6).[24]
- **BP should be reduced to as low a level as possible (typically <120 mm Hg)** without compromising organ perfusion.
  - BB therapy (i.e., esmolol, labetalol) is recommended to achieve a **target heart rate <70 beats per minute**.
  - Nondihydropyridine calcium channel blockers (i.e., diltiazem, verapamil) may be considered if BB therapy is contraindicated.
  - Care should be taken to **avoid vasodilators,** such as sodium nitroprusside in the absence of negative chronotropic medications, as they may induce reflex tachycardia and increase the dP/dt, which may extend the dissection.

Surgical Management

- **Emergent surgery is indicated when the ascending aorta (type A) is involved in the acute AD.**

TABLE 20-6	SELECTED PHARMACOLOGIC THERAPY FOR AORTIC DISSECTION[a]

IV β-blocker (preferred negative inotrope)

- **Esmolol**: Give 250–500 µg/kg IV bolus, then continuous IV infusion at 25–50 mg/kg/min, titrated to effect with maximum dose of 300 µg/kg/min. Short half-life allows rapid titration
- **Labetalol**: Give 20 mg IV over 2 minutes, then 20–80 mg IV every 10 minutes until adequate response (maximum 300 mg), then continuous IV infusion at 2–10 mg/min IV, titrated to effect
- **Metoprolol**: Give 2.5–15 mg IV followed by 2.5–15 mg IV every 3–6 hours

IV calcium channel blocker (secondary negative inotrope)

- **Diltiazem**: Initial bolus of 0.25–0.35 mg/kg IV bolus, then continuous IV infusion of 5–20 mg/h
- **Verapamil**: 5–10 mg IV and may repeat after 5–10 minutes

IV vasodilator (after initiation of negative inotrope)

- **Sodium nitroprusside**: Start continuous infusion with no bolus at 0.25–0.5 µg/kg/min, titrated to a maximum of 10 µg/min. **Use only in presence of β-blockers.** *Caution*: Thiocyanate toxicity may occur in patients with renal impairment or prolonged infusions
- **Nicardipine**: Give 2.5–5 mg/h and titrate up to a maximum of 15 mg/h
- **Clevidipine**: Give 1–2 mg/h with good response seen after 4–6 mg/h up to a maximum rate of 16 mg/h
- **Nitroglycerin**: Give 5–200 µg/min as IV an infusion
- **Enalaprilat**: Give 1.25–5 mg IV every 6 hours, titrated to effect
- **Fenoldopam**: Give 0.1 µg/kg/min and titrate up to a maximum of 1.6 µg/kg/min

[a]Goal of therapy is heart rate <70 beats/min and blood pressure as low as possible without compromising organ perfusion.

- Medical therapy alone is associated with 60% in-hospital mortality rate.[27]
- Surgery is associated with a 20-25% in-hospital mortality rate, with some single-center institutions reporting lower mortality.[6,22]
- Surgical repair involves excising the intimal tear, obliterating entry into the false channel proximally and distally, and placing a graft in an end-to-end manner to replace the ascending aorta.
- If significant AR complicates AD, the aortic valve is either resuspended or replaced, depending upon the underlying condition of the valve and aortic root. Composite valve graft placement or valve-sparing surgery may be required depending upon the circumstances.
- Endovascular repair for AD involving the ascending aorta is currently not performed outside compassionate use.
- Endovascular and surgical treatment for **descending (type B) AD**:
  - In the absence of complications (Table 20-7), type B ADs are initially managed medically.
  - Surgical intervention in the setting of an acute type B AD is associated with 23% mortality, compared to a mortality of about 9% for medical therapy alone.[6,22]
  - Uncomplicated type B ADs have a lower in-hospital mortality rate.
  - Malperfusion due to aortic and/or branch vessel occlusion may lead to life-threatening complications and is typically treated with TEVAR or other endovascular or catheter-based techniques.
  - Surgical or endovascular repair (generally TEVAR unless unable to be performed or in genetic syndromes) in acute type B AD is reserved for complications, such as end-organ ischemia, refractory pain, uncontrolled HTN, rupture, or a rapidly expanding aortic diameter.
  - Long-term complications of type B ADs include aneurysm formation, rupture, and retrograde dissection. Long-term follow-up requires surveillance by CT or MRI.

SPECIAL CONSIDERATIONS

Aortic Intramural Hematoma

- Aortic IMH is a variant of AD in which there is no visible intimal tear or false lumen, but instead a primary hematoma occurs in the aorta wall, possibly related to microscopic intimal disruption or rupture of the vasa vasorum.[28] See Figure 20-1.
- IMH may be focal or may propagate anterograde or retrograde through the aorta.
- Classification of location is the same as that of AD (types A and B).

TABLE 20-7	INDICATIONS FOR SURGICAL OR ENDOVASCULAR REPAIR FOR AORTIC DISSECTION

- Type A (or type I or II) dissection (emergency open surgical repair is recommended)
- Type B (or type III) dissection with[a]
  - Rupture
  - Branch vessel compromise/organ ischemia
  - Refractory hypertension
  - Aneurysmal dilation
  - Refractory pain

[a]Complications of type B dissection are typically treated with endovascular repair if suitable anatomy. Connective tissue disorders are typically treated with surgical repair if feasible.

- Symptoms are also similar to those of AD, predominantly sudden onset of severe chest or back pain.
- Complications include progression to classic AD, aortic rupture, hemopericardium, and AR.
- Natural history of IMH may include:
  - Progression to classic AD (in type A IMH, may be as high as 25-50%)[17]
  - Complete resolution of the hematoma
  - Persistence and stabilization of the hematoma
  - Progression to aortic aneurysm
  - Risk factors for progression include the presence of ulcer-like projections on imaging, IMH wall thickness, and aortic diameter.
- Diagnostic modalities include TEE, contrast CT, or MRI/MRA. The classic appearance is a smooth-walled lumen with a crescentic or circumferential thickening of the media (Figure 20-2B).
- Surgery is recommended for IMH involving the ascending aorta, and careful observation and medical management is recommended for IMH of the descending aorta. There are cases of type A IMH (predominantly from Asia) that have been managed successfully with medical therapy; however, there is significant morbidity associated with this strategy.

Penetrating Aortic Ulcer

- PAU results from an atherosclerotic plaque that penetrates the media and forms an ulceration or crater in the aortic wall.[28,29] See Figure 20-1.
- PAUs may be isolated, or associated with multiple atheroma and ulcers, and are most commonly located in the descending and abdominal aorta.
- Classically, PAUs occur in the elderly with significant atherosclerotic aortic and vascular disease and multiple coronary risk factors.
- Symptoms are very similar to classic AD, including sudden onset of chest, back, or abdominal pain. However, PAU may be an incidental finding on imaging.
- PAU may lead to aortic rupture, dissection, pseudoaneurysm, and late aneurysm formation. AD caused by PAU is likely to be a focal dissection, with a thick-walled intimal flap.
- Diagnostic modalities include TEE, CTA, MRI/MRA, and aortography.
  - The classic appearance is a focal, crater-like appearance of the atherosclerotic plaque and displacement of the intima.
  - Contrast studies will demonstrate an "outpouching" that constitutes the ulcer crater (Figure 20-2C).
- Surgical treatment is generally recommended for PAU in the ascending aorta.
- In the descending aorta, intervention is reserved for persistent pain, significant dilation of the aorta, rupture, or pseudoaneurysm formation.
  - In the descending and abdominal aorta, PAU and its complications are especially amenable to endovascular treatment, given the relatively short segment of the aorta that is usually affected.
  - Patients with PAU are often high-risk candidates for open surgical procedures.

REFERENCES

1. Guirguis-Blake JM, Beil TL, Senger CA, Whitlock EP. Ultrasonography screening for abdominal aortic aneurysms: a systematic evidence review for the U.S. Preventive Services Task Force. *Ann Intern Med.* 2014;160:321-9.
2. Chaikof EL, Dalman RL, Eskandari MK et al. The Society for Vascular Surgery practice guidelines on the care of patients with an abdominal aortic aneurysm. *J Vasc Surg.* 2018;67(1):2-77.
3. Moll FL, Powel JT, Fraedrich G, et al. Management of abdominal aortic aneurysms clinical practice guidelines of the European Society for Vascular Surgery. *Eur J Vasc Endovasc Surg.* 2011;41:S1-58.

4. U.S. Preventive Services Task Force. Screening for abdominal aortic aneurysm: recommendation statement. *Ann Intern Med.* 2014;161(4):281-90.
5. Habashi JP, Judge DP, Holm TM, et al. Losartan, an AT1 antagonist, prevents aortic aneurysm in a mouse model of Marfan syndrome. *Science.* 2006;312:117-21.
6. Braverman AC, Schermerhorn M. Diseases of the aorta. In: Zipes DP, Libby P, Bonow RO, Mann DL, Tomaselli GF, eds. *Braunwald's Heart Disease.* 11th ed. Elsevier; 2018:1295-327.
7. Schermerhorn ML, Buck DB, O'Malley AJ, et al. Long-term outcomes of abdominal aortic aneurysm in the Medicare population. *N Engl J Med.* 2015;373(4):328-38.
8. Andelfinger G, Loeys B, Dietz H. A decade of discovery in the genetic understanding of thoracic aortic disease. *Can J Cardiol.* 2016;32(1):13-25.
9. Gillis E, Van Laer L, Loeys BL. Genetics of thoracic aortic aneurysm: at the crossroad of transforming growth factor-β signaling and vascular smooth muscle cell contractility. *Circ Res.* 2013;113:327-40.
10. Lacro RV, Dietz HC, Sleeper LA, et al. Atenolol versus losartan in children and young adults with Marfan's syndrome. *N Engl J Med.* 2014;371(22):2061-71.
11. Loeys BL, Schwarze U, Holm T, et al. Aneurysm syndromes caused by mutations in the TGF-β receptor. *N Engl J Med.* 2006;355:788-98.
12. Hiratzka LF, Bakris GL, Beckman JA, et al. 2010 ACCF/AHA/AATS/ACR/ASA/SCA/SCAI/SIR/STS/SVM guidelines for the diagnosis and management of patients with thoracic aortic disease. *Circulation.* 2010;121(13):e266-369.
13. Erbel R, Aboyans V, Boileau C, et al. 2014 ESC guidelines on the diagnosis and treatment of aortic diseases: document covering acute and covering aortic diseases of the thoracic and abdominal aorta of the adult. The Task Force for the Diagnosis and Treatment of Aortic Diseases of the European Society of Cardiology (ESC). *Eur Heart J.* 2014;35(41):2873-926.
14. Ong KT, Perdu J, De Backer K, et al. Effect of celiprolol on prevention of cardiovascular events in vascular Ehlers–Danlos syndrome: a prospective randomized, open, blinded-endpoints trial. *Lancet.* 2010;376(9751):1476-84.
15. Braverman AC. The bicuspid aortic valve and associated aortic disease. In: Otto CM, Bonow RO, eds. *Valvular Heart Disease.* 4th ed. Saunders/Elsevier;2013:179.
16. Adamo L, Braverman AC. Surgical threshold for bicuspid aortic valve aneurysm: a case for individual decision making. *Heart.* 2015;101(17):1361-7.
17. Elefteriades JA, Farkas EA. Thoracic aortic aneurysm: clinically pertinent controversies and uncertainties. *Am Coll Cardiol.* 2010;55:841-57.
18. Kim JB, Kim K, Lindsay ME, et al. Risk of rupture or dissection in descending thoracic aortic aneurysm. *Circulation.* 2015;132(17):1620-9.
19. Braverman AC, Harris KM, Kovacs RJ, et al. Eligibility and disqualification recommendations for competitive athletes with cardiovascular abnormalities. Task Force 7: Aortic Disease, Including Marfan Syndrome. A scientific statement from the American Heart Association and American College of Cardiology. *Circulation.* 2015;132(22):e303-9.
20. Chaddha A, Eagle KA, Braverman AC, et al. Exercise and physical activity for the post-aortic dissection patient: the clinician's conundrum. *Clin Cardiol.* 2015;38(11):647-51.
21. Desai ND, Burtch K, Moser W, et al. Long-term comparison of thoracic endovascular aortic repair (TEVAR) to open surgery for the treatment of thoracic aortic aneurysms. *J Thorac Cardiovasc Surg.* 2012;144(3):604-9.
22. Booher AM, Isselbacher EM, Nienbaber CA, et al. The IRAD classification system for characterizing survival after aortic dissection. *Am J Med.* 2013;126(8):e719-30.
23. Nienaber CA, Eagle KA. Aortic dissection: new frontiers in diagnosis and management. Part I: from etiology to diagnostic strategies. *Circulation.* 2003;108:628-35.
24. Pape LA, Awais M, Woznicki EM, et al. Presentation, diagnosis, and outcomes of acute aortic dissection: 17 year trends from the International Registry of Acute Aortic Dissection. *J Am Coll Cardiol.* 2015;66(4):350-8.
25. Braverman AC. Acute aortic dissection: clinician update. *Circulation.* 2010;122:184-8.
26. Rogers AM, Hermann LK, Booher AM, et al. Sensitivity of the aortic dissection detection risk score, a novel guideline-based tool for identification of acute aortic dissection at initial presentation: results from the International Registry of Acute Aortic Dissection. *Circulation.* 2011;123(20):2213-8.
27. Evangelista A, Isselbacher EM, Bossone E, et al. Insights from the international registry of acute aortic dissection: a 20-year experience of collaborative clinical research. *Circulation.* 2018;137:1846-60.
28. Estrera A, Miller C, Lee T, et al. Acute type A intramural hematoma: analysis of current management strategy. *Circulation.* 2009;120:S287-91.
29. Braverman AC. Penetrating atherosclerotic ulcers of the aorta. *Curr Opin Cardiol.* 1994;9:591-7.

Aortic Valve Disease

21

Nishath Quader

Introduction

- Aortic valve (AV) disease, particularly aortic stenosis (AS), is common and increases in prevalence as the population ages.
- AS is present in 2% of people aged >65 years and in 4% of those aged >85 years.
- The AV is a trileaflet valve that permits unidirectional flow from the left ventricle (LV) into the aorta.
- AS is characterized by incomplete opening of the valve during systole, which limits antegrade flow, creating a systolic pressure gradient between the LV and the ascending aorta.
- Aortic regurgitation (AR) is caused by incompetence of the valve, allowing backward flow of blood from the aorta into the LV during diastole.

Aortic Stenosis

GENERAL PRINCIPLES

- Abnormality of the AV is the most common cause of flow obstruction from the LV into the aorta.
- Other causes of obstruction and the consequent pressure gradient between the LV and the aorta include obstruction above the valve (supravalvular) and below the valve (subvalvular). Subvalvular obstruction includes fixed obstruction (i.e., subaortic membrane) and dynamic obstruction (i.e., hypertrophic cardiomyopathy) with systolic anterior motion of the mitral valve along with basal septal hypertrophy).
- Aortic sclerosis is thickening of the AV leaflets, which causes turbulent flow through the valve and a murmur, but no gradient and, therefore, no stenosis. Aortic sclerosis is considered a risk factor for progression to stenosis.

Epidemiology

- AS is a progressive disease typically characterized by an asymptomatic phase until the valve area reaches a minimum threshold, generally <1.0 cm^2.
- In the absence of symptoms, patients with AS generally have a good prognosis with a risk of sudden death estimated to be <1% per year.
- Predictors of decreased event-free survival (free of aortic valve replacement [AVR] or death) include higher peak aortic jet velocity, extent of valve calcification, elevated B-type natriuretic peptide (BNP), and coexistent coronary artery disease (CAD).[1,2]
- Once patients experience symptoms, their average survival without treatment is 2 to 3 years, with an increased risk of sudden death.

Etiology

- **Calcific/degenerative:**
  - Most common cause of AS in the United States[3]
  - Progressive calcification and sclerosis to AS affects both trileaflet and bicuspid valves.

- Trileaflet calcific AS usually presents in the seventh through ninth decades of life (mean age mid-70s).
- Risk factors are similar to CAD, including age, male gender, smoking, and hypertension.[4]
- **Bicuspid**
  - Occurs in 1-2% of population (congenital lesion)
  - Usually presents in the fifth through seventh decades (mean age mid- to late-60s)
  - Approximately 50% of patients needing AVR for AS have a bicuspid valve.[5]
  - More prone to endocarditis than trileaflet valves
  - Associated with aortopathies (i.e., dissection, aneurysm)
- **Rheumatic:**
  - Most common cause worldwide and usually presents in the third through fifth decades
  - Almost always accompanied by mitral valve (MV) disease

Pathophysiology

The pathophysiology for symptoms in AS involves both the valve and the ventricular adaptation to the stenosis (see Figure 21-1).

DIAGNOSIS

Clinical Presentation

History
- Classic symptoms include:
  - Angina
  - Syncope
  - Heart failure
- Not infrequently, patients may limit their activity in ways that mask the presence of symptoms but indicate a progressive and premature decline in functional capacity. In the setting of severe AS and absence of other causes leading to a decline in function capacity, these patients are frequently classified as symptomatic.

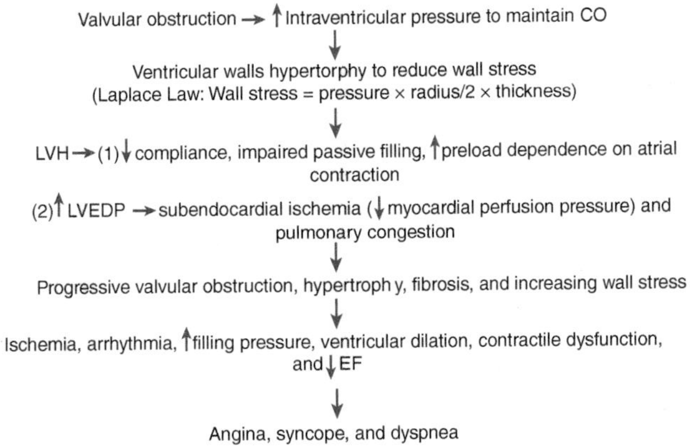

Valvular obstruction → ↑Intraventricular pressure to maintain CO

↓

Ventricular walls hypertorphy to reduce wall stress
(Laplace Law: Wall stress = pressure × radius/2 × thickness)

↓

LVH → (1)↓ compliance, impaired passive filling, ↑preload dependence on atrial contraction

(2)↑ LVEDP → subendocardial ischemia (↓myocardial perfusion pressure) and pulmonary congestion

↓

Progressive valvular obstruction, hypertroph y, fibrosis, and increasing wall stress

↓

Ischemia, arrhythmia, ↑filling pressure, ventricular dilation, contractile dysfunction, and ↓EF

↓

Angina, syncope, and dyspnea

FIGURE 21-1. Pathophysiology of aortic stenosis. CO, cardiac output; EF, ejection fraction; LVEDP, left ventricular end-diastolic pressure; LVH, left ventricular hypertrophy.

Physical Examination

- Harsh systolic crescendo–decrescendo murmur heard best at the right upper sternal border and radiating to both carotids; time to peak intensity correlates with severity (later peak = more severe).
- Diminished or absent A_2 (soft S_2) suggests severe AS.
- S4 reflects atrial contraction on a poorly compliant ventricle.
- Point of maximum impact (PMI) is sustained, diffuse and not displaced (unless the ventricle has dilated).
- Pulsus parvus et tardus: late peaking and diminished carotid upstroke in severe AS
- Gallavardin phenomenon is an AS murmur in which the musical element of the murmur is heard best at the apex (easily confused with mitral regurgitation [MR]).

Diagnostic Criteria

The diagnostic criteria for evaluation of AS are presented in Table 21-1.[3]

Diagnostic Testing

The standard evaluation of AS is presented in Table 21-2.[3]

TREATMENT

Medications

- See Table 21-3.
- There **are currently no medical treatments proven to decrease mortality or delay surgery.**
- Nevertheless, there are some guidelines for medical therapy in nonsurgical candidates, asymptomatic patients, or those with less severe stenosis.
- Hypertension:
  - Hypertension is very common in patients with AS.
  - Inadequate treatment of hypertension adds an additional load on the LV and contributes to the progression of symptoms.
  - Some data suggest that angiotensin-converting enzyme (ACE) inhibition may interfere with the valvular biology that leads to valve calcification.
  - Several clinical trials of patients with mild-to-severe AS failed to show any benefit with statins.[6-9] It is unknown if earlier intervention with statins (i.e., when the valve is sclerotic) would slow progression of the disease. It can be used for the prevention of atherosclerotic disease in these patients.
- Severe AS with decompensated heart failure:
  - Patients with severe AS may experience decompensated heart failure.
  - Depending on the clinical scenario, several options may help bridge the patient to valve replacement procedure:
    - Intra-aortic balloon pump (IABP) (contraindicated in patients with moderate AR or greater)
    - Sodium nitroprusside
    - Percutaneous aortic valvuloplasty
  - Each of the abovementioned measures provides some degree of afterload reduction, either at the level of the valve (valvuloplasty) or by reduction in systemic vascular resistance (IABP, nitroprusside); this afterload reduction can facilitate forward flow.
  - Operative mortality may decrease as heart failure improves and transient end-organ damage is reversed.

TABLE 21-1   STAGES OF AORTIC STENOSIS

Stage	Definition	Valve anatomy	Valve hemodynamics	Hemodynamic consequences	Symptoms
A	At risk of AS	BAV (or other congenital valve anomaly) Aortic valve sclerosis	Aortic V_{max} <2 m/s with normal leaflet motion	None	None
B	Progressive AS	Mild-to-moderate leaflet calcification/fibrosis of a bicuspid or trileaflet valve with some reduction in systolic motion or rheumatic valve changes with commissural fusion	Mild AS: aortic V_{max} 2.0–2.9 m/s or mean ΔP <20 mm Hg Moderate AS: aortic V_{max} 3.0–3.9 m/s or mean ΔP 20–39 mm Hg	Early LV diastolic dysfunction may be present Normal LVEF	None
C: Asymptomatic severe AS					
C1	Asymptomatic severe AS	Severe leaflet calcification/ fibrosis or congenital stenosis with severely reduced leaflet opening	Aortic V_{max} ≥4 m/s or mean ΔP ≥40 mm Hg AVA typically ≤1.0 cm^2 (or AVAi 0.6 cm^2/m^2), but not required to define severe AS Very severe AS is an aortic V_{max} ≥5 m/s or mean P ≥60 mm Hg	LV diastolic dysfunction Mild LV hypertrophy Normal LVEF	None Exercise testing is reasonable to confirm symptom status
C2	Asymptomatic severe AS with LV systolic dysfunction	Severe leaflet calcification/ fibrosis or congenital stenosis with severely reduced leaflet opening	Aortic V_{max} ≥4 m/s or mean ΔP ≥40 mm Hg AVA typically ≤1.0 cm^2 (or AVAi 0.6 cm^2/m^2), but not required to define severe AS	LVEF < 50%	None

D: Symptomatic severe AS

D1	Symptomatic severe high-gradient AS	Severe leaflet calcification/fibrosis or congenital stenosis with severely reduced leaflet opening	Aortic V_{max} ≥4 m/s or mean ΔP ≥40 mm Hg AVA typically ≤1.0 cm² (or AVAi 0.6 cm²/m²) but may be larger with mixed AS/AR	LV diastolic dysfunction LV hypertrophy Pulmonary hypertension may be present	Exertional dyspnea, decreased exercise tolerance, or HF Exertional angina Exertional syncope or presyncope
D2	Symptomatic severe low-flow, low-gradient AS with reduced LVEF	Severe leaflet calcification/fibrosis with severely reduced leaflet motion	AVA ≤1.0 cm² with resting aortic V_{max} <4 m/s or mean ΔP <40 mm Hg Dobutamine stress echocardiography shows AVA <1.0 cm² with V_{max} ≥4 m/s at any flow rate	LV diastolic dysfunction LV hypertrophy LVEF <50	HF Angina Syncope or presyncope
D3	Symptomatic severe low-gradient AS with normal LVEF OR paradoxical low-flow severe AS	Severe leaflet calcification/fibrosis with severely reduced leaflet motion	AVA ≤1.0 cm² (indexed AVA ≤0.6 cm²/m²) with an aortic V_{max} <4 m/s or mean ΔP <40 mm Hg AND Stroke volume index <35 mL/m² Measured when patient is normotensive (systolic blood pressure <140 mm Hg)	Increased LV relative wall thickness Small LV chamber with low stroke volume Restrictive diastolic filling LVEF ≥50%	HF Angina Syncope or presyncope

ΔP, pressure gradient between the LV and the aorta; AR, aortic regurgitation; AS, aortic stenosis; AVA, aortic valve area; AVAi, AVA indexed to body surface area; BAV, bicuspid aortic valve; HF, heart failure; LV, left ventricular; LVEF, left ventricular ejection fraction; V_{max}, maximum velocity (>4 m/s).

Reprinted from Otto CM, Nishimura RA, Bonow RO, et al. 2020 ACC/AHA guideline for the management of patients with valvular heart disease: a report of the American College of Cardiology/American Heart Association Joint Committee on Clinical Practice Guidelines. *J Am Coll Cardiol.* 2021;77(4):e25-197. Copyright © 2021 by the American College of Cardiology Foundation and the American Heart Association, Inc. With permission.

TABLE 21-2	RECOMMENDATION FOR DIAGNOSTIC TESTING IN AS

Class of recommendation	Recommendation
1	**TTE is indicated in assessment of AS; specifically evaluating hemodynamics, LV size and function**
1	In patients with low-flow, low-gradient AS and normal LVEF, optimization of blood pressure is needed before assessment of hemodynamics
2a	In patients with low-flow, low-gradient severe AS, dobutamine stress echo, invasive hemodynamics, and measurement of aortic calcium can be performed to further define severity
2a	**In asymptomatic patients with severe AS and normal LV function, exercise testing is reasonable to confirm the absence of symptoms**
3: Harm	Exercise testing is harmful in symptomatic patients with severe AS due to risk of hemodynamic collapse

AS, aortic stenosis; LV, left ventricle; LVEF, left ventricular ejection fraction; TTE, transthoracic echo.

Adapted from Otto CM, Nishimura RA, Bonow RO, et al. 2020 ACC/AHA guideline for the management of patients with valvular heart disease: a report of the American College of Cardiology/American Heart Association Joint Committee on Clinical Practice Guidelines. *J Am Coll Cardiol.* 2021;77(4):e25-197. Copyright © 2021 by the American College of Cardiology Foundation and the American Heart Association, Inc. With permission.

TABLE 21-3	MEDICAL THERAPY FOR AORTIC STENOSIS

Class of recommendation	Recommendation
1	**In patients at risk of developing AS, hypertension should be treated according to standard guidelines**
1	Statin therapy is recommended for primary and secondary prevention of atherosclerosis, but not for the prevention of AS progression
2b	ACEi or ARB may be considered to reduced long-term mortality after valve replacement

ACEi, angiotensin-converting enzyme inhibitor; ARB, angiotensin-receptor blocker; AS, aortic stenosis.

Surgical Management

- Therapeutic decisions are based on the presence of symptoms, LV dysfunction, and rate of progression of the disease (Table 21-4).[3,10]
- Treatment options include surgical (SAVR) and transcatheter (TAVR) aortic valve replacement.
- Symptomatic severe AS or severe AS associated with LV dysfunction requires prompt valve replacement.
- Certain associated high-risk features or the need for another cardiac surgical intervention may lead to the recommendation for an AVR even when the patient is asymptomatic or has less than severe stenosis.

TABLE 21-4	INDICATIONS FOR AORTIC VALVE REPLACEMENT FOR AORTIC STENOSIS (SURGICAL OR TRANSCATHETER)

Symptoms due to severe AS

Severe AS and LV ejection fraction < 50%

Low-flow, low-gradient severe AS

Asymptomatic patients with severe AS undergoing other cardiac surgery

Asymptomatic patients with severe AS and an abnormal exercise response

Asymptomatic patients with severe AS and rapid progression of disease, markedly elevated BNP, peak AV velocity > 5.0 m/s

AS, aortic stenosis; AV aortic valve; BNP, brain natriuretic peptide; LV, left ventricle.

Adapted from Otto CM, Nishimura RA, Bonow RO, et al. 2020 ACC/AHA guideline for the management of patients with valvular heart disease: a report of the American College of Cardiology/ American Heart Association Joint Committee on Clinical Practice Guidelines. *J Am Coll Cardiol.* 2021;77(4):e25-197.

- Operative mortality varies significantly depending on age, comorbidities, and concurrent surgical procedures to be performed. Operative mortality is calculated by using The Society of Therapeutic Surgeons (STS) risk calculator (www.sts.org).
- In young patients who need AVR, surgery maybe the best option if a mechanical AV is being considered. In general, mechanical AVs have been shown to have excellent longevity, but these do require life-long anticoagulation.

Transcatheter Aortic Valve Replacement
- TAVR has rapidly become the treatment choice for most patients and is approved for patients with severe AS (low-, moderate-, and high-risk patients).
- It requires careful preprocedural planning with a gated CT scan to assess annular size and access site. 3D TEE can also be used to assess annular size.
- Most patients may be eligible for TAVR unless there are unfavorable features. For example, extensive annular calcification poses a risk for significant paravalvular leak, heart block and aortic annular rupture.
- TAVR can be performed via transfemoral, transcarotid, subclavian approach. Transapical and transaortic approaches are less commonly utilized.
- Patients with bicuspid aortic valve (BAV) disease may also be eligible for a TAVR. Current-generation transcatheter AVs have been shown to be beneficial in this patient population with perhaps a higher rate of paravalvular insufficiency.
- Younger patients interested in TAVR require a careful multidisciplinary discussion highlighting pros and cons of TAVR versus SAVR; specifically focusing on the longevity of a TAVR valve versus mechanical AVR and valve morphology (trileaflet versus bicuspid).

Percutaneous Aortic Valvuloplasty
Valvuloplasty has a limited role in the management of AS; AV area increases modestly, and restenosis often occurs in weeks to months. It may be used:

- As a bridge to AVR in patients with decompensated heart failure (to improve end-organ function)
- As a palliative measure or "bridge-to-decision" in patients not undergoing valve replacement immediately (i.e., while a patient with unclear prognosis from cancer undergoes chemotherapy, or while an extremely frail or immobile patient rehabilitates)
- If urgent noncardiac surgery is needed in patients with severe symptomatic AS

Challenging Clinical Scenarios

- Asymptomatic severe AS with normal LV function—**is the patient really asymptomatic**?
  - Determine whether the patient is asymptomatic with an exercise stress test.
  - An elevated BNP may predict earlier symptom onset or worse outcome if surgery is delayed; these patients may benefit from AVR.
  - A CT scan to assess the extent of valve calcification can predict earlier symptom onset.
  - A mean gradient 60 mm Hg or rapidly progressing gradient is a marker of worse outcomes, and these patients may benefit from AVR before they develop symptoms.
- Concomitant CAD and moderate AS in a patient with angina—**what is causing the angina**?
  - Incorporate all data, including hemodynamic assessment of the coronary lesion and severity of AS, to guide management.
  - If AS is moderate and the coronary lesion is flow limiting, consider percutaneous coronary intervention to relieve angina. If there is no relief following percutaneous intervention, consider AVR.
- Combined AS/AR—**what if symptoms develop when AV disease is moderate?**
  - Generally, surgical timing is determined by the guidelines for isolated AS or AR.
  - However, patients with combined moderate AS and AR may develop symptoms and/or LV dysfunction before either lesion is severe.
  - It is reasonable to pursue AVR in combined moderate AS/AR when symptoms are present, LV function is reduced, or at the time of other cardiac surgery.
- Aortic root disease—**how does aortic root dilation influence the timing and extent of surgery?**
  - Almost 50% of patients with severe AS have a BAV.[5]
  - BAV is associated with an aortopathy that may predispose these patients to aortic dilation and dissection.
  - It is critical to evaluate the aortic dimensions in patients with BAV, as significant enlargement may indicate a need for surgery even before valve stenosis is severe. Regardless of which drives the timing of surgery (aortic dimension or AV disease), both may need to be addressed at the time of surgery.
  - All patients identified with a BAV should have imaging—CT or MRI—to evaluate for thoracic aortic pathology.
- LV dysfunction—**should surgery be done when the valve area suggests severe AS but the gradient is low?**
  - Dobutamine stress echo can be used to distinguish truly severe AS from pseudo-severe AS and to evaluate for the presence of stroke volume (SV) reserve.
  - Lack of SV reserve predicts an increased operative mortality.
  - Long-term survival is better with AVR than medical management in those with or without SV reserve.
  - Because of the high operative mortality in those with severe AS, LV dysfunction, and lack of SV reserve, TAVR is the preferred treatment in this group.

Aortic Regurgitation

GENERAL PRINCIPLES

- For the natural history of AR, see Table 21-5.[3,11]
- AR results from pathology of the AV with or without involvement of the aortic root.
- AR usually develops insidiously, but may be acute.
- **More common causes** include BAV, rheumatic disease, calcific degeneration, infective endocarditis, idiopathic dilatation of the aorta, myxomatous degeneration, systemic hypertension, dissection of the ascending aorta, and Marfan syndrome (MFS).

TABLE 21-5	NATURAL HISTORY OF AORTIC REGURGITATION
Asymptomatic patients with normal LV systolic function	
Progression to symptoms and/or LV dysfunction	<6% per year
Progression to asymptomatic LV dysfunction	<3.5% per year
Sudden death	<0.2% per year
Asymptomatic patients with LV dysfunction	
Progression to cardiac symptoms	>25% per year
Symptomatic patients	
Mortality rate	>10% per year

Reprinted from Bonow RO, Carabello BA, Chatterjee K, et al. ACC/AHA 2006 guidelines for the management of patients with valvular heart disease: a report of the American College of Cardiology/American Heart Association Task Force on Practice Guidelines. *Am Coll Cardiol.* 2006;48(3):e1-148. Copyright © 2006 American College of Cardiology Foundation and the American Heart Association, Inc. With permission.

- **Less common causes** include traumatic injury to the AV, collagen vascular diseases (e.g., ankylosing spondylitis, rheumatoid arthritis, reactive arthritis, giant cell aortitis, Whipple disease), syphilitic aortitis, osteogenesis imperfecta, Ehlers–Danlos syndrome (EDS), discrete subaortic stenosis, ventricular septal defect (VSD) with prolapse of an aortic cusp, and anorectic drugs.
- **Acute causes** are infective endocarditis, dissection of the ascending aorta, and trauma.
- The pathophysiology of acute and chronic AR is presented in Figures 21-2 and 21-3, respectively.

DIAGNOSIS

Clinical Presentation

- Acute: Patients with acute AR typically present with **pulmonary edema manifested by severe dyspnea**. Other presenting symptoms may be related to the causes of acute AR listed earlier. These patients generally have a normal LV function.

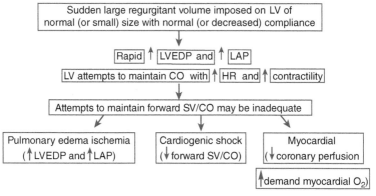

FIGURE 21-2. Pathophysiology of acute aortic regurgitation. CO, cardiac output; HR, heart rate; LAP, left atrial pressure; LV, left ventricle; LVEDP, left ventricular end-diastolic pressure; SV, stroke volume.

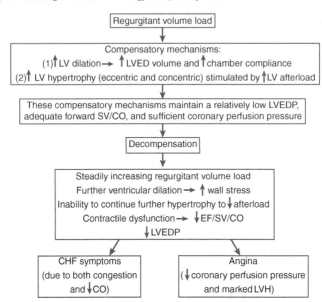

FIGURE 21-3. Pathophysiology of chronic aortic regurgitation. CHF, congestive heart failure; CO, cardiac output; EF, ejection fraction; HR, heart rate; LAP, left atrial pressure; LV, left ventricle; LVEDP, left ventricular end-diastolic pressure; LVH, left ventricular hypertrophy; SV, stroke volume.

- Chronic: **Symptoms depend on the presence of LV dysfunction and whether the patient is in the compensated versus decompensated stage.** Compensated patients are typically asymptomatic, whereas those in the decompensated stage may note decreased exercise tolerance, dyspnea, fatigue, and/or angina.

Physical Examination
- **Acute AR:**
  - Tachycardia
  - Wide-pulse pressure may not be present because forward SV (and, therefore, systolic blood pressure) is reduced.
  - A brief soft diastolic murmur heard best at the third left intercostal space (often not heard)
  - Systolic flow murmur (due to volume overload and hyperdynamic LV)
  - Diminished S_1 due to increased LV end-diastolic pressure (LVEDP) and premature MV closure
  - LV heave
  - Pulsus paradoxus (may suggest cardiac tamponade secondary to aortic dissection)
  - Measure blood pressure in both arms (a significant difference suggests aortic dissection).
  - Look for evidence of infective endocarditis.
  - Look for Marfanoid characteristics.
- **Chronic AR:**
  - LV heave
  - PMI is laterally displaced.
  - Diastolic decrescendo murmur heard best at lower sternal border (LSB) leaning forward at end-expiration (severity of AR correlates with duration, not intensity, of the murmur).

- ○ Systolic flow murmur (due mostly to volume overload; concomitant AS may also be present)
- ○ Austin Flint murmur—low-pitched diastolic murmur, heard best at the apex, caused by antegrade flow through a mitral orifice narrowed by severe AR, which restricts the motion of the anterior MV leaflet
- ○ S_3 is often heard as a manifestation of the volume overload and is not necessarily a sign of congestive heart failure (CHF).
- ○ Widened pulse pressure (often >100 mm Hg) with a low diastolic pressure
- ○ Characteristic signs related to wide-pulse pressure include:
  - Musset sign: head bobbing with each cardiac cycle
  - Corrigan pulse: rapid carotid upstroke followed by arterial collapse
  - Müller sign: pulsation of the uvula
  - Traube sign: pistol-shot murmur heard on the femoral artery
  - Duroziez sign: to-and-fro murmur over the femoral artery when partially compressed
  - Quincke pulse: visible capillary pulsation in the nail bed after holding the tip of the nail

Diagnostic Criteria

The diagnostic criteria for AR are presented in Table 21-6.[12]

Diagnostic Testing

The diagnostic evaluation will depend somewhat on the acuity of the presentation.

Electrocardiography
ECG findings include tachycardia, LV hypertrophy (LVH), and left atrial enlargement (LAE) (more common in chronic AR). New heart block may suggest an aortic root abscess.

Imaging
- **CXR:** look for pulmonary edema, widened mediastinum, and cardiomegaly.
- **Transthoracic echocardiography (TTE)**
  - ○ LV systolic function
  - ○ LV dimensions at end systole and end diastole
  - ○ Leaflet number and morphology
  - ○ Assessment of the severity of AR (see Table 21-6)[12]
  - ○ Look for evidence of endocarditis or aortic dissection.
  - ○ Dimension of aortic root
- **Transesophageal echocardiography (TEE)**
  - ○ Clarify valve morphology, if there is concern for a bicuspid valve on TTE
  - ○ Better sensitivity and specificity for aortic dissection than TTE
  - ○ Better for assessment of endocarditis and root abscess if unclear on TTE
  - ○ Better visualization of prosthetic AVs than TTE
- **MRI/CT**
  - ○ If echo assessment of the severity of AR is inadequate, MRI is useful for assessing the severity of AR.
  - ○ CT angiography (CTA) may be an alternative to cardiac catheterization to evaluate coronary anatomy before valve surgery.

Diagnostic Procedures
- Coronary angiography is performed in patients undergoing AVR who are at risk for CAD.
- Assessment of LV pressure, LV function, and severity of AR (via aortic root angiography) is indicated in symptomatic patients in whom the severity of AR is unclear on noninvasive imaging, or if imaging findings are discordant with clinical findings.

TABLE 21-6 GRADING THE SEVERITY OF CHRONIC AR WITH ECHOCARDIOGRAPHY

	AR severity		
	Mild	Moderate	Severe
Structural parameters			
Aortic leaflets	Normal or abnormal	Normal or abnormal	**Abnormal/flail or wide coaptation defect**
LV size	**Normal**[a]	Normal or dilated	Usually dilated[d]
Qualitative Doppler			
Jet width in LVOT, color flow	**Small in central jets**	Intermediate	**Large in central jets**; variable in eccentric jets
Flow convergence, color flow	**None or very small**	Intermediate	**Large**
Jet density, CW	Incomplete or faint	Dense	Dense
Jet deceleration rate, CW (PHT, ms)[b]	Incomplete or faint slow, >500	Medium, 500–200	**Steep, <200**
Diastolic flow reversal in descending aorta, PW	**Brief, early diastolic reversal**	Intermediate	**Prominent holodiastolic reversal**
Semiquantitative parameters[c]			
VCW (cm)	<0.3	0.3–0.6	>0.6
Jet width/LVOT width, central jets (%)	<25	25–45	46–64	≥65
Jet CSA/LVOT CSA, central jets (%)	<5	5–20	21–59	≥60
Quantitative parameters[c]			
RVol (mL/beat)	<30	30–44	45–59	≥60
RF (%)	<30	30–39	40–49	≥50
EROA (cm²)	<0.10	0.10–0.19	0.20–0.29	≥0.30

Reprinted from Zoghbi WA, Adams D, Bonow RO, et al. Recommendations for noninvasive evaluation of native valvular regurgitation: a report from the American Society of Echocardiography developed in collaboration from the Society for Cardiovascular Magnetic Resonance. J Am Soc Echocardiogr. 2017;30(4):303-71. Copyright © 2017 by the American Society of Echocardiography. With permission.

[a]Unless there are other reasons for LV dilation.
[b]PHT is shortened with increasing LV diastolic pressure and may be lengthened in chronic adaptation to severe AR.
[c]Quantitative parameters can subclassify the moderate regurgitation group.
[d]Specific in normal LV function, in absence of causes of volume overload. Exception: acute AR, in which chambers have not had time to dilate.

TREATMENT

Medications

- The role of medical therapy in patients with AR is limited. Randomized, placebo-controlled trials have not shown that vasodilator therapy delays the development of symptoms or LV dysfunction, warranting surgery.[13]
- **Vasodilator therapy** (i.e., nifedipine, ACE inhibitor, hydralazine) has a potential role in three situations:
  - Chronic therapy in patients with severe AR who have symptoms or LV dysfunction but are not surgical candidates
  - Short-term therapy to improve hemodynamics in patients with severe heart failure and severe LV dysfunction before surgery
  - Long-term therapy in asymptomatic patients with severe AR and are hypertensive.
- **β-Blockers** may be considered in the medical therapy of chronic severe AR.
  - β-Blockers may prolong the diastolic filling time by slowing the heart rate and thus make the AR worse.
  - While this is likely true in the case of acute severe AR, a recent observational study of patients with chronic severe AR showed a marked reduction in 1- and 5-year mortality in the patients treated with β-blockers.[14] Randomized trials will need to confirm this finding.

Surgical Management

- Surgery is indicated for any symptomatic patient with severe AR, regardless of LV systolic function (Table 21-7).[3]
- Acute, severe AR is almost always symptomatic.
- Valve repair may be feasible in a small subset of patients, usually those in whom aortic dissection is the cause of the AR.
- If the aortic root is dilated, it may be repaired or replaced at the time of AVR.
- AVR is often a better alternative than medical therapy in improving overall mortality and morbidity.
- Poor functional status based on the New York Heart Association (NYHA) functional class, LV dysfunction, and the chronicity of these abnormalities are predictors of higher operative and postoperative mortality.
- Short-term treatment with vasodilator therapy (i.e., nitroprusside) is reasonable to improve hemodynamics before surgery in the patient with decompensated heart failure.
- Currently, there are no approved transcatheter devices for the treatment of native AR with some investigational devices that maybe an option in the near future.

TABLE 21-7	INDICATIONS FOR AORTIC VALVE REPLACEMENT FOR AORTIC REGURGITATION

Severe symptomatic AR

Severe asymptomatic AR with LVEF ≤ 55%

Severe asymptomatic AR undergoing other cardiac surgery

Severe asymptomatic AR with LVEF > 55%; with LV end-systolic dimension 25 mm/m^2

Moderate AR undergoing other cardiac surgery

AR, aortic regurgitation; LV, left ventricle; LVEF, left ventricular ejection fraction.

Adapted from Otto CM, Nishimura RA, Bonow RO, et al. 2020 ACC/AHA guideline for the management of patients with valvular heart disease: a report of the American College of Cardiology/American Heart Association Joint Committee on Clinical Practice Guidelines. *J Am Coll Cardiol.* 2021;77(4):e25-197.

REFERENCES

1. Rosenhek R, Klaar U, Schemper M, et al. Mild and moderate aortic stenosis—natural history and risk stratification by echocardiography. *Eur Heart J.* 2004;25:199-205.
2. Rosenhek R, Binder T, Parenta G, et al. Predictors or outcome in severe, asymptomatic aortic stenosis. *N Engl J Med.* 2000;343:611-7.
3. Otto CM, Nishimura RA, Bonow RO, et al. 2020 ACC/AHA Guideline for management of patients with valvular heart disease: a report of the ACC/AHA joint committee on clinical practice guidelines. *Circulation.* 2020;143(5):e72-227.
4. Stewart BF, Siscovick DS, Lind BK, et al. Clinical factors associated with calcific aortic valve disease. *J Am Coll Cardiol.* 1997;29:630-44.
5. Roberts WC, Ko JM. Frequency by decades of unicuspid, bicuspid, and tricuspid aortic valves in adults having isolated aortic valve replacement for aortic stenosis, with or without associated aortic regurgitation. *Circulation.* 2005;111:920-5.
6. Chan KL, Teo K, Dumesnil JG, et al. Effect of lipid lowering with rosuvastatin on progression of aortic stenosis. *Circulation.* 2010;121:306-14.
7. Cowell SJ, Newby DE, Prescott RJ, et al. A randomized trial of intensive lipid lowering therapy in calcific aortic stenosis. *N Engl J Med.* 2005;352:2389-97.
8. Moura LM, Ramos SF, Zamorano JL, et al. Rosuvastatin Affecting Aortic Valve Endothelium to slow the progression of aortic stenosis (RAAVE). *J Am Coll Cardiol.* 2007;49:554-61.
9. Rossebo AB, Pedersen TR, Boman K, et al. Intensive lipid lowering with simvastatin and ezetimibe in aortic stenosis. *N Engl J Med.* 2008;359:1343-56.
10. Otto CM. Valvular aortic stenosis: disease severity and timing of intervention. *J Am Coll Cardiol.* 2006;47:2141-51.
11. Bonow RO, Carabello BA, Chatterjee K, et al. ACC/AHA 2006 Guidelines for the management of patients with valvular heart disease. *JACC.* 2006;48:e1-148.
12. Zoghbi WA, Adams D, Bonow RO, et al. Recommendations for noninvasive evaluation of native valvular regurgitation: a report from the American Society of Echocardiography developed in collaboration from the Society for cardiovascular magnetic resonance. *J Am Soc Echocardiogr.* 2017;30(4):303.
13. Evangelista A, Tornos P, Sambola A, et al. Long-term vasodilator therapy in patients with severe aortic regurgitation. *N Engl J Med.* 2005;353:1342-9.
14. Sampat U, Varadarajan P, Turk R, et al. Effect of beta-blocker therapy on survival in patients with severe aortic regurgitation. *J Am Coll Cardiol.* 2009;54:452-7.

Mitral Valve Disease

Jonathan D. Wolfe and Nishath Quader

22

Introduction

- The mitral valve (MV) permits unidirectional flow from the left atrium (LA) to the left ventricle (LV).
- The mitral apparatus is composed of an annulus, two leaflets, posteromedial and antero-lateral papillary muscles, and chordae tendineae. The latter two are considered part of the mitral subvalvular apparatus.
- Together with the LV, proper interaction between the mitral apparatus and the subvalvular apparatus is necessary for adequate function of the MV.

Mitral Stenosis

GENERAL PRINCIPLES

Etiology

- Mitral stenosis (MS) is characterized by incomplete opening of the MV during diastole, which limits anterograde flow and yields a sustained diastolic pressure gradient between the LA and the LV.
- MS is classified based on its etiology.
- Rheumatic heart disease is the predominant cause of MS worldwide, particularly in low- and middle-income countries. Rheumatic fever can cause fibrosis, thickening, and calcification, leading to fusion of the commissures, cusps, and/or chordae.
- Nonrheumatic calcific MS is found with increasing frequency in the elderly population. Calcific MS is the result of mitral annular calcification (MAC) that progresses to involve the base of the leaflets. Patients with end-stage renal disease are predisposed to MAC and calcific MS.[1]
- Other less common causes include radiation valvulopathy, congenital heart disease, carcinoid (in the setting of right-to-left shunt or pulmonary involvement), systemic lupus erythematosus, rheumatoid arthritis, and mucopolysaccharidoses.
- "Functional MS" may occur with obstruction of left atrial outflow due to any number of causes, including left atrial myxoma, left atrial thrombus, endocarditis with a large vegetation, congenital membrane of the LA (i.e., cor triatriatum), MV prosthesis dysfunction, an oversewn mitral annuloplasty ring, or after placement of an MV clip for mitral regurgitation (MR).

Pathophysiology

- Physiologic states that either increase the transvalvular flow (enhanced cardiac output) or decrease diastolic filling time (via tachycardia) can lead to elevation in LA pressure and increased symptoms at any given valve area.
- Pregnancy, exercise, hyperthyroidism, atrial fibrillation (AF) with rapid ventricular response, and fever are examples in which either or both of these conditions occur. Symptoms are often first noticed at these times (Figure 22-1).

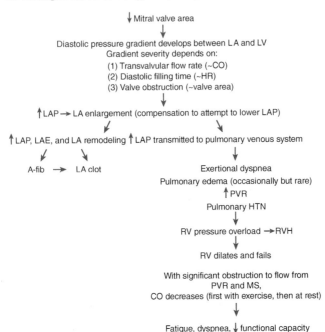

FIGURE 22-1. Pathophysiology of mitral stenosis. CO, cardiac output; HR, heart rate; HTN, hypertension; LA, left atrium; LAE, left atrial enlargement; LAP, left atrial pressure; MS, mitral stenosis; PVR, pulmonary vascular resistance; RV, right ventricle; RVH, right ventricular hypertrophy.

DIAGNOSIS

Clinical Presentation

- MS usually progresses slowly, with a long latent period (years) between rheumatic fever and the development of stenosis severe enough to cause symptoms (usually <2.5 cm² with exercise or <1.5 cm² at rest).
- A 10-year survival of untreated patients with MS depends on the severity of symptoms at presentation: asymptomatic or minimally symptomatic patients have an 80% survival of 10 years, whereas those with significant limiting symptoms have a 10-year survival of 0-15%.[2]
- Once severe pulmonary hypertension develops, mean survival is 3 years. Mortality in untreated patients is due (in order of frequency) to progressive pulmonary and systemic congestion, systemic embolism, pulmonary embolism, and infection.[2]
- Patients may present with any of the following symptoms: dyspnea, orthopnea and/or paroxysmal nocturnal dyspnea, fatigue, palpitations (often due to AF), systemic embolism, hemoptysis, chest pain, or signs and symptoms of infective endocarditis.

Physical Examination
- Findings on physical examination will depend on the severity of valve obstruction and the associated adaptations that have developed in response to it.
- Accentuation of S_1 may occur when the leaflets are flexible and becomes softer with increasing leaflet calcification.

- Opening snap (OS): caused by sudden tensing of the valve leaflets after they have completed their opening excursion; the S_2–O_S interval varies inversely with the severity of stenosis (shorter interval = more severe stenosis).
- Mid-diastolic rumble: low-pitched murmur heard best at the apex with the bell of the stethoscope; the severity of stenosis is related to the duration of the murmur, not intensity (more severe = longer duration).
- Irregularly irregular pulse may be present due to AF.
- MR murmur may be present.
- Loud P_2, tricuspid regurgitation (TR) murmur, and right ventricular (RV) heave can indicate pulmonary hypertension.
- Pulmonary rales, increased jugular venous pressure (JVP), hepatic congestion, and peripheral edema can indicate varying degrees of heart failure (HF).

Diagnostic Criteria

The stages of MS are defined by patient symptoms, valve anatomy, valve hemodynamics, and the cardiopulmonary sequelae of valve obstruction (Table 22-1).[1]

Diagnostic Testing

Recommendations for testing in the presence of MS are highlighted in Table 22-2.

Electrocardiography

The presence of P mitrale (P-wave duration in lead II $\geq$0.12 seconds, indicating left atrial enlargement [LAE]) is an important clue to the presence of MS. ECG signs of right ventricular hypertrophy (RVH) and AF may also be present.

Imaging

- **CXR**: Imaging with CXR will often reveal signs of LAE, enlargement of RA/RV and/or pulmonary arteries, and calcification of the MV and/or annulus.
- **Echocardiography**: Transthoracic (TEE) and transesophageal (TEE) echocardiography are critical tools to assess the etiology and severity of MS.
  - **Valve area** can be assessed by several methods (pressure half-time, continuity equation, direct planimetry by 2D or 3D visualization).
  - Echocardiography is the primary modality for determining mean **transmitral gradient**. The transmitral gradient is highly dependent on heart rate.
  - The severity of MS is best characterized by valve area. A mitral valve area (MVA) $\leq$1.5 cm^2 is considered severe and corresponds to a transmitral gradient of >5 to 10 mm Hg at normal heart rates. An MVA <1 cm^2 is considered critical.
  - Measurement of **pulmonary artery systolic pressure** (PASP) (using the TR jet velocity) is a crucial component of the echocardiographic examination of the patient with MS.
  - Measurement of **RV size and function** remains important for prognostic purposes.
  - Leaflet mobility, leaflet thickening, subvalvular thickening, and leaflet calcification are the determinants of the echocardiographic MV score (Wilkins score), which ranges from 0 to 16 and is important in determining candidacy for percutaneous mitral balloon valvotomy (PMBV).[3]
  - Exercise testing with echocardiography is helpful in clarifying hemodynamics for patients with MS whose symptoms are out of proportion to what is expected based on resting TTE. A mean transmitral gradient >15 mm Hg with exercise suggests severe MS.
  - TEE provides valuable adjunct information in the assessment of MS.
    - TEE is helpful when a more careful examination of MV morphology and hemodynamics is necessary for patients with MS for whom TTE was suboptimal.
    - TEE is a necessary imaging modality for patients being considered for PMBV in order to assess for the presence of LA thrombus and to evaluate the severity of MR.

TABLE 22-1 STAGES OF RHEUMATIC MITRAL STENOSIS

Stage	Definition	Valve anatomy	Valve hemodynamics	Hemodynamic consequences	Symptoms
A	At risk of MS	Mild valve doming during diastole	Normal transmitral flow velocity	None	None
B	Progressive MS	Rheumatic valve changes with commissural fusion and diastolic doming of the mitral valve leaflets Planimetered MVA > 1.5 cm²	Increased transmitral flow velocities Calculated MVA > 1.5 cm² Diastolic pressure half-time < 150 ms	Mild-to-moderate LA enlargement Normal pulmonary pressure at rest	None
C	Asymptomatic severe MS	Rheumatic valve changes with commissural fusion and diastolic doming of the mitral valve leaflets Planimetered MVA ≤ 1.5 cm²	Calculated MVA ≤ 1.5 cm² Diastolic pressure half-time ≥ 150 ms	Severe LA enlargement	None
D	Symptomatic severe MS	Rheumatic valve changes with commissural fusion and diastolic doming of the mitral valve leaflets Planimetered MVA ≤ 1.5 cm²	Calculated MVA ≤ 1.5 cm² Diastolic pressure half-time ≥ 150 ms	Severe LA enlargement Elevated PASP > 50 mm Hg	Decreased exercise tolerance Exertional dyspnea

LA, left atrium; MS, mitral stenosis; MVA, mitral valve area; PASP, pulmonary artery systolic pressure.

TABLE 22-2	**STANDARD EVALUATION OF MITRAL STENOSIS**
ECG	• LAE, atrial fibrillation, RVH
CXR	• Cardiomegaly; calcification of the aorta, AV, or coronaries
TTE	• Mitral valve leaflet number, morphology, and calcification
	• Measure valve area via planimetry in the parasternal short-axis view
	• Calculate valve area using PHT (valid in rheumatic MS): MVA = 220/PHT
	• Calculate valve area using continuity equation: MVA = (LVOT VTI × LVOT area)/MV VTI
	• The continuity equation is based on the principle that flow (velocity × area) is equal both distal to and at the level of the obstruction.
	• Transmitral mean gradients

AV, aortic valve; LAE, left atrial enlargement; LVOT, left ventricular outflow tract; MS, mitral stenosis; MVA, mitral valve area; PHT, pressure half-time; RVH, right ventricular hypertrophy; TTE, transthoracic echocardiogram; VTI, velocity time integral.

- ○ **3D echocardiography**: 3D echocardiography (with either TTE or TEE) provides greater accuracy in the measurement of MVA by planimetry than by 2D echocardiography.

Diagnostic Procedures

Cardiac catheterization: occasionally indicated
- To determine the severity of MS when clinical and echo assessments are discordant (see Figure 22-2).[4] Exercise testing with right heart catheterization (RHC) can also be performed.
- Can further characterize the etiology and severity of pulmonary hypertension when pulmonary pressures are out of proportion of the severity of MS as determined by noninvasive testing
- Typically performed in patients going for mitral valve replacement (MVR) with risk factors for coronary artery disease (CAD)

TREATMENT

Medications
- Medications may help with symptoms but do not change the natural history of MS.
- For HF symptoms, diuretics and a low-salt diet are helpful if there is evidence of pulmonary congestion.
- For patients who develop symptoms only with exercise (associated with tachycardia), negative chronotropic agents such as β-blockers or nondihydropyridine calcium channel blockers may be helpful.
- AF in rheumatic MS is considered valvular AF. Oral anticoagulation with vitamin K antagonist is recommended. The CHADS$_2$VASC score is used in nonvalvular AF.

Surgical Management
- Interventional and surgical treatment of MS[1,2]:
  - ○ For symptomatic patients with severe rheumatic MS and a favorable valve morphology, PMBV is recommended (Figure 22-3).[1,2]

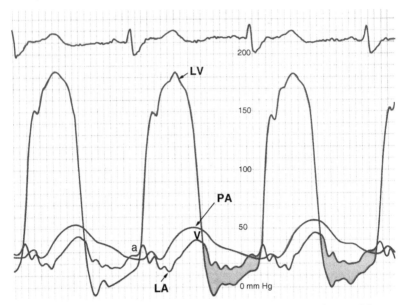

FIGURE 22-2. Hemodynamics observed in mitral stenosis. LA, left atrial; PA, pulmonary artery; V, venous. (Reprinted with permission from Murphy JG. Mayo *Clinic Cardiology Review*. 2nd ed. Lippincott Williams & Wilkins; 2000.)

- ○ PMBV is generally performed via a transseptal approach. After transseptal puncture of the interatrial septum, a catheter with a balloon is passed across the interatrial septum and the balloon is positioned across the MV. Balloon inflation separates the commissures and fractures some of the nodular calcium in the leaflets, yielding an increased valve area.
- ○ The transmitral pressure gradient usually decreases by 50-60%, cardiac output increases 10-20%, and a valve area >1.5 cm^2.
- ○ Contraindications to PMBV include LA thrombus, moderate or more MR, and a Wilkins score >8 (the latter is a relative contraindication) (Table 22-3).[5]
- ○ Complications include death (~1%), stroke, cardiac perforation, severe MR requiring surgical correction, and residual atrial septal defect requiring closure.
- ○ When done in those with favorable MV morphology, event-free survival (freedom from death, repeat valvotomy, or MVR) is 80-90% at 3 to 7 years.
- ○ This approach compares favorably with surgical mitral commissurotomy (open or closed) and is the procedure of choice in experienced centers for patients without contraindications.[1-3]
- • Indications for MV surgery in rheumatic MS are presented in Figure 22-3.[1]
- • Surgical treatment is usually reserved for those who are not the candidates for PMBV because of the presence of one or more contraindications to PMBV or because the percutaneous option is unavailable.
- • Surgical valvotomy is not widely performed in the US.
- • For patients with nonrheumatic calcific MS, valve intervention may be considered for patients with severe, symptomatic MS (MVA ≤ 1.5 cm). Patients with calcific MS are typically at high surgical risk due to extensive calcification, advanced age on average, and increased likelihood of multiple comorbidities.

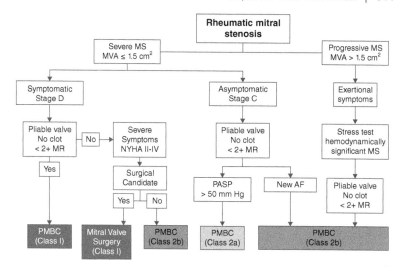

FIGURE 22-3. Treatment algorithm for intervention in rheumatic mitral stenosis. AF, atrial fibrillation; MR, mitral regurgitation; MS, mitral stenosis; MVA, mitral valve area; NYHA, New York Heart Association; PASP, pulmonary artery systolic pressure; PMBC, percutaneous mitral balloon commissurotomy. Adapted from Otto CM, Nishimura RA, Bonow RO, et al. 2020 ACC/AHA guideline for the management of patients with valvular heart disease: a report of the American College of Cardiology/ American Heart Association Joint Committee on Clinical Practice Guidelines. *J Am Coll Cardiol.* 2021;77(4):e25-197. Copyright © 2021 by the American College of Cardiology Foundation and the American Heart Association, Inc. With permission.

Mitral Regurgitation

GENERAL PRINCIPLES

Classification

- MR is caused by inadequate coaptation of the valve leaflets, allowing blood to flow backward from the LV into the LA during systole.
- **Primary MR** is caused by abnormalities of the valve leaflets and/or chordae tendineae (e.g., myxomatous degeneration, endocarditis, rheumatic).
- **Secondary or functional MR** refers to MR caused by annular dilatation from LV or LA enlargement resulting in incomplete coaptation of otherwise normal valve leaflets.

Etiology

- Primary MR:
  - Acute causes:
    - Ruptured papillary muscle may occur with a myocardial infarction (MI). This is often an inferior MI as the posteromedial papillary muscle is usually supplied only by the posterior descending artery. The single source of coronary blood supply makes the posteromedial papillary rupture more prone to injury in the setting of ischemia.
    - Ruptured chordae tendineae may occur spontaneously or with myxomatous valve disease.
    - Infective endocarditis may cause leaflet perforation or chordal rupture.

TABLE 22-3	WILKINS SCORE IN DETERMINING ELIGIBILITY FOR PERCUTANEOUS MITRAL BALLOON COMMISSUROTOMY			
Grade	Mobility	Subvalvular thickening	Thickening	Calcification
1	Highly mobile valve with only leaflet tips restricted	Minimal thickening just below the mitral leaflets	Leaflets near normal in thickness (4–5 mm)	A single area of increased echo brightness
2	Leaflet mid and base portions have normal mobility	Thickening of chordal structures extending up to one-third of the chordal length	Mid-leaflet normal, considerable thickening of margins (5–8 mm)	Scattered areas of brightness confined to leaflet margins
3	Valve continues to move forward in diastole, mainly from the base	Thickening extending to the distal third of the chords	Thickening extending through the entire leaflet (5–8 mm)	Brightness extending into the mid-portion of the leaflets
4	No or minimal forward movement of the leaflets in diastole	Extensive thickening and shortening of all chordal structures extending down to the papillary muscles	Considerable thickening of all leaflet tissue (>8–10 mm)	Extensive brightness throughout much of the leaflet tissue

Reproduced from Wilkins GT, Weyman AE, Abascal VM, et al. Percutaneous balloon dilatation of the mitral valve: an analysis of echocardiographic variables related to outcome and the mechanism of dilatation. *Br Heart J.* 1988;60(4):299-308 with permission from BMJ Publishing Group Ltd.

- **Mitral valve prolapse (MVP)/degenerative MR:**
  - Mitral valve prolapse (MVP) is defined on imaging as billowing of any portion of the mitral leaflets ≥2 mm above the annular plane.
  - Occurs in ~2.5% of the population (based on strict echocardiography criteria)
  - Female-to-male ratio is 2:1.
  - One or both leaflets may prolapse.
  - May occur as a primary condition (Barlow disease or fibroelastic deficiency) or associated with heritable connective tissue diseases, including Marfan syndrome, Ehlers–Danlos syndrome, and osteogenesis imperfecta
  - Primary MVP is associated with myxomatous degeneration of the MV leaflets and may be familial or nonfamilial.
- **Rheumatic MR:**
  - May be pure MR or combined MR/MS
  - Caused by thickening and/or calcification of the leaflets and chords
- **Infective endocarditis:** may cause destruction of the leaflet tissue (i.e., perforation), resulting in MR (acute or chronic)
- **Other causes:**
  - Congenital (cleft, parachute, or fenestrated MVs)
  - Infiltrative diseases (i.e., amyloid)

- Systemic lupus erythematosus (Libman–Sacks lesion)
- Hypertrophic cardiomyopathy with obstruction
- MAC
- Paravalvular prosthetic valve regurgitation
- Drug toxicity (e.g., fenfluramine/phentermine)
- Secondary MR:
  - **Ischemic MR:**
    - Ischemic MR refers to postinfarction MR.
    - The mechanism of MR usually involves one or both of the following:
      - Annular dilatation from ventricular enlargement
      - Local LV remodeling with papillary muscle displacement (both the dilatation of the ventricle and the akinesis or dyskinesis of the wall to which the papillary muscle is attached can prevent adequate leaflet coaptation)
  - **Dilated cardiomyopathy (DCM):**
    - Mechanism of MR due to both:
      - Annular dilatation from ventricular enlargement
      - Papillary muscle displacement due to ventricular enlargement and remodeling, which prevents adequate leaflet coaptation
    - May occur in the setting ischemic DCM or nonischemic DCM

DIAGNOSIS

Clinical Presentation

- The natural history and progression of MR depend on etiology, associated LV dysfunction, and severity of MR at the time of diagnosis.
- **MVP with little or no MR is most often associated with a benign prognosis and normal life expectancy**; a minority of these patients (10-15%) will go on to develop severe MR.
- The compensated asymptomatic phase of patients with severe organic MR (mostly degenerative but also due to rheumatic fever and endocarditis) with normal LV function is variable but may last several years.
- Patients with severe asymptomatic MR showed an event-free survival (free of death or an indication for surgery) of 10% at 10 years and 55% at 8 years. Factors independently associated with increased mortality after surgery include preoperative ejection fraction (EF) <60%, New York Heart Association (NYHA) functional class III to IV symptoms, age, associated CAD, AF, and effective regurgitant orifice (ERO) >40 mm^2.[6,7] Several of these factors and others are also associated with postoperative LV dysfunction and HF.
- The natural history of secondary MR is generally worse than for degenerative MR because of the associated comorbidities in these patients, such as CAD and LV dysfunction, with or without HF. Ischemic MR is independently associated with increased mortality after adjusting for MI; its impact on mortality increases with the severity of regurgitation.[8] The presence of MR in the setting of DCM is common (up to 60% of patients) and independently associated with increased mortality.[9]

History
- Acute MR (Figure 22-4):
  - The most prominent symptom is relatively rapid onset of significant dyspnea, which may progress quickly to respiratory failure.
  - Cardiogenic shock may occur depending on the patient's ability to compensate for the regurgitant volume.
- Chronic MR (Figure 22-5):
  - The etiology of MR and the time at which the patient presents will influence symptoms.

Acute Mitral Regurgitation

Sudden large volume load imposed on LA and LV of normal size and compliance

$\downarrow$

Rapid ↑LVEDP, ↑LAP

↑LV preload (from volume load) facilitates the attempt of LV to maintain forward SV/CO with ↑HR and ↑contractility via Frank–Starling mechanisms and catecholamines

$\downarrow$

Attempts to maintain forward SV/CO may be inadequate despite a supranormal EF because a large portion is ejected backward due to the lower resistance of the LA

↙   ↘

Pulmonary edema (↑LAP)   Hypotension (or shock) (↓forward SV/CO)

FIGURE 22-4. Pathophysiology of acute mitral regurgitation. HR, heart rate; LA, left atrium; LAP, left atrial pressure; LV, left ventricle; LVEDP, left ventricular end-diastolic pressure; SV/CO, stroke volume/cardiac output.

Chronic Mitral Regurgitation

Volume load imposed on LA and LV (usually it gradually increases over time)

$\downarrow$

↑LVEDP and ↑LAP

$\downarrow$

Compensatory dilatation of the LA and LV to accommodate volume load at lower pressures; this helps relieve pulmonary congestion
LV hypertrophy (eccentric) stimulated by LV dilatation (increased wall stress–Laplace Law)

$\downarrow$

↑Preload, LV hypertrophy, and reduced or normal afterload (low resistance LA provides unloading of LV) → large total SV (supranormal EF) and normal forward SV

$\downarrow$

"MR begets more MR" (vicious cycle in which further LV/annular dilatation ↑MR)

$\downarrow$

Contractile dysfunction→ ↓EF, ↑end-systolic volume → ↑LVEDP/volume, ↑LAP

↙   ↘

Pulmonary congestion and pHTN   Reduced forward SV/CO

FIGURE 22-5. Pathophysiology of chronic mitral regurgitation. EF, ejection fraction; LA, left atrium; LAP, left atrial pressure; LV, left ventricle; LVEDP, left ventricular end-diastolic pressure; MR, mitral regurgitation; pHTN, pulmonary hypertension; SV/CO, stroke volume/cardiac output.

- In MVP/degenerative MR that has progressed gradually, the patient may be asymptomatic even when the MR is severe.
- As compensatory mechanisms begin to fail, patients may develop dyspnea on exertion (which may be due to pulmonary hypertension and/or pulmonary edema exacerbated by increased regurgitant volume during exercise), palpitations (from AF), fatigue, volume overload, and other symptoms of HF.
- Patients with ischemic MR and MR due to DCM may have similar symptoms. In general, these patients tend to be more symptomatic because of associated LV dysfunction.

Physical Examination
- Acute MR:
  - Tachypnea with respiratory distress
  - Tachycardia
  - Systolic murmur, usually at the apex—may be minimal due to rapid equalization of pressures between the LV and the LA
  - S_3 and/or early diastolic flow rumble may be present due to rapid early filling of LV during diastole because of large regurgitant volume load in the LA.
  - Apical impulse may be hyperdynamic.
  - Crackles on lung examination
  - Hypotension/shock
- Chronic MR:
  - Apical holosystolic murmur that radiates to the axilla
  - Murmur may radiate to the anterior chest wall if the posterior leaflet is prolapsed or toward the back if the anterior leaflet is prolapsed.
  - In MVP, a midsystolic click is heard before the murmur.
  - The LV apical impulse is displaced laterally.
  - S_3 and/or early diastolic flow rumble may be present due to significant early antegrade flow over the MV during diastole; this does not necessarily indicate LV dysfunction.
  - Irregular rhythm of AF
  - Loud P_2 indicates pulmonary hypertension.
  - S_2 may be widely split due to an early A_2.
  - Other signs of HF (i.e., lower extremity edema, elevated central venous pressure, crackles, etc.)

Diagnostic Criteria
The qualitative and quantitative measures of MR severity are presented in Table 22-4.[10]

Diagnostic Testing
Electrocardiography
ECG may show the following:
- LAE, LV enlargement, and LVH
- Right atrial enlargement and RVH due to pulmonary hypertension
- AF
- Pathologic Q waves from a prior MI or ST-segment elevations in an acute MI, usually in the right coronary artery or circumflex distribution

Imaging
- **CXR:** Imaging with CXR will often reveal signs of LAE, pulmonary edema, enlarged pulmonary arteries, and/or cardiomegaly.
- **TTE:**
  - Used to assess the etiology of MR
  - LA size (should be increased in chronic, severe MR)

TABLE 22-4 GRADING OF MITRAL REGURGITATION SEVERITY

	Mild	Moderate	Severe
Structural parameters			
LA size	Normal[a]	Normal or dilated	Usually dilated[b]
LV size	Normal[a]	Normal or dilated	Usually dilated[b]
Mitral valve apparatus	Normal or abnormal	Normal or abnormal	Normal or abnormal
Doppler parameters			
Color-flow jet area (Nyquist limit of 50–60)	Small, central jet (usually <4 cm² or <20% of LA area)	Variable	Large central jet (usually >10 cm² or >40% of LA area) or variable size wall-impinging jet swirling in LA
Mitral inflow—PW	A wave dominant	Variable	E wave dominant
Jet density—CW	Incomplete or faint	Dense	Dense
Jet contour—CW	Parabolic	Usually parabolic	Early peaking triangular
Pulmonary vein flow	Systolic dominance	Systolic blunting	Systolic flow reversal
Quantitative parameters			
VC width (cm)	<0.3	0.3–0.69	≥0.7
Rvol (mL/beat)	<30	30–59	≥60
RF (%)	<30	30–49	≥50
EROA (cm²)	<0.2	0.2–0.39	≥0.40

CW, continuous wave Doppler; EROA, effective regurgitant orifice area; LA, left atrium; LV, left ventricle; PW, pulse wave Doppler; RF, regurgitant fraction; Rvol, regurgitant volume; VC, vena contracta.

[a] Unless there are other reasons for chamber enlargement.

[b] Exception: acute mitral regurgitation.

Adapted from Zoghbi WA, Enriquez-Sarano M, Foster E, et al. Recommendations for evaluation of the severity of native valvular regurgitation with two dimensional and doppler echocardiography. *J Am Soc Echocardiogr.* 2003;16(7):777-802. Copyright © 2003 American Society of Echocardiography. With permission.

- LV dimensions at end systole and end diastole (LV cavity should be dilated in chronic, severe MR of any etiology)
- LV systolic function should be hyperdynamic in the setting of severe MR. An EF ≤ 60% is considered relative LV systolic dysfunction.
- **TEE:**
  - Provides better visualization of the MV to help define anatomy and feasibility of repair
  - May help determine the severity of MR when TTE is nondiagnostic, particularly in the setting of an eccentric jet
  - Intraoperative TEE is indicated to guide repair and assess success.
- **3D echocardiography:** may provide additional and more accurate anatomic insights that can guide repair
- **Exercise testing with TTE:**
  - Helpful in clarifying functional capacity in cases where it is unclear if the patient is symptomatic
  - Assess the severity of MR with exercise in patients with exertional symptoms that seem discordant with the assessment of MR severity at rest
  - Assess PASP with exercise
- **Cardiac MRI:**
  - Assess EF in patients with severe MR but with an inadequate assessment of EF by echocardiography
  - Assess MR severity when echocardiography is nondiagnostic
  - Viability assessment may play a role in considering therapeutic strategy in ischemic MR.
- **Nuclear stress testing:**
  - Assess EF in patients with severe MR but with an inadequate assessment of EF by echocardiography
  - Viability assessment may play a role in considering therapeutic strategy in ischemic MR.
- **Coronary CT angiography:** may be an alternative to left heart catheterization to evaluate coronary anatomy before valve surgery

Diagnostic Procedures
Cardiac catheterization:
- RHC may be helpful to assess pulmonary pressures and pulmonary capillary wedge pressure. Large V waves in pulmonary capillary wedge pressure waveform suggest severe MR.
- Left heart catheterization may influence treatment strategy in ischemic MR and is used to evaluate for the presence of CAD in patients with risk factors before undergoing MV surgery.

TREATMENT

An outline of the treatment of primary MR is presented in Figure 22-6.[1]

Medications
- Acute MR:
  - In the setting of severe acute MR, surgical treatment is indicated. Medications may be used to stabilize patients.
  - **Aggressive afterload reduction** with IV vasodilators (often nicardipine or nitroprusside) or an intra-aortic balloon pump can promote forward flow and reduce pulmonary edema.
  - **Attempts to slow heart rate should be avoided** as cardiac output is heart rate dependent in these patients with reduced stroke volume.

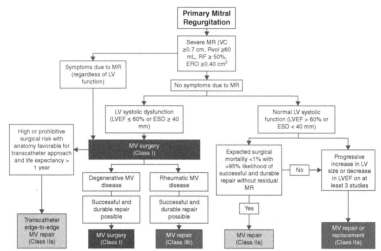

FIGURE 22-6. Treatment algorithm of chronic severe mitral regurgitation. ERO, effective regurgitant orifice; ESD, end-systolic dimension; LV, left ventricular; LVEF, left ventricular ejection fraction; MR, mitral regurgitation; RF, regurgitant fraction; Rvol, regurgitant volume; VC, vena contracta. Adapted from Otto CM, Nishimura RA, Bonow RO, et al. 2020 ACC/AHA guideline for the management of patients with valvular heart disease: a report of the American College of Cardiology/American Heart Association Joint Committee on Clinical Practice Guidelines. *J Am Coll Cardiol.* 2021;77(4):e25-197. Copyright © 2021 by the American College of Cardiology Foundation and the American Heart Association, Inc. With permission.

- Chronic MR: Patients with secondary MR should be treated as other patients with LV dysfunction. In this setting, angiotensin-converting enzyme (ACE) inhibitors/angiotensin-receptor blockers (ARBs), β-blockers, aldosterone antagonists, and/or sacubitril–valsartan are indicated and have been shown to reduce mortality and the severity of MR.[11-20] When indicated, cardiac resynchronization therapy reduces MR severity.[21-23]

Interventional and Surgical Treatment of Mitral Regurgitation

- Acute MR:
  - Prompt MV surgery, preferably MV repair if possible, is indicated in the setting of severe, acute MR and may be life-saving.
  - Percutaneous LA assist devices may be necessary to stabilize patients with acute severe MR and hemodynamic compromise before surgery.
- Chronic MR:
  - Primary MR: Indications for intervention in primary MR are presented in Table 22-5.
  - Surgery is indicated for patients with symptoms, relative systolic dysfunction (EF ≤ 60% or left ventricular end-systolic diameter [LVESD] ≥ 40 mm).[1,2]
  - MV repair is generally preferred to MVR. Freedom from reoperation or recurrent moderate or severe MR at 15 to 20 years is 80% and 60%, respectively, in patients treated with MV repair. These results are superior to the results of MVR.[1,2]
  - Surgery for asymptomatic patients with severe chronic primary MR may be considered if expected operative mortality is low (<1%) and the likelihood of a successful repair is high (>95%).[2]
  - For patients at prohibitive surgical risk who otherwise have an indication for intervention for chronic severe MR, transcatheter edge-to-edge repair (TEER) may be considered if anatomy is favorable.

TABLE 22-5 RECOMMENDATIONS FOR INTERVENTION IN CHRONIC PRIMARY MITRAL REGURGITATION

COR	LOE	Recommendations
1	B-NR	1. In symptomatic patients with severe primary MR, mitral valve intervention is recommended irrespective of LV systolic function.
1	B-NR	2. In asymptomatic patients with severe primary MR and LV systolic dysfunction (LVEF ≤ 60%, LVESD ≥ 40 mm), mitral valve surgery is recommended.
1	B-NR	3. In patients with severe primary MR for whom surgery is indicated, mitral valve repair is recommended in preference to mitral valve replacement with the anatomic cause of MR is degenerative disease, if a successful and durable repair is possible.
2a	B-NR	4. In asymptomatic patients with severe primary MR and normal LV systolic function (LVEF > 60%, LVESD < 40 mm), mitral valve repair is reasonable when the likelihood of a successful and durable repair without residual MR is >95% with an expected mortality of <1%, when it can be performed at a Comprehensive Valve Center.
2b	C-LD	5. In asymptomatic patients with severe primary MR and normal LV systolic function (LVEF > 60%, LVESD < 40 mm) but with a progressive increase in LV size or decrease in EF on ≥ 3 serial imaging studies, mitral valve surgery may be considered irrespective of the probability of a successful and durable repair.
2a	B-NR	6. In severely symptomatic patients with primary severe MR and high or prohibitive surgical risk, transcatheter edge-to-edge repair is reasonable if mitral valve anatomy is favorable for the repair procedure and patient life expectancy is at least 1 year.
2b	B-NR	7. In symptomatic patients with severe primary MR attributable to rheumatic disease, mitral valve repair may be considered at a Comprehensive Valve Center by an experienced team when surgical treatment is indicated, if a durable and successful repair is likely.
3: Harm	B-NR	8. In patients with severe primary MR where leaflet pathology is limited to less than half of the posterior leaflet, mitral valve replacement should not be performed unless mitral valve repair has been attempted at a Comprehensive Valve Center and was unsuccessful.

COR, class of recommendation; EF, ejection fraction; LD, limited data; LOE, level of evidence; LV, left ventricle; LVESD, left ventricular end-systolic diameter; MR, mitral regurgitation; NR, nonrandomized.

Adapted from Otto CM, Nishimura RA, Bonow RO, et al. 2020 ACC/AHA guideline for the management of patients with valvular heart disease: a report of the American College of Cardiology/American Heart Association Joint Committee on Clinical Practice Guidelines. *J Am Coll Cardiol.* 2021;77(4):e25-197. Copyright © 2021 by the American College of Cardiology Foundation and the American Heart Association, Inc. With permission.

- Secondary MR: Indications for intervention in secondary MR are presented in Table 22-6.
  - Generally, intervention for most patients with severe secondary MR is not indicated. Medical management for LV dysfunction is the mainstay of therapy.
  - For patients with severe secondary MR and persistent HF symptoms despite optimal guideline-directed medical therapy, TEER is reasonable if anatomy is favorable (LVEF 20-50%, LVESD ≤ 70 mm, PASP ≤ 70 mm Hg).[2]
  - MV surgery is reasonable in patients with severe secondary MR undergoing cardiac surgery for other indications.

TABLE 22-6		RECOMMENDATIONS FOR INTERVENTION IN CHRONIC SECONDARY MITRAL REGURGITATION
COR	**LOE**	**Recommendations**
2a	B-R	1. In patients with chronic severe secondary MR related to LV systolic dysfunction (EF < 50%) who have persistent symptoms (NYHA Class II, III, or IV) while on optimal GDMT for HF, TEER is reasonable in patients with appropriate anatomy as defined on TEE and with LVEF between 20% and 50%, LVESD ≤ 70 mm, and pulmonary artery systolic pressure ≤ 70 mm Hg.
2a	B-NR	2. In patients with severe secondary MR, mitral valve surgery is reasonable when CABG is undertaken for the treatment of myocardial ischemia.
2b	B-NR	3. In patients with chronic severe secondary MR from atrial annular dilation with preserved LV systolic function (LVEF ≥ 50%) who have severe persistent symptoms (NYHA class III or IV) despite therapy for HF and therapy for association AF or other comorbidities, mitral valve surgery may be considered.
2b	B-NR	4. In patients with chronic severe secondary MR related to LV systolic dysfunction (LVEF < 50%) who have persistent severe symptoms (NYHA class III or IV) while on optimal GDMT for HF, mitral valve surgery may be considered.
2b	B-R	5. In patients with CAD and chronic severe secondary MR related to LV systolic dysfunction (EF < 50%) who are undergoing mitral valve surgery because of severe symptoms (NYHA class III or IV) that persistent despite GDMT for HF, chordal-sparing mitral valve replacement may be reasonable to choose over downsized annuloplasty repair.

CABG, coronary artery bypass grafting; CAD, coronary artery disease; COR, class of recommendation; EF, ejection fraction; GDMT, guideline-directed medical therapy; HF, heart failure; LOE, level of evidence; LV, left ventricle; LVESD, left ventricular end-systolic diameter; MR, mitral regurgitation; NR, nonrandomized; NYHA, New York heart association; R, randomized; TEE, transesophageal echocardiography; TEER, transcatheter edge-to-edge repair.

Adapted from Otto CM, Nishimura RA, Bonow RO, et al. 2020 ACC/AHA guideline for the management of patients with valvular heart disease: a report of the American College of Cardiology/American Heart Association Joint Committee on Clinical Practice Guidelines. *J Am Coll Cardiol.* 2021;77(4):e25-197. Copyright © 2021 by the American College of Cardiology Foundation and the American Heart Association, Inc. With permission.

REFERENCES

1. Otto CM, Nishimura RA, Bonow RO et al. 2020 ACC/AHA Guideline for the Management of Patients With Valvular Heart Disease: a report of the American College of Cardiology/American Heart Association Joint Committee on Clinical Practice Guidelines. *Circulation.* 2021;143:e72-227.
2. Bonow RO, Carabello BA, Kanu C, et al. ACC/AHA 2006 Guidelines for the management of patients with valvular heart disease: a report of the American College of Cardiology/American Heart Association Task Force on Practice Guidelines (writing committee to revise the 1998 Guidelines for the Management of Patients With Valvular Heart Disease): developed in collaboration with the Society of Cardiovascular Anesthesiologists: endorsed by the Society for Cardiovascular Angiography and Interventions and the Society of Thoracic Surgeons. *Circulation.* 2006;114:e84-231.
3. Multicenter experience with balloon mitral commissurotomy. NHLBI Balloon Valvuloplasty Registry Report on immediate and 30-day follow-up results. The National Heart, Lung, and Blood Institute Balloon Valvuloplasty Registry Participants. *Circulation.* 1992;85:448-61.
4. Murphy JG. *Mayo Clinic Cardiology Review.* 2nd ed. Lippincott Williams & Wilkins; 2000.
5. Wilkins GT, Weyman AE, Abascal VM, et al. Percutaneous balloon dilatation of the mitral valve: an analysis of echocardiographic variables related to outcome and the mechanism of dilatation. *Br Heart J.* 1988;60:299-308.
6. Enriquez-Sarano M, Avierinos JF, Messika-Zeitoun D, et al. Quantitative determinants of the outcome of asymptomatic mitral regurgitation. *N Engl J Med.* 2005;352:875-83.
7. Rosenhek R, Rader F, Klaar U, et al. Outcome of watchful waiting in asymptomatic severe mitral regurgitation. *Circulation.* 2006;113:2238-44.
8. Grigioni F, Enriquez-Sarano M, Zehr KJ, et al. Ischemic mitral regurgitation: long-term outcome and prognostic implications with quantitative Doppler assessment. *Circulation.* 2001;103:1759-64.
9. Trichon BH, Felker GM, Shaw LK, et al. Relation of frequency and severity of mitral regurgitation to survival among patients with left ventricular systolic dysfunction and heart failure. *Am J Cardiol.* 2003;91:538-43.
10. Zoghbi WA, Adams D, Bonow RO, et al. Recommendations for noninvasive evaluation of native valvular regurgitation: a report from the American Society of Echocardiography developed in collaboration with the Society for Cardiovascular Magnetic Resonance. *J Am Soc Echocardiogr.* 2017;30:303-71.
11. Schön HR, Schröter G, Barthel P, Schömig A. Quinapril therapy in patients with chronic mitral regurgitation. *J Heart Valve Dis.* 1994;3:303-12.
12. Seneviratne B, Moore GA, West PD. Effect of captopril on functional mitral regurgitation in dilated heart failure: a randomised double blind placebo controlled trial. *Br Heart J.* 1994;72:63-8.
13. Wisenbaugh T, Sinovich V, Dullabh A, Sareli P. Six month pilot study of captopril for mildly symptomatic, severe isolated mitral and isolated aortic regurgitation. *J Heart Valve Dis.* 1994;3:197-204.
14. Høst U, Kelbaek H, Hildebrandt P, et al. Effect of ramipril on mitral regurgitation secondary to mitral valve prolapse. *Am J Cardiol.* 1997;80:655-8.
15. Marcotte F, Honos GN, Walling AD, et al. Effect of angiotensin-converting enzyme inhibitor therapy in mitral regurgitation with normal left ventricular function. *Can J Cardiol.* 1997;13:479-85.
16. Levine AB, Muller C, Levine TB. Effects of high-dose lisinopril-isosorbide dinitrate on severe mitral regurgitation and heart failure remodeling. *Am J Cardiol.* 1998;82:1299-301, a10.
17. Lowes BD, Gill EA, Abraham WT, et al. Effects of carvedilol on left ventricular mass, chamber geometry, and mitral regurgitation in chronic heart failure. *Am J Cardiol.* 1999;83:1201-5.
18. Capomolla S, Febo O, Gnemmi M, et al. Beta-blockade therapy in chronic heart failure: diastolic function and mitral regurgitation improvement by carvedilol. *Am Heart J.* 2000;139(4):596-608.
19. Ahmed MI, Aban I, Lloyd SG, et al. A randomized controlled phase IIb trial of beta(1)-receptor blockade for chronic degenerative mitral regurgitation. *J Am Coll Cardiol.* 2012;60:833-8.
20. Abraham WT, Fisher WG, Smith AL, et al. Cardiac resynchronization in chronic heart failure. *N Engl J Med.* 2002;346:1845-53.
21. St John Sutton MG, Plappert T, Abraham WT, et al. Effect of cardiac resynchronization therapy on left ventricular size and function in chronic heart failure. *Circulation.* 2003;107:1985-90.
22. Cleland JG, Daubert JC, Erdmann E, et al. The effect of cardiac resynchronization on morbidity and mortality in heart failure. *N Engl J Med.* 2005;352:1539-49.
23. van Bommel RJ, Marsan NA, Delgado V, et al. Cardiac resynchronization therapy as a therapeutic option in patients with moderate-severe functional mitral regurgitation and high operative risk. *Circulation.* 2011;124:912-9.

Tricuspid Valve Disease

23

Brittany M. Dixon and Homaa Ahmad

Introduction

- The tricuspid valve (TV) lies between the right atrium (RA) and right ventricle (RV).
- It has four components:
  - The three leaflets: anterior, posterior, and septal
  - The fibrous annulus
  - The papillary muscles
  - The chordal attachments
- Primary TV disease is relatively uncommon.

Tricuspid Stenosis

GENERAL PRINCIPLES

Definition

Tricuspid stenosis (TS) is characterized by incomplete opening of the TV during diastole, which limits anterograde flow and yields a sustained diastolic pressure gradient between the RA and the RV.[1]

Etiology

- **Rheumatic heart disease** (most common cause)[2]:
  - It is uncommon to have isolated rheumatic TS.
  - Usually, mitral valve (MV) and/or aortic valve disease are also present.
- Congenital abnormalities (i.e., congenital tricuspid atresia/stenosis, etc.). See Chapter 32 for further details.
- Infective endocarditis (i.e., TV vegetation)
- Carcinoid syndrome (more frequently causes tricuspid regurgitation [TR])
- RA mass/tumor may cause functional obstruction of the valve and mimic TS.
- Systemic rheumatic disease (i.e., Libman–Sacks endocarditis with systemic lupus erythematosus [SLE])[3]
- Hypereosinophilic syndromes (i.e., Löeffler endocarditis, endomyocardial fibrosis)
- Pacemaker lead (very uncommon; more frequently causes TR)[4]
- Extracardiac tumor (causing compression of TV)
- Radiation

DIAGNOSIS

Clinical Presentation

History
- As a result of the low cardiac output due to TV obstruction, patients typically note symptoms consistent with right heart failure: fatigue, peripheral edema, and increased abdominal girth (due to hepatomegaly and/or ascites). These symptoms may be more prominent than dyspnea alone.

- In a patient with known mitral stenosis (MS), the absence of pulmonary congestion should raise suspicion for possible TS.
- Patients may notice a "fluttering discomfort in neck" that corresponds to giant *a* wave in jugular venous pulse.
- Patients may also note palpitations due to atrial fibrillation.

Physical Examination

The physical examination findings of a patient with TS are similar to those seen in MS. Since MS and TS often coexist, the diagnosis of TS might be missed. Physical examination findings of TS include[1]:

- Low-frequency diastolic murmur with tricuspid "opening snap" heard best over left lower sternal border in the fourth intercostal space.
- Murmur and opening snap increase with increased flow across TV (i.e., with inspiration, leg raising, squatting, and exercise).
- Elevated jugular venous pulsations (JVPs) with a giant *a* wave and diminished rate of *y* descent.
- Clear lung fields
- Hepatomegaly with a pulsatile liver and often anasarca
- Edema in lower extremities

Diagnostic Testing

- **ECG:** may reveal tall, peaked P waves in lead II consistent with right atrial enlargement (RAE) or atrial fibrillation
- **CXR:** may reveal an enlarged right heart border
- **Transthoracic echocardiography (TTE) (see Table 23-1)[5]:**
  - Evaluate morphology/anatomy of valve:
    - In rheumatic disease of the TV, leaflets are thickened with fusion of commissures, and the subvalvular apparatus is thickened and retracted. This results in limited mobility with diastolic "doming" of the TV leaflets.
    - In carcinoid syndrome, serotonin-induced fibrosis causes short, thickened, and restricted "club" like leaflets that are fixed in an open position.
  - Determine the severity of stenosis (see Table 23-1):
    - Mean gradient: TV gradient >5 mm Hg supports severe TS.
    - Valve area: TV valve area <1.0 cm^2 supports severe TS. Note that the calculated valve area can be underestimated in the presence of severe TR.
  - Characterize associated TR or MV/aortic valve disease.
  - Assess for RAE.
  - A dilated inferior vena cava (IVC), often >2 cm, with no respiratory variation may be seen in severe TS.
  - Characterize any associated congenital abnormalities.
- **Transesophageal echocardiography (TEE):** provides better visualization of RA, the TV leaflets, and subvalvular apparatus
- **Right heart catheterization:** may be indicated to evaluate diastolic gradient between the RA and the RV in symptomatic patients with discordant clinical and noninvasive data

TREATMENT

Medications

Medical treatment consists mostly of **diuretic therapy** for volume overload in addition to strict sodium restriction. Further medical management depends on other medical comorbidities.

TABLE 23-1	ECHOCARDIOGRAPHIC FINDINGS OF HEMODYNAMICALLY SIGNIFICANT TRICUSPID STENOSIS
Specific findings of severe TS	• Mean pressure gradient $\geq$ 5 mm Hg • Inflow time–velocity integral > 60 cm • Pressure half-time $(T_{1/2}) \geq$ 190 ms • Valve area $\leq$ 1 cm^2 [a]
Supportive findings of severe TS	• Moderate or severely enlarged right atrium • Dilated IVC

IVC, inferior vena cava; TS, tricuspid stenosis.

[a] Valve area based on the continuity equation.

Adapted criteria from Baumgartner H, Hung J, Bermejo J, et al. Echocardiographic assessment of valve stenosis: EAE/ASE recommendations for clinical practice. *J Am Soc Echocardiogr.* 2009;22(1):1-23. Copyright © 2009 Elsevier. With permission.

Surgical Management/Percutaneous Interventions

• TV surgery is recommended for severe TS at the time of intervention for left-sided valvular lesions. Timing of surgical intervention is usually driven by the severity of the left-sided valvular lesions.[6,7]
• TV surgery is recommended for patients with isolated, symptomatic severe TS. This is because most cases of severe TS are accompanied by TR. TV replacement is preferably with a bioprosthesis due to low flow and higher risk of thrombosis.[6,7]
• Percutaneous balloon tricuspid commissurotomy might be considered in patients with isolated, symptomatic severe TS without accompanying TR. Tricuspid commissurotomy can result in increased TR.[6,7]
• For congenital TS, there may be other associated abnormalities that influence management and therapeutic decisions.

Tricuspid Regurgitation

GENERAL PRINCIPLES

Definition

• TR is caused by inadequate coaptation of the valve leaflets, allowing blood to flow backward from the RV into the RA during systole.
• Physiologic mild TR is normal and can be found in up to 70% of normal individuals.[8]

Etiology

• **Primary TR**
  ○ Acquired
    ■ Rheumatic
    ■ Nonrheumatic
      □ Myxomatous degeneration (Note: 20% of patients with MV prolapse also have TV prolapse)
      □ Infective endocarditis (frequently associated with IV drug abuse)

- □ Iatrogenic valve damage (e.g., from pacemaker/implanted cardioverter-defibrillator [ICD] lead or repeated RV biopsy after heart transplant)
- □ Carcinoid heart disease (also associated with TS)
- □ Drug-induced valvular heart disease (e.g., anorectic drugs such as methysergide, fenfluramine–phentermine)[9]
- □ Right-sided myocardial infarction (MI) causing papillary muscle dysfunction
- □ Endomyocardial fibrosis (seen in tropical Africa)
- □ Thoracic trauma
- □ Connective tissue disorders (e.g., Marfan syndrome)
- □ Autoimmune disorders (e.g., rheumatoid arthritis, SLE)
- □ Radiation-induced valvulitis
  - ○ Congenital (i.e., Ebstein anomaly, TV dysplasia, etc.); refer to Chapter 32.
- **Secondary (functional) TR** is caused by RAE and/or RV enlargement, which results in annular dilatation. This is the **most common cause of TR**.
  - ○ RV dysfunction
  - ○ Pulmonary hypertension
  - ○ Left heart disease (i.e., mitral regurgitation)
  - ○ RAE in the setting of permanent atrial fibrillation

Pathophysiology

- Severe TR leads to volume overload of the RV with resultant RV dilatation.
- Patients with severe TR and pulmonary hypertension typically develop right-sided congestion due to elevated RA and central venous pressure (CVP). Right-sided congestion may lead to peripheral edema, anasarca, and, in some cases, cardiac cirrhosis.[1]

DIAGNOSIS

Clinical Presentation

History
- In the absence of pulmonary hypertension, severe TR may initially present with minimal to no symptoms. Severe TR typically includes a prolonged asymptomatic period with progressive enlargement of right-sided chambers (RA and RV).[10,11]
- More recent data suggest that secondary TR does not regress after correction of the left-sided valve lesions.[10-12] Therefore, surgical intervention on TV is now also recommended in cases of severe TR (see later in this chapter).[6,7]
- As earlier, patients may complain of fatigue, lower extremity edema, increased abdominal girth (ascites), early satiety, or loss of appetite.

Physical Examination
Physical examination signs associated with TR may include:
- Elevated JVP with prominent *v* waves
- Holosystolic murmur heard best at the left lower sternal border that increases with inspiration (Carvallo sign). Note: the murmur of TR may be soft or absent in severe TR.
- Right-sided S_3 or increased P_2 intensity
- Pulsatile liver, hepatomegaly, lower extremity edema, and ascites

Diagnostic Testing

- **ECG:** may show RAE, atrial fibrillation, incomplete or complete right bundle branch block (RBBB), and right ventricular hypertrophy (RVH)
- **CXR:** may reveal an enlarged right heart border
- **TTE[8]:**

- ○ RAE, RV dilatation, and TV annular dilatation are usually present. In severe TR, TV annulus is dilated ≥40 mm, unless TR is acute.
- ○ Assess RV function as RV dysfunction may be present.
- ○ Evaluate morphology and motion of TV leaflets (e.g., malcoaptation of leaflets, flail leaflet, large perforation, severe retraction of leaflets).
- ○ Doppler evaluation of TR severity (see Table 23-2)[8]
- ○ A flattened septum with D-shaped LV cavity throughout the cardiac cycle is a sign of RV pressure and volume overload.
- ○ Pulmonary artery systolic pressure (PASP) is calculated using the Bernoulli equation (assuming no pulmonary stenosis): $PASP = V^2 + RAP$, where V is the TR jet velocity and RAP (RA pressure) is estimated by IVC size and collapsibility.
- ○ A dilated IVC, often >2 cm, with no respiratory variation may be seen in severe TR.
- ○ Assess pacemaker/defibrillator leads or catheters in right-sided chambers for vegetation or thrombus. Also assess for potential malcoaptation of TV leaflets resulting in TR.
- **TEE:** Better visualizes the RA, valve leaflets, and subvalvular apparatus and valvular regurgitation.
- **Cardiac MR (CMR) imaging:**
  - ○ Better visualize TV anatomy and function, especially when pathology is present. However, visualization of the TV can be limited by turbulent flow from TR.[8]
  - ○ Current gold standard for quantification of RV size and function[7]

TABLE 23-2	ECHOCARDIOGRAPHIC ASSESSMENT OF TRICUSPID REGURGITATION (TR)
	Severe TR
Structural findings	• Severe valve lesions (i.e., flail leaflet, severe retraction, large perforation) • Usually enlarged RV and RA, though can be normal in severe TR • IVC > 2.5 cm
Color-flow Doppler	• Large central jet or eccentric jet of variable size • **Jet area > 10 cm²** • **Vena contracta width ≥ 0.7 cm** • **PISA radius > 0.9 cm** • EROA ≥ 0.40 cm² or regurgitant volume ≥ 45 mL
Continuous-wave Doppler (CWD)/ pulsed-wave Doppler (PWD)	• **Dense, often triangular** jet with early systolic peak (CWD) • **Systolic flow reversal in hepatic vein** (PWD)

CWD, continuous-wave Doppler; EROA, effective regurgitant orifice area; IVC, inferior vena cava; PISA, proximal isovelocity surface area (with Nyquist limit >50–70 cm/s); PWD, pulsed-wave Doppler; RA, right atrium; RV, right ventricle; TR, tricuspid regurgitation.

Adapted from Zoghbi WA, Adams D, Bonow RO, et al. Recommendations for noninvasive evaluation of native valvular regurgitation: a report from the American Society of Echocardiography developed in collaboration from the Society for Cardiovascular Magnetic Resonance. *J Am Soc Echocardiogr.* 2017;30(4):303-71. Copyright © 2017 by the American Society of Echocardiography. With permission.

- **Right heart catheterization**
  - RAP tracing demonstrates prominent v waves with absent x descent; this indicates "ventricularization" of the atrial pressure.
  - Direct measurement of RAP, RV pressure, and PA pressure, which may help in diagnosing the etiology of TR. RAP and RV end-diastolic pressure are elevated.

TREATMENT

Medications

- Medical therapy is limited to **diuretics and medications to reduce PA pressures and pulmonary vasculature resistance**. This will decrease the severity of right-sided heart failure.
- TR is often secondary to some other process—pulmonary hypertension, left-sided heart failure, or other valvular abnormality. **Treating the underlying cause is the primary focus of treatment**.

Surgical Management/Percutaneous Interventions

- **The primary goal is to intervene before RV dysfunction develops.**
- Based on the most recent American Heart Association/American College of Cardiology (AHA/ACC) guidelines[6]:
  - TV surgery is recommended for patients with severe TR undergoing left-sided valve surgery (class I recommendation).
  - TV repair can be beneficial in patients with progressive TR with either annular dilatation or evidence of right-sided heart failure who are undergoing left-sided valve surgery (class IIa recommendation).
  - Surgery can be beneficial for symptomatic, severe primary TR that is unresponsive to medical therapy (class IIa recommendation).
  - Isolated TV surgery can be beneficial in patients with severe isolated secondary TR due to annular dilation (without pulmonary hypertension or left-sided heart disease) and right-sided heart failure (class IIa recommendation).
  - TV surgery may be considered for asymptomatic patients with severe primary TR and progressive RV dilation/systolic dysfunction (class IIb recommendation).
- "In patients with severe TR and right-sided heart failure who have previously undergone left-sided vale surgery, reoperation with isolated tricuspid valve surgery may be considered in the absence of severe pulmonary hypertension or severe RV systolic dysfunction (class IIb recommendation)."
- Note that TR may recur after repair.
- **If replacement is necessary, bioprosthetic valves are preferred** to mechanical valves due to the risk of thrombosis (lower pressure on the right side of the heart predisposes to thrombosis of mechanical valves).[6,7]
- Several ongoing clinical trials are examining the use of novel percutaneous devices to treat patients with severe TR.[13] Transcatheter TV replacement is also an emerging treatment for patients with TR.[14]

REFERENCES

1. Mann DL, Zipes DP, Libby P, Bonow RO. *Braunwald's Heart Disease: A Textbook of Cardiovascular Medicine.* 10th ed. Elsevier; 2015.
2. Yousof AM, Shafei MZ, Endrys G, et al. Tricuspid stenosis and regurgitation in rheumatic heart disease: a prospective cardiac catheterization study in 525 patients. *Am Heart J.* 1985;110:60-4.
3. Gur AK, Odabsi D, Kunt AG, Kunt AS. Isolated tricuspid valve repair for Libman–Sacks endocarditis. *Echocardiography.* 2014;31:E166-8.
4. Chang JD, Manning WJ, Ebrille E, Zimetbaum PJ. Tricuspid valve dysfunction following pacemaker or cardioverter-defibrillator implantation. *J Am Col Cardiol.* 2017;69:2331-9.

5. Baumgartner H, Hung J, Bermejo J, et al. Echocardiographic assessment of valve stenosis: EAE/ASE recommendations for clinical practice. *J Am Soc Echocardiogr.* 2009;22:1-23.
6. Otto CM, Nishimura RA, Bonow RO, et al. 2020 ACC/AHA guideline for the management of patients with valvular heart disease: a report of the American College of Cardiology/American Heart Association Joint Committee on Clinical Practice Guidelines. *J Am Coll Cardiol.* 2021;77:e25–197.
7. Baumgartner H, Falk V, Bax JJ, et al. 2017 ESC/EACTS Guidelines for the management of valvular heart disease: the task force for the management of valvular heart disease of the European Society of Cardiology (ESC) and the European Association for Cardio-Thoracic Surgery (EACTS). *Eur Heart J.* 2017;38:2739-91.
8. Zoghbi WA, Adams D, Bonow RO, et al. Recommendations for noninvasive evaluation of native valvular regurgitation: a report from the American Society of Echocardiography developed in collaboration with the Society for Cardiovascular Magnetic Resonance. *J Am Soc Echocardiogr.* 2017;30:303-71.
9. Bhattacharyya S, Schapira AH, Mikhailidis DP, Davar J. Drug-induced fibrotic valvular heart disease. *Lancet.* 2009;374:577-85.
10. Topilsky Y, Nkomo VT, Vatury O, et al. Clinical outcome of isolated tricuspid regurgitation. *JACC Cardiovasc Imaging.* 2014;7:1185-94.
11. Mas PT, Rodriguez-Palomares JF, Antunes MJ. Secondary tricuspid valve regurgitation: a forgotten entity. *Heart.* 2015;101:1840-8.
12. Kelly BJ, Ho Luxford JM, Butler CG, et al. Severity of tricuspid regurgitation is associated with long-term mortality. *J Thorac Cardiovasc Surg.* 2018;155:1032-8.
13. O'Neil BP, O'Neil WW. Tricuspid valve intervention. *J Am Col Cardiol.* 2016;68:10341036.
14. Krishnaswamy A, Navia J, Kapadia SR. Transcatheter tricuspid valve replacement. *Interv Cardiol Clin.* 2018;7:65-70.

Infective Endocarditis and Cardiac Device Infections

Courtney D. Chrisler, Justin M. Vader, Rugheed Ghadban, and Sandeep S. Sodhi

24

Infective Endocarditis

GENERAL PRINCIPLES

Definition

- Infective endocarditis (IE) is infection involving the endothelial surface of the heart.
- It is characterized by the presence of vegetations consisting of microorganisms, inflammatory cells, and platelet–fibrin deposits.
- Valves are the most common location of infection, although IE can also occur at ventricular septal defect (VSD) and atrial septal defect (ASD), chordae tendineae, or damaged mural endocardium.
- Multiple organisms can cause IE (Table 24-1).[1]

Classification

IE may be categorized according to the following (see Table 24-2):

- Type of presentation
- Underlying valve characteristics
- Predisposing factors

Epidemiology

- In a multinational review of 15 studies, incidence of IE was found to be 1.4 to 6.2 cases per 100,000 patient-years, with mortality ranging from 14% to 46%.[2]
- In developed countries, the proportion of IE cases in patients with underlying rheumatic heart disease has markedly decreased.
- A higher incidence of IE is now seen in the setting of IV drug use, cardiac and vascular prostheses, and nosocomial infections.

Pathophysiology

The pathophysiology of IE is outlined in Figure 24-1.

Risk Factors

- The major risk factor for the development of IE is a structural abnormality of a heart valve, often causing a stenotic or regurgitant lesion (e.g., bicuspid aortic valve, myxomatous mitral disease).
- Predisposing risk factors for native valve endocarditis (NVE) include **degenerative valve disease**, **age**, **IV drug use**, **poor dental hygiene**, **long-term hemodialysis**, and **diabetes mellitus**.

| TABLE 24-1 | FREQUENCY OF VARIOUS ORGANISMS CAUSING INFECTIVE ENDOCARDITIS | | | |

Organism	NVE (%)	IV drug abusers (%)	Early PVE (%)	Late PVE (%)
Streptococci	60	15–25	5	35
S. viridans	35	5–10	<5	25
S. gallolyticus (bovis)	10	<5	<5	<5
Enterococcus faecalis	10	10	<5	<5
Staphylococci	25	50	50	30
Coagulase positive	23	50	20	10
Coagulase negative	<5	<5	30	20
Gram-negative aerobic bacilli	<5	5	20	10
Fungi	<5	<5	10	5
Culture-negative endocarditis	5–10	<5	<5	<5

NVE, native valve endocarditis; PVE, prosthetic valve endocarditis.

Republished with permission of McGraw Hill LLC from O'Rourke RA, Fuster V, Alexander RW, eds. *Hurst's the Heart.* 10th ed. McGraw-Hill; 2000:596; permission conveyed through Copyright Clearance Center, Inc.

| TABLE 24-2 | CLASSIFICATION OF ENDOCARDITIS |

Acute bacterial endocarditis (ABE)	• Highly infective and particularly toxic • Develops within 1–2 days • Can cause significant valvular destruction and embolic infections • Most commonly caused by *Staphylococcus aureus*
Subacute bacterial endocarditis (SBE)	• More indolent course than ABE • Develops within weeks to months • More often associated with immunologic phenomena • Often caused by streptococcal organisms, particularly *Streptococcus viridans*; also HACEK organisms and other gram-negative bacilli • *Streptococcus gallolyticus (bovis)* is often associated with colon cancer and polyps.
Native valve endocarditis (NVE)	• Often predisposed by an abnormal native heart valve (e.g., mitral valve prolapse, bicuspid aortic valve) • Common organisms: *S. viridans, S. aureus, S. gallolyticus (bovis)*, and *Enterococcus*
Prosthetic valve endocarditis (PVE)	• Increased incidence in recent decades accounting for 10–30% of all IE • *Early* if it occurs within 2 months of valve replacement (early PVE often involves coagulase-negative staphylococci)

TABLE 24-2	CLASSIFICATION OF ENDOCARDITIS *(continued)*
	• *Late* if it occurs after 2 months (late PVE involves the usual NVE pathogens such as *S. viridans*, *S. aureus*, and *Enterococcus*)
	• Fungal endocarditis (*Candida* and *Aspergillus*) is more common in PVE than in NVE.
	• Greatest risk of IE within 6 months of valve replacement
	• Rates of infection appear to be similar between mechanical and bioprosthetic valves.
Right-sided endocarditis	• Often seen in IV drug users; almost always involves the *tricuspid valve*
	• Most common pathogen is *S. aureus* (60%).
Nonbacterial thrombotic endocarditis (NBTE)	Requires endothelial injury and a hypercoagulable state:
	• *Marantic endocarditis*, when associated with cancer
	• Libman–Sacks endocarditis, often with lupus
	• Antiphospholipid antibody syndrome
	• Often related to prior antibiotic treatment
Culture-negative endocarditis	• Incidence may be as high as 5–10%
	• Caused by fastidious or slow-growing organisms such as *HACEK*, fungi, anaerobes, *Legionella*, *Chlamydia psittaci*, *Coxiella*, *Brucella*, and *Bartonella*
CIED-related endocarditis	• Increased incidence due to increased indications for implantation
	• Often caused by *S. aureus* or coagulase-negative staphylococci
Fungal endocarditis	• Often involves *Candida* or *Aspergillus*
	• Due to prosthetic valves, indwelling intravascular devices, immunosuppression, or IV drug use
HIV-related endocarditis	• *S. aureus* is the most common pathogen.
	• Usually related to IV drug use or indwelling IV catheters

HACEK, *Haemophilus aphrophilus, Haemophilus parainfluenzae*, and *Haemophilus paraphrophilus*; *Actinobacillus actinomycetemcomitans*; *Cardiobacterium hominis*; *Eikenella corrodens*; and *Kingella kingae*; IE, infective endocarditis.

DIAGNOSIS

Clinical Presentation

• The clinical spectrum can range from subtle, indolent manifestations of subacute infection presenting as a fever of undetermined origin (FUO) to extensive valve destruction and fulminant heart failure (HF).
• The most common clinical features of IE are **fever and a new heart murmur**.
• Fever may not be present in the elderly, the immunocompromised, patients with HF, or those with chronic renal disease.

History

A thorough history should take into account a detailed assessment of conditions that may predispose a patient to IE as noted earlier.

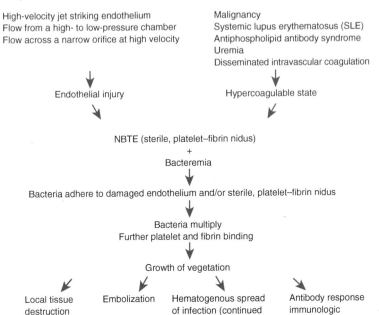

High-velocity jet striking endothelium
Flow from a high- to low-pressure chamber
Flow across a narrow orifice at high velocity

Malignancy
Systemic lupus erythematosus (SLE)
Antiphospholipid antibody syndrome
Uremia
Disseminated intravascular coagulation

Endothelial injury

Hypercoagulable state

NBTE (sterile, platelet–fibrin nidus)
+
Bacteremia

Bacteria adhere to damaged endothelium and/or sterile, platelet–fibrin nidus

Bacteria multiply
Further platelet and fibrin binding

Growth of vegetation

Local tissue destruction

Embolization

Hematogenous spread of infection (continued bacteremia)

Antibody response immunologic sequelae

FIGURE 24-1. Pathophysiology of infective endocarditis. NBTE, nonbacterial thrombotic endocarditis.

Physical Examination
- The physical examination is an important component of the evaluation of a patient with IE, and several organ systems may be involved (Table 24-3).
- Particular emphasis should be placed on searching for immunologic and embolic findings that may support the diagnosis of IE.

Diagnostic Criteria

There are several proposed criteria for the diagnosis of IE. The Duke criteria are shown in Tables 24-4 and 24-5.[3]

Diagnostic Testing

Laboratories
- **Blood cultures**: Draw at least two sets from different sites and over a period of time (at least 1 hour between the first and last sets, ideally at least 24 hours) before administering antibiotics; obtain fungal cultures if fungal endocarditis is suspected. Culture yield is dependent upon the volume of blood obtained, so attention should be paid to obtaining adequate samples.
- **Complete blood count** (CBC): Evaluate for leukocytosis, thrombocytosis (acute-phase reactant), thrombocytopenia (sepsis, microangiopathy), and anemia (anemia of chronic disease, hemolytic anemia).
- **Blood urea nitrogen** (BUN), **creatinine**, and urinalysis to evaluate for evidence of immune-complex glomerulonephritis

TABLE 24-3	PHYSICAL EXAMINATION FINDINGS IN ENDOCARDITIS
Organ system	**Findings**
Neurologic	• Range of clinical presentations (e.g., confusion, decreased alertness, focal deficit) • May occur due to embolic stroke, hemorrhagic stroke (transformed embolic stroke or mycotic aneurysm rupture), cerebritis from microabscesses, or meningitis • Any neurologic finding is associated with increased mortality
Cardiac	• Assess for new or worsening murmur due to valvular destruction, ruptured chordae tendineae, or obstruction due to large vegetation • Congestive heart failure • Irregular and/or bradycardic rhythm may indicate the presence of heart block
Abdominal	• Abdominal pain due to emboli and subsequent intestinal, splenic, and/or renal ischemia/infarcts • Splenomegaly may be present, more commonly in subacute IE
Skin and extremities	• Assess for signs of IV drug use • Noteworthy peripheral manifestations include: • **Petechiae:** usually found on conjunctivae, buccal and palatal mucosa, and behind ears • **Osler nodes:** tender SC nodules often found at the pulp of the fingers • **Janeway lesions:** painless, blanchable, macular red spots on the palms and soles • **Splinter hemorrhages:** dark linear streaks seen at the nail bed
Ophthalmologic	• **Roth spots:** round retinal hemorrhages with a pale center

- **Erythrocyte sedimentation rate** (ESR), **C-reactive protein** (CRP), and **rheumatoid factor** (RF) are usually elevated.
- Serologic testing for *Brucella, Legionella, Bartonella, Coxiella burnetii, Mycoplasma*, and *Chlamydia* species as indicated by epidemiology for culture-negative endocarditis
- Occasionally, polymerase chain reaction (PCR) testing of explanted valve tissue is useful to identify unusual or fastidious organisms in culture-negative cases.

Electrocardiography
- An ECG should be obtained to assess for conduction abnormalities (such as varying and progressive degrees of atrioventricular [AV] block) suggestive of aortic root abscess formation, which can be seen with aortic valve endocarditis.
- Ischemic/infarct changes suggestive of coronary emboli

Imaging
- **CXR**
  - Evidence of HF (pulmonary edema)
  - Septic emboli, particularly in IV drug users with suspected right-sided endocarditis

TABLE 24-4	DEFINITION OF TERMS USED IN THE PROPOSED MODIFIED DUKE CRITERIA FOR THE DIAGNOSIS OF IE

Major criteria

Blood culture positive for IE

Typical microorganisms consistent with IE from two separate blood cultures;

Viridans streptococci, *Streptococcus gallolyticus (bovis)*, HACEK group, *Staphylococcus aureus*; or

Community-acquired enterococci, in the absence of a primary focus; or

Microorganisms consistent with IE from persistently positive blood cultures, defined as follows:

At least two positive cultures of blood samples drawn >12 hours apart; or

All of three or a majority of four or more separate cultures of blood (with first and last sample drawn at least 1 hour apart)

Single positive blood culture for *Coxiella burnetii* or antiphase I IgG antibody titer >1:800

Evidence of endocardial involvement

Echocardiogram positive for IE (TEE recommended for patients with prosthetic valves, rated at least "possible IE" by clinical criteria, or complicated IE [paravalvular abscess]: TTE as first test in other patients) defined as follows:

Oscillating intracardiac mass on valve or supporting structures, in the path of re-gurgitant jets, or on implanted material in the absence of an alternative anatomic explanation; or

Abscess; or

New partial dehiscence of prosthetic valve

New valvular regurgitation (worsening or changing of preexisting murmur not sufficient)

Minor criteria

Predisposition, predisposing heart condition, or injection drug use

Fever, temperature >38°C

Vascular phenomena, major arterial emboli, septic pulmonary infarcts, mycotic an-eurysm, intracranial hemorrhage, conjunctival hemorrhages, and Janeway lesions

Immunologic phenomena: glomerulonephritis, Osler nodes, Roth spots, and rheumatoid factor

Microbiological evidence: positive blood culture but does not meet a major criterion as noted earlier or serologic evidence of active infection with organism consistent with IE

Echocardiographic minor criteria eliminated

HACEK, *Haemophilus aphrophilus, Haemophilus parainfluenzae, and Haemophilus paraphro-philus; Actinobacillus actinomycetemcomitans; Cardiobacterium hominis; Eikenella corro-dens; and Kingella kingae*; IE, infective endocarditis; TEE, transesophageal echocardiogram; TTE, transthoracic echocardiogram.

From Li JS, Sexton DJ, Mick N, et al. Proposed modifications to the Duke criteria for the diagnosis of infective endocarditis. *Clin Infect Dis.* 2000;30(4):633-8. Reproduced by permission of the Infectious Diseases Society of America.

TABLE 24-5	DEFINITION OF IE ACCORDING TO THE PROPOSED MODIFIED DUKE CRITERIA

Definite IE
- Pathologic criteria:
  - Microorganisms demonstrated by culture or histologic examination of a vegetation, a vegetation that has embolized, or an intracardiac abscess specimen; or
  - Pathologic lesions: Vegetation or intracardiac abscess confirmed by histologic examination showing active endocarditis
- Clinical criteria[a]:
  - Two major criteria; or
  - One major criterion and three minor criteria; or
  - Five minor criteria

Possible IE
- One major criterion and one minor criterion; or
- Three minor criteria

Rejected
- Firm alternate diagnosis explaining evidence of IE; or
- Resolution of IE syndrome with antibiotic therapy for ≤4 days; or
- No pathologic evidence of IE at surgery or autopsy, with antibiotic therapy for ≤4 days; or
- Does not meet criteria for possible IE, as earlier

IE, infective endocarditis; TEE, transesophageal echocardiography; TTE, transthoracic echocardiography.

[a] Excludes single positive cultures for coagulase-negative staphylococci and organisms that do not cause endocarditis.

From Li JS, Sexton DJ, Mick N, et al. Proposed modifications to the Duke criteria for the diagnosis of infective endocarditis. *Clin Infect Dis.* 2000;30(4):633-8. Reproduced by permission of the Infectious Diseases Society of America.

- **Transthoracic echocardiography** (TTE):
  - TTE is a mainstay of the initial evaluation of a patient with suspected IE.
  - TTE is used to assess for valvular vegetations and to characterize the hemodynamic severity of valvular lesions in patients with IE.
  - It can also assess for other complications of IE (e.g., abscesses, perforation, shunts).
  - TTE can be used to reassess high-risk patients (e.g., those with a virulent organism, clinical deterioration, persistent or recurrent fever, new murmur, or persistent bacteremia).
  - TTE can be considered a reasonable option:
    - To diagnose IE of a prosthetic valve in the presence of persistent fever without bacteremia or a new murmur
    - For the reevaluation of prosthetic valve endocarditis (PVE) during antibiotic therapy in the absence of clinical deterioration
  - High-risk features on transthoracic echo that should be further evaluated by transesophageal echocardiography (TEE):
    - Large vegetation(s)
    - Moderate-to-severe valvular regurgitation or stenosis

- Suggestion of perivalvular extension (i.e., abscess, pseudoaneurysm, fistula)
- Evidence of ventricular dysfunction
  - Repeat TTE is generally not recommended to reevaluate uncomplicated (including no regurgitation on baseline echocardiogram) NVE during antibiotic treatment in the absence of clinical deterioration, new physical findings, or persistent fever.
- **TEE**
  - TEE is a more invasive, more costly, but more sensitive tool to assist in the diagnosis and management of IE.
  - TEE is often used in clinical settings where TTE is nondiagnostic or lacks adequate sensitivity, for instance:
    - If TTE does not confirm diagnoses of IE in setting of high clinical suspicion (e.g., persistent staphylococcal bacteremia without a known source)
    - If TTE cannot adequately characterize or assess the severity of a particular valvular abnormality
    - If there is concern for cardiac abscess or other complication that cannot readily be seen on TTE
  - TEE is preferred to TTE to diagnose PVE and assess for associated complications.
  - TEE may be useful in preoperative evaluation in patients with known IE, and intraoperative TEE is recommended for patients undergoing valve surgery for IE.
- **Coronary CT angiography (CCTA)** is a useful alternative to left heart catheterization to evaluate coronary anatomy, particularly in less stable patients and those with complicated AV endocarditis.
- **Brain CT/MRI**
  - Assess any new neurologic symptoms.
  - MRI may be needed to assess the severity of damage and the presence of hemorrhage caused by emboli to the brain.
  - MR angiography (MRA) may be needed to evaluate for cerebral mycotic aneurysms.

Diagnostic Procedures
Cardiac catheterization may be done to evaluate coronary anatomy in patients with risk factors for coronary artery disease (CAD) needing valve surgery.

TREATMENT
Medications

- Effective treatment involves a coordinated multidisciplinary approach, including cardiology, infectious diseases, and cardiac surgery. See Table 24-6 for recommended antibiotic regimens.[4]
- **Empiric antibiotic coverage** for the most likely organisms (*Staphylococcus aureus*, gram-negative bacilli, *Streptococcus* spp., and *Enterococcus* spp.) is appropriate once adequate samples for blood cultures have been drawn.
  - Acute NVE is more likely to be caused by staphylococci, whereas subacute NVE is more likely to be caused by streptococci or enterococci.
  - Initial antimicrobial regimen should also take into account any antibiotic allergies or intolerances, potential for antibiotic toxicities (e.g., nephrotoxicity), and other clinical factors, including any need for antibiotic penetration to protected sites (e.g., central nervous system [CNS], lung).
  - Infectious diseases consultation should be considered for assistance with constructing an appropriate empiric antibiotic regimen for each individual patient.
  - Commonly utilized antibiotics may include:
    - Vancomycin, dosed for weight and renal function, with a goal trough level of 15 to 25 µg/mL (for methicillin-resistant *Staphylococcus aureus* [MRSA], methicillin-resistant coagulase-negative staphylococci, or susceptible enterococci)

TABLE 24-6	RECOMMENDED ANTIBIOTIC REGIMENS FOR SELECTED CAUSES OF IE

Native valve IE

Pathogen	Antibiotic regimen
Streptococcus viridans and *Streptococcus gallolyticus (bovis)* Highly PCN susceptible – PCN **MIC** $\leq$**0.12 µg/mL**	• IV PCN G or ceftriaxone for 4 weeks • IV PCN G or ceftriaxone plus gentamicin for 2 weeks • Vancomycin for 4 weeks, if unable to tolerate β-lactam
S. viridans and *S. gallolyticus (bovis)* Relatively PCN resistant – PCN MIC **(MIC >0.12–<0.5 µg/mL)**	• IV PCN G or ceftriaxone for 4 weeks plus gentamicin for 2 weeks • Vancomycin for 4 weeks, if unable to tolerate β-lactam plus gentamicin
S. viridans, resistant to PCN (MIC > 0.5), other streptococci, *Abiotrophia defectiva, Granulicatella*	• Seek infectious diseases consultation
Enterococcus spp. Susceptible to PCN, gentamicin, vancomycin	• Ampicillin or IV PCN G plus gentamicin for 4–6 weeks • Ceftriaxone bid plus ampicillin for 6 weeks • Vancomycin plus gentamicin for 6 weeks, if unable to tolerate β-lactam
Enterococcus spp. Resistant to PCN or vancomycin	• Seek infectious diseases consultation
Staphylococcus (*S. aureus*, coagulase negative)	Methicillin susceptible: • Nafcillin or oxacillin for 6 weeks • Cefazolin for 6 weeks Methicillin resistant • Vancomycin for 6 weeks • Daptomycin for 6 weeks
HACEK	• Ceftriaxone or ampicillin–sulbactam or ciprofloxacin for 4 weeks
Culture negative	• Seek infectious diseases consultation
Bartonella	• Doxycycline plus gentamicin for 2 weeks, then doxycycline for 3 months
Candida spp.	• Seek infectious diseases consultation • Amphotericin B or echinocandin followed by long-term suppressive therapy with an oral azole

(continued)

TABLE 24-6	RECOMMENDED ANTIBIOTIC REGIMENS FOR SELECTED CAUSES OF IE (*continued*)

Prosthetic valve IE

Pathogen	*Antibiotic regimen*
S. viridans and *S. gallolyticus (bovis)* Highly PCN susceptible – PCN **MIC ≤0.12 µg/mL**	• IV PCN G or ceftriaxone for 6 weeks with or without gentamicin for 2 weeks • Vancomycin for 6 weeks, if unable to tolerate β-lactam
S. viridans and *S. gallolyticus (bovis)* Relatively PCN resistant – PCN MIC **(MIC >0.12)**	• IV PCN G or ceftriaxone plus gentamicin for 6 weeks • Vancomycin for 6 weeks, if unable to tolerate β-lactam plus gentamicin
Staphylococcus (*S. aureus*, coagulase negative)	Methicillin susceptible: • Nafcillin or oxacillin plus rifampin for 6 weeks + gentamicin for 2 weeks Methicillin resistant: • Vancomycin plus rifampin for 6 weeks plus gentamicin for 2 weeks

HACEK, *Haemophilus aphrophilus, Haemophilus parainfluenzae and Haemophilus paraphrophilus, Actinobacillus actinomycetemcomitans, Cardiobacterium hominis, Eikenella corrodens, Kingella kingae;* IE, infective endocarditis; MRSA, methicillin-resistant *Staphylococcus aureus;* MSSA, methicillin-sensitive *Staphylococcus aureus;* PCN, penicillin.

Source: American Heart Association, Inc.

- Oxacillin or nafcillin 2 g IV q4h (for methicillin-sensitive *Staphylococcus aureus* [MSSA] or susceptible coagulase-negative staphylococci)
- Ampicillin 2 g IV q4h (for susceptible streptococci or enterococci)
- Gentamicin 1 mg/kg IV q8h (for synergy against some streptococci, enterococci, or staphylococcal prosthetic valve infection)
- Ceftriaxone 2 g IV q24h (for susceptible streptococci or HACEK gram-negative organisms)
- Rifampin 300 mg PO/IV q8h may be used as adjunct therapy with vancomycin or oxacillin or nafcillin if concern for staphylococcal prosthetic valve IE.
  - Antimicrobial therapy should be tailored appropriately once the causative pathogen is identified.
- Anticoagulation
  - There is no clear role for antiplatelet or anticoagulant agents in preventing thromboemboli.
  - In patients with an indication for anticoagulation (e.g., mechanical valve), warfarin should be changed to unfractionated heparin in anticipation of possible surgery and/or for easy reversal if neurologic symptoms develop.

Surgical Management

- Advances in surgical technique and a growing understanding that surgery may improve the natural history of the disease have made early surgical involvement crucial.
- In general, surgery is performed in any patient with hemodynamic instability, HF, complicated IE, or IE caused by a highly resistant organism.[5-7]
- Prompt surgical intervention should be initiated for hemodynamic instability and/ or HF.
- For patients with embolism to the brain or intracranial hemorrhage, timing of surgery is more difficult, as early surgery can worsen neurologic function and increase mortality. Urgent or emergent surgery may be considered in patients with NVE or PVE who exhibit mobile vegetations >10 mm in length with evidence of embolic phenomena despite appropriate antimicrobial treatment.
- **Surgical indications for native valve IE**
  - Acute IE that presents with valve stenosis or regurgitation resulting in HF
  - Acute IE that presents with aortic regurgitation (AR) or mitral regurgitation (MR) with hemodynamic evidence of elevated left ventricular (LV) end-diastolic or left atrial pressures (e.g., premature closure of mitral valve [MV] with AR, rapid decelerating MR signal by continuous-wave Doppler, or moderate-to-severe pulmonary hypertension)
  - IE caused by fungal or other highly resistant organisms
  - If heart block, annular or aortic abscesses, or destructive penetrating lesions are present
  - Recurrent emboli and persistent vegetations despite appropriate antibiotic therapy
- **Suggested indications for early surgical intervention in PVE indications for prosthetic valve IE**
  - HF from valve dysfunction or damage from infection—valve dehiscence, intracardiac fistula, severe regurgitation
  - IE complicated by heart block, annular abscess, or destructive penetrating lesions
  - Persistent bacteremia despite appropriate antibiotic therapy for 5 to 7 days and in whom other sites of infection have been excluded
  - PVE caused by fungi or highly resistant organisms
  - PVE complicated by recurrent embolic events
  - Relapsing PVE
  - PVE with mobile vegetations > 10 mm may be considered for early surgical intervention.
  - Routine surgery is not always indicated for patients with uncomplicated IE of a prosthetic valve caused by the first infection with a sensitive organism.

SPECIAL CONSIDERATIONS

In 2008, the recommendations for **endocarditis prophylaxis** were revised (Tables 24-7 to 24-9).[8]

OUTCOME/PROGNOSIS

- Several factors have been shown to independently predict increased mortality, including advanced age, the presence of congestive heart failure (CHF), prosthetic valve, organism (*S. aureus*), type 2 diabetes mellitus, renal insufficiency, and larger vegetation size. A risk stratification score for mortality has been developed for patients with complicated left-sided NVE (see Table 24-10).[9]
- Complications significantly contribute to the morbidity and mortality of IE and can include valvular dysfunction and HF, abscess formation (which can lead to heart block or fistulas between various chambers of the heart), emboli, and uncontrolled infection.

TABLE 24-7	AHA GUIDELINES—CARDIAC CONDITIONS FOR WHICH INFECTIVE ENDOCARDITIS PROPHYLAXIS IS RECOMMENDED

- Patients with prosthetic cardiac valve or prosthetic material used for cardiac valve repair
- Previous IE
- CHD
  - Unrepaired cyanotic CHD, including palliative shunts and conduits
  - Completely repaired congenital heart defect with prosthetic material or device, whether placed by surgery or by catheter intervention, during the first 6 months after the procedure
  - Repaired CHD with residual defects at the site of or adjacent to the site of a prosthetic patch or prosthetic device (which inhibits endothelialization)
- Cardiac transplantation recipients with valve regurgitation due to a structurally abnormal valve

AHA, American Heart Association; CHD, congenital heart disease; IE, infective endocarditis.
Source: American Heart Association, Inc.

TABLE 24-8	AHA GUIDELINES—SCENARIOS IN WHICH INFECTIVE ENDOCARDITIS PROPHYLAXIS IS RECOMMENDED

- The following recommendations only apply to patients with the cardiac conditions listed in Table 24-7.
- All dental procedures that involve manipulation of gingival tissues or periapical region of teeth or perforation of oral mucosa.
- Prophylaxis against infective endocarditis is **not recommended for nondental procedures** (such as transesophageal echocardiogram, esophagogastroduodenoscopy, or colonoscopy) in the absence of active infection.

AHA, American Heart Association; IE, infective endocarditis.
Source: American Heart Association, Inc.

Infections of Implantable Cardiac Devices

GENERAL PRINCIPLES

- Implanted cardiac devices can become infected, similar to any other foreign body.
- Examples of such devices include permanent pacemakers (PPMs), implantable cardioverter-defibrillators (ICDs), cardiac stents, left ventricular assist devices (LVADs), and intra-aortic balloon pumps (IABPs).
- Most device infections are associated with cardiac implantable electrophysiologic devices (CIEDs), such as PPMs and ICDs.
- The use of CIED therapy is increasing with the improvement in technology. As a result, CIED-related infections are also increasing and have become a significant clinical problem.
- Symptoms and signs, presentation, consequences, and treatment vary according to the device type, the location of the infected part(s) of the device, the extent of infection, and the clinical characteristics of the patient.

TABLE 24-9 AHA GUIDELINES—REGIMENS FOR A DENTAL PROCEDURE

Situation	Agent	Regimen: Single dose 30–60 minutes before the procedure	
		Adults	**Children**
Oral	Amoxicillin	2 g	50 mg/kg
Unable to take oral medication	Ampicillin OR	2 g IM or IV	50 mg/kg IM or IV
	Cefazolin or ceftriaxone	1 g IM or IV	50 mg/kg IM or IV
Allergic to penicillins or ampicillin, oral	Cephalexin[a,b] OR	2 g	50 mg/kg
	Clindamycin OR	600 mg	20 mg/kg
	Azithromycin or clarithromycin	500 mg	15 mg/kg
Allergic to penicillins or ampicillin and unable to take oral medication	Cefazolin or ceftriaxone[b] OR	1 g IM or IV	50 mg/kg IM or IV
	Clindamycin	600 mg IM or IV	20 mg/kg IM or IV

[a] Or other first- or second-generation oral cephalosporin in equivalent adult or pediatric dosage.

[b] Cephalosporins should not be used in an individual with a history of anaphylaxis, angioedema, or urticaria with penicillins or ampicillin.

Reprinted with permission from Wilson W, Taubert KA, Gewitz M, et al. Prevention of infective endocarditis: guidelines from the American Heart Association: a guideline from the American Heart Association Rheumatic Fever, Endocarditis, and Kawasaki Disease Committee, Council on Cardiovascular Disease in the Young, and the Council on Clinical Cardiology, Council on Cardiovascular Surgery and Anesthesia, and the Quality of Care and Outcomes Research Interdisciplinary Working Group. *Circulation.* 2007;116(15):1736-54. Copyright ©2007 American Heart Association, Inc.

Epidemiology

- The incidence of cardiac device infection is difficult to determine due to the lack of a comprehensive registry or mandatory reporting. Reported rates have varied between 0.2% and 5.8%.
- Infection in CIED is associated with a twofold increase in mortality.

Pathophysiology

- CIED contamination and secondary infection happen at the time of implant or during subsequent manipulation of the device (e.g., generator changes).
- The surgical pocket can also become infected in the setting of bacteremia or fungemia.
- Staphylococcal species account for 60-80% of infections, particularly coagulase-negative *Staphylococcus* and *S. aureus.*[10]
- Gram-negative bacilli, *Propionibacterium (Cutibacterium) acnes, Corynebacterium,* and *Candida* spp. are other, less common causes of CIED-related infections.

TABLE 24-10	PROGNOSIS WITH COMPLICATED LEFT-SIDED ENDOCARDITIS			
Parameter	**Points**			
Mental status				
Alert	0			
Lethargy or disorientation	4			
Charlson comorbidity scale score				
0–1	0			
≥2	3			
Congestive heart failure[a]				
None or mild	0			
Moderate or severe	3			
Microbiology				
Viridans streptococci	0			
Staphylococcus aureus	6			
Other[b]	8			
Treatment				
Surgery	0			
Medical	5			
Total points	≤6	7–11	12–15	>15
6-Month mortality	9%	25%	39%	63%

[a] None or mild: absence of rales, no shortness of breath at rest, and no pulmonary edema; moderate or severe: presence of at least one.

[b] Includes other streptococci, *Enterococcus*, coagulase-negative staphylococci, Enterobacteriaceae, other gram-negative bacilli, *Haemophilus aphrophilus, Haemophilus parainfluenzae and Haemophilus paraphrophilus, Actinobacillus actinomycetemcomitans, Cardiobacterium hominis, Eikenella corrodens, Kingella kingae* (HACEK), fungi, and culture-negative endocarditis.

Data from Hasbun R, Vikram HR, Barakat LA, et al. Complicated left-sided native valve endocarditis in adults–risk classification for mortality. *JAMA.* 2003;289:1933–40.

Risk Factors[10]

- Diabetes mellitus
- HF
- Renal failure
- Previous generator replacement
- Underlying malignancy
- Dermatologic disorders
- Urgent placement of device
- Fever within 24 hours
- Use of periprocedural temporary pacing
- Low procedural volume

Prevention[10]

- Strict aseptic technique
- Prophylactic antibiotics
  - Administered 60 minutes before starting the procedure
  - 1 to 2 g of cefazolin IV
  - Vancomycin if the patient has had MRSA or is allergic to penicillin
- Avoiding implantation in patients with signs of clinical infection

DIAGNOSIS

Clinical Presentation

- Symptoms and signs are dependent on the organism, the presence of bacteremia, and the degree and specific site of infection.
- **Generator pocket infection[10]**
  - Generator pocket infection typically involves pain, swelling, and/or erythema over the area of infection.
  - If severe, pocket erosion and discharge can be noted.
  - Generator pocket infection is sometimes difficult to differentiate from isolated superficial incisional infection—which presents as pain, swelling, erythema and/or stitch abscess, and possible wound dehiscence and discharge localized to the superficial surgical incision.
  - Occasionally, deep-seated pocket infections can present with pain in the pocket and no other systemic signs or symptoms.
  - Pocket erosion can also occur without major systemic signs or symptoms and must be treated as a pocket infection.
- **Infection of PPM or ICD leads (CIED-related endocarditis)**
  - May be isolated or in association with generator pocket infection
  - Systemic signs include fevers, rigors, malaise, anorexia, and even hemodynamic compromise.
  - Signs and symptoms of endocarditis are often seen, such as infective and thrombotic embolization, mostly affecting the right-sided valves. Patients may present with tricuspid regurgitation (TR), tricuspid stenosis (TS), pulmonary emboli, and pneumonia.
  - The clinical presentation can be acute or subacute and seldom involves signs of left-sided endocarditis.

Diagnostic Testing

- A high index of clinical suspicion is necessary, and the diagnosis should be considered in patients with devices and underlying fever.
- No single test is specific or sensitive enough to make the diagnosis.
- At least two sets of blood cultures should be collected before antimicrobial therapy is initiated (Table 24-11).[10]
- Positive blood cultures often confirm the diagnosis, particularly in *Staphylococcus* spp.
- Other findings that may aid in the diagnosis of CIED-related infections include leukocytosis, elevated CRP, and ESR.
- **TEE is the test of choice to exclude endocarditis** and should be performed in all patients with suspected CIED infection who have positive blood cultures or who have negative blood cultures with antimicrobial therapy administered before cultures, and in patients with suspected CIED-related endocarditis.
- 18-Flourodeoxyglucose (F-FDG) positron emission (PET)/CT scanning can be helpful when diagnosis of CIED pocket or lead infection is uncertain. CXR, pulmonary CTA, and ventilation–perfusion pulmonary scintigraphy may also be helpful adjunctive tests.

TABLE 24-11	AHA GUIDELINES FOR DIAGNOSIS OF CIED INFECTION AND ASSOCIATED COMPLICATIONS

Class I

1. All patients should have at least two sets of blood cultures drawn at the initial evaluation before prompt initiation of antimicrobial therapy for CIED infection. (*Level of Evidence: C*)
2. Generator pocket tissue Gram stain and culture and lead-tip culture should be obtained when the CIED is explanted. (*Level of Evidence: C*)
3. Patients with suspected CIED infection who either have positive blood cultures or have negative blood cultures but have had recent antimicrobial therapy before blood cultures were obtained should undergo TEE for CIED infection or valvular endocarditis. (*Level of Evidence: C*)
4. All adults suspected of having CIED-related endocarditis should undergo TEE to evaluate the left-sided heart valves, even if transthoracic views have demonstrated lead-adherent masses. In pediatric patients with good views, TTE may be sufficient. (*Level of Evidence: B*)

Class IIa

1. Patients should seek evaluation for CIED infection by cardiologists or infectious disease specialists if they develop fever or bloodstream infection for which there is no initial explanation. (*Level of Evidence: C*)

Class III

1. Percutaneous aspiration of the generator pocket should not be performed as part of the diagnostic evaluation of CIED infection. (*Level of Evidence: C*)

AHA, American Heart Association; CIED, cardiac implantable electrophysiologic device; TTE, transthoracic echocardiography.

Reprinted with permission from Baddour LM, Epstein AE, Erickson CC, et al. Update on cardiovascular implantable electronic device infections and their management: a scientific statement from the American Heart Association. *Circulation.* 2010;121(3):458-77. Copyright ©2010 American Heart Association, Inc.

- Gallium and radiolabeled leukocyte scintigraphy are neither sensitive nor specific for device infection.
- Cultures of the generator, surgical pocket, and lead tips at the time of device removal can be potentially helpful to determine the causative microorganism.
- **Percutaneous aspiration of the CIED pocket should not be performed** because of poor diagnostic yield and the potential to introduce pathogens into the surgical pocket.[10]

TREATMENT

Medications

- **Antimicrobial therapy is largely adjunctive to CIED removal.**[10]
  - Intensity and duration of antibiotics are dependent upon the extent of infection, presence of bacteremia, lead vegetation, endocarditis, and pathogen.
  - Antibiotics should be chosen based on in vitro antibiotic sensitivity.
  - Blood cultures should be obtained, and, if positive, parenteral antibiotic therapy should be given as mandated for appropriate management of bacteremia.
- **Superficial or incisional infections** that do not involve the surgical pocket or the device itself do not require removal of the device.[10]

- ○ Managed with **antibiotics that cover *Staphylococcus* spp.**, such as oral cephalexin or dicloxacillin for 7 to 14 days
- ○ Can be very difficult to distinguish from early deep infection
- ○ A wound swab and culture should be performed to help direct antimicrobial treatment.
- ○ Patients should be closely monitored, and management escalated if needed, including alternative broader spectrum antibiotics or prolonged duration of treatment, and consideration of device removal if the infection does not resolve.
- **Generator pocket infections** without evidence of endocarditis require the removal of the entire CIED system, including generator, suture sleeves, sutures, and leads.
- Initial antibiotic therapy should cover staphylococci (e.g., vancomycin).
- Duration of antibiotic therapy should be at least 2 weeks.
- **CIED-related endocarditis should be treated with device removal and a full course of antibiotics, as for NVE.**[11]
  - ○ Complete removal of the CIED system including generator, suture sleeves, sutures, and leads in cases where infection is strongly suspected or established is the goal in most cases.
  - ○ This applies to all CIED infections other than superficial or incisional wound infections.
  - ○ Recurrence of infection is high if any components are retained.
  - ○ Erosion of any part of the CIED components implies contamination of the entire system and necessitates extraction of the entire system.
  - ○ If there is lead involvement alone but no vegetations noted on the heart valves, the duration of antibiotic therapy is 2 to 4 weeks.
  - ○ With evidence of valvular vegetation, antibiotic course should be extended to 4 to 6 weeks.
- **Patients with positive blood cultures but no evidence of local infection in the CIED** pose difficult management scenario.
  - ○ CIED infection may be present and can be indicated by persistent bacteremia and/or relapsed bacteremia after an appropriate period of antibiotic treatment when no other source of bacteremia is identified. Infectious disease consultation should be obtained.
  - ○ All non-CIED sources of infection should be removed (i.e., central and peripheral lines, catheters, etc.).
- *S. aureus* bacteremia carries a particularly high risk of CIED infection and warrants careful evaluation for device infection and consideration for device removal.

Nonpharmacologic Therapy

- **Percutaneous CIED lead extraction** has become the preferred method to remove leads due to improved technologies, including excimer laser, cautery, and rotational dissection systems.[10]
- The procedure has significant risks, including tamponade, hemothorax, pulmonary embolism, lead migration, pneumonia, and death.
- Nonetheless, in experienced centers, complete percutaneous lead removal can be performed relatively safely with a high success rate (97%) and a low rate of major complications (2%) and mortality rate (<1%).[12,13]
- Surgical management should be considered when percutaneous management has failed or when hardware is retained.
- Should not be postponed due to the timing of antimicrobial therapy. Extraction within 3 days of hospitalization is shown to be associated with lower mortality.[14]

SPECIAL CONSIDERATIONS

- **CIED reimplantation after extraction**
  - ○ Every patient should be evaluated for the need for CIED reimplantation after extraction of an infected device.

○ Device reimplantation, when necessary, should be performed on the contralateral side. If this is not possible, then the leads should be tunneled to a device placed SC elsewhere, such as in the abdomen. Epicardial systems or subcutaneous ICD (S-ICD) should be considered, if clinically appropriate.

○ There are limited data regarding the optimal timing of reimplantation, but guidelines recommend waiting a minimum of 72 hours with negative blood cultures following device explant. In cases where valvular vegetations are seen, a minimum of 2 weeks from negative blood cultures is recommended.

- **LVAD infections**
  ○ Durable LVADs are surgically implanted continuous-flow circulatory pumps connected to an external power source via an electric drive line. LVADs are used in patients with end-stage HF as either a bridge to heart transplant or destination therapy.
  ○ Infection may occur in the pump, pump pocket, outflow conduit, or driveline.
  ○ Infection is a frequent complication of LVAD placement and is a significant source of morbidity and mortality.[15]
  ○ Incidence of infection has been highly variable among different surveys, reported to range between 13% and 80%.
  ○ LVAD infections are a significant cause of morbidity and mortality among this patient population, with driveline infections being the most common source of infection.
  ○ Bloodstream infections among LVAD patients are less frequently reported than driveline or pocket infections but are generally linked to poorer outcomes.
  ○ **Types of infection**
    ▪ **Driveline infection is the most common** type of LVAD-related infection and usually presents with local inflammation and drainage at the driveline exit site in the abdomen.
    ▪ **Pocket infections** may present with local inflammatory change in the upper abdomen or chest wall or with bacteremia and sepsis.
    ▪ Less commonly, **infection of the pump** itself may occur. No imaging technique permits visualization of the internal components of the pump—the diagnosis is clinical and should be suspected with bacteremia and no other local source.
    ▪ More than one component of the LVAD system may become infected simultaneously.
  ○ **Organisms**
    ▪ The organisms involved depend on the location of infection and on whether there is an associated bloodstream infection.
    ▪ Staphylococci are the most common, followed by gram-negative bacilli (including *Pseudomonas aeruginosa* and *Escherichia coli*), *Enterococcus*, *Corynebacterium*, and *Candida* spp.
    ▪ Device-related infections usually involve gram-positive cocci (*Staphylococcus* or *Enterococcus* spp.), although gram-negative infections also occur (*P. aeruginosa*, *Enterobacter*, *Klebsiella*).
  ○ Patient-level **risk factors** include diabetes and obesity. Operative risk factors for infection include bleeding, blood product transfusion, thrombosis, and surgical reexploration.
  ○ **The clinical presentation** may include fever, leukocytosis, and/or local signs of infection. LVAD pump infections can present with fever, bacteremia, embolic events, and valvular vegetations.
  ○ **Treatment** is centered on antimicrobial therapy targeted at the causative organism. Secondary prevention of infection recurrence is an area of uncertainty. Many centers maintain patients on long-term suppressive antibiotics.
  ○ Surgical debridement of infected tissue surrounding the LVAD driveline is performed in patients with driveline infection and refractory pain, drainage, or systemic signs of infection. In certain cases, the driveline position may be moved to encourage healing.

In cases of extensive infection, plastic surgery may be required to provide adequate tissue coverage.

○ LVAD device explant is rarely performed due to the high morbidity of such a procedure in patients with extremely compromised cardiac function. Transplant should be considered in eligible patients with recent severe and/or chronic LVAD infection.

- **Coronary artery stent infections**
  ○ Infections of intracoronary stents are rare but are often fatal due to severe damage to the arterial wall.
  ○ They occur secondary to contamination of stent at the time of implantation or due to subsequent bacteremia. Infection can occur within 4 weeks of placement.
  ○ Fever, phlebitis, local infection, and bacteremia occur in <1% of all procedures.
  ○ *S. aureus* and *P. aeruginosa* are most common pathogens.
  ○ There may also be findings of associated abscess, suppurative pancarditis, and pericardial empyema.
  ○ Brachial artery access has been associated with a 10-fold higher incidence of infectious complications, due to a cutdown approach. Repeated puncture of ipsilateral femoral artery or indwelling sheaths postprocedure is associated with an increased incidence of infection.
  ○ Prevention strategies should involve sterile technique, avoidance of access through endovascular grafts, avoidance of access ipsilateral to a prosthetic hip, and minimization of indwelling catheters after the procedure.
  ○ Treatment should involve broad-spectrum empiric antibiotics until culture results are obtained.

- **IABP infections**
  ○ Infections of IABPs are uncommon, and the rate of infection is related to the duration of therapy.
  ○ Local wound infections are the most common, and bacteremia is usually secondary to contamination from a colonized or infected insertion site.
  ○ Risk factors for infection include contamination of the femoral site, especially in obese patients, and emergent placement performed outside the operating room or catheterization laboratory.
  ○ Treatment should be with appropriate antimicrobial therapy, local wound care, and removal of the IABP whenever possible.

REFERENCES

1. O'Rourke RA, Fuster V, Alexander RW, eds. *Hurst's the Heart*. 10th ed. McGraw-Hill; 2000:596.
2. Tleyjeh IM, Abdel-Latif A, Rahbi H, et al. A systematic review of population-based studies of infective endocarditis. *Chest*. 2007;132:1025-35.
3. Li JS, Sexton DJ, Mick N, et al. Proposed modifications to the Duke criteria for the diagnosis of infective endocarditis. *Clin Infect Dis*. 2000;30:633-8.
4. Baddour LM, Wilson WR, Bayer AS, et al. AHA guidelines—infective endocarditis in adults: diagnosis, antimicrobial therapy, and management of complications: a scientific statement for healthcare professionals from the American Heart Association. *Circulation*. 2015;132:1435-86.
5. Bonow RO, Carabello BA, Chatterjee K, et al. American College of Cardiology/American Heart Association Task Force on Practice Guidelines. 2008 focused update incorporated into the ACC/AHA 2006 guidelines for the management of patients with valvular heart disease. *J Am Coll Cardiol*. 2008;52:e1-142.
6. Kang DH, Kim YJ, Kim SH, et al. Early surgery versus conventional treatment for infective endocarditis. *N Engl J Med*. 2012;366(26):2466-73.
7. Pettersson GB, Coselli JS, Hussain ST, et al. 2016 American Association for Thoracic Surgery (AATS) consensus guidelines: surgical treatment of infective endocarditis: executive summary. *J Thorac Cardiovasc Surg*. 2017;153:1241-58.
8. Wilson W, Taubert KA, Gewitz M, et al. Prevention of infective endocarditis guidelines from the American Heart Association. *Circulation*. 2007;116:1736-54.

9. Hasbun R, Vikram HR, Barakat LA, et al. Complicated left-sided native valve endocarditis in adults–risk classification for mortality. *JAMA*. 2003;289:1933-40.

10. Baddour LM, Epstein AE, Erickson CC, et al. Update on cardiovascular implantable electronic device infections and their management: a scientific statement from the American Heart Association. *Circulation*. 2010;121:458-77.

11. Kusomoto FM, Schoenfeld MH, Wilkoff BL. 2017 HRS Expert consensus statement on cardiovascular implantable electronic device lead management and extraction. *Heart Rhythm*. 2017;14(12):e503-51.

12. Fu H, Huang X, Zhong LI, et al. Outcomes and complications of lead removal: can we establish a risk stratification schema for a collaborative and effective approach? *Pacing Clin Electrophysiol*. 2015;38(12):1439-47.

13. Sood N, Martin DT, Lampert R, et al. Incidence and predictors of perioperative complications with transvenous lead extractions: real-world experience with national cardiovascular data registry. *Circ Arrhythm Electrophysiol*. 2018;11(2):e004768.

14. Viganego F, O'Donoghue S, Eldadah Z, et al. Effect of early diagnosis and treatment with percutaneous lead extraction on survival in patients with cardiac device infections. *Am J Cardiol*. 2012;109(10):1466-71.

15. O'Horo JC, Abu Saleh OM, Stulak JM, et al. Left ventricular assist device infections: a systematic review. *ASAIO J*. 2018;64(3):287-94.

Basic Electrocardiography

25

Elizabeth M. Riddell and Timothy W. Smith

GENERAL PRINCIPLES

- Even though the ECG is one of the most widely used and important tests in the hospital, ECG interpretation is often seen as an esoteric skill and approached with trepidation. Contributing factors may include poor instruction in ECG basics as well as large gaps in time between ECG teaching and practice. This chapter is not meant to serve as a complete guide to ECG interpretation but will, we hope, be a helpful start to bridging the knowledge gap. For a more complete review, see the suggested readings at the end of this chapter.
- Important advice for improving your ECG interpretation skills include:
  - **Same way every time**. By approaching ECG interpretation the same way each time, you will become more efficient and accurate. You will also be less likely to miss subtle diagnoses.
  - **Practice, practice, practice**. Review online tutorials. Obtain a book of unknown ECG tracings with answers. Examine ECGs from patients on cardiology services. Attend cardiology/ECG conferences. Avoid gaps in time without ongoing ECG practice.
  - **Keep a file** of interesting ECGs. By collecting ECGs, you maintain a sense of vigilance. You will begin to recognize certain patterns of disease. Your collection will also be useful when asked to give a conference with limited notice.

DIAGNOSIS

The Practical Five-Step Method: Rate, Rhythm, Axis, Intervals, Injury

- **Rate:**
  - The first method for determining rate is the easiest but potentially the least reliable: Look at the top of the ECG for the computer interpretation (though often correct, it is best to corroborate).
  - Another method to determine the rate is to divide 300 by the number of "big" boxes (5-mm boxes) between QRS complexes.
    - For example, if the distance between two QRS complexes is five "big" boxes, the ventricular rate is 300 (big boxes/minute) divided by 5 big boxes/cycle, which equals **60** cycles (beats) per minute (bpm).
    - The following series of numbers are the rates for each additional "big" box between QRS complexes starting with one box... 1:**300 bpm,** 2:**150 bpm,** 3:**100 bpm,** 4:**75 bpm,** 5:**60 bpm,** 6:**50 bpm**... It is easy to count boxes between waves (e.g., between QRS's): Instead of saying "1, 2, 3, 4, 5...," memorize and say: "300, 150, 100, 75, 60, 50, (43)."
  - The rate can also be calculated using one of the following equations:
    - RATE = 1500/(mm between similar waves)
    - RATE = (Cycles/6-second strip) × 10
    - Also, **RATE = Cycles/10-second strip × 6. Note: Common full-page 12-lead ECG formats are 10 seconds long.**

○ Common rates associated with particular rhythms include:
 ▪ 60 to 100 bpm: normal sinus rhythm
 ▪ 40 to 60 bpm: junctional escape rhythm
 ▪ 20 to 40 bpm: ventricular escape rhythm
 ▪ 150 bpm: atrial flutter with 2:1 conduction
• **Rhythm** (refer to Figure 25-1):
 ○ Normal conduction
  ▪ Sinus rhythm is a cardiac rhythm in which the impulse for conduction starts at the sinus node. This impulse then spreads to depolarize both atria, thus forming the P wave seen on ECG.
  ▪ Normal conduction then leads to activation of the atrioventricular (AV) node, which conducts more slowly than normal myocardium. This is represented by the PR segment, the isoelectric (flat) segment between the P wave and the QRS. Note that the PR interval is composed of the P wave and the PR segment.
  ▪ The electrical impulse then travels to the ventricles using the rapidly conducting His-Purkinje system, which allows for coordinated ventricular depolarization. The QRS complex represents ventricular depolarization on the ECG.
 ○ When determining the rhythm on an ECG, look for the sequence of components in a normally conducted heartbeat: P wave … PR interval … QRS complex.

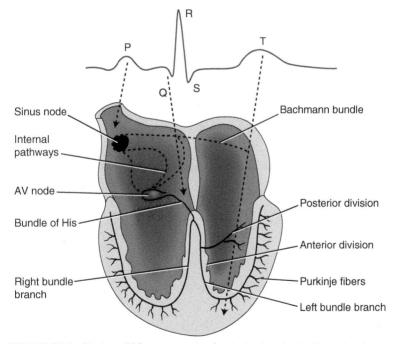

FIGURE 25-1. Rhythm: ECG components of a single sinus beat with anatomic correlation. The P wave reflects atrial activation from the sinus node. The PR interval is the time during which the signal is passing through the atrioventricular (AV) node. The narrow QRS complex represents the coordinated ventricular activation through the His-Purkinje system. The T wave signifies ventricular repolarization.

○ Sinus P waves occur at regular intervals. With normal conduction, there should be one P wave for every QRS and one QRS for every P wave.

■ Variation in P-wave interval or shape throughout an ECG is usually the result of one or more ectopic atrial foci (e.g., multifocal atrial tachycardia).

■ Absence of a P wave with irregular QRS occurrences usually means atrial fibrillation; however, atrial standstill can occur with severe hyperkalemia or extensive atrial fibrosis.

○ The PR interval (normal: 120 to 200 ms) represents the time for the electrical impulse to conduct through the atria and AV node. If the PR interval changes, some type of AV block is usually the culprit.

○ A narrow QRS (<100 ms) implies that the ventricle is being activated by normal conduction through the AV node and His-Purkinje system.

○ A wide QRS (>120 ms) is an indication of slow or blocked conduction through the normal conduction system in the ventricles. It can also be the result of abnormal conduction through the ventricles that does not use the normal conduction system. Examples include:

■ Left bundle branch block (LBBB)
■ Right bundle branch block (RBBB)
■ Intraventricular conduction delay (IVCD)
■ Ventricular ectopic beat or an impulse that originates from the ventricle (e.g., premature ventricular contraction or ventricular tachycardia)
■ Electrical signal that passes through an accessory pathway between the atrium and ventricles rather than through the AV node

• **Axis** (Figure 25-2)[1] is the major direction of electrical wave progression. It usually refers to ventricular activation (QRS complex), but the concept of axis may be applied to P waves or even T waves. The normal direction is inferior and to the patient's left (−30 degrees to +90 degrees; see Figure 25-2). Leads I and II are helpful in determining QRS axis.

○ In Figure 25-2, lead I runs from the patient's right to left arm across the top of the diagram. If the QRS is predominantly positive in lead I, the electrical signal is heading in the direction of lead I or toward the patient's left (anywhere from −90 degrees to +90 degrees).

○ Lead II runs from the patient's right arm to left leg. If it is predominantly positive, we know that the electrical signal is heading in the direction of lead II (leftward and inferior; anywhere from −30 degrees to +150 degrees).

○ If the QRS is positive in **both** lead I and lead II, the axis direction falls in the area where the two leads overlap (between −30 degrees and +90 degrees), which is considered normal axis (see Figure 25-2).

○ What is the axis if the QRS deflection is mostly positive in lead I but negative in lead II? A positive deflection in lead I means the electrical signal is moving from the patient's right to left, but a negative deflection in lead II means the signal is moving in the opposite direction (rightward and superior). This puts the axis between −30 degrees and −90 degrees, consistent with left-axis deviation (LAD).

○ What is the axis if the QRS deflection is mostly negative in lead I but positive in lead II? A negative deflection in lead I means that the electrical signal is moving from left to right. The positive deflection in lead II means the signal is moving from superior to inferior. This puts the axis between +90 degrees and +150 degrees consistent with right-axis deviation (RAD).

• **Intervals** (Figure 25-3)[1]:
○ **P waves**:
■ Lead V1 lies directly over the atria, so it is useful for evaluating atrial enlargement.
■ A normal P wave is biphasic in lead V1 and monophasic in lead II.
■ With **left atrial enlargement** (LAE), the P wave in lead V1 has an abnormally large and wide terminal negative component. In lead II, a "notched" P wave with duration >120 ms also suggests LAE.

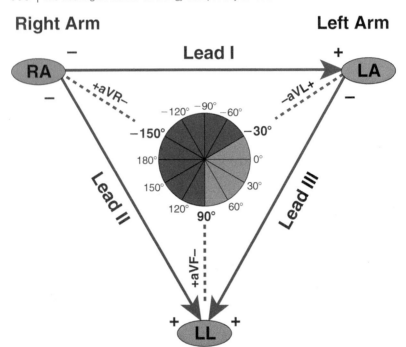

FIGURE 25-2. Axis: Einthoven triangle and normal QRS axis (−30 degrees to +90 degrees). (Reprinted with permission from Frank G. Yanowitz, MD. ECG Learning Center. https://ecg.utah.edu/.)

- With **right atrial enlargement** (RAE), the P wave in lead V1 has a large, often peaked, initial positive component. In lead II, a tall P wave (exceeding 2.5 mm) also suggests RAE.
  - **PR interval:**
    - Time from the onset of the P wave to the start of the QRS complex
    - A normal PR interval is 120 to 200 ms (three to five "small" boxes).
    - If the PR interval is constant but long (>200 ms), it is consistent with first-degree AV block.
    - If the baseline PR interval is prolonged, but then varies and prolongs further before a subsequent QRS complex is dropped, it is consistent with second-degree AV block, Mobitz type I (also known as Wenckebach), which usually represents conduction block within the AV node.
    - If the PR intervals are normal for conducted QRS complexes but some P waves fail to conduct, this is consistent with second-degree AV block, Mobitz type II, which is generally associated with a block in the Purkinje fibers (His bundle or bundle branches). An exception to this would be abnormal P waves that come early in the cardiac cycle, or *premature atrial complexes* (PACs). These P waves may not be conducted to the ventricles, due to reaching the AV node at a time when it is refractory.
    - Third-degree AV block is a total or complete block of conduction from the atria to the ventricles, resulting in AV dissociation on the ECG. P-wave rate is usually superimposed on a slower, independent QRS rate.

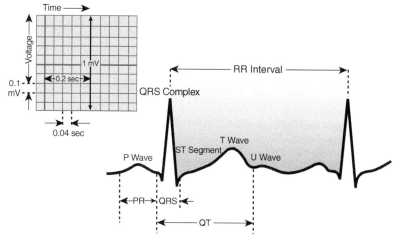

FIGURE 25-3. Intervals: Defining the intervals and segments on the ECG and identifying specific pathology to look for in each interval or segment. **P wave size:** Look for atrial enlargement (LAE in V1, RAE in lead II). **PR interval:** Look for AV block (PR >200 ms) or ventricular preexcitation (PR <40 ms). **QRS size:** Large voltage suggests LVH, and small voltage suggests pericardial effusion. **QRS interval:** Wide QRS (>120 ms) signifies a poorly coordinated beat due to LBBB, RBBB, IVCD, or ventricular beats. **QT interval:** LQT intervals can be due to many causes, including "hypo's," "anti's," congenital syndromes, intracerebral hemorrhage, or cardiac ischemia (see text). AV, atrioventricular; IVCD, intraventricular conduction delay; LAE, left atrial enlargement; LBBB, left bundle branch block; RAE, right atrial enlargement; RBBB, right bundle branch block. (Reprinted with permission from Frank G. Yanowitz, MD. ECG Learning Center. https://ecg.utah.edu/.)

- A short PR interval (<120 ms) suggests preexcitation (the presence of an accessory pathway between the atria and ventricle; e.g., **Wolff–Parkinson–White (WPW) syndrome**—characterized by short PR, broad QRS, and a δ wave, which is a slurred upstroke to the QRS complex, along with symptoms suggesting paroxysmal supraventricular tachycardia).
  ○ **QRS complex:**
    - Width: The normal QRS width is between 80 and 120 ms. If it is >120 ms, it is an indication of abnormal electrical conduction through the ventricles. (See examples in the Rhythm section.)
    - Voltage: The height and depth of the QRS complex can indicate the presence of **left ventricular hypertrophy** (LVH). Many criteria have been established for determining LVH, one of which is the Sokolov–Lyon criteria. This method involves adding the depth of lead V1 with the height of lead V5 or V6. A sum >35 mm (3.5 mV) is consistent with LVH. Small voltages (<5 mm [0.5 mV] in the limb leads, <10 mm [1.0 mV] in the precordial leads) can occur when a poorly conductive material is present between the heart and the ECG lead. Examples include air (hyperinflated lungs in chronic obstructive pulmonary disease), fluid (pericardial effusion), or fat. Low voltages can also be observed with infiltrative diseases of the myocardium (e.g., cardiac amyloid).
  ○ **QT interval:**
    - The QT interval should be corrected for the underlying heart rate by using the formula: QTc = QT (ms)/square root of R-R interval (s).

- Normal QTc is up to 440 ms for men and 460 ms for women. The ECG machine is generally reliable at measuring and calculating the QTc; however, there is no substitute for determining the QT interval yourself, especially if QT prolongation is a concern.
- Long QT (LQT) is associated with torsade de pointes, a potentially lethal ventricular rhythm. The five causes of LQT can be grouped into as follows:
  - **Hypo's:** hypokalemia, hypomagnesemia, hypothermia
  - **Medications:** Examples include antibiotics, antiarrhythmics, antihistamines, and antipsychotics. For a more comprehensive list of medications associated with LQT, visit CredibleMeds.org.
  - **Congenital:** LQT syndromes
  - **Intracerebral hemorrhage:** also characterized by diffuse, deep, symmetric, large inverted T waves ("cerebral T waves")
  - **Cardiac ischemia:** in the form of "Wellens waves," which are biphasic T waves with a terminal negative portion, or deep, symmetric, inverted T waves, particularly seen in leads V1 to V3, classically associated with proximal left anterior descending disease
- **Injury (ischemia/infarction)** (Figure 25-4):
  - **ST-segment elevation:** classically described in acute myocardial infarction (MI). The differential also includes LVH, pericarditis, and ventricular aneurysms. ST elevation associated with MI is an **acute injury pattern** until Q waves (see later) have developed.

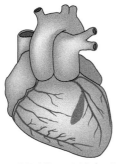

V1, V2 septal infarct

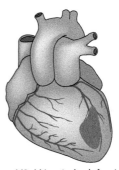

V3, V4 anterior infarct

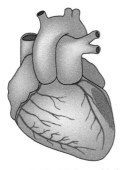

I, aVL, V5, V6 lateral infarct

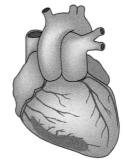

II, III, aVF inferior infarct

FIGURE 25-4. Injury: ECG leads and coronary artery distributions. ST-segment elevations in specific leads reflect a myocardial injury (infarction or ischemia) in certain anatomic locations, as shown.

The ECG criteria for MI require >1 mm elevation in two contiguous limb leads or >2 mm elevation in lead V2 or V3.

○ **ST-segment depression:** classically described with myocardial ischemia. The differential also includes LVH, digoxin effect (ST "scooping" may occur with digoxin therapy and does not necessarily signify toxicity), and WPW syndrome. It is important to remember that ST depressions can represent ST elevations on the opposite side of the heart. This is why ST depression (known as reciprocal changes) can be seen in the leads (coronary territories) not involved in the acute MI (leads with ST elevation).

○ **T-wave inversions:** generally nonspecific; however, Wellens waves (described earlier) are more suspicious for significant ischemia.

○ **Q waves:** signify a prior infarct that has subsequently developed scar

○ The distribution of the particular findings should be noted, as changes consistent throughout a specific coronary artery territory are more likely to indicate a true area of infarction (Figure 25-4).

  ▪ Inferior (usually right coronary artery territory): leads II, III, aVF
  ▪ Anterior (usually left anterior descending territory): leads V2 to V4
  ▪ Lateral (usually left circumflex artery territory): leads V5 to V6, I, aVL

• **Put It All Together: When you are initially learning how to read an ECG, talk out loud and say what you see** (Figure 25-5)**:**

○ Rate/rhythm/axis: "The rate is (300, 150, 100, 75, 60) slightly more than five big boxes, so about 55 bpm and the rhythm is sinus, so sinus bradycardia. The second QRS complex comes early and has a different preceding P-wave morphology, consistent with a PAC. The QRS axis is positive in leads I and II, so normal axis."

○ Intervals: "The terminal negative portion of the P wave in lead V1 is slightly >1 mm, so there is LAE. PR interval is <200 msec, which is normal. QRS is <120 msec, which is normal. No LVH. QTc interval is 420 milliseconds, which is normal."

○ Injury: "I do not see any ST elevation. There are slightly down sloping ST segments and T-wave inversions in V1 to V2, which can be normal. There are no Q waves that would suggest an old MI."

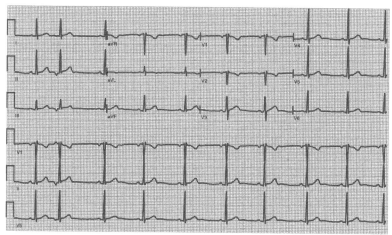

FIGURE 25-5. Sample ECG for interpretation.

REFERENCE

1. Yanowitz FG. ECG learning center. Accessed 8/31/21. https://ecg.utah.edu/

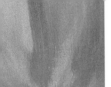

Advanced Electrocardiography: ECG 201

26

Curtis M. Steyers III and Timothy W. Smith

DIAGNOSIS

Myocardial Infarction

- Clinically, myocardial infarction (MI) can be divided into ST-segment elevation myocardial infarction (STEMI) and non–ST-segment elevation myocardial infarction (NSTEMI) subtypes. STEMI is characterized by ST-segment elevations, while NSTEMI can have variable ECG appearances. This section focuses on the ECG features of STEMI.
- STEMI is defined by the presence of new ST-segment elevations in at least two contiguous leads of >2 mm in men (>1.5 mm in women) in leads V2 to V3 or >1 mm in other leads.
- Occasionally, hyperacute T waves may be the only ECG finding early in an evolving STEMI.
- The diagnosis is further confirmed by the identification of **reciprocal changes**, which are characterized by ST-segment depressions in leads representing anatomic locations opposite the infarct.[1]

Infarct Localization and Anatomy-Specific Considerations

- In STEMI, the infarct-related artery and region of myocardial injury can often be identified by ECG. ST elevations generally occur in leads corresponding to the anatomic location of infarction.
- **Inferior STEMI** is characterized by ST-segment elevation >1 mm in two of leads II, III, and aVF. Depending on the patient's anatomy and the site of coronary obstruction, there may be associated posterior (ST depression in leads V2 to V3) or lateral (ST elevation in leads I, aVL, V5, and V6) infarction and associated ECG changes.
  - Reciprocal ST depressions are often seen in lead aVL.
  - Inferior MI is usually caused by occlusion of the right coronary artery (RCA). The RCA supplies the atrioventricular (AV) node in most people, so **PR prolongation or AV block** is often found with inferior MI.
  - The RCA also supplies the right ventricle (RV) through RV marginal arteries. Occlusion of the RCA proximal to these branch arteries can cause *RV infarction.*
    - One should always consider RV infarction when the diagnosis of inferior STEMI is made, as these patients may be particularly susceptible to hypotensive effects of preload-reducing interventions, such as nitrates and diuretics.
    - RV infarction is suggested with **ST elevation in lead V1** and when **ST elevations are greater in lead III than in lead II.**
    - Diagnosis can be made using right-sided ECG leads (Figure 26-1), looking for **any ST elevation in right-sided V4 (V4R).**
- **Anterior STEMI** is associated with several distinct patterns of ST elevation corresponding to the level of occlusion of the left anterior descending (LAD) or left main (LM) coronary artery. In general, there must be ST elevations in two contiguous precordial leads. There must be >2 mm (1.5 mm in women) elevations in leads V2 to V3 due to

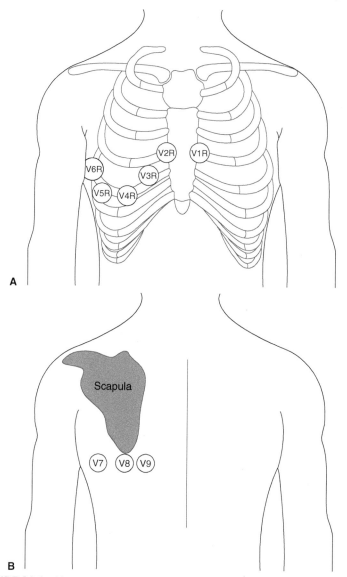

FIGURE 26-1. Alternate positions for ECG leads. **(A)** Right-sided leads (V1R to V6R) for diagnosing a right ventricular infarct. **(B)** Posterior leads (V7 to V9) for diagnosing a posterior infarct.

higher baseline voltages. Patterns include **septal** (V1 to V2), **anterior** (V2 to V5), and **anterolateral** (V3 to V6, I, aVL) infarction.

- ○ Because the left bundle branch is supplied by septal and diagonal branches of the LAD, proximal LAD occlusion can occasionally present with **new left bundle branch block (LBBB).** This is usually clinically dramatic, with severe chest pain, hypotension, and signs and symptoms of heart failure.
- ○ Patients presenting with chest pain and preexisting LBBB pose a diagnostic challenge. The **modified Sgarbossa criteria** are useful for the diagnosis of STEMI in the context of LBBB[2,3]:
  - ST elevation ≥1 mm concordant with QRS
  - ST depression ≥1 mm in lead V1, V2, or V3 concordant with QRS
  - ST elevation excessively discordant with QRS, defined as ≥25% of the amplitude of the preceding S wave
- **Posterior STEMI** is often difficult to detect with ECG. The posterior left ventricular myocardium is usually supplied by branches of the distal left circumflex coronary artery (LCx) and is not well represented with traditional ECG lead placement. The diagnosis of posterior MI requires a high degree of clinical suspicion and can often be recognized by several findings:
  - ○ Reciprocal ST depressions and pronounced R waves in the anterior precordial leads (V1 to V3)
  - ○ ST elevations in dedicated posterior leads (V7 to V9) (Figure 26-1)
- **Lateral STEMI** often occurs in the context of infarction of another territory (e.g., anterolateral, inferolateral). However, isolated lateral or "high lateral" STEMI can also occur when there is occlusion of an obtuse marginal, diagonal, or ramus intermedius branch. Involvement of the lateral left ventricular wall is recognized by ST elevations in leads I, aVL, V5, and V6.
- There are several ECG patterns corresponding to critical proximal LAD or LM stenosis that require more urgent management that do not meet traditional clinical criteria for STEMI. These patients are often unstable or at risk for hemodynamic deterioration, making rapid identification and triage important.
  - ○ **Wellens syndrome** is characterized by symmetric, deeply inverted or biphasic T-wave inversions in the anterior precordial leads (usually V2 to V3) without Q waves or ST-segment elevations. This syndrome represents critical proximal LAD stenosis and impending anterior wall infarction. Clinical presentation is usually consistent with acute coronary syndrome, and patients should generally be managed in an urgent manner.[4]
  - ○ **ST elevation in lead aVR** and **diffuse precordial ST depressions** are often indicative of severe LM disease. In some cases, it may represent severe three-vessel disease. These findings are likely secondary to diffuse subendocardial ischemia with reciprocal ST elevation in aVR. In the correct clinical scenario, these findings can be interpreted and managed as an STEMI equivalent.[5]

Alternative Causes of ST-Segment Elevation

There are many causes of ST elevation beyond ischemia; thus, **ST elevation is not synonymous with MI.**[6] These causes range from benign to life-threatening. It is important to recognize these ST elevation variants and distinguish them from STEMI. Consideration of the clinical context is critical.

- Many young adult men have especially **rapid or "early" ventricular repolarization,** which causes concave ST elevations, usually largest in lead V2. This is a normal pattern for young males.
- An **early repolarization pattern** has been described with a notched J point (immediately after the QRS complex) and tall, upright T waves, most pronounced in lead V4.
- LBBB is associated with ST-segment deviation in the direction opposite (discordant) the major QRS deflection.

- Hyperkalemia, pulmonary embolism (PE), and left ventricular hypertrophy (LVH) can cause ST elevations in distinct ways.
- The Brugada pattern is characterized by rSR' pattern with downsloping ST elevations in leads V1 and V2.
- A common mimic of MI is **acute pericarditis**. Patients with either disease can present with significant chest pain and have ST elevations on ECG. Several important clinical and ECG distinctions are outlined in Table 26-1.

Tachycardias

- The ECG is the most important diagnostic tool for evaluation of tachycardia. A systematic approach is essential in order to establish the correct diagnosis and appropriately manage the patient. Management of patients with various tachyarrhythmias is outlined in Chapter 40.
- Our approach to the ECG analysis of tachyarrhythmias is summarized in Figure 26-2.[7]
- Tachycardias can be classified as either **narrow complex or wide complex**, based on QRS duration of less than or greater than 120 ms, respectively.

Wide-Complex Tachycardias

- Wide-complex tachycardia (WCT) is defined as tachycardia with QRS duration >120 ms. The differential diagnosis for WCT is broad, so care must be taken to consider all possible mechanisms during initial ECG analysis. Establishing the mechanism of WCT has important prognostic and therapeutic implications.

TABLE 26-1	FEATURES TO HELP DISTINGUISH PERICARDITIS FROM MYOCARDIAL INFARCTION	
	MI	**Pericarditis**
History	Risk factors of prior CAD, advanced age, diabetes, hypertension, hypercholesterolemia, tobacco use, early family history of CAD	Recent viral illness History of chest radiation History of cancer
Chest pain characteristics	Variable, but classically "constant, severe squeezing" in the substernal area, with or without radiation to the left jaw and arm.	Variable, but worse with respiration and lying down. Improved with sitting forward.
Physical examination	Variable, but dyspnea, diaphoresis, rales more specific for MI	Variable, but friction rub is specific for pericarditis.
ECG characteristics	ST elevations in an "anatomic" distribution. Reciprocal ST-segment depressions	Diffuse ST elevations. PR depression.
Cardiac-specific biomarkers (troponin)	With large MI, markedly elevated biomarkers	Mild to absent elevation of biomarkers
Echocardiogram	Wall motion abnormalities in the distribution of the infarcting artery	No wall motion abnormalities

CAD, coronary artery disease; MI, myocardial infarction.

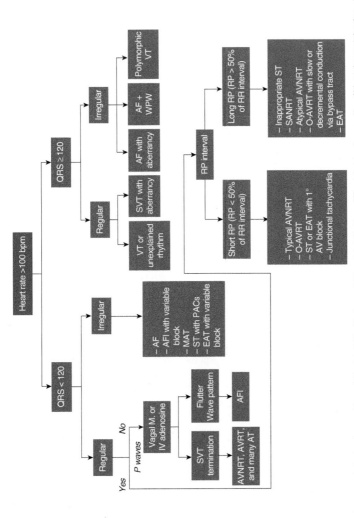

FIGURE 26-2. Approach to tachycardias. AF, atrial fibrillation; AFL, atrial flutter; AT, atrial tachycardia; AV, atrioventricular; AVNRT, atrioventricular nodal reentrant tachycardia; AVRT, atrioventricular reentrant tachycardia; EAT, ectopic atrial tachycardia; MAT, multifocal atrial tachycardia; O-AVRT, orthodromic atrioventricular reentrant tachycardia; PAC, premature atrial contraction; SANRT, sinoatrial nodal reentrant tachycardia; ST, sinus tachycardia; SVT, supraventricular tachycardia; VT, ventricular tachycardia; WPW, Wolff–Parkinson–White. (Reprinted with permission from Sharma S, Cooper DH, Faddis MN. Cardiac arrhythmias. In: Foster C, Mistry NF, Peddi PF, et al, eds. *The Washington Manual of Medical Therapeutics.* 33rd ed. Wolters Kluwer Health/Lippincott Williams & Wilkins; 2010:201-48.)

- When encountering a wide QRS complex, one must first consider the three potential causes: **ventricular origin, aberrant conduction**, or **preexcitation** (also discussed in Chapters 30 and 40).
  - Rhythms originating from the ventricles include **ventricular tachycardia (VT)** and **ventricular pacing**.
  - Any **supraventricular tachycardia (SVT)** conducted aberrantly through the native conduction system will appear as a WCT. This includes sinus tachycardia (ST), atrial fibrillation, atrial tachycardia (AT), atrial flutter (AFL), junctional tachycardia, AV nodal reentrant tachycardia (AVNRT), and atrioventricular reentrant tachycardia (AVRT).
  - Patients with an **accessory pathway** capable of antegrade conduction may develop WCT secondary to (1) **antidromic AVRT** or (2) any SVT conducting to the ventricles at least partially via the accessory pathway—**preexciting the ventricles**—a situation in which the accessory pathway is considered a bystander (not necessary for maintenance of the arrhythmia).
- The most important initial distinction to make when a patient presents with WCT is whether the rhythm is VT or SVT (either conducted aberrantly or preexcited). This distinction will profoundly affect prognosis and management decisions. Clinical and ECG clues that favor VT versus SVT are outlined in Table 26-2.
  - If the patient is hemodynamically unstable, **immediate cardioversion** is indicated regardless of the mechanism of WCT.
  - The baseline ECG, if available, should always be reviewed.
    - The presence of **bundle branch block during sinus rhythm** may help identify aberrantly conducted SVT if the QRS morphology during WCT is identical to the sinus rhythm morphology.

TABLE 26-2	**CLINICAL CLUES TO DISTINGUISH BETWEEN VENTRICULAR AND SUPRAVENTRICULAR TACHYCARDIAS FOR A WIDE-COMPLEX TACHYCARDIA**	

Clinical clue	Ventricular tachycardia	Supraventricular tachycardia with aberrancy
History	Structural heart disease present	No structural heart disease
Initiation	VPD initiates	APD initiates
P-wave timing	AV dissociation	Consistent AV relationship
QRS morphology	Fusion beats or capture beats	Characteristic QRS morphology for aberrant conduction (V1, V6)
	QRS concordance (positive or negative)	
	QRS duration >140 ms if RBBB	
	QRS duration >160 ms if LBBB	
	Extreme axis (−90 to −180 degrees), monophasic R wave in aVR	

APD, atrial premature depolarization; AV, atrioventricular; LBBB, left bundle branch block; RBBB, right bundle branch block; VPD, ventricular premature depolarization.

- The presence of **Wolff–Parkinson–White (WPW) pattern** (short PR, wide QRS with slurred upstroke) during sinus rhythm increases the likelihood of antidromic AVRT or preexcited SVT as the mechanism of WCT.
  - Several classical ECG findings during WCT can be rapidly identified that are highly specific for VT, obviating the need for more complex discrimination algorithms.
    - The presence of **VA dissociation** during WCT is diagnostic of VT. This is identified by recognizing P waves at regular intervals throughout the tachycardia with no relationship to the QRS complexes.
    - Negative (and, to a lesser degree, positive) **concordance of the QRS complexes** in the precordial leads is highly specific for VT. Pure QS complexes from V1 to V6 during WCT reflect ventricular activation (VA) arising from near the apex of the heart, which virtually excludes any SVT mechanism.
    - **Capture beats** (narrow QRS complexes preceded by a P wave during an episode of WCT) reflect transient conduction of a sinus impulse via the native conduction system with capture of the ventricular myocardium between wide-complex beats and are virtually diagnostic of VT.
    - **Fusion beats** (slightly narrower QRS complexes than during WCT but wider than during sinus rhythm) result from collision of a natively conducted sinus impulse with an impulse of ventricular origin and are equivalent to capture beats in specificity for VT.
  - If these findings are not identified upon initial review of the ECG, there are multiple algorithms to help distinguish discriminate VT from SVT (Figure 26-3).
- Patients with accessory pathways capable of antegrade conduction may develop **preexcited atrial fibrillation**. This can be life-threatening due to the potential for degeneration into ventricular fibrillation. It should be suspected if the WCT is **fast, bizarre, and irregular ("FBI")**, particularly in patients with known WPW syndrome.
  - Rapid identification of this rhythm is critical, as the initial therapy of choice is generally electrical cardioversion.
  - **AV node-slowing agents (calcium channel blockers, β-blockers, digoxin)** should be avoided during preexcited atrial fibrillation, due to their potential to accelerate the frequency of conduction over the accessory pathway, increase the ventricular rate, and precipitate ventricular fibrillation.

Narrow-Complex Tachycardias
- Narrow-complex tachycardia (NCT) is defined as any fast rhythm with QRS duration <120 ms. The differential diagnosis is broad. However, all NCTs share a common feature: the ventricular myocardium is activated via the native His-Purkinje system.
- A useful diagnostic approach to NCTs is outlined in Figure 26-2. In general, the initial evaluation of an NCT should seek to answer the following questions:
  - Is the tachycardia **regular or irregular?**
  - Is there **discernable atrial activity?**
  - What is the **VA (RP) relationship?**
- Analysis of the VA relationship: One of the most diagnostically useful distinctions to make in the analysis of NCT is to determine the VA relationship or the RP relationship on ECG. In general, NCTs can be divided into long RP and short RP tachycardias.
  - **Short RP tachycardia:** P waves occur during the first half of the R-R interval. Differential diagnosis includes:
    - Typical AVNRT (RP < 70 ms)
    - Orthodromic atrioventricular reentrant tachycardia (O-AVRT) (RP > 70 ms)
    - Junctional tachycardia
  - **Long RP tachycardia:** P waves occur during the second half of the R-R interval. Implies very slow retrograde VA conduction during reentry or rapid AV conduction during 1:1 conduction of a focal tachycardia.
    - ST

- Focal AT
- Atypical AVNRT (retrograde conduction via slow pathway)
- Response to adenosine: In stable patients with NCT, administration of adenosine can be both diagnostic and therapeutic. By profoundly depressing conduction in the AV node, adenosine can produce the following effects[8]:
  - **Slowing of the ventricular rate**, allowing better visualization of the atrial activity. If the tachycardia continues with a slower ventricular rate, AVNRT and O-AVRT can be effectively excluded. Often, P waves (AT), flutter waves (AFL), or fibrillatory waves (AF) can be seen between QRS complexes.

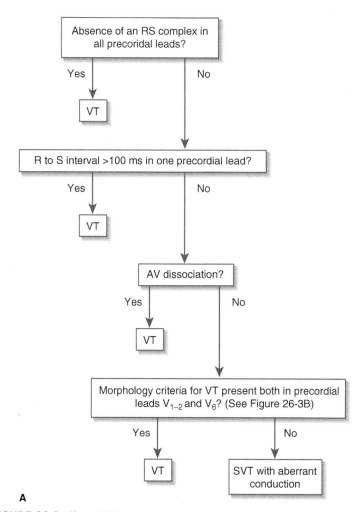

A

FIGURE 26-3. (**A** and **B**) Brugada criteria for distinguishing ventricular tachycardia from supraventricular tachycardia with aberrancy in wide-complex tachycardias.

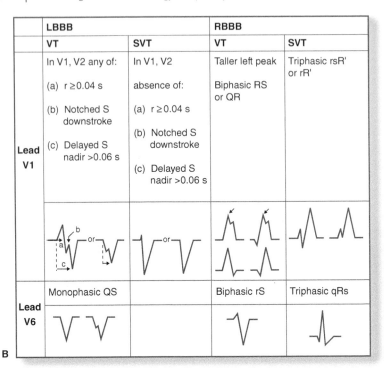

	LBBB		RBBB	
	VT	**SVT**	**VT**	**SVT**
Lead V1	In V1, V2 any of: (a) r ≥0.04 s (b) Notched S downstroke (c) Delayed S nadir >0.06 s	In V1, V2 absence of: (a) r ≥0.04 s (b) Notched S downstroke (c) Delayed S nadir >0.06 s	Taller left peak Biphasic RS or QR	Triphasic rsR' or rR'
Lead V6	Monophasic QS		Biphasic rS	Triphasic qRs

FIGURE 26-3. *(continued)*

- ○ **Termination of the tachycardia,** primarily in NCTs utilizing the AV node as a critical limb of the circuit (AVNRT, O-AVRT). This **suggests but does not prove** the diagnosis of AVNRT or O-AVRT. **Caveat: Some ATs will terminate with adenosine.**
- **Atrial fibrillation:** The most common sustained tachyarrhythmia is discussed as a separate topic in Chapter 28.
- **AFL:** Defined mechanistically as a **macroreentrant AT**, generally characterized on ECG by a fast, regular atrial rhythm lacking an isoelectric interval between deflections.
  - ○ The second most common atrial arrhythmia. Associated with advanced age and structural heart disease
  - ○ Ventricular rate during AFL is dependent on the degree and pattern of conduction block in the AV node. Most commonly, AFL presents as a **regular rhythm** with 2:1 AV block, but can be **irregularly irregular** when associated with variable AV block.
  - ○ AFL can be divided into **typical** and **atypical** subtypes. This distinction reflects the mechanism of arrhythmia and has important therapeutic implications.
    - ■ **Typical AFL** is a macroreentrant AT whose circuit is contained entirely within the right atrium, rotating in a counterclockwise (or sometimes clockwise) direction around the tricuspid annulus.
      - □ The atrial rate is usually 240 to 340 beats per minute, corresponding to a ventricular rate around 150 beats per minute during 2:1 AV conduction. **Suspect typical AFL when the ventricular rate is 150 beats per minute during an NCT.**

- In its usual clockwise form, **"sawtooth" flutter waves** with sharp negative deflections can be seen in leads II, III, and aVF, while there are positive deflections in lead V1.
- The **cavotricuspid isthmus** provides a zone of slow conduction necessary for reentry and is the target for ablation of typical AFL.
  - **Atypical AFL** comprises all other macroreentrant ATs *not* using the typical flutter circuit. Difficult to distinguish from focal AT on ECG.
    - Because atypical AFL is a heterogeneous group of ATs arising from either atrium with widely varying anatomic substrates, there is no common atrial rate or P-wave morphology.
    - Commonly arises in patients with congenital heart disease or after AF ablation, MAZE procedure, or any cardiac surgical procedure during which an atriotomy is made

- **Focal AT:** rapid, regular atrial rhythm originating from a focal source of atrial myocardium outside the sinus node (sinoatrial [SA] node) region. Often difficult to distinguish from atypical AFL based on ECG alone
  - Distinguished mechanistically from AFL by the absence of a macroreentrant circuit. Instead, AT is thought to reflect one of the following:
    - Enhanced automaticity
    - Triggered activity
    - Microreentry
  - AT can be paroxysmal (short bursts) or sustained (less common). Often discovered incidentally on ambulatory cardiac monitors.
  - ECG: fast, regular rhythm with P waves of a single morphology preceding each QRS complex, with **a discrete isoelectric interval between deflections**. Atrial rate is usually 130 to 240 beats per minute. Ventricular rate depends on AV conduction. AT often conducts 1:1, presenting as a **long RP tachycardia**.
- **Multifocal atrial tachycardia (MAT):** an **irregularly irregular** rhythm that may be difficult to distinguish from sinus rhythm with frequent premature atrial contraction (PAC) or atrial fibrillation
  - Represents chaotic atrial activity with rapid impulse formation arising from several distinct ectopic atrial foci
  - Usually seen in elderly hospitalized patients with severe cardiopulmonary disease. Strong association with chronic obstructive pulmonary disease (COPD) and heart failure
  - ECG shows rapid, irregular rhythm with **at least three distinct P-wave morphologies.**
  - Treatment is generally directed at the underlying disease process.
- **ST:** the most common **long RP tachycardia**
  - Most often, ST is a normal physiologic response to hyperadrenergic states (e.g., fever, pain, hypovolemia, anemia, hypoxia) but can also be induced by illicit drugs (e.g., cocaine, amphetamines, methamphetamine) and prescription drugs (e.g., theophylline, atropine, β-adrenergic agonists).
  - **Inappropriate ST** refers to persistently elevated sinus rates in the absence of an identifiable physiologic stimulus.
- **AVNRT:** common reentrant tachycardia whose circuit exists within the AV node and perinodal atrial tissue. Occurs in patients with dual AV nodal physiology, wherein the AV node is functionally dissociated into "slow" and "fast" pathways
  - Strong female predominance (2:1)
  - Common in younger patients without structural heart disease
  - Usually 1:1 AV relationship; however, rarely, there can be 2:1 block below the AV node
  - Divided into typical and atypical subtypes:

- **Typical AVNRT** is most common.
  - □ Defined by antegrade conduction over the slow pathway and retrograde conduction up the fast pathway, producing a **short RP tachycardia**
  - □ ECG: P waves hidden in QRS complexes or buried at the end of QRS complexes creating a **pseudo-r′ (V₁) or a pseudo-s′ (II)**. Compare QRS in tachycardia and sinus rhythm to identify retrograde P waves
  - **Atypical AVNRT**: includes "fast-slow" and "slow-slow" variants, all of which involve retrograde conduction up the slow pathway, resulting in **long RP tachycardia**
- **AVRT:** group of reentrant tachycardias utilizing an **accessory pathway** for conduction directly between the atria and the ventricles in either antegrade or retrograde manner. In AVRT, the atria, ventricles, accessory pathway, and AV node are all critical participants in the reentrant circuit.
  - ○ Most common in children, adolescents, and young adults. Less common in the elderly
  - ○ By definition, there is a 1:1 AV relationship. **AV block during tachycardia excludes AVRT**.
  - ○ **O-AVRT:** accounts for about 95% of all AVRT and is the most common mechanism of SVT in patients with the WPW syndrome.
    - Antegrade conduction to the ventricles occurs via the AV node and retrograde conduction to the atria via the accessory pathway.
    - ECG: **short RP tachycardia**, with retrograde P waves often visible outside the QRS complex (RP > 70 ms)
    - **Preexcitation** may or may not be present during sinus rhythm, and its presence does not affect the likelihood that an SVT is O-AVRT. Preexcitation during sinus rhythm is referred to as the **WPW pattern**, characterized by short PR interval and a wide QRS preceded by a **δ wave**.
    - In order for preexcitation to be present during sinus rhythm, the accessory pathway must be capable of antegrade conduction (**manifest pathway**). Many accessory pathways are **concealed**, meaning they are only capable of retrograde conduction and will not cause ventricular preexcitation.
  - ○ Antidromic AVRT involves antegrade conduction over the accessory pathway, leading to a WCT. This is discussed in section Wide-Complex Tachycardia.
- **Junctional tachycardia:** arises from enhanced automaticity within the AV junction. In a manner similar to AVNRT, there is nearly simultaneous activation of the atria and ventricles. This manifests on ECG as retrograde P waves buried within QRS complex.

SPECIAL CONSIDERATIONS

The following are several classic ECG findings associated with common clinical scenarios:
- **Hyperkalemia:** Multiple ECG findings are seen as potassium levels rise, including peaked T waves, QRS widening, PR prolongation, P-wave flattening, and, eventually, "sine wave" pattern.
- **Digitalis effect:** Downsloping, curved ST segments are seen with a characteristic "up-tick" T wave.
- **Digitalis toxicity:** Because digitalis increases the automaticity of the atrial and ventricular tissues while slowing the SA and AV nodes, two common ECG findings with digitalis toxicity are AT with AV block and bidirectional VT.
- **Osborne waves:** Also called J waves, these are seen as additional notching at the end of the QRS complex and are associated with profound hypothermia.

- **LVH:** There are multiple ECG criteria that predict with varying success the presence of LVH on echocardiography. In general, these criteria are specific but insensitive (Table 26-3).[9,10]
- **Pulmonary disease pattern:** Because of hyperinflated lungs, more vertical orientation of the heart within the chest, and elevated pulmonary artery pressures, patients with COPD may have reduced QRS amplitude, right-axis deviation, incomplete right bundle branch block (RBBB) in V1 (rSR′ pattern), right atrial enlargement, and delayed R-wave transition in the precordial leads.
- **PE:** Acute obstruction of the pulmonary arterial system leading to RV strain can cause a series of ECG changes.
  - ST is the most common finding in acute PE.
  - Atrial arrhythmias (AFL, AF, AT) may be present.
  - Complete or incomplete RBBB pattern
  - S1Q3T3 pattern (S wave in lead I, Q wave in lead III, and inverted T wave in lead III), while often cited, is uncommon.
- This chapter concludes with several unknown ECG tracings (with interpretations, Figures 26-4 through 26-8) to exercise your ECG analysis skills.

TABLE 26-3	VARIOUS ELECTROGRAPHIC CRITERIA FOR DETERMINING THE PRESENCE OF LEFT VENTRICULAR HYPERTROPHY	
Criteria	**Measurement**	**Points**
Cornell voltage	S in V3 + R in aVL >28 mm (men) S in V3 + R in aVL >20 mm (women)	
Framingham	R in aVL >11 mm, R in V4 to V6 >25 mm S in V1 to V3 >25 mm S in V1 or V2 + R in V5 or V6 >35 mm R in I + S in III >25 mm	
Sokolow–Lyon index	S in V1 + R in V5 or V6 >35 mm	
Romhilt–Estes point score	Any limb lead R wave or S wave ≥20 mm or S in V1/V2 ≥30 mm or R in V5/V6 ≥30 mm	3
	ST-T-wave abnormality (with or without digitalis)	1 or 3
	Left atrial abnormality	3
	Left-axis deviation	2
	QRS duration ≥90 ms	1
	Intrinsicoid deflection in V5/V6 ≥50 ms	1
	Definite LVH = 5 or more points; probable LVH = 4 points	
Peguero–Lo Presti	Depth of deepest S wave in any lead + depth of S wave in V4 ("$S_D+S_{V_4}$"). LVH if ≥28 mm (men) or ≥23 mm (women)	

LVH, left ventricular hypertrophy.

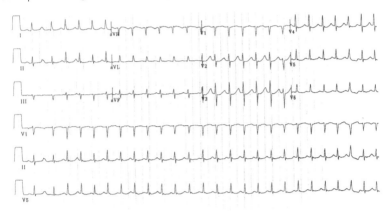

FIGURE 26-4. ECG tracing for interpretation. **Rate:** 160 beats per minute. **Rhythm:** Regular rhythm with a narrow QRS and **no obvious P waves**. This is a narrow-complex tachycardia. Differential diagnosis includes atrioventricular nodal reentrant tachycardia (AVNRT), atrioventricular reentrant tachycardia (AVRT), automatic atrial tachycardia, atrial flutter, and atrial fibrillation. **Axis:** Up in lead I and up in lead II, so normal axis. **Intervals:** Without a P wave, there is no PR interval. QRS is narrow, and there is no LVH. QT interval is <400 ms. **Injury:** No significant ST-segment elevation no depression. No significant Q waves. **Putting it all together:** narrow-complex tachycardia, likely due to **AVNRT**. Note that the retrograde P waves are likely buried within the QRS complex.

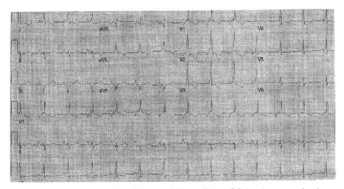

FIGURE 26-5. ECG tracing for interpretation. **Rate:** 80 beats per minute. **Rhythm:** Sinus rhythm. **Axis:** Up in lead I and down in lead II, so left-axis deviation. **Intervals:** P waves are markedly negative in lead V1 left atrial enlargement (LAE) and markedly positive in lead II right atrial enlargement (RAE). **PR interval is <120 ms**, seen best in the precordial leads. QRS is wide, but only at the initial upstroke (**δ wave**). No left ventricular hypertrophy. QT intervals are normal. **Injury:** Neither significant ST-segment deviations nor *true* Q waves (there are negative δ waves in leads III and aVF, a "pseudo-infarct" pattern), but **marked T-wave inversions V2 to V3**. **Putting it all together:** With a short PR interval, a δ wave, and localized T-wave inversions, this patient has ventricular preexcitation through an accessory pathway.

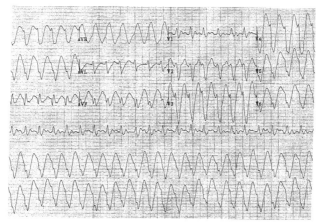

FIGURE 26-6. ECG tracing for interpretation. **Rate:** 150 beats per minute. **Rhythm:** No obvious P waves. Wide, regular QRS complex. This is a wide-complex tachycardia. Differential diagnosis includes ventricular tachycardia, supraventricular tachycardia with aberrancy, ventricular preexcitation. **Axis:** Down in lead I and down in lead II. This is **extreme left-axis deviation. Intervals:** No P waves, so no PR interval. **QRS is markedly wide (200 ms).** It is neither an LBBB nor RBBB morphology, so it is termed **idioventricular conduction delay (IVCD).** Left ventricular hypertrophy and QT intervals cannot be assessed in this wide-complex tachycardia. **Injury:** Difficult to assess in this wide-complex rhythm. **Putting it all together:** Using the various tools available, including Brugada criteria, this is a ventricular tachycardia. Because the QRS is extremely wide and of IVCD morphology (neither a true RBBB nor LBBB), suspect **hyperkalemia** as well. LBBB, left bundle branch block; RBBB, right bundle branch block.

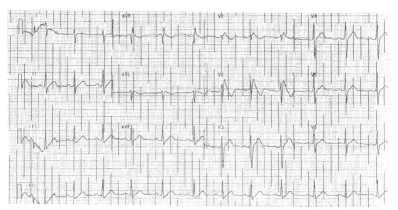

FIGURE 26-7. ECG tracing for interpretation. **Rate:** 70 beats per minute. **Rhythm:** Sinus. **Axis:** Down in lead I and up in lead II. Right-axis deviation. **Intervals:** P wave and PR intervals are normal. QRS is narrow without left ventricular hypertrophy. **QT interval is short** (QTc = 340 ms). **Injury: Large, rapidly downsloping ST-segment elevations in leads V1 and V2.** No reciprocal changes or Q waves. **Putting it all together:** This is a classic ECG of a patient with **Brugada syndrome,** with coved ST elevations in leads V1 to V2 and an incomplete right bundle branch block pattern.

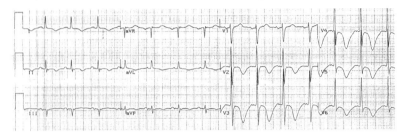

FIGURE 26-8. ECG tracing for interpretation. **Rate:** 90 beats per minute. **Rhythm:** Sinus. **Axis:** Up in lead I and up in lead II. Normal axis. **Intervals:** P wave and PR intervals are normal. QRS is narrow. Left ventricular hypertrophy by Sokolow–Lyon criteria (S in lead I + R in lead V5 is >35 mm). **QT interval is long** (QTc >600 ms). Differential diagnosis (see Chapter 25) includes hypo's, anti's, congenital, cerebral causes, or impending infarction (Wellens waves). **Injury:** No significant ST-segment deviations. Isolated Q wave in lead III is generally normal. **Large, deep, symmetric T-wave inversions, primarily in the precordial leads. Putting it all together:** This is a classic ECG of a patient with **Wellens waves** due to a critical proximal left anterior descending artery lesion.

REFERENCES

1. Zimetbaum PJ, Josephson ME. Use of the electrocardiogram in acute myocardial infarction. *N Engl J Med.* 2003;348:933-40.
2. Sgarbossa EB, Pinski SL, Barbagelata A, et al. Electrocardiographic diagnosis of evolving acute myocardial infarction in the presence of left-bundle branch block. *N Engl J Med.* 1996;334:481-87.
3. Smith SW, Dodd KW, Henry TD, et al. Diagnosis of ST-elevation myocardial infarction in the presence of left bundle branch block with the ST-elevation to S-wave ratio in a modified Sgarbossa rule. *Ann Emerg Med.* 2012;60(6):766-76.
4. Zwaan C, Bar F, Wellens H. Characteristic electrocardiographic pattern indicating a critical stenosis high in left anterior descending coronary artery in patients admitted because of impending myocardial infarction. *Am Heart J* 1982;103(4 pt 2):730-6.
5. Task Force on the management of ST-segment elevation acute myocardial infarction of the European Society of Cardiology (ESC), Steg PG, James SK, et al. ESC guidelines for the management of acute myocardial infarction in patients presenting with ST-segment elevation. *Eur Heart J.* 2012;33(20):2569-619.
6. Wang K, Asinger RW, Marriott HJL. ST-segment elevation in conditions other than acute myocardial infarction. *N Engl J Med.* 2003;349:2128-35.
7. Sharma S, Cooper DH, Faddis MN. Cardiac arrhythmias. In: Foster C, Mistry NF, Peddi PF, Sharma S, eds. *The Washington Manual of Medical Therapeutics.* 33rd ed. Lippincott Williams & Wilkins; 2010:201-48.
8. Delacretaz E. Supraventricular tachycardia. *N Engl J Med.* 2006;354:1039-51.
9. Hancock EW, Deal BJ, Mirvis DM, et al. AHA/ACCF/HRS recommendations for the standardization and interpretation of the electrocardiogram: part V: electrocardiogram changes associated with cardiac chamber hypertrophy. *J Am Coll Cardiol.* 2009;53:992-1002.
10. Peguero JG, Lo Presti S, Perez J, et al. Electrocardiographic criteria for the diagnosis of left ventricular hypertrophy. *J Am Coll Cardiol.* 2017;69(13):1694-703.

Bradyarrhythmias and Permanent Pacemakers

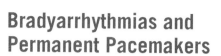

Prashanth D. Thakker and Amit Noheria

GENERAL PRINCIPLES

Definition

- The normal resting heart rate ranges from 60 to 100 beats per minute (bpm). **Bradycardia** is defined as a ventricular rate <60 bpm. Bradycardia can be a physiologic response to increased vagal tone.
- **A bradyarrhythmia** is a nonphysiologic bradycardia that can be attributed to dysfunction at different levels within the native conduction system. Therefore, a review of conduction during normal sinus rhythm, the vascular supply of the conduction system, and the intrinsic and extrinsic influences on the conduction system (Table 27-1) is useful.

Sinoatrial Node

- The sinoatrial (SA) or sinus node is a collection of specialized pacemaker cells located in the high right atrium, specifically in the subepicardial **sulcus terminalis**.
- The sinus node demonstrates **regular spontaneous diastolic depolarization** that initiates the electrical impulse to generate the normal sinus rhythm. The electrical impulse then sequentially activates the right and left atria to produces atrial systole.
- The autonomic tone to the sinus node, controlled by the sympathetic and parasympathetic inputs, determines the resting **sinus node rate, usually 60 to 100 bpm.**
- Arterial blood is supplied to the sinus node via the **sinus node artery**. The sinus node artery originates from the proximal right coronary artery in ~65% people; proximal left circumflex artery in 25%; or dual in 10%. From its origin, the sinus node artery courses posteriorly in the superior interatrial groove and travels anterior or posterior to the superior vena cava or bifurcates to form a peri-superior vena cava ring to reach the sulcus terminalis and supply the sinus node.[1-3]

Atrioventricular Node

- Activation spreads from the atrium through specific atrionodal tracts (commonly referred to as the fast and slow pathways) to another grouping of specialized cells, the atrioventricular (AV) node.
- The AV node is an atrial structure located in the AV septum between the annular right atrium and the left ventricle. In developmentally normal hearts, the AV node is situated within the **triangle of Koch,** which is defined as bounded by the attachment of the septal tricuspid valve leaflet, the tendon of Todaro, and the orifice of the coronary sinus.[3]
- In developmentally mature hearts, the AV node should serve as the only electrical connection between the atria and the ventricles. AV node demonstrates **slow conduction**, producing a delay typically in the range of 50 to 120 ms that accounts for the majority of the PR interval measured on ECG. The autonomic tone to the AV node modulates the conduction through the AV node, with parasympathetic inputs slowing conduction and sympathetic inputs accelerating conduction.

TABLE 27-1	CAUSES OF BRADYCARDIA

Intrinsic
Idiopathic degeneration (aging)
Surgical trauma: valve surgery and transplantation
Congenital disease (may present later in life)
Cardiomyopathies including neuromuscular diseases
Ischemia or infarction
Infiltrative disease: sarcoidosis, amyloidosis, hemochromatosis
Infectious/inflammatory disease: endocarditis, Lyme disease, Chagas disease, myocarditis
Systemic inflammatory disease: systemic sclerosis, systemic lupus erythematosus

Extrinsic
Neurocardiogenic (vasovagal) syncope
Carotid sinus hypersensitivity
Increased vagal tone: coughing, vomiting, micturition, defecation, intubation
Drugs: β-blockers, calcium channel blockers, digoxin, antiarrhythmic agents
Hypothyroidism
Hypothermia
Neurologic and autonomic disorders
Electrolyte imbalances: hyperkalemia, hypermagnesemia, hypocalcemia
Obstructive sleep apnea
Sepsis

- The AV node, like the sinus node, possesses inherent pacemaking properties and, in the absence of an overdriving faster sinus rhythm, usually generates an escape **junctional rhythm at 40 to 50 bpm**.
- The AV node is supplied by the **AV nodal artery**, which typically originates from the distal right coronary artery (80%), a dominant distal left circumflex artery (10%), or both (10%). In addition, the AV node receives collateral arterial flow from the proximal left anterior descending artery.[1-3]

Infranodal Conduction System or His-Purkinje System
- Conduction fibers converge into the compact AV node at the apex of the triangle of Koch and continue as a discrete AV bundle (also referred to as the **bundle of His**). The AV bundle is an insulated structure that penetrates though the fibrous annular tissue at the central fibrous body. The penetrating AV bundle travels through the membranous septum and reaches the crest of the muscular interventricular septum branching into the insulated **right and left bundle branches**. The right and left bundles themselves then branch out into subendocardial **Purkinje network** that interfaces with and activates the ventricular myocardium.[3]
- The penetrating AV bundle of His and the right bundle branch receive blood via the AV nodal artery and from septal perforators off the left anterior descending artery. The left bundle branch has a variable anatomy but can be classified into an anterior and a posterior fascicle on the left side of the interventricular septum. The anterior fascicle is supplied by septal perforators from the left anterior descending artery, and the posterior fascicle is supplied by the septal branches of both the posterior descending artery and the left anterior descending artery.

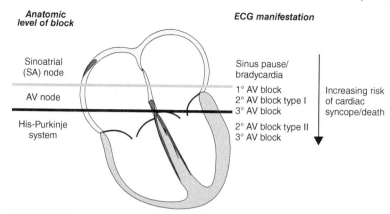

Anatomic level of block

ECG manifestation

Sinoatrial (SA) node — Sinus pause/ bradycardia

AV node — 1° AV block / 2° AV block type I / 3° AV block

His-Purkinje system — 2° AV block type II / 3° AV block

Increasing risk of cardiac syncope/death

FIGURE 27-1. Diagram detailing the anatomic level of block. The column on the left describes the anatomic levels of the conduction system. The column on the right describes associated rhythm as assessed by ECG. Block below the level of the atrioventricular (AV) node (lower line) portends a high risk of syncope/death.

Classification

Bradyarrhythmias are classified based on the location of the pathology (Figure 27-1), which then determines the clinical prognosis and guides therapy.

Sinus Node Dysfunction

- Sinus node disease is often a degenerative process due to aging but can be accelerated in younger patients with structural heart disease, cardiac surgery, ischemia, or systemic inflammatory diseases. Symptomatic sinus node dysfunction (**sick sinus syndrome**) is the most common reason for pacemaker implantation in the US. Sinus node dysfunction can manifest in several ways (Figure 27-2):
- **Sinus bradycardia** is defined as a regular rhythm with QRS complexes preceded by sinus P waves (upright P waves in II, III, aVF; terminal negative in V1) at a rate <60 bpm. Sinus bradycardia can be benign and is frequently seen in conditioned athletes and during sleep.
- **Sinus arrest** or sinus pause refers to failure of the sinus node to depolarize, which manifest as periods of atrial asystole (no P waves). This may be accompanied by ventricular asystole or escape beats from AV junction or ventricle. Pauses of 2 to 3 seconds can be seen in healthy, asymptomatic patients, especially during sleep. Pauses >3 seconds, particularly during daytime hours, raise concern for sinus node dysfunction.
- **SA exit block** represents the appropriate depolarization of the sinus node but failure to engage the atrial myocardium, often due to fibrosis in the perinodal tissue. As sinus node activity is not registered on the surface ECG, sinus exit block is nearly indistinguishable from sinus arrest, except that PP interval during sinus exit block may be a multiple of the PP interval immediately preceding the bradycardia.
- **Tachy–brady syndrome** occurs when tachycardia alternates with bradycardia. A classic example can be seen in the termination of atrial fibrillation (AF) (tachycardia), where a long pause may occur before the sinus node recovers (bradycardia). Sinus node dysfunction and AF mechanistically share the underlying atriopathy, and a patient who has AF may have symptomatic sinus bradycardia at other times.
- **Chronotropic incompetence** is the inability to increase the sinus rate appropriately in response to increased physiologic demand, for example, with exercise.

Sinus bradycardia

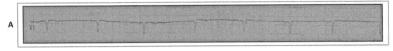

Sinoatrial node exit block

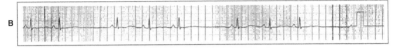

Sinus rhythm with blocked premature atrial complexes

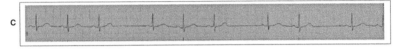

Tachy-brady syndrome with prolonged sinus pause

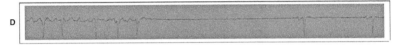

FIGURE 27-2. Examples of sinus node dysfunction. **(A)** Sinus bradycardia. The sinus rate is ~45 bpm. **(B)** Sinoatrial exit block. Note that the PP interval for the pause is exactly twice that of the nonpaused PP interval. **(C)** Blocked premature atrial complexes. This rhythm is often misinterpreted as sinus node dysfunction or atrioventricular block. Note the premature, nonconducted P waves inscribed in the T wave that resets the sinus node leading to the observed pauses. **(D)** Tachy–brady syndrome. Note the termination of atrial fibrillation followed by a prolonged 4.5-sec pause before the first sinus beat.

Atrioventricular Conduction Disturbances or Heart Block
- AV conduction can be prolonged (first-degree block), periodically interrupted (second-degree block), mostly interrupted (advanced or high-degree block), or completely absent (third-degree block) (Figure 27-3).
- **First-degree AV block** describes a conduction delay, usually localized to the AV node, that results in a PR interval >200 ms on ECG. "Block" is a misnomer because, by definition, there are no blocked beats (i.e., there is a QRS complex for every P wave).
- **Second-degree AV block** is present when there are periodic interruptions (i.e., dropped beats) in AV conduction. Distinction between Mobitz type I and Mobitz type II is important because they have a different natural history of progression to higher degrees of heart block.
  - **Mobitz type I block (Wenckebach)** is represented by a progressive prolongation in PR interval with successive atrial impulses until an impulse fails to conduct, followed by reiterations of the sequence. Type I block is usually localized to the AV node with an intact reliable junctional escape focus. This portends a **benign natural history**. On ECG, classic type I block manifests as:
    - Progressive prolongation of the PR interval before a nonconducted P wave. Correspondingly, the first PR interval after the nonconducted P wave is shorter than the last PR interval before the nonconducted P wave.
    - Shortening of each subsequent RR interval before the dropped beat. The RR interval encompassing the dropped beat will be less than twice the shortest RR interval.
    - A regularly irregular grouping of QRS complexes (group beating)

First-degree AV block

A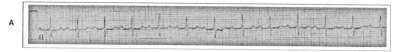

Second-degree AV block-mobitz type I (Wenckebach block)

B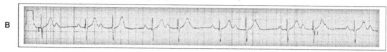

Second-degree AV block-mobitz type II

C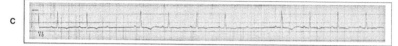

2:1 Second-degree AV block

D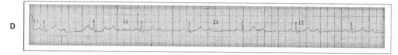

Third-degree (Complete) AV block

E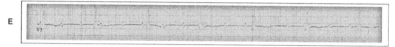

FIGURE 27-3. Examples of atrioventricular (AV) block. **(A)** First-degree AV block. There are no dropped beats, and the PR interval is >200 ms. **(B)** Second-degree 3:2 AV block Mobitz type I. Note the "group beating" and the prolonging PR interval before the dropped beat. There are regular P waves through this tracing with every third P wave inscribed in the terminal part of the preceding T wave. **(C)** Second-degree AV block Mobitz type II. Note the abrupt AV conduction block without evidence of progressive conduction delay. **(D)** Second-degree 2:1 AV block. This cannot be classified as Mobitz type I or II due to the absence of two consecutive conducted P waves. However, note the narrow QRS complex, which supports a more proximal origin of block (type I mechanism). A wider QRS with concomitant bundle branch or fascicular block would suggest a type II mechanism. **(E)** Complete heart block. Note the independent regularity of both the atrial and ventricular rhythms (junctional escape), which have no clear association with each other throughout the rhythm strip.

○ **Mobitz type II block** is often a marker of infranodal level of conduction block and may coexist with bundle branch or bifascicular block. Type II block is characterized by an abrupt AV conduction block without the progressive PR prolongation that is characteristic of block in the AV node. PR intervals remain unchanged preceding and following the nonconducted P wave. **Type II block carries an unfavorable prognosis** and is associated with high incidence of progression to complete heart block without a reliable junctional escape rhythm.

○ A **2:1 block** is characterized by conducted P waves alternating with blocked P waves. Due to the absence of two consecutive conducted P waves, a distinction between

Mobitz type I (prolonging PR intervals) and Mobitz type II (fixed PR intervals) cannot be made. The block may be inferred to be benign at the AV node level if the PR interval of the conducted beats is long (suggesting slow conduction within the AV node), there is absence of bundle branch block, and the same patient demonstrates Mobitz I (Wenckebach) block at other times. See Table 27-2 on how provocative measures can help distinguish the level of block, that is, intra-AV nodal versus infra-AV nodal.

- **Third-degree or complete heart block** is present when all atrial impulses fail to conduct to the ventricles. There is complete dissociation between the atria and the ventricles. In the absence of an artificial pacemaker, the patient will either have a dissociated regular escape junctional/ventricular rhythm or will be asystolic.

- **Advanced or high-degree AV block** is present when third-degree heart block is predominantly present, but occasionally, a P wave will conduct to the ventricle. Unlike complete AV block, the RR intervals will have some irregularity due to intermittent conduction.

- **Paroxysmal AV block:** Some patients with normal AV conduction at most times can have paroxysmal high-grade or complete AV block, often associated with presyncope or syncope. Paroxysmal AV block can be subcategorized as[4]:
  - **Intrinsic AV block** (cardiac syncope/Stokes–Adams attack): Intrinsic AV block is often associated with evidence of infranodal disease like bundle branch block and occurs in the elderly population. AV block can occur without any prodromal symptoms and has risk of progression to persistent AV block. An episode of AV block may be triggered by a compensatory pause following a premature ventricular or supraventricular complex.
  - **Extrinsic vagal AV block** (neurally mediated/reflex syncope): Vagally mediated AV block occurs at the level of AV node in setting of normal infranodal conduction (narrow QRS complex at baseline). AV block is often preceded by a brief vagal prodrome characterized by feeling warm, lightheaded, diaphoretic, and/or nauseated. Vagal AV block can be provoked by emotional stress, dehydration, prolonged standing, visual, auditory or olfactory stimuli, pain, cough, micturition, defecation, or carotid sinus pressure. Due to parasympathetic overactivity, the AV block is preceded by PR prolongation and is associated with slowing of the sinus rate (prolongation of PP intervals).
  - **Extrinsic adenosine-sensitive AV block**: Adenosine-sensitive AV block also occurs at the level of AV node, often in setting of normal infranodal conduction. However, as opposed to vagal block, this is not associated with changes in PR or PP intervals. Often, there is a long history of recurrent syncope without prodrome in a patient generally over age 40 years. Adenosine-sensitive block has been associated with low circulating levels of adenosine and exquisite AV node sensitivity to exogenous adenosine.

DIAGNOSIS

Clinical Presentation

- The clinical manifestations of bradyarrhythmias are variable, ranging from asymptomatic to nonspecific (e.g., lightheadedness, fatigue, weakness, exercise intolerance) to overt (i.e., syncope). The physician should try to delineate a **direct temporal relationship**

TABLE 27-2	RESPONSE OF ATRIOVENTRICULAR (AV) BLOCK WITH AUTONOMIC MANEUVERS	
Maneuver	**Block at level of AV node**	**Block at infranodal level**
Exercise/atropine	Improves conduction	Worsens conduction
Carotid sinus massage	Worsens conduction	Improves conduction

between bradycardia and symptoms. A summary of the approach to management of bradyarrhythmia is provided in Figure 27-4.

- The initial focus in evaluating a patient with bradycardia should be on assessing the **hemodynamic stability** of the arrhythmia. If the patient is demonstrating signs of poor end-organ perfusion (e.g., hypotension, altered mental status, cyanosis, acidosis), administration of atropine or IV catecholaminergic drugs and emergent transcutaneous or transvenous pacing may be required.

- If the patient is hemodynamically stable, a more thorough **history and physical examination** can be obtained, with emphasis on the following:

  ○ **Coronary ischemia**, especially involvement of the right coronary artery, can precipitate bradyarrhythmias, including sinus bradycardia and different degrees of AV block. Acute coronary syndrome should be considered in acute presentations with bradyarrhythmia.

  ○ Triggers that are known to elicit parasympathetic vagal outflow preceding episodes of presyncope/syncope suggest a **neurally mediated** etiology. A vagal response can occur by elicitation of neurocardiogenic/vasovagal reflex with emotional/orthostatic stress or unpleasant stimuli, or triggered by micturition, defecation, coughing, or carotid sinus pressure.

  ○ Tachyarrhythmias like AF suppress the sinus node. Pharmacologic drugs used to treat tachyarrhythmias generally further suppress the sinus node. The termination of a tachycardia episode in a patient with underlying sinus node disease may, therefore, be followed by sinus pauses (**tachy–brady syndrome**). The patient may have symptoms of palpitations, followed by lightheadedness or syncope.

  ○ Bradyarrhythmias may be a manifestation of an **underlying condition** like hypothyroidism, obstructive sleep apnea, connective tissue disorders, systemic inflammatory diseases, infections (e.g., endocarditis, Lyme disease, Chagas disease), congenital heart disease, infiltrative cardiomyopathies (e.g., sarcoidosis, amyloid, hemochromatosis), specific genetic cardiomyopathies (e.g., laminopathies, sodium channel mutations), neuromuscular diseases (e.g., Steinert myotonic dystrophy, Emery–Dreifuss muscular dystrophy, Kearns–Sayre syndrome), or prior cardiac surgery (Table 27-1).

  ○ Many **medications** (e.g., calcium channel blockers, β-blockers, digoxin, antiarrhythmic drugs, sedatives) or supplements can lead to bradycardia.

  ○ **Iatrogenic**

    ▪ **Catheter ablation** of the heart or **surgical maze** can lead to bradyarrhythmias, including sinus node dysfunction and AV block. Complete heart block can develop in <1% of patients undergoing atrial flutter ablation, 1-2% of AV nodal reentry tachycardia (AVNRT) ablation, and a higher rate for septal accessory pathway ablation and surgical maze.[5-7]

    ▪ **Surgical aortic valve replacement** can cause AV conduction abnormalities attributable to debridement of the right fibrous trigone and membranous septum with the calcified aortic annulus, resulting in trauma to the AV conduction system.[8] Postsurgical AV block may spontaneously resolve usually within 5 days. The incidence of permanent pacemaker (PPM) implantation after surgical aortic valve replacement is ~3-4%.[8,9]

    ▪ **Transcatheter aortic valve replacement (TAVR)** has a higher risk of AV conduction abnormalities. The incidence of complete heart block is device dependent. Self-expanding valves have a higher incidence of complete heart block, ~25%. Balloon-expanded valves have an incidence around 6%.[10] There is a small risk of paroxysmal intrinsic AV block late after TAVR, causing syncope or death.

    ▪ Other procedures such as ventricular septal defect closures (either transcatheter or surgical), mitral and tricuspid valve surgery, alcohol septal ablations, and congenital heart surgery have been known to cause AV conduction abnormalities.

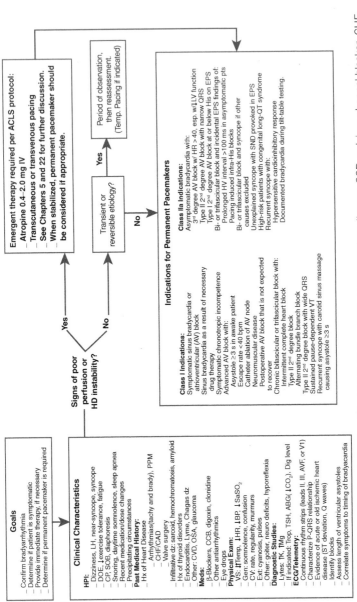

Goals
- Confirm bradyarrhythmia
- Determine if patient is symptomatic
- Provide immediate therapy, if necessary
- Determine if permanent pacemaker is required

Clinical Characteristics

HPI:
- Dizziness, LH, near-syncope, syncope
- DOE, ↓ exercise tolerance, fatigue
- CP, SOB, diaphoresis
- Snoring, daytime somnolence, sleep apnea
- Recent medication/dose changes
- Precipitating circumstances

Past Medical History:
- Hx of Heart Disease
  - Arrhythmias(tachy and brady), PPM
  - CHF/CAD
  - Valve surgery
- Infiltrative dz: sarcoid, hemochromatosis, amyloid
- Hx of thyroid disorders
- Endocarditis, Lyme, Chagas dz
- Other: CVD, OSA, glaucoma

Meds:
- β-Blockers, CCB, digoxin, clonidine
- Other antiarrhythmics
- Eye drops

Physical Exam:
- VS: ↑Temp, ↓HR, ↓BP, ↓SaO₂
- Gen: somnolence, confusion
- CV: rate, regularity, murmurs
- Ext: cyanosis, pulses
- Other: goiter, neuro deficits, hyporeflexia

Diagnostic Studies:
- Lytes: ↑K, ↑Mg
- If indicated: Trop, TSH, ABG (↓CO₂), Dig level

ECG/Telemetry:
- Continuous rhythm strips (leads II, III, AVF, or V1)
- Characterize P-QRS relationship
- Evidence of acute or old ischemic heart disease (ST deviation, Q waves)
- Identify blocks
- Assess length of ventricular asystoles
- Correlate symptoms to timing of bradycardia

Signs of poor perfusion or HD instability?

Yes → **Emergent therapy required per ACLS protocol:**
- Atropine 0.4–2.0 mg IV
- Transcutaneous or transvenous pacing
- See Chapters 5 and 22 for further discussion.
- When stabilized, permanent pacemaker should be considered if appropriate.

No → **Transient or reversible etiology?**

Yes → Period of observation, then reassessment. (Temp. Pacing if indicated.)

No →

Indications for Permanent Pacemakers

Class I Indications:
- Symptomatic sinus bradycardia or atrioventricular (AV) block
- Sinus bradycardia as a result of necessary drug therapy
- Symptomatic chronotropic incompetence
- Advanced AV block with:
  - Asystole ≥3 s in awake patient
  - Escape rate <40 bpm
  - Catheter ablation of AV node
  - Neuromuscular disease
  - Postoperative AV block that is not expected to recover
- Chronic bifascicular or trifascicular block with:
  - Intermittent complete heart block
  - Type II 2nd degree block
  - Alternating bundle branch block
- Type II 2nd degree block with wide QRS
- Sustained pause-dependent VT
- Recurrent syncope with carotid sinus massage causing asystole ≥3 s

Class IIa Indications:
- Asymptomatic bradycardia with:
  - 3rd degree AV block w/ HR >40, esp. w/↓LV function
  - Type II 2nd degree AV block with narrow QRS
  - Bi- or trifascicular AV block at or below His on EPS
- Incidental EPS findings of:
  - Prolonged HV interval >100 ms in asymptomatic pts
  - Pacing induced infra-His blocks
- Bi- or trifascicular block and syncope if other causes excluded
- Unexplained syncope with SND provoked in EPS
- High-risk patients with congenital long-QT syndrome
- Recurrent syncope with:
  - Hypersensitive cardioinhibitory response
  - Documented bradycardia during tilt-table testing.

FIGURE 27-4. Approach to bradyarrhythmias. AF, atrial fibrillation; CAD, coronary artery disease; CCB, calcium channel blocker; CHF, congestive heart failure; CP, chest pain; CVD, cerebrovascular disease; DOE, dyspnea on exertion; EPS, electrophysiologic study; HD, hemodynamic; LH, lightheadedness; OSA, obstructive sleep apnea; PPM, permanent pacemaker; SND, sinus node dysfunction; SOB, shortness of breath; VT, ventricular tachycardia; ↓BP, hypotension; ↓HR, bradycardia; ↓SaO₂, hypoxia; ↑K, hyperkalemia; ↑Mg, hypermagnesemia.

• A travel and social history may help identify a patient at risk for bradycardia due to infectious causes like Lyme or Chagas disease, or endocarditis, and family history could identify genetic causes.
• **Physical examination** should focus on identification of any findings suggesting systemic disorders such as thyroid abnormalities, systemic sclerosis, and neuromuscular disease. Physical examination correlates of bradycardia is a slow pulse and heart rate, first-degree AV block is a soft first heart sound, and complete heart block is cannon A waves on jugular venous pulse.

Diagnostic Testing
Electrocardiography
• **12-Lead ECG** is the cornerstone diagnostic tool in evaluation of bradycardia. It is prudent to examine rhythm strips from ECG leads that reveal discrete P waves (often easiest to see in leads II and/or V1).
• The analysis of ECG in the setting of bradycardia should focus on localizing the **level of dysfunction in the conduction system**. Sinus node function can be assessed by evaluating the PP intervals, AV conduction from P-R relationship, and bundle branch blocks from QRS duration and morphology. In addition to correlating symptoms to the bradyarrhythmia, the level of block will help determine risk of syncope/death (Figure 27-1).
• ECG features suggesting old and acute manifestations of **coronary artery disease** (e.g., ST elevations, T-wave inversions, pathologic Q waves) should be sought in addition to changes attributable to any cardiomyopathy, for example, low voltages with amyloidosis.

Laboratories and Imaging
• Laboratory studies should include **electrolytes** and **thyroid function tests** in most patients. Digoxin or other drug levels, cardiac enzymes to evaluate for myocardial injury or myocarditis, and Lyme serologies should be checked when clinically appropriate.
• **Echocardiogram** should be considered to evaluate systolic and valvular function, a transesophageal echocardiogram may be required to exclude endocarditis, and cardiac MRI may identify structural cardiomyopathies and myocarditis.

Rhythm Monitoring
• A routine 10-second ECG may not be sufficient if the arrhythmia is episodic and transient. In these circumstances, some form of continuous monitoring is indicated. In the inpatient setting, **continuous telemetry monitoring** can be utilized. In the outpatient setting, 24- or 48-hour **Holter monitor** is useful for patients with frequent symptom episodes. If the symptoms are infrequent, a 30-day **event recorder** or an **implantable loop recorder** (2-4 years) should be considered. Patients should be counseled to log symptoms during monitoring to establish a rhythm–symptom temporal correlation.
• **Smartphone ECG monitoring** systems work by having the patient use the thumb or finger on both hands to contact the case that allows recording of bipolar lead I single-lead ECG. This can be stored, viewed, and transmitted using the smartphone.[11] An important limitation is that the single-lead ECG is patient triggered and there is potential to miss the arrhythmia. Other smart devices like smart watches and pulse rate monitors can provide a log of pulse rate trends, with newer devices incorporating ECG capabilities.
• Evaluation of the pulse rate before and after walking the patient in the hallway or up a flight of stairs is an easy and inexpensive way to evaluate for the chronotropic response to exercise. A treadmill or bicycle **exercise ECG** can also be used to assess chronotropic response or elicit infranodal AV block exacerbated by an increase in sinus rate.

Electrophysiology Study
• An invasive electrophysiology (EP) study using transvenous catheters may be indicated in patients with AV conduction disturbance or unexplained syncope to evaluate the conduction system.[12]

• During an EP study, the His-Purkinje reserve is measured and provocative testing is performed to assess for impaired infranodal conduction. Normally, the **His-ventricular (HV) interval** is 35 to 55 ms. HV interval >70 ms demonstrates infranodal conduction disease. HV interval >100 ms, or presence of intra-/infra-Hisian block represents evidence of high-risk disease. Sodium channel blockers (ajmaline, flecainide, or procainamide) may be required to unmask high-risk AV conduction disease. If atrial pacing <150 to 170 bpm produces second- or third-degree block within the His-Purkinje system, this is considered abnormal and concerning for high-risk AV block.

• An EP study can also be used to study SA node function, but this is rarely of any clinical utility, and management decisions are primarily based on clinical symptoms.

TREATMENT

• Bradyarrhythmias that lead to hemodynamic instability are considered cardiovascular emergencies and should be managed as outlined in **acute cardiac life support (ACLS)** guidelines. See Chapters 40 and 41 for a more in-depth discussion of **temporary pacing** and management of severe, hemodynamically unstable bradycardia.

• Any **reversible causes** for bradycardia should be appropriately addressed. Medication list should be reviewed, and any medications exacerbating bradycardia should be evaluated for clinical need or discontinued.

Medications

• **Atropine** is an anticholinergic agent that given in doses of 0.5 to 2.0 mg IV is the cornerstone pharmacologic agent for the emergent treatment of bradycardia.

• IV **dopamine** (5 to 10 μg/kg/minute) or **epinephrine** (2 to 10 μg/minute) infusion may be used for symptomatic bradycardia unresponsive to atropine and is considered equally effective to external pacing as a temporizing measure. IV **isoproterenol** (2 to 20 μg/minute) infusion is a reasonable alternative.

• **Theophylline** is a noncompetitive adenosine-receptor antagonist and can be used PO (600 mg daily) to treat bradycardia, especially paroxysmal adenosine-sensitive AV block with syncope.

Temporary Pacing

• Temporary pacing is indicated for **Mobitz type II second-degree AV block or complete heart block** that causes syncope, presyncope, or occurs in the setting of an acute process, such as myocardial infarction (MI) or myocarditis.

• Sinus bradycardia, Mobitz type I second-degree AV block, or AF with a slow ventricular response may require temporary pacing only if significant symptoms or **hemodynamic instability** occur.

• Temporary pacing is achieved preferably via insertion of a **transvenous pacemaker,** usually from internal jugular or femoral venous access.

• External **transcutaneous pacing** is less preferable due to the lack of reliability of capturing the heart and patient discomfort. Transcutaneous pacing is contraindicated for hemodynamically stable patients with bradycardia as pacing may suppress intrinsic electrical activity and render them pacemaker dependent or may provoke malignant tachyarrhythmias, for example, in patients with hypothermia.

Permanent Pacing

• Once hemodynamic stability has been confirmed or reestablished as earlier, the focus turns to determining whether the patient's condition warrants placement of a PPM.

• In symptomatic patients, key determinants favoring PPM include **temporal correlation** of symptoms to the arrhythmia and **lack of reversible causative factors**.

- In asymptomatic patients, the key determinant indicating need for PPM is based on whether the conduction abnormality has a **natural history of progression to higher degrees of heart block**.

Permanent Pacemaker

- **Indications** for permanent pacing are listed in Figure 27-4.[13,14]
- Permanent pacing involves the placement of anchored, electronic pacing lead(s) in the atrium and/or the ventricle via central veins (or epicardial lead placement during cardiac surgery). The pacing leads are connected to the pacemaker generator that is commonly placed SC in the prepectoral region.
- Infrequent **complications** of PPM placement include pneumothorax, cardiac perforation with tamponade, lead dislodgement, device infection, deep venous thrombosis, and bleeding.
- Most pacemakers are programmed to provide electrical stimulation to the heart whenever the rate drops below a preprogrammed **lower rate limit**. Therefore, the ECG appearance of a pacemaker depends on pacemaker programming relative to the patient's intrinsic heart rate.
- A pacing system can be **single chamber** if one functional pacing lead is present in either the atrium or the ventricle, or **dual chamber** if leads are present in both the atrium and the ventricle.
- Contemporary PPMs can mimic normal physiology through maintenance of **AV synchrony** and **rate-adaptive programming** for chronotropic response.
- **Pacing artifacts/spikes** can be seen on surface ECG and if immediately followed by the generated P wave or QRS complex indicate capture of the chamber (Figure 27-5A).
- Atrial leads are typically placed in the right atrial appendage. Ventricular leads are usually placed at the right ventricular apex; therefore, the paced QRS complexes often assume a left bundle branch block (starting activation in the right ventricle) like morphology, with left superior axis (negative in the inferior leads II, III, and aVF) and negative precordial concordance. Chronic right ventricular pacing, like left bundle branch block, may have a deleterious hemodynamic effect and lead to adverse cardiac remodeling or **pacing-mediated cardiomyopathy**.
- Before PPM implantation, the patient must be free of any active infections, and anticoagulation issues must be considered. Hematomas in the pacemaker pocket develop most commonly in patients who are receiving IV heparin or SC low-molecular-weight heparin. In severe cases, surgical evacuation is required.

Leadless Pacemaker

- Leadless pacemakers are single-chamber ventricular pacemakers with the entire pacing system including the electrode, circuitry, and battery miniaturized in a large-drug-capsule-sized device with no need for leads (Figure 27-6). The entire pacemaker is implanted in the right ventricle using a delivery system inserted through the femoral vein.[15]
- The single-chamber ventricular leadless pacemaker is a solution for patients with permanent AF/flutter and slow intrinsic ventricular rates.[16]
- **Benefits**: Leadless pacemaker is feasible and minimizes risks in patients with limited vascular access, for example, patients on dialysis, and those at high risk of infections at conventional pacemaker surgical site.
- **Drawbacks**: Currently, leadless pacemakers are available only with single-chamber ventricular pacing capability and unable to provide dual-chamber pacing to maintain AV synchrony.

Cardiac Resynchronization Therapy

- Cardiac resynchronization therapy (CRT) involves placement of a pacemaker system with a specialized left ventricular lead often implanted in a posterior/lateral cardiac vein through the coronary sinus.[17-19] Dual-site pacing including a site on the posterior/lateral left ventricular wall is **hemodynamically superior** to single-site pacing from the right ventricle or intrinsic conduction with left bundle branch block.

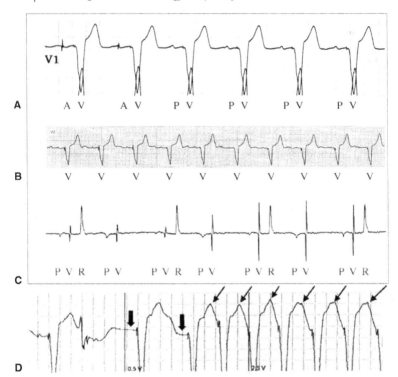

FIGURE 27-5. Pacemaker rhythms. **(A)** Normal dual-chamber (DDD) pacing. First two complexes are atrioventricular (AV) sequential pacing, followed by sinus with atrial sensing (P) and ventricular pacing (V). **(B)** Normal single-chamber (VVI) pacing. The underlying rhythm is atrial fibrillation (no distinct P waves), with ventricular pacing (V) at 60 bpm. **(C)** Pacemaker malfunction. The underlying rhythm is sinus (P) at 80 bpm with 2:1 heart block (R). Ventricular pacing spikes (V) are seen after each P wave, demonstrating appropriate sensing and tracking of the P waves but without ventricular capture. **(D)** Pacemaker-mediated tachycardia. Two ventricular-paced events (vertical arrows) lead to atrial sensed events (angled arrows). Each atrial sensed event is followed by ventricular pacing, which causes another atrial sensed event, and the cycle continues. (**A** to **C**: Reprinted with permission from Cooper DH, Faddis MN. Cardiac arrhythmias. In: Cooper DH, Krainik AJ, Lubner SJ, et al, eds. *The Washington Manual of Medical Therapeutics.* 32nd ed. Wolters Kluwer Health/Lippincott Williams & Wilkins; 2007:193-223.)

- CRT is recommended in **chronic systolic heart failure** patients and left bundle branch block with wide QRS complex or high-grade AV block requiring chronic ventricular pacing.
- **Benefits**: CRT is known to decrease ventricular dyssynchrony and promotes favorable reverse cardiac remodeling and improvement in cardiac function.
- **Drawbacks**: CRT is associated with longer procedure time, and it may not always be feasible due to the inability to appropriately place the left ventricular lead due to technical reasons. The left ventricular lead in a coronary vein is also prone to dislodgement, may

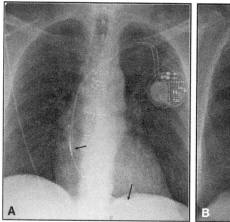
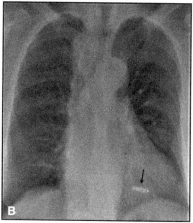

FIGURE 27-6. CXRs in posteroanterior projections showing, in part A, a transvenous dual-chamber pacemaker with right atrial and right ventricular leads (arrows), and in part B, a leadless pacemaker system in the right ventricle (arrow).

have suboptimal electrical parameters, and may cause extracardiac stimulation, such as left phrenic nerve stimulation. Further, the beneficial response to CRT may be unpredictable in an individual patient.

His Bundle Pacing
- His bundle pacing involves mapping the location of the penetrating AV bundle of His and placing an electrode to stimulate the His and the proximal left bundle branch in order to attain ventricular resynchrony with a narrow QRS complex.[20]
- **Benefits**: His bundle pacing can potentially be used for patients who may have a high burden of pacing to prevent right ventricular pacing–induced cardiomyopathy. It is valuable for heart failure patients in whom left ventricular lead placement for CRT has failed or proven futile.
- **Drawbacks**: Currently, the constraints with His bundle pacing include technical difficulty in implantation, lead instability, high pacing capture thresholds, and inability to circumvent distal conduction disease.

Biologic Pacemakers
- Two forms of biologic pacing are being developed and may become available for clinical use in the future.[21] **Gene therapy** with transcription factors transforms somatic ventricular myocytes to cells with increased automaticity and autonomically modulated pacemaking function. **Cell-based** approaches generate cells with pacemaker-like properties or use cells to deliver genes to form pacemaker units.

Pacing Modes
- Pacemakers are programmed to function in a specific manner described as a pacing modes designated by a naming system with a sequence of three to five letters.[22]
  - **Position I** denotes the chamber that is **paced**: A for atria, V for ventricle, D for dual (A and V), or O for none.
  - **Position II** refers to the chamber that is **sensed**: A for atria, V for ventricle, D for dual (A and V), or O for none.

- **Position III** denotes the type of **response** that the pacemaker will have to a sensed signal: I for inhibition, T for triggering, D for dual (I and T), or O for none.
  - **Position IV** is used to signify the presence of **rate-adaptive pacing** (R) in response to increased metabolic need.
  - **Position V** specifies the chamber(s) with multisite pacing: A for atria, V for ventricle, D for dual (A and V), or O for none.
  - The pacing mode is often designated with the **first three letters,** respectively, for chamber paced, chamber sensed, and the response function (e.g., VVI, DDD, or AAI), and the fourth letter R can be added when rate-adaptive pacing is enabled.
- There are several variables to consider in choosing the most appropriate pacing system and mode for a patient—the primary indication for placement, the responsiveness of the sinus node, the state of AV conduction, the presence of comorbid tachyarrhythmias, and the patient's activity level.
- The most common pacing modes are **VVI(R)**, **DDD(R)**, and **AAI(R)**.[23] In general, an exclusive single-chamber atrial system (AAI) is used only for pure sinus node dysfunction in the absence of any AV conduction abnormalities. The presence or possibility of AV conduction disease makes a dual-chamber device (DDD) more appropriate. Patients with permanent AF warrant a single-chamber ventricular device (VVI).
- Dual-chamber pacemakers have the capability of **mode switching**. When a patient with a pacemaker operating in DDD mode develops AF or flutter, the pacemaker switches to a nontracking DDI mode to avoid rapid ventricular pacing from tracking the atrial arrhythmia. It will return to DDD when the tachyarrhythmia resolves.
- There are a variety of algorithms for dual-chamber pacemakers to promote native AV conduction and **avoid ventricular pacing** and its attendant adverse effects on hemodynamics and cardiac remodeling. These include:[24]
  - Some algorithms function in a **single-chamber atrial mode** (ADI mode) and switch to DDD on the detection of AV block, including Managed Ventricular Pacing (MVP™, Medtronic), Rhythmiq™ (Boston Scientific), and I-Opt™ (Biotronik). The pacemaker will revert back to ADI once AV conduction has recovered.
  - **AV hysteresis** prolongs AV delay so long as AV conduction is present to promote intrinsic conduction. If intrinsic conduction fails to prevent ventricular pacing, pacing is delivered with a shorter and more physiologic AV delay. The algorithm periodically checks for return of intrinsic conduction by prolonging the AV delay for one beat.

Pacemaker Malfunction

- Pacemaker malfunction is a potentially life-threatening situation, particularly for patients who are pacemaker dependent. The workup of suspected malfunction should begin with a 12-lead ECG (Figure 27-5).
- If no pacing activity is seen, a **magnet** can be placed over the pacemaker generator to assess for ability to deliver pacing output and capture and resume pacing. Application of a magnet switches most pacemakers to an **asynchronous pacing mode** such as VVI becomes VOO (asynchronous ventricular pacing) and DDD becomes DOO (asynchronous sequential AV pacing). It usually does not affect pacing function in implanted defibrillators where a magnet is used to disable ventricular tachyarrhythmia detection and defibrillator shock function.
- If malfunction is obvious or if the ECG is unrevealing and malfunction is still suspected, then a formal **pacemaker interrogation** should be done. Patients should carry a card identifying the make and model of the device.
- A CXR (two views) should also be obtained to assess for evidence of overt lead abnormalities (dislodgement, fracture, migration).
- General categories of pacemaker malfunction include oversensing, failure to output, failure to capture, undersensing, and pacemaker-mediated tachycardia.

○ **Oversensing** refers to situations where a pacemaker **does not deliver a stimulus when it should**. It generally occurs when the pacemaker senses an inappropriate signal as cardiac activity. Inappropriate signal could be cardiac, such as T-wave oversensing and crosstalk (sensing QRS complexes on atrial lead); extracardiac, such as pectoralis or diaphragmatic myopotential oversensing; noise from lead malfunction (conductor fracture or insulation break); or external electromagnetic interference. An example can be seen during surgery when electrocautery on the torso can be oversensed, leading to inappropriate inhibition of pacing. In patients who are pacemaker dependent, temporarily programming the pacemaker in asynchronous mode is recommended.

○ **Failure to output** can be occasionally seen if a patient fails to undergo timely generator replacement and battery reaches end of life. Pure generator or battery malfunction resulting in failure to output is quite rare.

○ **Undersensing** occurs when intrinsic cardiac activity falls below the programmed sensing threshold and is not identified by the pacemaker. This may lead to pacing output spikes on top of native P, QRS, or T complexes and can occasionally provoke tachyarrhythmia by pacing at inappropriately short coupling interval from undersensed intrinsic systole.

○ **Failure to capture** refers to situations where the pacing stimulus is delivered but fails to recruit the paced chamber, that is, failure to generate P or QRS complex. Elevation in the threshold voltage required to initiate a depolarization wave can occur due to changes in the tissue surrounding the electrode (i.e., fibrosis), antiarrhythmic drugs, electrolyte/metabolic abnormalities, lead fractures, or micro/macro lead dislodgement.

○ **Pacemaker-mediated tachycardia** or endless loop tachycardia occurs due to continuous tracking of retrograde atrial impulses created by the previous ventricular-paced beat, resulting in ventricular pacing at pacemaker upper rate limit (Figure 27-5D).

SPECIAL CONSIDERATIONS

Acute myocardial infarction

• Bradyarrhythmias and conduction abnormalities in the setting of MI are common. Careful consideration must be given to the artery involved, the extent of infarct, prior conduction disease, and success of reperfusion to best determine whether the arrhythmia will be self-limiting or irreversible.

• **Inferior MI** can result in AV block that is typically at the level of the **AV node**. In the first 24 hours, AV nodal block can result from a heightened vagal tone (Bezold–Jarisch reflex) and may be responsive to atropine. Adenosine released from ischemic myocardium may be responsible AV node block for 1 to 2 weeks and is responsive to theophylline or aminophylline. Due to dual circulation to the AV node, it is generally resistant to infarction and conduction abnormalities usually resolve without need for permanent pacing.

• **Anterior MI** is more likely to cause conduction abnormalities due to necrosis of the **infranodal** His bundle or proximal bundle branches that are less likely to respond and may be worsened with atropine. Post MI infranodal block is likely to be irreversible and requires permanent pacing.

Cardiac Transplantation

• **Cardiac denervation** and withdrawal of the neural autonomic regulation to the heart following cardiac transplantation generally result in donor's heart to revert to elevated inherent sinus rates usually 80 to 110 bpm.

• **Sinus node dysfunction** can also occur and is the most common bradyarrhythmia presentation.[25,26] Causes include surgical trauma, perioperative ischemia, residual effect of pretransplant amiodarone, and rejection. Bicaval anastomosis, now more common than biatrial anastomosis, decreases the likelihood of surgical trauma to the sinus node or sinus node artery and, therefore, sinus node dysfunction.

- AV conduction block is rare after cardiac transplant. Incident **AV block** should prompt high suspicion for **allograft rejection or vasculopathy**.
- **Right bundle branch block** is a common finding in post-transplant patients and is thought to be a consequence of periodic endomyocardial biopsies of the right ventricular septum to ensure appropriate immunosuppression.

Infectious Causes of Bradyarrhythmias

- Although infections and febrile illness typically cause resting tachycardia, some infectious syndromes can be complicated by bradyarrhythmias.
- In patients with suspected or known **endocarditis**, ECGs should be ordered and carefully reviewed daily for prolongation of the PR interval or higher degree AV block, which can signal the presence of an underlying or developing aortic root abscess.
- **Lyme disease**, a tick-borne illness caused by *Borrelia burgdorferi* and endemic to the northeastern US, can present with a constellation of findings that includes myocarditis, conduction abnormalities, and, rarely, left ventricular failure. Dynamically evolving first-degree AV block with PR prolongation and higher degrees of AV conduction blocks can be seen.[27] Marked PR prolongation (>300 ms) predicts progression to complete heart block.[28] These dysrhythmias typically resolve within days to weeks with appropriate antibiotic therapy, rarely requiring permanent pacing.
- **Chagas disease**, a protozoan illness endemic to South America, presents with cardiac involvement in over 90% of cases. In addition to heart failure, patients can present with all degrees of AV block.

Bradycardia Due to Neurologic Causes

- Increased intracranial pressure causes stretch of the brainstem and results in a reflex vagally mediated bradycardic response.
  - The presence of **bradycardia**, **hypertension**, and **respiratory depression** (Cushing triad or reflex) should raise suspicion for intracranial hypertension.
  - Clinical situations that could lead to intracranial hypertension include hepatic failure, central nervous system tumors, trauma, and hydrocephalus. These medical emergencies require immediate treatment to avoid catastrophic neurologic compromise.
- Injury to the central nervous system, especially transection of the spinal cord, can lead to **autonomic lability** and transient episodes of bradycardic or asystolic hemodynamic collapse. This may respond to parasympatholytic agents such as atropine and catecholaminergic agents such as dopamine or theophylline, but may on occasion require pacing support.
- Systemic autonomic disorders (e.g., multiple system atrophy, inflammatory demyelinating neuropathies, diabetes mellitus, amyloidosis) can lead to varied syndromes encompassing orthostatic hypotension, postural tachycardia syndrome, and reflex bradycardia.
- **Neurally mediated reflex syncope** is generally a benign condition that includes carotid sinus hypersensitivity, situational syncope (cough, micturition, defecation), and neurocardiogenic (vasovagal) syncope.
  - Unopposed parasympathetic vagal outflow provoked by stimulation of stretch receptors (carotid sinuses or cardiac mechanoreceptors activated due to reduced blood return) results in transient hypotension due peripheral vasodilatation and bradycardia.
  - Triggers include dehydration, unpleasant visual or olfactory stimuli, and prolonged standing, and treatment generally involves adequate hydration, trigger avoidance, and fall prevention.

Drug Toxicity

- **Digoxin** toxicity should be suspected in any patient taking digoxin, the elderly, patients with renal insufficiency, or interacting medications such as amiodarone. Digoxin toxicity classically presents with enhanced automaticity and increased AV block, classically paroxysmal atrial tachycardia with AV block. Therapy is supportive, with temporary pacing and discontinuation of digoxin.

- ○ In life-threatening situations, **digoxin-specific antibodies** (Digibind and DigiFab) can be used as an antidote to bind to digoxin and making it unavailable for toxic effects.[29]
- ○ Digoxin-specific antibodies can precipitate heart failure and severe hypokalemia and carries significant expense. It should be reserved for situations where significant overdose (>10 mg) is suspected, extreme serum digoxin levels (>10 ng/mL) are discovered, or life-threatening bradyarrhythmias are present.

- If **β-blocker** toxicity is suspected, **atropine** (up to 2 mg IV), IV fluids, and **glucagon** (50 to 150 µg/kg IV over 1 minute, followed by 1 to 5 mg/hour in 5% dextrose) can be used to bypass the β-adrenergic receptor blockade and act downstream to improve contractility and heart rate.
  - ○ If bradycardia and hypotension persist, escalation of management would sequentially include IV insulin/glucose, calcium, isoproterenol, and vasopressors (norepinephrine or dopamine).
  - ○ Hemodialysis may be useful with sotalol, atenolol, acebutolol, and nadolol, but not with metoprolol, propranolol, or timolol. Temporary transvenous pacing can be used for high-grade AV block unresponsive to initial management.

- If **calcium channel blocker** overdose is suspected, **glucagon** and **calcium** should be administered. Calcium channel blocker toxicity tends to be less responsive to atropine.
  - ○ The nondihydropyridines (diltiazem and verapamil) are more likely to cause bradycardia, sinus pauses, and high-grade AV block. Dihydropyridines (amlodipine, nifedipine, and nicardipine) will cause hypotension and, more commonly, a reflex tachycardia.
  - ○ Transvenous temporary pacing can be used for heart block refractory to noninvasive management.

REFERENCES

1. Mangrum JM, DiMarco JP. The evaluation and management of bradycardia. *N Engl J Med.* 2000;342:703-9.
2. Pejković B, Krajnc I, Anderhuber F, Kosutić D. Anatomical aspects of the arterial blood supply to the sinoatrial and atrioventricular nodes of the human heart. *J Int Med Res.* 2008;36:691-8.
3. Anderson RH, Yanni J, Boyett MR, et al. The anatomy of the cardiac conduction system. *Clin Anat.* 2009;22:99-113.
4. Aste M, Brignole M. Syncope and paroxysmal atrioventricular block. *J Arrhythm.* 2017;33:562-7.
5. Belhassen B, Glick A, Rosso R, et al. Atrioventricular block during radiofrequency catheter ablation of atrial flutter: incidence, mechanism, and clinical implications. *Europace.* 2011;13:1009-14.
6. Hindricks G. Incidence of complete atrioventricular block following attempted radiofrequency catheter modification of the atrioventricular node in 880 patients. Results of the Multicenter European Radiofrequency Survey (MERFS) The Working Group on Arrhythmias of the European Society of Cardiology. *Eur Heart J.* 1996;17:82-8.
7. Schwagten B, Knops P, Janse P, et al. Long-term follow-up after catheter ablation for atrioventricular nodal reentrant tachycardia: a comparison of cryothermal and radiofrequency energy in a large series of patients. *J Interv Card Electrophysiol.* 2011;30:55-61.
8. Erdogan HB, Kayalar N, Ardal H, et al. Risk factors for requirement of permanent pacemaker implantation after aortic valve replacement. *J Card Surg.* 2006;21:211-5; discussion 216-7.
9. Nagaraja V, Raval J, Eslick GD, Ong ATL. Transcatheter versus surgical aortic valve replacement: a systematic review and meta-analysis of randomised and non-randomised trials. *Open Heart.* 2014;1:e000013.
10. Lee MY, Yeshwant SC, Chava S, Lustgarten DL. Mechanisms of heart block after transcatheter aortic valve replacement–cardiac anatomy, clinical predictors and mechanical factors that contribute to permanent pacemaker implantation. *Arrhythm Electrophysiol Rev.* 2015;4:81-5.
11. Walsh JA 3rd, Topol EJ, Steinhubl SR. Novel wireless devices for cardiac monitoring. *Circulation.* 2014;130(7):573-81.

12. Katritsis DG, Josephson ME. Electrophysiological testing for the investigation of bradycardias. *Arrhythm Electrophysiol Rev.* 2017;6:24-8.

13. Epstein AE, DiMarco JP, Ellenbogen KA, et al. ACC/AHA/HRS 2008 guidelines for device-based therapy of cardiac rhythm abnormalities: a report of the American College of Cardiology/American Heart Association task force on practice guidelines. *J Am Coll Cardiol.* 2008;51:e1-62.

14. Epstein AE, DiMarco JP, Ellenbogen KA, et al. 2012 ACCF/AHA/HRS focused update incorporated into the ACCF/AHA/HRS 2008 guidelines for device-based therapy of cardiac rhythm abnormalities. *J Am Coll Cardiol.* 2013;61:e6-75.

15. Ritter P, Duray GZ, Steinwender C, et al. Early performance of a miniaturized leadless cardiac pacemaker: the Micra Transcatheter Pacing Study. *Eur Heart J.* 2015;36:2510-9.

16. Gillis AM, Russo AM, Ellenbogen KA. et al. HRS/ACCF expert consensus statement on pacemaker device and mode selection. *J Am Coll Cardiol.* 2012;60:682-703.

17. Abraham WT, Fisher WG, Smith AL, et al. Cardiac resynchronization in chronic heart failure. *N Engl J Med.* 2002;346:1845-53.

18. Curtis AB. Biventricular pacing for atrioventricular block and systolic dysfunction. *N Engl J Med.* 2013;369:579.

19. Cleland JG, Daubert JC, Erdmann E, et al. The effect of cardiac resynchronization on morbidity and mortality in heart failure. *N Engl J Med.* 2005;352:1539-49.

20. Ellenbogen KA, Padala SK. His bundle pacing: the holy grail of pacing? *J Am Coll Cardiol.* 2018;71:2331-4.

21. Boink GJ, Christoffels VM, Robinson RB, Tan HL. The past, present, and future of pacemaker therapies. *Trends Cardiovasc Med.* 2015;25:661-73.

22. Bernstein AD, Daubert JC, Fletcher RD, et al. The revised NASPE/BPEG generic code for antibradycardia, adaptive-rate, and multisite pacing. North American Society of Pacing and Electrophysiology/British Pacing and Electrophysiology Group. *Pacing Clin Electrophysiol.* 2002;25:260-4.

23. Lamas GA, Ellenbogen KA. Evidence base for pacemaker mode selection: from physiology to randomized trials. *Circulation.* 2004;109:443-51.

24. Auricchio A, Ellenbogen KA. Reducing ventricular pacing frequency in patients with atrioventricular block: is it time to change the current pacing paradigm? *Circ Arrhythm Electrophysiol.* 2016;9:e004404.

25. Thajudeen A, Stecker EC, Shehata M, et al. Arrhythmias after heart transplantation: mechanisms and management. *J Am Heart Assoc.* 2012;1:e001461.

26. Leonelli FM, Pacifico A, Young JB. Frequency and significance of conduction defects early after orthotopic heart transplantation. *Am J Cardiol.* 1994;73:175-9.

27. McAlister HF, Klementowicz PT, Andrew C, et al. Lyme carditis: an important cause of reversible heart block. *Ann Intern Med.* 1989;110:339-45.

28. Steere AC, Batsford WP, Weinberg M, et al. Lyme carditis: cardiac abnormalities of Lyme disease. *Ann Intern Med.* 1980;93:8-16.

29. Antman EM, Wenger TL, Butler VP Jr, et al. Treatment of 150 cases of life-threatening digitalis intoxication with digoxin-specific Fab antibody fragments. Final report of a multicenter study. *Circulation.* 1990;81:1744-52.

Atrial Fibrillation

28

Curtis M. Steyers III and Mitchell N. Faddis

GENERAL PRINCIPLES

- Atrial fibrillation (AF) is the most common sustained arrhythmia, accounting for over one-third of hospitalizations for cardiac arrhythmias.
- AF is associated with thromboembolic stroke, heart failure, and increased all-cause mortality.
- AF can be classified by frequency and duration of symptoms into paroxysmal, persistent, long-standing persistent, and permanent categories.
- The management for AF includes rate control, rhythm control, and anticoagulation to prevent thromboembolism.
- Rate control is achieved with β-blockers, calcium channel blockers, or digoxin.
- Rhythm control is achieved with antiarrhythmic drugs and synchronized direct current (DC) cardioversion. Surgical and catheter-based therapies are available for selected patients.
- The overall goal of preventing thromboembolic events with oral anticoagulation must be balanced against the bleeding risks. The $CHADS_2VASC$ risk score estimates yearly stroke risk based on underlying risk factors in patients with nonvalvular AF.[1,2]

Definition

- AF is a supraventricular arrhythmia characterized by rapid, uncoordinated, chaotic electrical activity in the atria and deterioration of normal atrial mechanical function, with an irregular ventricular response.
- Mechanism of AF is likely multifactorial; however, it primarily involves focal electrical "triggers" that originate predominantly from the pulmonary veins (PVs) and an anatomic substrate capable of initiation and perpetuation of AF.

Classification[3,4]

- Current classification of AF focuses on timing and duration of AF episodes and may not accurately identify subtypes of AF pathophysiology. This classification scheme more directly reflects decisions made by patients and physicians regarding medical interventions. For example, an individual patient may have either paroxysmal or persistent AF, depending on the timing of a planned electrical cardioversion.
- **Paroxysmal AF:** AF episodes terminate spontaneously or with intervention <7 days after onset.
- **Persistent AF:** Continuous AF lasting >7 days or requiring electrical or pharmacologic cardioversion. Episodes may occur rarely and terminate easily with electrical cardioversion or may persist for many years (long-standing persistent AF).
- **Long-standing persistent AF**: Continuous AF lasting >1 year
- **Permanent AF:** Long-standing persistent AF wherein a decision has been made not to pursue restoration of sinus rhythm by any means, including electrical cardioversion, antiarrhythmic drug therapy, catheter, or surgical ablation
- **Nonvalvular AF:** Occurring in the absence of rheumatic mitral stenosis, prosthetic heart valve, or mitral valve repair

Epidemiology

- AF afflicts up to 6 million people in North America alone, but it is frequently asymptomatic and diagnosed only after a complication, such as a stroke. AF often coexists with other conditions, including hypertension, heart failure, coronary heart disease, and valvular/structural heart disease.[5-8]
- AF is strongly associated with increasing age. The estimated prevalence of AF is ~1% in the general population, with a wide range from 0.1% among adults <55 years to over 9% among octogenarians.[5-8]
- The lifetime risk of developing AF is nearly one in four.[5-8]

Etiology

In the overwhelming majority of cases, AF occurs in the context of multiple risk factors, most of which are common chronic diseases. Rarely, initiation of AF may be more directly and causally linked to an underlying disease or exposure, which may be at least partially reversible. The **mnemonic PIRATES** can be a helpful way to remember some of these causes and risk factors (Table 28-1).

Pathophysiology

- The pathophysiology of AF can be broadly organized into **triggers**, responsible for initiation of AF, and **maintenance**, responsible for perpetuation of AF.
- In most cases, AF is triggered by repetitive firing from sleeves of atrial myocardium at the PV ostia extending into the PVs. Occasionally, AF can be triggered by other organized supraventricular tachycardia (SVT) mechanisms such as atrial flutter or atrioventricular nodal reentrant tachycardia (AVNRT).[9-11]
- There are multiple proposed mechanisms for AF maintenance, including **multiple reentrant wavelets, spiral wave reentry and high-frequency rotors** in the body of the left atrium.[9-11]
- Maintenance of AF is thought to be dependent on an anatomic substrate capable of supporting one of several proposed mechanisms discussed earlier. The conduction properties of the atrium are influenced by multiple chronic disease states, such as hypertension, diabetes mellitus, obesity, cardiomyopathy, and obstructive sleep apnea, and likely arise from atrial fibrosis, inflammation, and mechanical stretch.
- Restoration of sinus rhythm has a higher success rate when it is achieved rapidly; there is increasing stability of AF with the longer the arrhythmia is present.
- The axiom "a-fib begets a-fib" refers to **atrial electrical remodeling that reinforces the mechanisms underlying AF,** such as shortening of the atrial action potential duration and refractory period.

TABLE 28-1	FACTORS THAT PREDISPOSE PATIENTS TO ATRIAL FIBRILLATION ("PIRATES" MNEMONIC)

P—pericarditis, pulmonary disease, pulmonary embolism, postoperative
I— ischemia, infection
R—rheumatic heart disease (particularly mitral valve disease)
A—alcohol ("holiday heart"), atrial myxoma
T—thyrotoxicosis, theophylline
E—enlargement (particularly left atrial enlargement)
S—systemic hypertension, sick sinus syndrome, sleep apnea, and size (obesity)

DIAGNOSIS

Clinical Presentation

History

- Common symptoms include **palpitations, shortness of breath, fatigue, decreased exertional capacity**, and **chest discomfort**.
- Less commonly, orthopnea and edema from heart failure can occur. In the presence of sinus node dysfunction, patients may have conversion pauses >4 seconds and present with syncope.
- An embolic event can cause focal neurologic symptoms or organ/limb ischemia.
- **Many episodes of AF are asymptomatic.**[11]
- It is important to determine the clinical pattern of AF, including time of onset, precipitating cause, and duration and frequency of symptoms, along with complications and coexisting disorders. In addition, a past medical history can assess for underlying cardiac disease, and social habits can be helpful to identify risk factors.

Physical Examination

- Significant findings may be absent if AF is paroxysmal. If present, there can be an irregular pulse, tachycardia, or the absence of the *a* wave in the jugular venous pulsation. For more severe cases, heart failure signs may be present.
- It is important to identify possible etiologies such as valvular murmurs or wheezing for underlying pulmonary disease. A goiter may be present, indicating hyperthyroidism. Other findings may include focal neurologic deficits demonstrating recent thromboembolism.

Diagnostic Testing

Laboratories

If appropriate, thyroid function tests and cardiac biomarkers should be checked.

Electrocardiography

- AF can be identified on ECG or rhythm strip as an **irregularly irregular ventricular rhythm without discrete P waves.** The atrial activity can vary widely, from coarse fibrillatory waves similar to atrial flutter to very fine, sometimes indiscernible baseline undulations between QRS complexes (Figure 28-1).

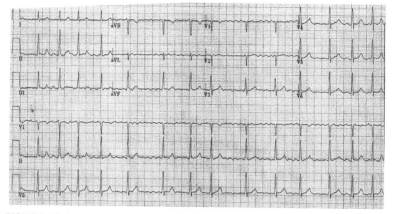

FIGURE 28-1. Typical ECG demonstrating atrial fibrillation. Note the irregular ventricular rhythm and fibrillatory waves that have replaced P waves.

- The ventricular rate during AF can be highly variable and reflects the state of the AV node (AVN) and distal conduction system. Younger patients can conduct extremely rapidly, sometimes with rates >200 beats per minute, while older patients may have normal ventricular rates due to diseased AVNs. Autonomic tone and medications can further modulate the AVN response. Patients with accessory pathways can conduct extremely rapidly, bypassing the AVN, and may be at risk for ventricular fibrillation.
- AF may occur with additional arrhythmias, including atrial flutter and focal atrial tachycardias.
- The **Ashman phenomenon** refers to wide-complex beats that arise due to transient block in one bundle branch—usually right bundle branch block—of the atrial impulses at varying cycle lengths, characteristically preceded by a "long–short" interval.
- Ambulatory cardiac rhythm monitoring is indicated for outpatients in whom AF is suspected. It is helpful to identify the frequency and duration of paroxysmal AF.

Imaging
- CXR can be helpful to identify intrinsic pulmonary pathology and assess cardiac borders.
- Echocardiography:
  - The transthoracic echocardiogram can evaluate ventricular size and function, atrial size, and the presence of structural heart disease.
  - Transesophageal echocardiography (TEE) is much more sensitive for identifying thrombi in the left atrium and left atrial appendage. TEE is used to assess left atrial and left atrial appendage thrombi before cardioversion in patients without appropriate duration of preceeding anticoagulation.[3]
  - Echocardiographic features associated with the development of AF include mitral regurgitation, left atrial enlargement, left ventricular (LV) hypertrophy, and reduced LV fractional shortening.[12]

TREATMENT

- Patients with new-onset AF can often be managed on an outpatient basis. Indications for hospital admission include signs, symptoms, or ECG findings concerning for ongoing ischemia; difficult to control ventricular rate; advanced age with frailty; decompensated heart failure; hemodynamic compromise; or the need for the initiation of QT-prolonging antiarrhythmic medications.
- There are three main goals in the management of AF:
  - **Rate control**
  - **Rhythm control**
  - **Anticoagulation to prevent thromboembolism**
- The appropriate choice of therapy is tailored to each patient based on the type of AF, safety factors, symptoms, and patient preference. Refer to the management overview and algorithm for evaluating newly diagnosed AF, recurrent paroxysmal AF, recurrent persistent AF, and permanent AF (Figures 28-2 through 28-4).[13]

Rate Control

- Ventricular rate control allows for adequate filling during diastole, improved hemodynamics, reduces symptoms associated with AF, and may prevent development of tachycardia-induced cardiomyopathy.
- Strict rate control (<80 beats per minute at rest or <110 beats per minute during 6-minute walk) is not superior to lenient rate control (resting heart rate <110 beats per minute) in patients with persistent AF who have ejection fraction >40%.[14,15]
- In hospitalized patients, correction of acute medical problems (hypovolemia, hypoxia, infection, pain, thyrotoxicosis) dramatically improves the success of rate control.

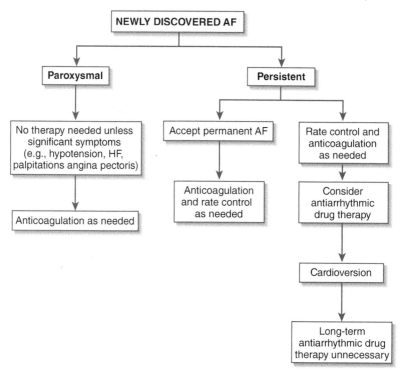

FIGURE 28-2. Management overview and algorithm with pharmacologic therapy for patients with newly diagnosed atrial fibrillation (AF). HF, heart failure. (Reprinted from Fuster V, Rydén LE, Cannom DS, et al. 2011 ACCF/AHA/HRS focused updates incorporated into the ACC/AHA/ESC 2006 guidelines for the management of patients with atrial fibrillation: a report of the American College of Cardiology Foundation/American Heart Association Task Force on Practice Guidelines developed in partnership with the European Society of Cardiology and in collaboration with the European Heart Rhythm Association and the Heart Rhythm Society. *J Am Coll Cardiol.* 2011;57(11):e101-98. Copyright © 2011 American College of Cardiology Foundation, the American Heart Association, Inc., and the European Society of Cardiology. With permission.)

- **Pharmacologic rate control is achieved by modulating conduction through the AVN.** There are four classes of agents available for routine use: **β-blockers, nondihydropyridine calcium channel blockers, digoxin, and amiodarone.**[3]
- **β-Blockers:**
  - First-line agent for rate control in most patients with AF. Preferred drug for AF associated with thyrotoxicosis, acute myocardial infarction, and high adrenergic tone in the postsurgical state
  - IV formulations can be used for acute rate control for inpatients.
  - Use with caution in patients with acute decompensated heart failure or reactive airway disease
- **Calcium channel blockers** (nondihydropyridine):
  - Another first-line agent for rate control in most patients with AF
  - IV diltiazem or verapamil given as a continuous infusion is effective for acute rate control in hospitalized patients who fail to respond to initial bolus dosing of β-blockers or calcium channel blockers.
  - Avoid use in patients with systolic heart failure and hypotension.

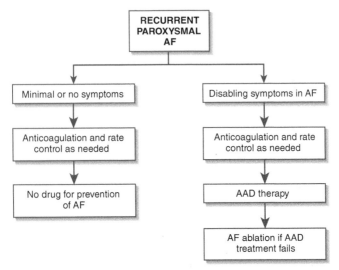

FIGURE 28-3. Management overview and algorithm with pharmacologic therapy for patients with recurrent paroxysmal atrial fibrillation (AF). AAD, antiarrhythmic drug. (Reprinted from Fuster V, Rydén LE, Cannom DS, et al. 2011 ACCF/AHA/HRS focused updates incorporated into the ACC/AHA/ESC 2006 guidelines for the management of patients with atrial fibrillation: a report of the American College of Cardiology Foundation/American Heart Association Task Force on Practice Guidelines developed in partnership with the European Society of Cardiology and in collaboration with the European Heart Rhythm Association and the Heart Rhythm Society. *J Am Coll Cardiol.* 2011;57(11):e101-98. Copyright © 2011 American College of Cardiology Foundation, the American Heart Association, Inc., and the European Society of Cardiology. With permission.)

- **Digoxin:**
  - Reduces AVN conduction directly and by increasing vagal activity
  - Reserved for patients with AF and symptomatic heart failure with reduced ejection fraction who cannot tolerate negative inotropic and hypotensive effects of β-blockers and calcium channel blockers
  - Ineffective in patients with uncontrolled ventricular rates during exercise (sympathetically driven)
  - Renally excreted; avoid use in patients with significant renal dysfunction
  - Less effective than first-line options mentioned earlier.
- **Amiodarone:**
  - Class III antiarrhythmic that also decreases AVN conduction through its effect on calcium channels and β-adrenergic receptors
  - Considered a **second-line** agent for rate control, used primarily in critically ill patients with hypotension or decompensated heart failure
  - Potential for pharmacologic cardioversion and attendant risk of thromboembolism in patients with prolonged AF who are not anticoagulated
  - Inhibits warfarin metabolism often requiring dose reduction of warfarin to maintain stable international normalized ratio (INR)
- In patients in whom maintenance of sinus rhythm has been abandoned or is not achievable and pharmacologic rate control has been inadequate, **AVN ablation** can be considered as a last-resort option to control ventricular rate. **Requires permanent pacemaker implantation** at the time of the procedure, if not already present.

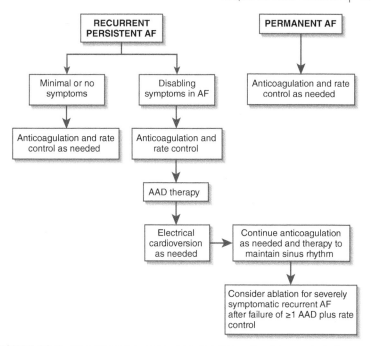

FIGURE 28-4. Management overview and algorithm with pharmacologic therapy for patients with recurrent persistent or permanent atrial fibrillation (AF). AAD, antiarrhythmic drug. (Reprinted from Fuster V, Rydén LE, Cannom DS, et al. 2011 ACCF/AHA/HRS focused updates incorporated into the ACC/AHA/ESC 2006 guidelines for the management of patients with atrial fibrillation: a report of the American College of Cardiology Foundation/American Heart Association Task Force on Practice Guidelines developed in partnership with the European Society of Cardiology and in collaboration with the European Heart Rhythm Association and the Heart Rhythm Society. *J Am Coll Cardiol.* 2011;57(11):e101-98. Copyright © 2011 American College of Cardiology Foundation, the American Heart Association, Inc., and the European Society of Cardiology. With permission.)

Rhythm Control

- Restoration and maintenance of sinus rhythm can be achieved in the following ways:
  - **Antiarrhythmic medications**
  - **Electrical cardioversion**
  - **Catheter ablation**
  - **Surgical ablation (Cox-Maze)**
- For most patients, a combination of several interventions (antiarrhythmic medication and DC cardioversion) is required to maintain sinus rhythm. Patients generally require lifelong follow-up and often require repeated interventions over time.
- After successful DC cardioversion, only 20-30% of patients maintain sinus rhythm for 1 year without additional antiarrhythmic therapy.
- Risk factors for recurrence: advanced age, heart failure, left atrial enlargement, rheumatic heart disease, and hypertension[3-5]
- Two large randomized controlled trials comparing a rhythm control strategy with anti-arrhythmic medications and DC cardioversion versus rate control strategy in AF **failed**

to **demonstrate mortality benefit** for the rhythm control strategy. Furthermore, there was **no reduction in stroke or heart failure** end points with rhythm control strategy.[14-19]

- Despite the absence of evidence for improvement in hard outcomes with a pharmacologic rhythm control strategy, many patients with symptomatic AF prefer restoration and maintenance of sinus rhythm to improve quality of life. In general, **the decision to pursue a rhythm control strategy should be driven by symptoms.**[4,20]
- In selected patients with AF and symptomatic heart failure with reduced ejection fraction, emerging evidence suggests that restoring and maintaining sinus rhythm with catheter ablation may prevent worsening heart failure, improve ejection fraction, and reduce all-cause mortality compared to a rate control strategy.[20-22]

Antiarrhythmic Medications

- There are multiple antiarrhythmic medications available to restore and maintain sinus rhythm; appropriate selection is guided primarily by an understanding of the patient's comorbidities and safety profile of each agent. See Figure 28-5.[13] The following medications are currently recommended for routine use in AF[3,20,23]:
  - Vaughan-Williams class Ic: **flecainide, propafenone**
  - Vaughan-Williams class III: **dofetilide, sotalol, amiodarone, dronedarone**
- For every patient, one must consider the following comorbid conditions before selecting an antiarrhythmic agent:
  - Coronary artery disease
  - LV systolic dysfunction

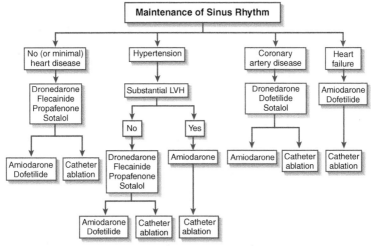

FIGURE 28-5. Management overview and algorithm for antiarrhythmic therapy to maintain normal sinus rhythm, based on various disease states, for patients with recurrent paroxysmal or persistent atrial fibrillation. LVH, left ventricular hypertrophy. (Adapted from Fuster V, Rydén LE, Cannom DS, et al. 2011 ACCF/AHA/HRS focused updates incorporated into the ACC/AHA/ESC 2006 guidelines for the management of patients with atrial fibrillation: a report of the American College of Cardiology Foundation/American Heart Association Task Force on Practice Guidelines developed in partnership with the European Society of Cardiology and in collaboration with the European Heart Rhythm Association and the Heart Rhythm Society. *J Am Coll Cardiol.* 2011;57(11):e101-98. Copyright © 2011 American College of Cardiology Foundation, the American Heart Association, Inc., and the European Society of Cardiology. With permission.)

- ○ LV hypertrophy
- ○ Prolonged QT interval or history of torsades de pointes
- ○ Renal or hepatic dysfunction
- Pharmacologic cardioversion is less effective than DC cardioversion, although pretreatment with certain antiarrhythmic medications (e.g., amiodarone, flecainide, ibutilide, propafenone, sotalol) can enhance the success of DC cardioversion.[3,20,22]
- **Proarrhythmia** is the most important risk associated with antiarrhythmic agents. Antiarrhythmic drugs that prolong the QT interval increase the risk of torsades de pointes and are often initiated and titrated on an inpatient basis with continuous telemetry monitoring and routine ECGs.[3]
- Several antiarrhythmic agents are associated with **organ toxicity** and require regular outpatient follow-up with laboratory monitoring.
- Amiodarone in particular should be reserved for patients with refractory AF who have failed or cannot tolerate alternative agents, or for patients of advanced age in whom the risk of long-term organ toxicity is not as relevant.

Cardioversion

- Cardioversion can be performed with **synchronized DC electrical current and/or antiarrhythmic medications**.[3,20]
- Because of the increased risk of thromboembolic events in the first several weeks after cardioversion, elective cardioversions should generally be performed with therapeutic anticoagulation and continued for a minimum of 4 weeks thereafter.[3,20]
- If the patient is hemodynamically unstable, urgent synchronized DC cardioversion is warranted without anticoagulation.[3,20]
- Other situations in which cardioversion can be considered without anticoagulation include short-duration AF (<48 hours) or after a TEE demonstrates the absence of a left atrial thrombus.[3,20]
- In the stable patient, if the AF has lasted >48 hours, is of unknown duration, or there is coexisting mitral stenosis or a history of a thromboembolism, cardioversion should be delayed until anticoagulation can be maintained at appropriate levels (INR of 2.0 to 3.0 with warfarin, consistent uninterrupted use of a novel oral anticoagulant) for 3 to 4 weeks or until TEE evaluation for thrombi of the left atrial appendage is performed.[3,20]

Ablation

- **Catheter ablation**:
  - ○ Catheter ablation of AF is a rapidly evolving field. As new techniques and technologies are developed and new literature emerges, the role of catheter ablation in the management of AF is likely to change significantly.
  - ○ **Pulmonary vein isolation (PVI)** is the most common form of AF ablation and is based on the observation that AF is triggered, in the majority of cases, by rapidly firing foci in the ostia of the PVs.[3,10,20]
  - ○ During PVI, catheters are advanced into the left atrium via a transseptal approach after percutaneous femoral venous access. Radiofrequency energy, or in some cases cryothermal energy, is applied in a pattern that encircles and electrically isolates the antra of the PVs, preventing PV triggers from initiating AF.
- Catheter ablation has the following advantages over alternative rhythm control strategies[3,20-24]:
  - ○ **More effective than antiarrhythmic medications** at maintaining sinus rhythm
  - ○ Potential to **avoid toxicities** associated with long-term use of antiarrhythmic medications
  - ○ **Lower procedural morbidity and mortality** than surgical AF ablation (Cox-Maze)
- The main disadvantages of catheter ablation are procedural complications and lower efficacy than surgical AF ablation.

- The efficacy of AF ablation varies significantly across studies (50-88%) and is dependent upon several variables[3,24]:
  - Pattern of AF (paroxysmal vs. persistent)
  - Presence or absence of structural heart disease and left atrial enlargement
  - End point of interest (burden of AF, quality of life, symptoms)
- Although the indications for catheter ablation continue to evolve, it can currently be considered in the following scenarios[3,20]:
  - **For symptom relief** in symptomatic patients with paroxysmal or persistent AF refractory to or intolerant of at least one class I or III antiarrhythmic medication
  - **For symptom relief** in symptomatic patients with paroxysmal or persistent AF without prior trial of antiarrhythmic medication when avoidance of medication is desired
  - **For prevention of worsening heart failure and death** in symptomatic patients with persistent AF and systolic heart failure (New York Heart Association [NYHA] classes II to III)
- **Surgical ablation:**
  - The gold-standard surgical treatment for AF is the **Cox-Maze procedure**, which aims to eliminate all macroreentrant circuits that may develop in the atria.[3,20]
  - Initially, this procedure involved many surgical incisions across both the right and left atria ("cut and sew"), but more refined variations have used linear ablation lines with various energy systems, including radiofrequency energy, microwave, cryoablation, laser, and high-intensity–focused ultrasound. Long-term success is reported to be 70% to >95%.[3,20]
  - Often used in patients undergoing concomitant cardiac surgery (mitral valve surgery) but can be considered as a stand-alone procedure and in selected patients who have been refractory to catheter ablation or in patients for whom catheter ablation is expected to be unsuccessful

Lifestyle/Risk Modification

- For obese patients, weight loss can reduce the burden of AF.
- Sleep-disordered breathing can trigger AF, and evaluation with a sleep study is appropriate in select patients.
- Activity restriction has not been shown to reduce AF burden.

PREVENTION OF ISCHEMIC STROKE

Risk Stratification

- Perhaps the most important tenet of AF management is risk stratification and prevention of thromboembolic ischemic stroke.
- AF independently increases the risk of ischemic stroke by a number of mechanisms. Thrombus formation is promoted by a loss of coordinated mechanical contraction in the fibrillating left atrium, leading to stasis of blood. The left atrial appendage is particularly susceptible thrombus formation.
- The annual risk of stroke from AF has been estimated at 1.5% in patients aged 50 to 59 years and 23.5% in patients aged 80 to 89 years.[25]
- The risk of thromboembolism should be routinely assessed for all patients with nonvalvular AF using the **CHA_2DS_2-VASc** scoring system (Table 28-2). Patients with valvular AF are at elevated risk of thromboembolism and should not be risk stratified using the CHA_2DS_2-VASc score.[2,3,20]
- The decision to initiate antithrombotic therapy in AF must weigh the risk of thromboembolic events against the risk of major bleeding and should be **independent** of the pattern of AF, or the decision to pursue a rhythm versus rate control strategy.
- The decision to initiate antithrombotic therapy must be individualized for each patient. General recommendations are shown in Table 28-2.

TABLE 28-2 **STROKE RISK IN PATIENTS WITH NONVALVULAR ATRIAL FIBRILLATION**

CHA_2DS_2-VASc Risk Criteria[1-3]	Points
Congestive Heart Failure/LV Dysfunction	1
Hypertension	1
Age >75 Years	2
Diabetes Mellitus	1
Prior **S**troke, TIA, thromboembolism	2
Peripheral **V**ascular Disease or Coronary Artery Disease	1
Age 65–74 Years	1
Sex Category (i.e., Female Sex)	1

CHA2DS2-VASc Score	Recommended therapy
0	No therapy preferred
1	Aspirin, 81–325 mg daily, or oral anticoagulant[a]
≥2	Oral anticoagulant[b]

Score	Adjusted stroke rate (% per year) based on CHA2DS2-VASc score 2–3
0	0
1	1.3
2	2.2
3	3.2
4	4.0
5	6.7
6	9.8
7	9.6
8	6.7
9	15.2

AF, atrial fibrillation; INR, international normalized ratio; LV, left ventricular; TIA, transient ischemic attack.

[a]No therapy is acceptable for patients <65 years old and no heart disease (lone AF).

[b]If warfarin is the oral anticoagulant used, INR should be 2.0–3.0, with a target of 2.5. INR <2.0 is not effective at preventing strokes. If mechanical valve, target INR >2.5.

Antithrombotic Therapy

- **Warfarin**
  - Warfarin inhibits vitamin K–dependent coagulation factor synthesis in the liver.
  - The anticoagulation effect of warfarin is highly variable with genetic polymorphisms, oral intake of vitamin K, and interactions with other drugs.

○ The anticoagulation effect can be monitored with the INR blood test, which is a standardized way to report the prothrombin time (PT). In most patients, the goal INR is 2.0 to 3.0, although a higher INR target may be warranted in specific clinical scenarios.

○ Warfarin is the oldest and most extensively studied antithrombotic agent available. In the following clinical situations, it is the only recommended agent due to an absence of safety data with novel oral anticoagulants[3,20]:

  ▪ Patients with **mechanical prosthetic heart valves**
  ▪ Patients with **end-stage renal disease on hemodialysis**
  ▪ **Pregnancy**

• **Direct-oral anticoagulants (DOACs):**

  ○ For important considerations, see Table 28-3.
  ○ Novel agents directly inhibit specific downstream enzymes in the coagulation cascade, including:
  ○ Direct thrombin inhibitors: **dabigatran**
  ○ Direct factor Xa inhibitors: **rivaroxaban, apixaban, edoxaban**

    ▪ As a rule, DOACs do not require laboratory testing for monitoring of anticoagulation effect. This feature makes DOACs highly desirable for most patients and physicians.
    ▪ Because all DOACs are **renally excreted**, dose adjustment based on estimated glomerular filtration rate is critical.
    ▪ An important limitation of many DOACs is the lack of widely available reversal agents. Agents such as prothrombin complex concentrate (PCC) or recombinant factor VIIa (rFVIIa) may be considered, but these have not been studied in clinical trials.

TABLE 28-3	ANTITHROMBOTIC THERAPY FOR PATIENTS WITH ATRIAL FIBRILLATION			
	Dabigatran	*Apixaban*	*Rivaroxaban*	*Edoxaban*
Mechanism of Action	**Direct thrombin inhibitor**	**Direct factor Xa inhibitor**	**Direct factor Xa inhibitor**	**Direct factor Xa inhibitor**
Dosing (PO)	75–150 mg bid[a]	2.5–5 mg bid[b]	15–20 mg qday[c]	30–60 mg qday[d]
Renal clearance	85%	~27%	~33%	50%
Mean half-life ($t_{1/2}$)	14–17 hours	~12 hours	5–13 hours	10–14 hours
Time to peak effect	0.5–2 hours	3–4 hours	2–4 hours	1–2 hours

[a]150 mg bid for patients with CrCl >30 mL/min; 75 mg bid for patients with CrCl 15–30 mL/min. Discontinue use in patients who develop acute renal failure. Do not use in patients with mechanical heart valves.

[b]5 mg bid is recommended dose. 2.5 mg bid is recommended for patients with at least two of the following: age of 80 years or older, body weight of 60 kg or less, SCr of 1.5 mg/dL or more. Not recommended for use in patients with severe hepatic impairment.

[c]20 mg with evening meal for patients with CrCl >50 mL/min; 15 mg with evening meal for patients with CrCl 15–50 mL/min. Do not use in patients with moderate and severe hepatic impairment or with hepatic disease associated with coagulopathy.

[d]30 mg once daily for patients with CrCl <30 mL/min.

Data from individual drug package inserts.

- **Idarucizumab** is a humanized anti-dabigatran monoclonal antibody available for patients taking dabigatran who develop intractable or life-threatening bleeding.
- **Andexanet alfa** is a recombinant, catalytically inactive form of factor Xa that acts as a reversal agent for factor Xa inhibitors. This agent is not currently widely available.
  ○ Dabigatran:
    - Direct thrombin inhibitor approved to reduce the risk of stroke and systemic embolism in patients with nonvalvular AF based largely on a head-to-head trial comparing dabigatran to warfarin (RE-LY)[26]
    - The 150-mg bid dose was superior to warfarin for stroke prophylaxis, though it had similar rates of important bleeding events.
    - The 110-mg bid dose (not currently available in the United States) was noninferior to warfarin for stroke prevention, with lower rates of bleeding events.
    - The 75-mg bid dose that is currently available was not formally studied.
    - The most common side effect is dyspepsia or gastric ulcers, attributed to the acidic nature of the medication.
  ○ Apixaban:
    - Oral factor Xa inhibitor approved to reduce the risk of stroke and systemic embolism in patients with nonvalvular AF
    - In the pivotal ARISTOTLE trial, apixaban was superior to warfarin for prevention of stroke or systemic embolism, bleeding events, and mortality.[27]
    - The standard dose is 5 mg bid. Dose reduction to 2.5 mg bid should be considered if patients meet **two of the following criteria**:
      □ Body mass <60 kg
      □ Age >80 years
      □ Serum creatinine >1.5 mg/dL
  ○ Rivaroxaban:
    - Oral factor Xa inhibitor approved to reduce the risk of stroke and systemic embolism in patients with nonvalvular AF
    - In ROCKET AF, its pivotal clinical trial, rivaroxaban was noninferior to warfarin for prevention of stroke or systemic embolism, with similar overall major bleeding events and fewer intracranial and fatal bleeding events.[28]
    - Rivaroxaban is marketed for **once-daily dosing**. It **should be taken with the evening meal** for adequate absorption.
    - Dose reduction is necessary for renal impairment. Patients with creatinine clearance <50 mL/min should receive 15 mg instead of the standard 20-mg dose.
  ○ Edoxaban:
    - Oral factor Xa inhibitor approved to reduce the risk of stroke and systemic embolism in patients with nonvalvular AF
    - Edoxaban was **noninferior to warfarin** for prevention of stroke or systemic embolization and was superior to warfarin with respect to bleeding and cardiovascular death in the ENGAGE AF-TIMI 48 trial leading to its approval.[29]
    - Longer half-life allows for **once-daily dosing.**
    - Dose reduction from 60 to 30 mg once daily is required for patients with creatinine clearance <30 mL/min.

Left Atrial Appendage Exclusion

- The left atrial appendage is thought to be the most common location of thrombus formation, leading to systemic embolization and stroke in patients with AF. Mechanical exclusion of the left atrial appendage from the body of the left atrium may reduce the risk of stroke or systemic embolization.

- Although most patients with AF should receive oral antithrombotic therapy, the risk of major bleeding occasionally precludes the use of these agents.
  - Patients with **recurrent falls** resulting in injury
  - Patients with recurrent severe **gastrointestinal hemorrhage**
  - Patients with prior **intracranial hemorrhage**
  - Patients with inherited or acquired **coagulation disorders** associated with bleeding
- There are two major approaches to left atrial appendage exclusion: **surgical** and **percutaneous**.
- **Surgical** excision or ligation of the appendage can be performed at the time of surgery for other indications. Common scenarios include mitral valve surgery or Maze procedure.
- Several techniques have been used for **percutaneous** left atrial appendage exclusion. The most widely used device is currently the **WATCHMAN** device, a self-expandable nitinol cage covered with a permeable polytetrafluoroethylene (PTFE) membrane that is implanted in the left atrial appendage via a transseptal approach.
  - Two randomized trials comparing WATCHMAN to long-term warfarin therapy led to the device's Food and Drug Administration (FDA) approval.
    - The PROTECT AF study demonstrated noninferiority of the WATCHMAN device with respect to its primary efficacy end point of stroke, major bleeding, or cardiovascular death.[30]
    - The subsequent PREVAIL study did not meet prespecified noninferiority criteria; however, event rates were similar.[31]
    - The WATCHMAN device is currently FDA approved for patients with nonvalvular AF who have indications for long-term anticoagulation but for whom there are reasons to avoid long-term anticoagulation. Importantly, **patients must be fully anticoagulated for at least 6 weeks postimplantation.**

SPECIAL CONSIDERATIONS

- Wolff–Parkinson–White (WPW) syndrome[3]:
  - **Preexcited AF can be life-threatening** due to the potential for rapid antegrade conduction over an accessory pathway and degeneration into ventricular fibrillation.
  - **Calcium channel blockers are contraindicated** in patients with WPW, due to their effect of promoting antegrade conduction over the accessory pathway.
  - Hemodynamically unstable patients with preexcited AF should be electrically cardioverted. Alternatively, stable patients may respond to IV procainamide or amiodarone infusion. **Avoid diltiazem and verapamil** in this scenario as noted earlier.
- Sinus node dysfunction:
  - Patients with AF associated with sinus node dysfunction often have prolonged pauses when AF converts to sinus rhythm.
  - Sinus pauses and sinus bradycardia may preclude the use of AVN blocking agents and poses a challenge when attempting to achieve adequate rate control in AF. **Permanent pacemaker implantation** is often required in this situation.[3]

REFERENCES

1. Gage BF, Waterman AD, Shannon W, et al. Validation of clinical classification schemes for predicting stroke: results from the National Registry of Atrial Fibrillation. *JAMA.* 2001;285:2864-70.
2. Lip GY, Nieuwlaat R, Pisters R, Lane DA, Crijns HJ. Refining clinical risk stratification for predicting stroke and thromboembolism in atrial fibrillation using a novel risk factor-based approach: the Euro Heart Survey on Atrial Fibrillation. *Chest.* 2010;137:263-72.
3. January CT, Wann LS, Alpert JS, et al. 2014 ACCF/AHA/HRS guideline for the management of patients with atrial fibrillation: a report of the American College of Cardiology/American

Heart Association Task Force on Practice Guidelines and the Heart Rhythm Society. *Circulation.* 2014;130:e199-267.

4. Calkins H, Kuck KH, Cappato R, et al. 2012 HRS/EHRA/ECAS expert consensus statement on catheter and surgical ablation of atrial fibrillation: recommendations for patient selection, procedural techniques, patient management and follow-up, definitions, endpoints, and research trial design. *Heart Rhythm.* 2012;9:632-96.

5. Kornej J, Börschel CS, Benjamin EJ, Schnabel RB. Epidemiology of atrial fibrillation in the 21st century: novel methods and new insights. *Circ Res.* 2020;127:4-20.

6. Cameron A, Schwartz MJ, Kronmal RA, et al. Prevalence and significance of atrial fibrillation in coronary artery disease (CASS Registry). *Am J Cardiol.* 1988;61:714-7.

7. Go AS, Hylec, EM, Philips KA, et al. Prevalence of diagnosed atrial fibrillation in adults: national implications for rhythm management and stroke prevention: the Anticoagulation and Risk Factors in Atrial Fibrillation (ATRIA) study. *JAMA.* 2001;285:2370-5.

8. Krahn AD, Manfreda J, Tate RB, et al. The natural history of atrial fibrillation: incidence, risk factors, and prognosis in the Manitoba follow-up study. *Am J Med.* 1995;98:476-84.

9. Chen SA, Hsieh MH, Tai CT, et al. Initiation of atrial fibrillation by ectopic beats originating from the pulmonary veins: electrophysiological characteristics, pharmacological responses, and effects of radiofrequency ablation. *Circulation.* 1999;100:1879-86.

10. Haïssaguerre M, Jais P, Shah DC, et al. Spontaneous initiation of atrial fibrillation by ectopic beats originating in the pulmonary veins. *N Engl J Med.* 1998;339:659-66.

11. Page RL, Wilkinson WE, Clair WK, et al. Asymptomatic arrhythmias in patients with symptomatic paroxysmal atrial fibrillation and paroxysmal supraventricular tachycardia. *Circulation.* 1994;89:224-7.

12. Vaziri SM, Larson MG, Benjamin EJ, Levy D. Echocardiographic predictors of nonrheumatic atrial fibrillation. The Framingham Heart Study. *Circulation.* 1994;89:724-30.

13. Fuster V, Rydén LE, Cannom DS, et al. 2011 ACCF/AHA/HRS focused updates incorporated into the ACC/AHA/ESC 2006 guidelines for the management of patients with atrial fibrillation. *J Am Coll Cardiol.* 2011;57:e101-98.

14. Van Gelder IC, Groenveld HF, Crijns HJ, et al. Lenient versus strict rate control in patients with atrial fibrillation. *N Engl J Med.* 2010;362:1363-73.

15. Van Gelder IC, Hagens VE, Bosker HA, et al. A comparison of rate control and rhythm control in patients with recurrent persistent atrial fibrillation. *N Engl J Med.* 2002;347:1834-40.

16. Wyse DG, Waldo AL, DiMarco JP, et al. A comparison of rate control and rhythm control in patients with atrial fibrillation. The Atrial Fibrillation Follow-up Investigation of Rhythm Management (AFFIRM) investigators. *N Engl J Med.* 2002;347:1825-33.

17. Carlson J, Miketic S, Wendeler J, et al. Randomized trial of rate-control versus rhythm-control in persistent atrial fibrillation: the Strategies of Treatment of Atrial Fibrillation (STAF) study. *J Am Coll Cardiol.* 2003;41:1690-6.

18. Opolski G, Torbicki A, Kosior DA, et al. Rate control vs rhythm control in patients with nonvalvular persistent atrial fibrillation: the results of the Polish How to Treat Chronic Atrial Fibrillation (HOT CAFE) Study. *Chest.* 2004;126:476-86.

19. Honloser SH, Kuck KH, Lilienthal J. Rhythm or rate control in atrial fibrillation—Pharmacological Intervention in Atrial Fibrillation (PIAF): a randomised trial. *Lancet.* 2000;356:1789-94.

20. Anderson JL, Halperin JL, Albert NM, et al. Management of patients with atrial fibrillation (compilation of 2006 ACCF/AHA/ESC and 2011 ACCF/AHA/HRS recommendations): a report of the American College of Cardiology/American Heart Association Task Force on Practice Guidelines. *J Am Coll Cardiol.* 2013;61:1935-44.

21. Prabhu S, Taylor AJ, Costello BT. Catheter ablation versus medical rate control in atrial fibrillation and systolic dysfunction: the CAMERA-MRI Study. *J Am Coll Cardiol* 2017;70:1949-61.

22. Marrouche NF, Brachmann J, Andresen D, et al. Catheter ablation for atrial fibrillation with heart failure. *N Engl J Med.* 2018; 378:417-27.

23. Nichol G, McAlister F, Pham B, et al. Meta-analysis of randomized controlled trials of the effectiveness of antiarrhythmic agents at promoting sinus rhythm in patients with atrial fibrillation. *Heart.* 2002;87:535-43.

24. Terasawa T, Balk E, Chung M. Systematic Review: Comparative effectiveness of radiofrequency catheter ablation for atrial fibrillation. *Ann Intern Med.* 2009;151:191-202.

25. Wolf PA, Abbott RD, Kannel WB. Atrial fibrillation as an independent risk factor for stroke: the Framingham Study. *Stroke.* 1991;22:983-8.

26. Connolly SJ, Ezekowitz MD, Yusuf S, et al. Dabigatran versus warfarin in patients with atrial fibrillation. *N Engl J Med.* 2009;361:1139-51.

27. Granger CB, Alexander JH, McMurray JJ, et al. Apixaban versus warfarin in patients with atrial fibrillation. *N Engl J Med.* 2011;365:981-92.

28. Patel MR, Mahaffey KW, Garg J, et al. Rivaroxaban versus warfarin in nonvalvular atrial fibrillation. *N Engl J Med.* 2011;365:883-91.

29. Giugliano RP, Ruff CT, Braunwald EB, et al. Edoxaban versus warfarin in patients with atrial fibrillation. *N Engl J Med.* 2013;369:2093-104.

30. Reddy VY, Sievert H, Halperin J, et al. Percutaneous left atrial appendage closure vs warfarin for atrial fibrillation. *JAMA.* 2014; 312:1988-98.

31. Holmes DR, Kar S, Price MJ, et al. Prospective randomized evaluation of the WATCHMAN left atrial appendage closure device in patients with atrial fibrillation versus long-term warfarin therapy: the PREVAIL trial. *J Am Coll Cardiol.* 2014;64:1-12.

Approach to Syncope

Krasimira M. Mikhova, J. Ernesto
Betancourt, and Daniel H. Cooper

29

GENERAL PRINCIPLES

- The evaluation of syncope can be daunting as there are myriad circumstances that can cause or mimic this common clinical problem.
- It is a presentation that requires a consistent approach with realization that a clear precipitating etiology is not diagnosed in half of events.
- Our role as consultants is to help risk stratify patients for future events via diagnostic testing, as appropriate, and to recommend therapy to prevent recurrences and reduce the risk of injury or death.

Definition

- The term "syncope" should be applied to situations where there is:
  ○ **Temporary, transient loss of consciousness (TLOC)**
  ○ Complete and, typically, rapid recovery
  ○ Global **cerebral hypoperfusion** as the final common pathway, regardless of etiology
- Otherwise, the episode should be referred to as transient loss of consciousness (TLOC) so as to include nonsyncopal etiologies in the differential diagnosis (Table 29-1).

Epidemiology

- The prevalence of syncope is 19-50%, depending on the population studied, with a higher incidence in women.[1-3]
- The age distribution of syncope illustrates three peaks[4].
  ○ The first around 20 years of age (women > men)
  ○ Then in patients around 60 years of age
  ○ Finally around 80 years of age
- Syncope accounts for ~1% of emergency department visits in the US, with 27-35% of those visits resulting in hospital admission.[5,6]

TABLE 29-1	CAUSES OF NONSYNCOPAL TLOC	
No loss of consciousness	**Partial or complete loss of consciousness**
Falls	Epilepsy
Cataplexy/drop attacks	Intoxication
Psychogenic pseudosyncope	Metabolic disorders (hypoglycemia and hypoxemia)
TIA	TIA
CAD	Vertebrobasilar disease

CAD, carotid artery disease; TIA, transient ischemic attack; TLOC, transient loss of consciousness.

Etiology

- Syncope first must be differentiated from nonsyncopal events involving real or apparent TLOC, such as seizures and falls (Table 29-1).
- Further subdivision of true syncope is based on specific pathophysiologic etiologies that include the following four general categories (Table 29-2) in descending order of frequency:
  - Neurally mediated (reflex) syncope
  - Orthostatic syncope
  - Primary cardiac arrhythmias
  - Structural cardiac or cardiopulmonary disease

DIAGNOSIS

Clinical Presentation

- Initial evaluation of syncope utilizes the **history**, **physical examination**, and **ECG** to classify presumed causes and identify patients who are at high risk for death. There are three key questions that need to be answered with the initial evaluation:
  - Is loss of consciousness attributable to syncope or not?
  - Is heart disease present or not?
  - Are there important clinical features in the history that suggest the diagnosis?
- In addition, consideration of inpatient versus outpatient evaluation should depend on comorbidities and initial findings. In general, patients with the following should be admitted to avoid delay and adverse outcomes:
  - Elderly (age > 65 years)
  - Known structural heart disease
  - Symptoms suggestive of primary cardiac syncope
  - Abnormal ECG
  - Severe orthostatic hypotension
  - Focal neurologic deficits
  - Family history of sudden death
  - Exertional syncope
  - Syncope causing severe injury
  - Syncope while driving

History

- Often, the diagnosis of syncope is evident from a comprehensive history.
- Aspects of the history that need to be explored in order to aid diagnosis and further categorize the event include a prodrome **before** the attack, **eyewitness** accounts during the event, the patient's recollection immediately **after** the attack, **circumstances** that may have played a causative role in the event, and general questions about the patient's medical **history**.
- A helpful mnemonic is: "I passed out on the BEACH" (Table 29-3).
- **For patients with recognizable reflex or orthostatic syncope that occurs infrequently or as an isolated episode, no further workup is necessary.** These patients generally have a good prognosis and can be managed as outpatients with treatments listed below.
- **In patients with a suspected cardiac etiology, an inpatient cardiac evaluation is warranted.** Features on history that may suggest cardiac etiology include syncope during exertion or while supine, little or no prodrome, quick recovery (unless prolonged unconsciousness), personal history of structural heart disease, or family history of sudden unexplained death.

Physical Examination

- The examination should include assessment of orthostatic vital signs and careful neurologic, pulmonary, and cardiovascular assessment.

TABLE 29-2   CLASSIFICATION AND CLASSIC PRESENTATIONS OF SYNCOPE

Types of syncope	Classic presentations
Reflex (neurally mediated)	Combination of reflex bradycardia and vasodilation, most common cause of syncope
Vasovagal	Precipitated by emotional stress, prolonged standing. Prodrome often includes diaphoresis, warmth, pallor, and/or nausea.
Carotid sinus	Precipitated by carotid artery manipulation
Situational	Related to micturition, defecation, or coughing
Orthostatic hypotension	Posture changes result in symptoms and/or a drop in systolic blood pressure >20 mm Hg
Volume depletion	Heat exposure, decreased oral intake, diuretic use
Autonomic failure	Parkinson disease, diabetes, cardiac amyloidosis
Drug induced	Nitrates, α-blockers, clonidine, other antihypertensives
Cardiac arrhythmia	Insufficient cardiac output to meet systemic demands due to either bradycardia or tachycardia Often preceded by palpitations
Sinus node dysfunction	Symptomatic bradycardia, sick sinus syndrome with AF
AV conduction disease	β-Blockers, calcium channel blockers, Lenègre disease
Tachycardias	SVT or VT
Long QT	Congenital and/or drug induced. Current use of certain antiarrhythmic, antihistamine, antibiotic, antipsychotic, antidepressant medications
Cardiopulmonary disease	Insufficient cardiac output to meet systemic demands due to abnormalities in the structure or function of the heart Clues include known cardiac disease, exertional syncope, family history of sudden death, and syncope while supine
Valvular heart disease	Severe aortic stenosis
Acute ischemia/infarction	Particularly right ventricular infarct
HCM	Often exercise-induced syncope
Pulmonary hypertension or embolism	Acute decrease in LV filling
Vascular steal	Subclavian steal syndrome, with increased arterial blood flow to upper extremity causing a reversal of blood flow in the Circle of Willis

AF, atrial fibrillation; AV, atrioventricular; HCM, hypertrophic cardiomyopathy; LV, left ventricular; SVT, supraventricular tachycardia; VT, ventricular tachycardia.

TABLE 29-3	ESSENTIAL QUESTIONS TO EVALUATE HISTORY OF SYNCOPE
Before	Nausea, vomiting, feeling cold, sweating, dizziness, visual changes
Eyewitness	Duration of transient loss of consciousness, movements (tonic, clonic, other), description of patient falling
After	Confusion, muscle aches, incontinence, nausea, vomiting, sweating, pallor
Circumstances	Position (supine, standing), activity (rest, exercise, rising to stand, cough, urination), possible precipitants (fear, pain, prolonged standing)
History	Prior syncopal episodes, known cardiac, neurologic, or metabolic disease, known history or symptoms of obstructive sleep apnea, medications (including over the counter), alcohol or illicit drug use, family history of sudden cardiac death

- Proper orthostatic vital signs include:
  - After patient lies supine for at least 5 minutes, check the blood pressure (BP) in both arms.
  - After standing for 3 minutes, check the BP again.
  - Classic orthostatic hypotension = 20 mm Hg decrease in systolic BP and/or 10 mm Hg decrease in diastolic BP.
- Cardiovascular findings that may point to cardiogenic syncope include:
  - Arrhythmias (tachyarrhythmias, bradyarrhythmias, and irregularity)
  - Murmurs (especially aortic stenosis or hypertrophic obstructive cardiomyopathy)
  - Evidence for heart failure (S_3, S_4, edema, and elevated jugular venous distention [JVD])
- Neurologic findings are often absent, but might include evidence of autonomic neuropathy (e.g., inappropriate sweating, lack of heart rate [HR] variability, extreme orthostatic BP changes).
- If carotid sinus hypersensitivity is suspected, carotid sinus massage may reproduce symptoms.
  - This maneuver can be performed safely at the bedside with the patient lying recumbent on telemetry monitoring and appropriate bradycardia treatments readily available.
  - Pressure is applied to the carotid sinus (usually inferior to the angle of the mandible over the carotid artery) on each side, sequentially.
  - The test is considered positive if it results cardioinhibitory response with ventricular pause of >3 seconds, or if there is a marked vasodepressor response with >50 mm Hg drop in systolic BP.
  - Neurologic complications are rare, but the procedure should be avoided in patients with known carotid disease, carotid bruits, or a recent transient ischemic attack (TIA)/cerebrovascular accident.

Diagnostic Testing

- Standard diagnostic testing in the evaluation of syncope includes a resting 12-lead ECG. Any additional diagnostic testing should be guided by the comprehensive history, physical examination, and baseline ECG obtained.
- The 2006 American Heart Association (AHA)/American College of Cardiology (ACC) algorithm for cardiac evaluation of syncope is outlined in Figure 29-1.[7]

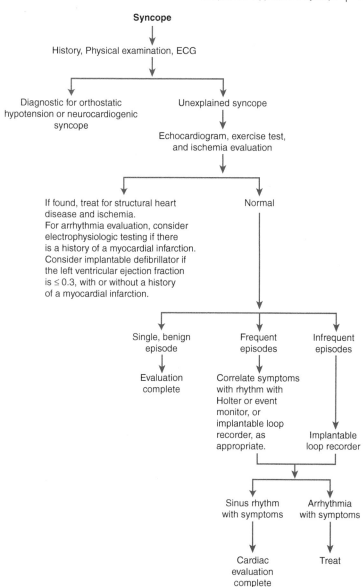

FIGURE 29-1. Algorithm for the evaluation of syncope. (Reprinted from Strickberger SA, Benson DW, Biaggioni I, et al. AHA/ACCF scientific statement on the evaluation of syncope: from the American Heart Association Councils on Clinical Cardiology, Cardiovascular Nursing, Cardiovascular Disease in the Young, and Stroke, and the Quality of Care and Outcomes Research Interdisciplinary Working Group; and the American College of Cardiology Foundation In Collaboration With the Heart Rhythm Society. *J Am Coll Cardiol.* 2006;47(2):473-84. Copyright © 2006 American College of Cardiology Foundation. With permission.)

Electrocardiography

Specific abnormalities to look for on ECG include:

- Evidence of sinus node dysfunction
- Evidence of atrioventricular conduction abnormalities
- Tachyarrhythmias (supraventricular tachycardia [SVT], ventricular tachycardia [VT], atrial fibrillation [AF])
- Evidence of ventricular preexcitation (δ waves)
- Evidence of underlying structural heart disease includes:
  - Q waves suggestive of prior myocardial infection
  - Wide QRS (>120 milliseconds)
  - Left ventricular (LV) hypertrophy pattern suggestive of hypertrophic cardiomyopathy (HCM)
  - Anterior precordial T-wave inversions and/or epsilon waves suggestive of arrhythmogenic right ventricular dysplasia (ARVD)
- Evidence of channelopathy includes:
  - Long or short QT
  - Right bundle branch block with down-sloping ST elevation and T-wave inversion in V1–V3 (Brugada pattern)

Imaging

- If structural heart disease is suspected, an expanded cardiac evaluation can include an **echocardiogram, exercise testing, and an ischemic evaluation**.
  - In appropriate patients, an exercise stress echo would be sufficient to complete all three aspects of testing (baseline imaging followed by exercise protocol and stress imaging).
  - The echocardiogram alone may be diagnostic in cases of valvular heart disease, cardiomyopathy, or congenital heart disease.
  - Exercise testing is preferable to pharmacologic stress and should be symptom limited. Aside from risk stratification for ischemic coronary artery disease, it can be useful in establishing cause if syncope was exertional.
  - If there is evidence of ischemia or previously unrecognized infarction, noninvasive testing for ischemia should be followed by **cardiac catheterization**.
- Cardiac MRI may be helpful in the evaluation of structural heart disease, including HCM, ARVD, or coronary anomalies. Coronary CT angiography (CCTA) can also identify coronary anomalies.

Monitoring and Additional Provocative Testing

- If an arrhythmic cause is suspected, but not evident on the initial workup or on expanded cardiac evaluation, **ambulatory cardiac rhythm monitoring** can be achieved via one of the following modalities[8]:
  - Holter monitor (24 to 48 hours of continuous recording)
  - Event recorder (1 month of patient-activated or patient-triggered recordings to temporally correlate with symptoms)
  - Mobile Continuous Outpatient Telemetry (MCOT) for up to 1 month of continuous monitoring
  - Implantable loop recorder (years of continuous recording)
  - The choice of monitoring is dependent on the frequency of symptoms and type of suspected arrhythmia. Even in a highly selected population, the diagnostic yield of ambulatory cardiac monitoring is relatively low.
- **Tilt table testing** has been used traditionally as a diagnostic tool to characterize a patient's hemodynamic response to controlled postural change from supine to upright state to aid in the diagnosis of a reflex-mediated (neurocardiogenic) syncope.
  - Physiologically, there is a large volume shift during repositioning, with 500 to 1000 mL of blood moving from the thorax to the distensible venous system below the diaphragm within the first 10 seconds.

○ The hydrostatic pressures created by the upright position result in a similar volume of fluid moving to the interstitial space within 10 minutes.

○ Autonomic vasoconstriction is the key reflex to counter this orthostatic stress, and failure of the vasoconstriction mechanism at any point may result in syncope.

○ An under-filled right ventricle will trigger a strong vagal response, leading to bradycardia and hypotension.

○ Results are classified as primarily vasodepressor, cardioinhibitory, or mixed.

○ Unfortunately, **the test has a low sensitivity and reproducibility with frequent false-positive results (virtually everyone will have syncope given an adequate hemodynamic stress)**. It is our institutional bias that a tilt table test adds very little to a thorough history, physical examination, and standard cardiac workup of syncope.

• **Electrophysiology studies (EPSs)** can be useful in selected patients. Indications for EPS include:

○ Abnormal ECG suggestive of conduction system cause

○ Syncope during exertion or while supine or in the presence of structural heart disease

○ Syncope with associated palpitations

○ Family history of sudden death

○ To define/ablate identified arrhythmias in patients with high-risk occupations

TREATMENT

• Treatment of syncope can be broadly defined as **preventing recurrences** and **reducing the risk of injury or death**.

• Treatment is tailored to treat the suspected underlying etiology of the syncope. More comprehensive guideline-directed therapies should be referenced for cardiogenic or arrhythmic causes of syncope.[9]

• Various approaches to treating the four etiologies of syncope are shown in Table 29-4.

Nonpharmacologic Therapies

• For reflex syncope, effective treatment may be as simple as avoiding syncopal precipitants.

TABLE 29-4	TAILORED TREATMENT OF SYNCOPE
Reflex	Avoid precipitants (prolonged standing, overheating); adequate hydration; isometric muscle contraction during prodrome to abort episodes; cardiac pacing for carotid sinus syncope with bradycardia; compression stockings; salt supplementation; fludrocortisone; midodrine
Orthostatic	Adequate hydration; eliminate offending drugs; stand slowly; support stockings; consider salt supplementation, fludrocortisone, or midodrine
Arrhythmia	Cardiac pacing for sinus node dysfunction or high-degree AV block; discontinue QT-prolonging drugs; ICD for documented VT without correctable cause; endocardial ablation procedure in select patients
Cardiopulmonary	Correction of underlying disorder (valve replacement, revascularization); ICD for syncope with EF <35% even in the absence of documented arrhythmia (presumed VT)

AV, atrioventricular; ICD, implantable cardioverter-defibrillator; EF, ejection fraction; VT, ventricular tachycardia.

- When such precipitants cannot be avoided, coping strategies can be helpful. Physical counterpressure maneuvers (leg crossing, handgrip, or arm tensing) can improve venous return and abort frank syncope in patients with a recognizable prodrome.[10]
- Volume expansion with liberalized salt and fluid intake can decrease susceptibility to reflex syncope and orthostatic hypotension.
- Compression garments (thigh high and above) can improve orthostatic symptoms.

Medications

- In the setting of vasovagal syncope and orthostatic hypotension, the most common pharmacologic options for preventing venous pooling and aiding intravascular volume expansion include:
  - **Midodrine** (2.5 to 10 mg PO tid)[11,12]
    - Peripheral α-agonist causing both arterial and venous constriction
    - Adverse effects include paresthesias, piloerection, pruritus, and supine hypertension.
    - Avoid in patients with carotid artery disease (CAD), peripheral arterial disease, and acute renal failure
    - The only drug shown effective in trials for orthostatic hypotension and reflex-mediated syncope
  - **Fludrocortisone** (start 0.1 mg PO daily, can increase by 0.1 mg weekly to maximum of 1.0 mg PO daily)
    - Synthetic mineralocorticoid causing sodium retention and volume expansion
    - Adverse effects include hypertension, peripheral edema, and hypokalemia.[13]
    - The benefit of fludrocortisone in preventing vasovagal syncope was not statistically significant in the Second Prevention of Syncope Trial (POST-2).[14]
  - β-Blockers were not shown to be effective compared to placebo in the treatment of vasovagal syncope in the POST.[15]

Lifestyle/Risk Modification

- In patients with unexplained syncope, driving restrictions should be discussed when appropriate.
- In general, in patients with a serious episode of syncope that is not cleared due to a reversible etiology, guidelines recommend driving restriction for 3 to 6 syncope-free months.
- Recommendations currently vary depending on etiology, underlying disease, type of license held (private vs. commercial), and adequacy of treatment. Also, federal law and variable state law pertinent to licensure in these individuals exist and should be consulted when applicable.
- If the cause of syncope is an active cardiac arrhythmia, patients should be instructed not to drive until successful treatment has been initiated and the patient has received permission from the treating physician.

OUTCOME/PROGNOSIS

- Approximately one-fifth of patients who present to the emergency department for syncope will have recurrence within 2 years.[16] This does not account for the meaningful proportion of patients who do not seek medical attention after an episode of TLOC.
- Select subgroups of patients with noncardiac syncope have an excellent prognosis. Young, otherwise healthy individuals with a normal ECG and without identifiable heart disease have essentially no increased risk of death relative to the population at large.
- Reflex syncope is not associated with an increased risk of mortality.
- Syncope from orthostatic hypotension has an excellent prognosis if the underlying abnormality is easily identified and treated.

- In contrast, syncope with an identifiable cardiac etiology carries a higher risk of mortality, due to the underlying disease process. This is true particularly in patients with advanced heart failure, where mortality approaches 45% at 1 year for those with syncope and LV ejection fraction <20%.[17]

REFERENCES

1. Kenny RA, Bhangu J, King-Kallimanis BL. Epidemiology of syncope/collapse in younger and older western patient populations. *Prog Cardiovasc Dis.* 2013;55:357-63.
2. Chen LY, Shen W-K, Mahoney DW, et al. Prevalence of syncope in a population aged more than 45 years. *Am J Med.* 2006;119:1088.e1-7.
3. Ganzeboom KS, Mairuhu G, Reitsma JB, et al. Lifetime cumulative incidence of syncope in the general population: a study of 549 Dutch subjects aged 35–60 years. *J Cardiovasc Electrophysiol.* 2006;17:1172-6.
4. Ruwald MH, Hansen ML, Lamberts M, et al. The relation between age, sex, comorbidity, and pharmacotherapy and the risk of syncope: a Danish nationwide study. *Europace.* 2012;14:1506-14.
5. Probst MA, Kanzaria HK, Gbedemah M, et al. National trends in resource utilization associated with emergency department visits for syncope. *Am J Emerg Med.* 2015;33:998-1001.
6. Sun BC, Emond JA, Camargo CA. Characteristics and admission patterns of patients presenting with syncope to U.S. emergency departments, 1992–2000. *Acad Emerg Med.* 2004;11:1029-34.
7. Strickberger AS, Benson WD, Biaggioni I, et al. AHA/ACCF scientific statement on the evaluation of syncope. *Circulation.* 2006;113:316-27.
8. Subbiah R, Gula LJ, Klein GJ, et al. Syncope: review of monitoring modalities. *Curr Cardiol Rev.* 2008;4:41-8.
9. Shen W, Sheldon RS, Benditt DG, et al. 2017 ACC/AHA/HRS guideline for the evaluation and management of patients with syncope. *J Am Coll Cardiol.* 2017;70:e39-110.
10. van Dijk N, Quartieri F, Blanc J-J, et al. Effectiveness of physical counterpressure maneuvers in preventing vasovagal syncope: the Physical Counterpressure Manoeuvres Trial (PC-Trial). *J Am Coll Cardiol.* 2006;48:1652-7.
11. Low PA, Gilden JL, Freeman R, Sheng KN, McElligott MA. Efficacy of midodrine vs placebo in neurogenic orthostatic hypotension: a randomized, double-blind multicenter study. *JAMA.* 1997;277:1046-51.
12. Wright RA, Kaufmann HC, Perera R, et al. A double-blind, dose-response study of midodrine in neurogenic orthostatic hypotension. *Neurology.* 1998;51:120-4.
13. Chobanian AV, Volicer L, Tifft CP, et al. Mineralocorticoid-induced hypertension in patients with orthostatic hypotension. *N Engl J Med.* 1979;301:68-73.
14. Sheldon R, Raj SR, Rose MS, et al. Fludrocortisone for the prevention of vasovagal syncope: a randomized, placebo-controlled trial. *J Am Coll Cardiol.* 2016;68(1):1-9.
15. Sheldon R, Connolly S, Rose S, et al. Prevention of Syncope Trial (POST). *Circulation.* 2006;113:1164-70.
16. Solbiati M, Casazza G, Dipaola F, et al. Syncope recurrence and mortality: a systematic review. *Europace.* 2015;17:300-308.
17. Middlekauff HR, Stevenson WG, Stevenson LW, Saxon LA. Syncope in advanced heart failure: high risk of sudden death regardless of origin of syncope. *J Am Coll Cardiol.* 1993;21:110-16.

Sudden Cardiac Death

Andrew E. Berdy and Marye J. Gleva

30

GENERAL PRINCIPLES

Definition

- **Sudden cardiac death** (SCD)[1,2] is defined as sudden and unexpected death that occurs within 1 hour of symptom onset, or within 24 hours of being witnessed alive and asymptomatic.
- **Sudden cardiac arrest** (SCA)[1,2] is defined as the sudden cessation of cardiac activity such that the victim becomes unresponsive, with gasping or absent respirations, and no evidence of circulation without other known or identifiable cause.
- These two terms are generally used interchangeably. However, there are data suggesting that only about half of SCD cases are due to SCA,[3,4] and so more precise definitions with more meaningful separation of these terms are likely to be needed in the future.

Classification

- Ventricular arrhythmias
  - Monomorphic ventricular tachycardia (VT)
  - Polymorphic VT
  - Ventricular fibrillation (VF)
- Bradyarrhythmias
  - Asystole
  - Pulseless electrical activity (PEA)

Epidemiology

- **SCD is responsible for up to 15% of overall deaths in the US, a total of between 230,000 and 350,000 deaths annually.**[1,4,5]
  - Responsible for as much as 50% of cardiac deaths
  - **First presentation of cardiac disease in as many as 25% of patients**
- **The majority of SCD occurs outside the hospital and is associated with a 6-10% survival rate. In-hospital arrest is associated with a 24% survival rate.**
- SCD is more common in[4,6,7]:
  - Increasing age
  - Males than females
  - African Americans than Caucasians, Hispanics, and Asians
  - Coronary artery disease (CAD)
  - Increasing cardiac mass in the absence of CAD
  - Lower socioeconomic status
  - Lower education levels
  - Lower income levels
- While the incidence of SCD is higher in high-risk populations—such as CAD, cardiomyopathy, and channelopathy—over two-thirds of those who do suffer SCD are in low risk, or no known risk, populations.[8] See Figure 30-1 for absolute numbers and event rates in specific subpopulations.[8]

Etiology

- Ventricular tachyarrhythmias are most commonly associated with diseases of the ventricular myocardium.
- CAD remains the most common cause of SCD, associated with 40-80% of cases (see Figure 30-2); however, the relative incidence of SCD due to ischemic heart disease appears to be decreasing.
- Myocardial fibrosis, myocardial inflammation, myocardial hypertrophy, or infiltrative diseases
- Inherited channelopathies or acquired derangements of myocardial repolarization
- Hemodynamic derangements seen in patients with repaired or unrepaired congenital heart disease
- Bradyarrhythmic arrests are associated with single or multisystem organ failure as well as tension pneumothorax and cardiac tamponade.

Pathophysiology

A "perfect storm" of structural abnormalities, biochemical alterations, and electrical instability bring about the arrhythmias that cause SCD. See Figure 30-3.[9]

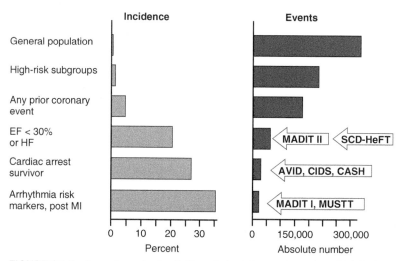

FIGURE 30-1. Annual event rates (left) and absolute event numbers (right) of sudden cardiac death in the general population as well as in specific subpopulations. Clinical trials that include specific subpopulations of patients are shown on the right side. General population refers to an unselected population aged 35 years or older. High-risk subgroups include those with multiple risk factors for a first coronary event. AVID, antiarrhythmics versus implantable defibrillators; CASH, Cardiac Arrest Study Hamburg; CIDS, Canadian Implantable Defibrillator Study; EF, ejection fraction; HF, heart failure; MADIT, Multicenter Automatic Defibrillator Implantation Trial; MI, myocardial infarction; MUSTT, Multicenter UnSustained Tachycardia Trial; SCD-HeFT, Sudden Cardiac Death in Heart Failure Trial. (Modified with permission from Myerburg RJ, Kessler KM, Castellanos A. Sudden cardiac death. Structure, function, and time-dependence of risk. *Circulation*. 1992;85(1 Suppl):I2-10.)

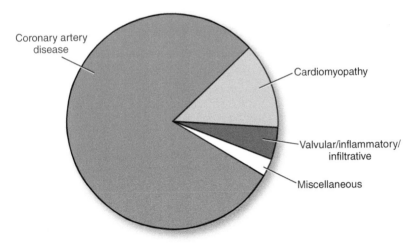

FIGURE 30-2. Etiology of sudden cardiac death.

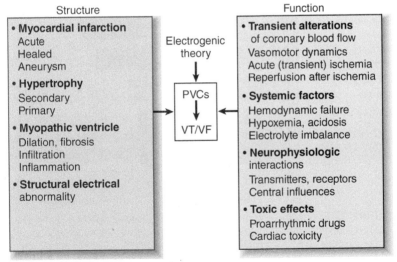

FIGURE 30-3. Biologic model of sudden cardiac death (SCD). Structural cardiac abnormalities are commonly defined as the causative basis for SCD. However, functional alterations of the abnormal anatomic substrate are usually required to alter stability of the myocardium, thus permitting a potentially fatal arrhythmia to be initiated. In this conceptual model, short-term or long-term structural abnormalities interact with functional modulations to influence the probability that premature ventricular contractions initiate ventricular tachycardia or fibrillation. (Adapted from Myerburg RJ, Kessler KM, Basset AL, et al. A biological approach to sudden cardiac death: structure, function, and cause. *Am J Cardiol.* 1989;63(20):1512-16. Copyright © 1989 Elsevier. With permission.)

Risk Factors

- **Overall, current risk stratification models are inadequate to identify individuals who will, or will not, suffer SCD.**
- While there are high-risk findings, conditions, and populations—which are discussed later—currently, there are no robust models for individualize risk stratification.
- The majority of SCD occurs in those with no identifiable risk factors.
- The strongest risk factor for SCD is having a previously survived SCD or SCA or having had hemodynamically significant VT or VF.
- Additional risk factors for SCD:
  ○ Reduction of left ventricular ejection fraction (LVEF) <35%
  ○ CAD
  ○ LV hypertrophy, only a risk factor in the absence of CAD
  ○ Premature ventricular contractions (PVCs) and nonsustained VT (NSVT)
  ○ Hypertension
  ○ Chronic obstructive pulmonary disease
  ○ Diagnosis with conditions addressed in section Associated Conditions

Prevention

- Prevention of SCD is divided into two broad categories: primary and secondary prevention.
  ○ Primary prevention therapy prevents SCD from occurring in an individual who is at high risk for SCD but has not had SCD.
  ○ Secondary prevention therapy prevents subsequent SCD from occurring in an individual who has already suffered SCD.
- Aside from specific ventricular tachyarrhythmia syndromes, **there is only one treatment that has been definitively and consistently proven to reduce the incidence of SCD— an implantable cardioverter-defibrillators (ICD).**[10-12]
- Data supporting the use of ICD for both primary and secondary prevention are presented in Table 30-1.
- The different types of ICDs are discussed subsequently in section Surgical Management.
- The use of radiofrequency catheter ablation in ICD patients reduces ICD shocks but does not improve survival.[13,14]

Associated Conditions

- See Table 30-2 for abnormalities associated with SCD.[22]
- Ischemic cardiomyopathy (ICM):
  ○ Primary prevention in ICM is driven by key clinical trials and long-term trial participant follow-up (Table 30-1).
  ○ Primary prevention ICD indicated in those with LVEF ≤35%.
    ▪ Benefits of primary prevention device are highest in those with good functional status.
    ▪ ICM benefits more than nonischemic patients.[15]
    ▪ Survival benefit seen as far out as 10 years.[15]
  ○ In the setting of acute coronary syndrome (ACS), guidelines recommend implantation 40 days after myocardial infarction or 90 days after revascularization.[1]
  ○ Arrhythmic death was not reduced by the wearable cardioverter-defibrillator (WCD) after ACS.[18]
  ○ All ICM patients should be on maximally tolerated doses of optimal medical therapy with β-blocker, angiotensin-converting enzyme inhibitor (ACEI) or angiotensin-receptor blocker (ARB), mineralocorticoid-receptor antagonist, appropriate antiplatelet therapy, and appropriate lipid-lowering therapy.
  ○ Primary prevention ICD should not be implanted until after 90 days of optimal medical therapy.[1]

○ Antiarrhythmic drugs (AADs) have only been shown to reduce ICD discharges and arrhythmia episodes, not mortality.

○ Secondary prevention ICD should be placed in patients with ICM, so long as SCD event is not attributed to ACS. Revascularization is the indicated treatment for SCD occurring in the setting of ACS.

TABLE 30-1	TEN KEY AND COMMONLY CITED TRIALS FOR CARDIOVERTER-DEFIBRILLATOR USE ORGANIZED BY TYPE OF SCD PREVENTION	
	SCD-HeFT[10]	2521 patients with NYHA classes II–III HF and LVEF ≤35% ICD (78%) versus amiodarone (72%) versus placebo (71%) alive at 45 months	23% RRR mortality (P = NS, 0.007)
	SCD-HeFT 10-year follow-up[15]	1855 patients with NYHA classes II–III HF and LVEF ≤35% ICD (47.5%) versus amiodarone (47.3%) versus placebo (47.3%) alive at 10 years Overall survival benefit seen at 6 years, but gone at 10 ICD (55.4%) versus placebo (47.9%) alive at 10 years in NYHA class II HF ICD (41%) versus placebo (32%) in ICM alive at 10 years	(P = NS) 14% RRR mortality (P = 0.001) 12.7% RRR mortality (P = 0.009)
Primary Prevention	MADIT I[11]	196 patients with prior myocardial infarction, LVEF ≤35%, NYHA classes I–III HF, NSVT, inducible VT on EPS ICD (84.2%) versus conventional therapy (61.4%) alive average 27 months	54% RRR mortality (P = 0.009)
	MADIT II[12]	1232 patients with prior myocardial infarction and LVEF ≤30% ICD (85.8%) versus conventional therapy (80.2%) alive average 20 months	31% RRR mortality (P = 0.016)
	MADIT II 8-year follow up[16]	1232 patients with prior myocardial infarction and LVEF ≤35% ICD (51%) versus conventional therapy (38%) alive at 8 years	21% RRR mortality (P < 0.001)
	PRAETO-RIAN[17]	849 patients with a class I or IIa indication for primary prevention ICD and no indication for pacing S-ICD (15.1%) versus ICD (15.7%) had device complication at 49 months	(P = NS)
	VEST[18]	2302 patients after acute myocardial infarction with LVEF ≤35% WCD (1.6%) versus medical therapy (2.4%) had arrhythmic death at 3 months.	(P = NS)

TABLE 30-1	TEN KEY AND COMMONLY CITED TRIALS FOR CARDIOVERTER-DEFIBRILLATOR USE ORGANIZED BY TYPE OF SCD PREVENTION (continued)

Secondary Prevention	AVID[19]	1016 patients resuscitated from VF or sustained VT with syncope or other serious cardiac symptoms with LVEF ≤40% ICD (75.4%) versus antiarrhythmic drugs (64.1%) alive at 3 years	31% RRR mortality ($P = 0.02$)
	CASH[20]	288 survivors of cardiac arrest due to ventricular arrhythmias ICD (65.4%) versus amiodarone or metoprolol (55.6%) alive average 57 months	23% RRR mortality ($P = NS$, 0.08)
	CIDS[21]	659 survivors of cardiac arrest or syncope secondary to arrhythmia ICD (76.7%) versus amiodarone (73%) alive at 3 years	20% RRR mortality, P-NS, 0.142)

AVID, Antiarrhythmic Drug versus Defibrillator; CASH, cardiac arrest survival in Hamburg; CIDS, Canadian Implantable Defibrillator Study; EPS, electrophysiology study; HF, heart failure; ICD implantable cardioverter-defibrillator; LVEF, left ventricular ejection fraction; MADIT Multicenter Automatic Defibrillator Implantation Trial; NSVT, nonsustained ventricular tachycardia; NYHA, New York Heart Association; PRAETORIAN, Prospective Randomized Comparison of Subcutaneous and Transvenous Implantable Cardioverter Defibrillator; SCD-HeFT, Sudden Cardiac Death in Heart Failure; S-ICD, subcutaneous ICD; VEST, Vest Prevention of Early Sudden Death Trial; VF, ventricular fibrillation; VT, ventricular tachycardia; WCD, wearable cardioverter-defibrillator.

TABLE 30-2	ABNORMALITIES ASSOCIATED WITH SUDDEN CARDIAC DEATH

Myocardial disease
- Ischemic cardiomyopathy
  - Acute myocardial infarction
  - Chronic myocardial ischemic disease
- Nonischemic cardiomyopathy
  - Dilated cardiomyopathy
  - Alcoholic cardiomyopathy
  - Postpartum cardiomyopathy

Coronary artery
- Coronary atherosclerosis
- Coronary arteritis
- Coronary vasospasm
- Spontaneous coronary artery dissection
- Coronary artery embolism
- Congenital coronary abnormalities

Hypertrophic states
- Hypertensive heart disease
- Obstructive and nonobstructive hypertrophic cardiomyopathy
- Hypertensive heart disease
- Pulmonary hypertension

(continued)

TABLE 30-2	ABNORMALITIES ASSOCIATED WITH SUDDEN CARDIAC DEATH (*continued*)

Valvular abnormalities
- Native valvular regurgitation or stenosis
- Infective endocarditis
- Prosthetic valve dysfunction

Inflammatory, infiltrative, neoplastic, and degenerative processes
- Cardiac amyloidosis
- Arrhythmogenic right ventricular cardiomyopathy
- Chagas disease
- Hemochromatosis
- Cardiac sarcoidosis
- Infectious myocarditis
- Neuromuscular disorders—muscular dystrophy, myotonic dystrophy, Friedreich ataxia

Congenital heart disease
- Residual shunts
- Postsurgical repair

Electrophysiologic abnormalities
- Conduction system abnormalities
- Accessory pathways
- Inherited channelopathies

Commotio cordis

Central nervous system
- Intracranial hemorrhage

Stress and neurohumoral abnormalities
- Catecholamine outflow

Drug induced
- Class I and III antiarrhythmics
- QT prolonging agents

Sudden infant death syndrome

Toxin/metabolic disturbances
- Magnesium
- Potassium
- Calcium
- Acid/base
- Sympathomimetics

Other conditions
- Pericardial tamponade
- Aortic dissection
- Hemorrhage
- Massive pulmonary embolism

Modified from Myerberg RJ, Castellanos A. Cardiac arrest and sudden cardiac death. In: Bonow RO, Mann DL, Zipes DP, et al, eds. *Braunwald's Heart Disease: A Textbook of Cardiovascular Medicine.* 9th ed. Elsevier; 2012:845-84. Copyright © 2012 Elsevier. With permission.

- Nonischemic cardiomyopathy (NICM):
  - The data to support implantation of primary prevention ICD in NICM[10] are less robust compared to data in ICM.
  - Primary prevention devices are recommended in ICM if LVEF remains ≤35% after 90 days of optimal medical therapy.
  - The primary treatment for NICM is guideline-directed medical therapy for heart failure, including a combination of β-blocker, ACEI/ARB/angiotensin receptor-neprilysin inhibitor (ARNI), and aldosterone antagonist.
  - Additional evaluation is recommended in NICM to evaluate for other conditions such as genetic, inflammatory, or infiltrative cardiomyopathies. Discovery of one of these conditions changes the risk profile, medication recommendations, and ICD recommendations.
- Hypertrophic cardiomyopathy (HCM)[23]:
  - HCM is covered in detail in Chapter 16.
  - Younger patients with HCM are at higher risk of SCD than older patients. There is no difference in SCD risk based on sex or race.
  - SCD risk assessment should be performed annually as the risk remains and changes over times. Noninvasive risk assessment includes the following:
    - Personal history of ventricular arrhythmias or cardiac arrest, arrhythmogenic suspected syncope
    - Family history of SCD, premature HCM–related SCD in a first-degree relative or close family member aged 50 years or older, or sustained ventricular arrhythmias
    - Imaging findings including LV apical aneurysm, maximal wall thickness ≥ 30 mm, and/or LV systolic function ≤ 50%
    - NSVT episodes on continuous ambulatory ECG monitoring
  - Compared to cardiac magnetic resonance imaging (CMR), echocardiography may underestimate maximal LV wall thickness and may not detect a LV apical aneurysm. Extensive myocardial fibrosis, ≥ 15% of LV mass detected by CMR late gadolinium enhancement, is associated with increased risk of SCD.
  - ICD placement should be considered in patients with one or more risk factors. ICD placement in patients without risk factors and for the sole or purpose of participating in competitive sports is not recommended.
- Arrhythmogenic right ventricular cardiomyopathy (ARVC)[24-26]
  - ARVC is a genetic condition leading to fibrofatty replacement of right ventricular, and eventually LV, myocardium.
  - Multiple gene mutations have been identified, which lead to abnormalities of the desmosome.
  - Diagnosis is made based on criteria from imaging, ECG, arrhythmia history, family history, and pathology.
  - Increased risk of VT causing SCD
  - Commonly associated with SCD in young individuals or with exercise since VT is catecholamine sensitive
  - Responsible for 5% of overall SCD and 4% of death in young athletes during exertion. It may present with monomorphic VT, PVC, syncope, or heart failure. Symptoms and arrhythmias are often provoked and occur with exertion.
  - ICD placement reduces the risk of SCD.
  - Primary prevention ICD should be implanted in ARVC if:
    - Survived SCD event
    - Sustained VT
    - RVEF or LVEF ≤35%
  - Secondary prevention ICD regardless of risk factors
  - Should have treatment with β-blocker and avoid strenuous exercise

- Catecholaminergic polymorphic ventricular tachycardia (CPVT):
  - Exercise induced, bidirectional VT
  - First-line treatment is β-blocker or calcium channel blocker.
  - ICD is recommended if VT or syncope despite maximally tolerated medical therapy. ICD shocks may increase catecholamine surges and exacerbate ventricular arrhythmias.
- Cardiac sarcoidosis:[27]
  - Sarcoidosis is a granulomatous inflammatory disease. Approximately 5-27% have cardiac involvement.
  - Arrhythmia is common in cardiac sarcoidosis, including VT, VF, complete heart block, and supraventricular tachyarrhythmias. SCD in cardiac sarcoidosis may be due to tachyarrhythmias or bradyarrhythmias.
  - Arrhythmia in cardiac sarcoidosis is thought to be due to inflammation and scar.
  - Patients with cardiac sarcoidosis are at increased risk for SCD. Patients with cardiac sarcoidosis and arrhythmias are at higher risk for SCD than those without.[28]
  - ICD is recommended for primary prevention in those with LVEF ≤35%, VT, inducible VT by electrophysiology study (EPS), and scar by CMR or positron emission tomography.
  - ICD also recommended for secondary prevention.
  - Immunosuppressive therapy can reduce VT if inflammation is present.
- Cardiac amyloidosis[29]:
  - Cardiac amyloid is a systemic disease of deposition of amyloid fibrils. Cardiac involvement occurs if there is deposition in myocardial extracellular space.
  - VT, VF, complete heart block, and supraventricular tachyarrhythmias are common. SCD may be due to tachyarrhythmias or bradyarrhythmias.
  - 50% of cardiac amyloid patients die suddenly.
  - PVC, NSVT, and VT all increase the risk of SCD.
  - **ICD implantation does not improve overall survival**.
  - There are no specific guidelines regarding ICD placement for both primary and secondary prevention, as it is still controversial at the time of writing. The decision for ICD implantation should be individualized.
  - Tafamidis, a new drug that has been approved for transthyretin amyloidosis, has not been studied with regard to SCD.
- Inflammatory and infiltrative cardiomyopathies:
  - Heterogeneous group of conditions caused by myriad causes
  - Treatment typically limited to the underlying cause and optimal medical therapy for heart failure.
  - ICD indications are the same as those for NICM.
- Brugada syndrome[30,31]:
  - Inherited channelopathy resulting in loss of function in sodium channel, most commonly SCN5A. Brugada syndrome is eight times more common in males than females, most prevalent in those of Southeast Asian descent, most commonly presents in the fifth decade.
  - Accounts for 4-12% of SCD worldwide, and 20-50% of SCD in those without structural heart disease
  - **ECG shows right bundle branch block and coved ST-segment elevation in leads V1-V3.**
  - Presents with syncope, palpitations, VT/VF, SCD, and nocturnal agonal breathing. Symptoms worse with sleep, fever, and alcohol consumption.
  - Specific sodium channel–blocking agents, such as flecainide, can be used to diagnose Brugada syndrome.
  - ICD implantation is recommended for SCD, documented VT, or documented VF.

- ○ ICD implantation can be considered in the setting of syncope suspected to be due to an arrhythmia.
- ○ Quinidine can be considered in VT storm, or in those who are unwilling, or unable, to have ICD implanted.
- ○ The role for radiofrequency ablation is emerging.
- Inherited arrhythmia syndromes and channelopathies:
  - ○ Long QT syndrome
  - ○ Short QT syndrome
  - ○ Idiopathic VF
  - ○ Early repolarization syndrome
  - ○ ICD generally recommended for secondary prevention, if unable to tolerate medical therapy, or if VT or syncope despite maximal medical therapy.
- Commotio cordis[32]:
  - ○ Low-impact trauma to the anterior chest wall during a vulnerable period in the cardiac cycle causing VF and SCD
  - ○ Typically seen in athletes during competition involving high-speed projectiles
  - ○ Sudden collapse after apparently incidental impact
  - ○ Rapid cardiopulmonary resuscitation and defibrillation are imperative to good outcomes.

DIAGNOSIS

Clinical Presentation

- Prodromal symptoms of chest pain, palpitations, dyspnea, and fatigue are common in the days and hours, leading to SCD event.
- Onset is sudden, from seconds to hours from initial symptoms to loss of consciousness and cardiac activity.
- Knowledge of the circumstances of the SCD, as well as the **presenting rhythm** (VT/VF or PEA) is critical to successful resuscitation and treatment of SCD.

Differential Diagnosis

- Must consider other causes of hypotension, such as the different forms of shock, to explain cardiovascular collapse
- Consider primary neurologic conditions, such as hemorrhage, cerebrovascular accident, and seizure, to explain change in neurologic status

Diagnostic Testing

Laboratory Testing

- Cardiac arrest and systemic hypoperfusion will cause significant laboratory derangements, which limit specificity of laboratory testing.
- Primary use is retrospective, or if already resulted. Treatment should not be delayed awaiting laboratory results.
- Cardiac biomarkers, such as troponin, will be elevated after any SCD; however, signifiant elevation with ischemic findings on EKG can indicate acute myocardial infarction as the etiology.
- Significant electrolyte and pH derangements can cause SCD, and if identified by lab work should be immediately corrected.

Electrocardiography

- 12-lead ECG or telemetry should be obtained immediately in SCD.
- Determination of the culprit rhythm is paramount in directing resuscitation and further treatment.

Echocardiography
- Resuscitation should not be delayed to allow for transthoracic echocardiography.
- Low sensitivity, however, can identify signs concerning for ACS, pulmonary embolism, chamber dilation, and significant structural abnormalities.
- Important for the evaluation of pericardial tamponade
- Can confirm PEA.

Imaging
CXR imaging can identify significant pulmonary pathology, such as tension pneumothorax.

TREATMENT

- **Acute management of SCD[33]:**
  - The key to successful management and resuscitation from SCD is correct identification of the causative rhythm and restoration of a normal, perfusing rhythm.
  - If outside the hospital, after assessing for scene safety, lack of responsiveness, and lack of pulse, basic life support should begin immediately with the use of an automated external defibrillator for rapid defibrillation. Availability of advanced cardiac life support measures may vary by community.
  - New guidelines continue to reiterate the importance of early defibrillation both in and out of the hospital.
  - Inside the hospital, advanced cardiac life support should be initiated immediately, in accordance with the most up-to-date algorithms.
  - Once stabilized, obtain diagnostic studies to determine the cause of SCD.
  - Presenting rhythm, electrolytes, and corrected QT interval on ECG can assist with selection of antiarrhythmic therapy.
  - CAD is the most common cause of SCD, so assessment and evaluation for urgent coronary angiography is often appropriate.
- Once stabilized, the focus of care switches from resuscitation to identification of the cause of SCD, improvement of neurologic outcomes, and prevention of further episodes with secondary prevention strategies.
  - Targeted temperature management improves neurologic outcomes after survived SCD.
  - Treatment of reversible causes: electrolyte repletion or removal, thrombolytics for pulmonary embolism, revascularization for ACS

Medical Therapy[33]
- Acute management of hemodynamically unstable tachyarrhythmias:
  - Amiodarone
    - The most commonly used antiarrhythmic
    - Given as a 150 or 300 mg bolus followed by infusion at 1 mg/min for 6 hours, then 0.5 mg/min for 18 hours
  - Lidocaine
    - Second-line therapy for VT
    - Particularly effective if VT is due to myocardial ischemia
  - Magnesium: effective for torsades de Pointes and polymorphic VT with long QT intervals
  - β-Blockers
    - More commonly used in long-term, as opposed to acute, management of arrhythmia
    - Of particular benefit if concomitant ACS
    - Avoid if decompensated heart failure or hemodynamically unstable
- Chronic management of hemodynamically unstable tachyarrhythmias:
  - β-Blockers are effective for VT from all causes, particularly for ACS and CPVT.

○ Amiodarone and sotalol are the class III agents that are effective against VT.
○ Mexiletine is a class I agent effective against VT.
○ They reduce episodes of VT and ICD shocks, but not mortality or the occurrence of SCD.

Surgical Therapy

• **ICD:**
  ○ Implantable device that recognizes life-threatening tachyarrhythmias and delivers therapy to restore normal sinus rhythm
  ○ Can deliver antitachycardia pacing as well as defibrillation shocks
  ○ Transvenous ICDs also function as a pacemaker to provide stimulus in the face of bradycardia.
  ○ **ICDs should only be implanted if the patient's survival is estimated to be >1 year. This is true for all indications for ICD therapy and all types of ICD devices.**[1]
  ○ There are multiple varieties of ICD. The broadest division is transvenous and subcutaneous.
  ○ Transvenous ICDs can be single lead, dual lead, or cardiac resynchronization devices (colloquially known as a "BiV ICD").
  ○ Transvenous leads allow for pacing support and antitachycardia pacing, but are associated with a chronic risk of infection and lead malfunction.
  ○ Subcutaneous ICDs are noninferior to transvenous with regard to survival and are associated with a lower rate of infection and lead malfunction. However, subcutaneous devices cannot provide any pacing therapies.[17]
  ○ ICDs are successful in terminating VT and VF in >95% of cases and are standard of care in the secondary prevention of SCD.
• Catheter ablation:
  ○ Adjuvant therapy to reduce episodes of VT or ICD shocks
  ○ Does not replace ICD therapy, and ICD implantation should not be delayed to allow for ablation[13]

SPECIAL CONSIDERATIONS

• CAD is still the most common cause of SCD. However, it represents a far smaller proportion of SCD than it has previously.[4]
• An external, temporary WCD is available. The use of this device has not been shown to improve mortality when used as a bridge to implantation of primary prevention ICD after ACS.[18] However, it is used as a bridge therapy when ICDs, particularly if placed for secondary prevention, have to be removed for any reason.

Structural and Social Determinants of Health[4,7]

• Race, socioeconomic status, ethnicity, social support, culture, language, access to care, and living environment all effect the incidence of SCD, the treatment received for SCD, and the outcomes of SCD.
• While a population-wide problem, certain populations have higher rates of SCD as well as worse outcomes.

OUTCOME/PROGNOSIS

• Patient outcomes in SCD are poor, even in hospitalized patients. Survival is as low as 6% and as high as 24%.[4,5]
• This is often because patients who suffer SCD are brought to medical attention until after their condition is no longer reversible.

- In addition, even in those who survive SCD myriad and numerous neurologic, functional, and cardiopulmonary are extremely common and often severely limiting.[33]
- Long-term prognosis for survivors is directly related to the underlying condition that caused SCD.

REFERENCES

1. Al-Khatib SM, Stevenson WG, Ackerman MJ, et al. 2017 AHA/ACC/HRS guideline for management of patients with ventricular arrhythmias and the prevention of sudden cardiac death: executive summary a report of the American College of Cardiology/American Heart Association Task Force on Clinical Practice Guidelines and the Heart Rhythm Society. *Heart Rhythm.* 2018;15:e190-252.
2. Stiles MK, Wilde AAM, Abrams DJ, et al. 2020 APHRS/HRS expert consensus statement on the investigation of decedents with sudden unexplained death and patients with sudden cardiac arrest, and of their families. *Heart Rhythm.* 2020;18:e1-50.
3. Tseng ZH, Olgin JE, Vittinghoff E, et al. Prospective countywide surveillance and autopsy characterization of sudden cardiac death: POST SCD Study. *Circulation.* 2018;137:2689-700.
4. Steinhaus DA, Vittinghoff E, Moffatt E, et al. Characteristics of sudden arrhythmic death in a diverse, urban community. *Am Heart J.* 2012;163:125-31.
5. Zheng ZJ, Croft JB, Giles WH, Mensah GA. Sudden cardiac death in the United States, 1989 to 1998. *Circulation.* 2001;104:2158-63.
6. Reinier K, Stecker EC, Vickers C, et al. Incidence of sudden cardiac arrest is higher in areas of low socioeconomic status: a prospective two year study in a large United States community. *Resuscitation.* 2006;70:186-92.
7. Havranek EP, Mujahid MS, Barr DA, et al. Social determinants of risk and outcomes for cardiovascular disease: a scientific statement from the American Heart Association. *Circulation.* 2015;132:873-98.
8. Myerburg RJ, Kessler KM, Castellanos A. Sudden cardiac death. Structure, function, and time-dependence of risk. *Circulation.* 1992;85:I2-10.
9. Myerberg RJ, Kessler KM, Bassett AL, et al. A biological approach to sudden cardiac death: structure, function and cause. *Am J Cardiol.* 1989;63:1512-16.
10. Bardy GH, Lee KL, Mark DB, et al. Amiodarone or an implantable cardioverter–defibrillator for congestive heart failure. *N Engl J Med.* 2005;352:225-37.
11. Moss AJ, Hall WJ, Cannom JP, et al. Improved survival with an implanted defibrillator in patients with coronary disease at high risk for ventricular arrhythmia. *N Engl J Med.* 1996;335:1933-40.
12. Moss AJ, Zareba W, Hall WJ, et al. Prophylactic implantation of a defibrillator in patients with myocardial infarction and reduced ejection fraction. *N Engl J Med.* 2002;346:877-83.
13. Willems S, Tilz RR, Steven D, et al. Preventive or deferred ablation of ventricular tachycardia in patients with ischemic cardiomyopathy and implantable defibrillator (BERLIN VT): a multicenter randomized trial. *Circulation.* 2020;141:1057-67.
14. Reddy VY, Reynolds WR, Neuzil P, et al. Prophylactic catheter ablation for the prevention of defibrillator therapy. *N Engl J Med.* 2007;357:2657-65.
15. Poole JE, Olshansky B, Mark DB, et al. Long-term outcomes of implantable cardioverter-defibrillator therapy in the SCD-HeFT. *J Am Coll Cardiol.* 2020;76:405-15.
16. Goldenberg I, Gillespie J, Moss AJ, et al. Long-term benefit of primary prevention with an implantable cardioverter-defibrillator: an extended 8-year follow-up study of the Multicenter Automatic Defibrillator Implantation Trial II. *Circulation.* 2010;122:1265-71.
17. Knops RE, Olde Nordkamp LRA, Delnoy PPHM, et al. Subcutaneous or transvenous defibrillator therapy. *N Engl J Med.* 2020;383:526-36.
18. Olgin JE, Pletcher MJ, Vettinghoff E, et al. Wearable cardioverter–defibrillator after myocardial infarction. *N Engl J Med.* 2018;379:1205-15.
19. Zipes DP, Wyse DG, Friedman PL, et al. Comparison of antiarrhythmic-drug therapy with implantable defibrillators in patients resuscitated from near-fatal ventricular arrhythmias. *N Engl J Med.* 1997;337:1576-84.
20. Kuck KH, Cappato R, Siebels J, Rüppel R. Randomized comparison of antiarrhythmic drug therapy with implantable defibrillators in patients resuscitated from cardiac arrest: the Cardiac Arrest Study Hamburg (CASH). *Circulation.* 2000;102:748-54.
21. Connolly SJ, Gent M, Roberts RS, et al. Canadian implantable defibrillator study (CIDS): a randomized trial of the implantable cardioverter defibrillator against amiodarone. *Circulation.* 2000;101:1297-302.

22. Myerberg RJ, Castellanos A. Cardiac arrest and sudden cardiac death. In: Bonow RO, Mann DL, Zipes DP, Libby P, Braunwald E, eds. *Braunwald's Heart Disease: A Textbook of Cardiovascular Medicine.* 9th ed. Elsevier; 2012:845-84.

23. Ommen SR, Mital S, Burke MA, et al. 2020 AHA/ACC guideline for the diagnosis and treatment of patients with hypertrophic cardiomyopathy: a report of the American College of Cardiology/ American Heart Association Joint Committee on Clinical Practice Guidelines. *J Am Coll Cardiol.* 2020;76:e159-240.

24. Corrado D, Leoni L, Link MS, et al. Implantable cardioverter-defibrillator therapy for prevention of sudden death in patients with arrhythmogenic right ventricular cardiomyopathy/dysplasia. *Circulation.* 2003;108:3084-91.

25. Gemayel C, Pelliccia A, Thompson PD. Arrhythmogenic right ventricular cardiomyopathy. *J Am Coll Cardiol.* 2001;38:1773-81.

26. Marcus FI, McKenna WJ, Sherrill D, et al. Diagnosis of arrhythmogenic right ventricular cardiomyopathy/dysplasia: proposed modification of the task force criteria. *Circulation.* 2010;121: 1533-41.

27. Okada DR, Smith J, Derakhshan A, et al. Ventricular arrhythmias in cardiac sarcoidosis. *Circulation.* 2018;138:1253-64.

28. Desai R, Kakumani K, Fong HK et al. The burden of cardiac arrhythmias in sarcoidosis: a population-based inpatient analysis. *Ann Transl Med.* 2018;6:330-9.

29. Giancaterino S, Urey MA, Darden D, Hsu JC. Management of arrhythmias in cardiac amyloidosis. *JACC Clin Electrophysiol.* 2020;6:351-61.

30. Brugada P, Brugada J. Right bundle branch block, persistent ST segment elevation and sudden cardiac death: a distinct clinical and electrocardiographic syndrome. A multicenter report. *J Am Coll Cardiol.* 1992;20:1391-6.

31. Priori SG, Napolitano C, Gasparini M, et al. Natural history of Brugada syndrome: insights for risk stratification and management. *Circulation.* 2002;105:1342-7.

32. Link MS, Estes NA. Mechanically induced ventricular fibrillation (commotio cordis). *Heart Rhythm.* 2007;4:529-32.

33. Panchal AR, Bartos JA, Cabañas JG, et al. Part 3: adult basic and advanced life support: 2020 American Heart Association guidelines for cardiopulmonary resuscitation and emergency cardiovascular care. *Circulation.* 2020;142:S366-468.

QT Syndromes

31

Krasimira M. Mikhova, Geoffrey Joseph Orme, and Daniel H. Cooper

GENERAL PRINCIPLES

- The QT interval on the surface ECG represents the action potential duration of ventricular myocytes.
- The **cardiac action potential** is determined by the transmembrane flux of ion currents through specific channels, especially the inward flow of Na^+ and Ca^{2+} currents and the outward flow of K^+ currents (Figure 31-1).[1]
- Abnormal lengthening or shortening of this interval suggests dysfunction of ion channels responsible for action potential duration and can predispose to arrhythmias. This dysfunction can be acquired or congenital.
- **Congenital long QT syndrome** (LQTS) refers to a group of inherited **cardiac ion channelopathies** manifested by ECG findings (QT prolongation, T-wave abnormalities) and ventricular arrhythmic events (most notably **torsades de pointes [TdP]**).[2]
- **Acquired LQTS**, in contrast, represents alteration of a functioning ion channel by an **exogenous factor**, typically a drug or electrolyte abnormality, which can predispose to ventricular arrhythmias.
- **Short QT syndrome** (SQTS) refers to a group of very rare inherited channelopathies that manifest with QT shortening, T-wave abnormalities, and atrial and ventricular arrhythmias.
- Congenital LQTS and SQTS are suggested, but not exclusively defined by, QT interval duration.
- The QT interval is the time in milliseconds (ms) from the onset of the QRS complex to the end of the T wave on the 12-lead surface ECG (Figure 31-2).[1]
  - The QT is usually measured in lead II or lead V_5 but should reflect the **longest QT interval found in any lead**.
  - Because of the direct influence of heart rate on the QT, it is advisable to correct the measurement (QTc), as with **Bazett formula** (QTc = QT/$\sqrt{RR}$). This method, however, is known to underestimate the QT interval in bradycardia and to overestimate the QT interval in tachycardia.
  - QRS prolongation (due to aberrancy or pacing) can confound QTc calculation. A suggested way to adjust for this is to normalize the QRS duration to 100 or 110 ms. This can be done by subtracting the difference between the actual QRS and normalized QRS from the QT, before calculating QTc.
- The 99th percentile QTc value for adults is estimated to be 470 ms for men and 480 ms for women. For both, a QTc >500 ms is considered unequivocally abnormal.[3] A **shorthand rule for estimating QTc** has been described: At heart rates of $\geq$70, the QTc is not prolonged if the QT is less than one-half of the RR interval.[4]
- **Lower limit of normal** for the QTc interval is 360 ms in males and 370 ms in females.

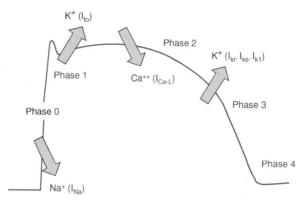

FIGURE 31-1. Phases of the cardiac action potential with associated ion currents. Downward-facing arrows indicate inward (depolarizing) currents, and upward-facing arrows indicate (repolarizing) outward currents. (Adapted from Morita H, Wu J, Zipes DP. The QT syndromes: long and short. *Lancet*. 2008;372(9640):750-63. Copyright © 2008 Elsevier. With permission.)

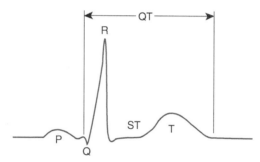

FIGURE 31-2. Surface ECG with identified deflections and measurement of the QT interval. (Adapted from Morita H, Wu J, Zipes DP. The QT syndromes: long and short. *Lancet*. 2008;372(9640):750-63. Copyright © 2008 Elsevier. With permission.)

Long QT Syndrome

GENERAL PRINCIPLES

- The first cases of LQTS were reported in 1957 by Jervell and Lange-Nielsen, who described arrhythmogenic prolongation of the QT interval in association with congenital deafness, inherited in an autosomal recessive manner (**Jervell** and **Lange-Nielsen syndrome**). Subsequently, Romano and Ward described the complex in the presence of normal hearing, inherited in an autosomal dominant manner (**Romano–Ward syndrome**).
- Before genotyping, two additional syndromes, **Andersen–Tawil syndrome** and **Timothy syndrome**, were classified as LQTS, though with vastly different clinical features.

- The genetic basis of LQTS was determined in the 1990s, when mutations in cardiac Na$^+$ and K$^+$ channels were found to result in prolongation of the QT interval.[5]
- The mechanism of arrhythmia and sudden cardiac arrest is similar in both forms.

Definition

- While QT prolongation refers to a measured QT interval that is greater than the upper limit of normal, the criteria to make a diagnosis of LQTS are more specific and include ruling out causes of acquired QT prolongation (see section on Diagnostic Criteria).
- LQTS may also be defined by the **presence of mutations in specific ion channels** (see section on Classification), even with a normal QT interval. A subset of patients (20-40%) are thought to have **"concealed" LQTS**, where prolongation of the QT is seen only with sympathetic stimulation, exercise, or specific triggers.

Classification

- The congenital LQTS are categorized by the specific genetic mutation identified (see section on Diagnostic Testing). There are at least 17 genes reported to cause LQTS, though only three are currently considered definitively causative in typical LQTS—*KCNQ1*, *KCNH2*, and *SCN5A* corresponding to LQT1, LQT2, and LQT3, respectively.[6] Each of these have characteristic ECG findings (Figure 31-3).[7] Taken together, these account for 75-95% of cases.

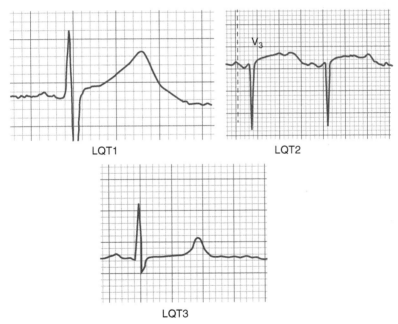

FIGURE 31-3. Characteristic ECG appearance of LQTS. A broad T wave suggests LQT1, a notched T wave suggests LQT2, and a long isoelectric ST segment and T wave suggest LQT3. (Reprinted with permission from Zimetbaum P, Buxton A, Josephson M. Sudden death syndromes. In: *Practical Clinical Electrophysiology.* 2nd ed. Wolters Kluwer; 2018:228.)

- While historically LQTS classification used a successive numbering approach, this is becoming reserved for LQT1, LQT2, and LQT3, with further variants named for their specific gene as the number and clinical significance of discovered mutations are still evolving.[6]

Epidemiology

- Initial estimates of the **prevalence** of congenital LQTS ranged from 1:5000 to 1:10,000. However, with the development of mutation-specific genotyping, recent studies have suggested significantly higher rates, with one study of neonates suggesting a prevalence approaching 1:2000.[8]
- The **incidence** of sudden cardiac death occurring between birth and age 40 in patients diagnosed with LQTS depends is estimated at 3-4%.[9] Individual risk is influenced by genetic locus, gender, and QTc interval (see section on Diagnostic Testing).[10]

Pathophysiology

- Clinically, prolongation of the QT interval is a reflection of prolonged cardiac action potentials caused by either a **loss of function of potassium channels** or a **gain of function of sodium channels**.
  - Lengthening of the action potential, which is often inhomogeneous, can lead to perturbation of repolarization in the form of **early afterdepolarizations** (EADs).
  - EADs can initiate a triggered activity, which may stimulate neighboring myocytes and lead to a ventricular premature depolarization (VPD). Such a VPD occurring very early can create local reentrant excitation.
  - In a heart with QT prolongation and dispersion of repolarization, such a local reentrant excitation can then propagate into **polymorphic ventricular tachycardia,** often in the form of **TdP.**[11]
- TdP is usually seen following a sequence of **long–short RR interval,** where a VPD (the short interval) follows a pause (the long interval), which may be compensatory, following another VPD (Figure 31-4).[12]
- Another phenomenon connected to TdP is beat-to-beat amplitude variation in the T waves **(T-wave alternans)**. It can occur a variable time before the arrhythmic event and is a sign of a high risk of TdP.
- **Repolarization reserve** is a concept that has been proposed to explain the interplay of congenital and acquired factors in determining the variable penetrance and clinical manifestations of the syndrome.[13]

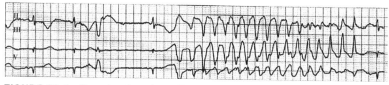

FIGURE 31-4. Torsades de pointes. The arrhythmia in the middle of the strip is preceded by a long–short RR interval. (Reprinted with permission from Bigatello LM. *Critical Care Handbook of the Massachusetts General Hospital.* 5th ed. Wolters Kluwer Health/Lippincott Williams & Wilkins; 2009:286.)

○ It suggests that redundancy in ion channels and their respective currents involved in repolarization provides a measure of safety.

○ Patients with "poor" repolarization reserve may be especially susceptible to arrhythmias when exposed to QT-prolonging agents or sympathetic stimulation.

DIAGNOSIS

Clinical Presentation

• Increasingly, due to improved awareness and ECG utilization, most patients are identified in the absence of symptomatic manifestations.

• Symptomatic patients with LQTS may present in adolescence and early adulthood with variable complaints related to ventricular arrhythmia, often with **unexplained syncope** and **sudden cardiac arrest**.

• A history of seizures, often representing a missed diagnosis of ventricular fibrillation, should increase suspicion.

• Congenital LQTS is now known, via postmortem molecular genetic studies, to affect a significant portion of infants who die unexpectedly (sudden infant death syndrome).[14]

• Obtaining a thorough family history, including unexpected sudden cardiac death, syncope, diagnoses of LQTS, and defibrillator implantation, is necessary.

Diagnostic Criteria

Per expert consensus guidelines,[2] LQTS can be diagnosed:

• In the presence of QTc ≥500 ms on repeated 12-lead ECGs in the absence of secondary causes

• In the presence of QTc between 480 and 499 ms on repeated 12-lead ECGs in a patient with unexplained syncope in the absence of a secondary cause

• In the presence of an unequivocally pathogenic mutation in one of the *LQTS* genes

• In the presence of an LQTS risk score ≥3.5 (Figure 31-5).[15] This scoring system otherwise known as the "Schwartz score" was developed before the advent of genetic testing.

Clinical History

	Points
Syncope (with stress)	2
Syncope (without stress)	1
Congenital Deafness	0.5

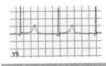

ECG Findings

	Points
QTc > 480 msec	3
QTc 460-470 msec	2
QTC > 450 msec (men)	2
Torsades de pointes	2
T-wave alternans	1
Notched T waves (three leads)	1
Low heart rate (for age)	0.5

Family History

	Points
Family Member with definite long QT Syndrome	1
Unexplained Sudden Cardiac Death before age 30 in immediate family members	0.5

FIGURE 31-5. Diagnostic Criteria for Long QT Syndrome. (Derived from Schwartz PJ, Moss AJ, Vincent GM, Crampton RS. Diagnostic criteria for the long QT syndrome. An update. *Circulation*.1993;88:782–4)

Diagnostic Testing

- Repeated ECGs and clinical history are the starting points for testing and diagnosis as earlier.
  - Notably, patients who are genetically affected may have normal QTc on ECG (36% in LQT1, 19% in LQT2, 10% in LQT3 in one study).[10]
  - If a patient is with intermediate probability (LQTS risk score 1.5 to 3 points) or the index of suspicion remains high, ambulatory monitoring, exercise treadmill testing, or epinephrine infusion can be used to identify concealed LQTS.[16,17]
- Causes of acquired QT prolongation should be excluded (see section on Acquired Prolongation of the QT Interval).
- **Genetic testing (comprehensive or LQT1, LQT2, and LQT3 targeted)** is commercially available and should be considered in patients with appropriate ECG criteria and history.
  - In patients with *clinically diagnosed* LQTS, genetic counseling and genetic testing are recommended by guidelines.[16] This allows for mutation-specific counseling and screening of family members, if mutation is identified.
  - In patients with *suspected* LQTS, genetic testing can make the diagnosis (see section on Diagnostic Criteria), as well as inform patient and family counseling.
- While at least 17 genes are currently implicated in LQTS, only three are definitively causative for typical LQTS (*KCNQ1*, *KCNH2*, and *SCN5A* corresponding to LQT1, LQT2, and LQT3, respectively, phenotypically described later), four are definitive for LQTS with atypical features (*CALM1*, *CALM2*, *CALM3*, and *TRDN*), one has moderate evidence, and the rest are classified as having limited or disputed evidence in causing LQTS.[6]
  - **LQT1 is the most common genetic variant** of LQTS, comprising ~40-55% of genotyped cases.[18]
    - It is associated with a **loss-of-function** mutation in gene *KCNQ1* encoding the α-subunit of the ion channel responsible for the **slowly activating delayed rectifier potassium current** I_{Ks}. Mutations in KCNQ1 can be inherited in an autosomal dominant or autosomal recessive pattern. The autosomal recessive form is sometimes associated with profound deafness; this is referred to as the Jervell and Lange-Nielsen syndrome.
    - Clinical features involve syncope and **adrenergic-triggered arrhythmia** including **exercise**, as I_{Ks} is responsible for shortening QT interval with increased sympathetic tone including exercise. **Swimming** is a commonly reported situation preceding events. Because of the association with adrenergic stimulation, epinephrine infusion may be particularly useful in "unmasking" patients with latent LQT1 for diagnostic purposes.
    - The characteristic T wave in LQT1 is **broad based** and **monophasic**.
  - **LQT2 is the second most common genetic variant**, comprising 30-45% of genotyped patients.[18]
    - It is associated with **loss-of-function** mutation in *KCNH2* (sometimes referred to as *HERG*), encoding the α-subunit of the ion channel responsible for the **rapidly activating delayed rectifier potassium current** I_{Kr}. Normally, the I_{Kr} current is involved in the terminal portion of the action potential and allows protection against EADs.
    - Clinically, events are often triggered by **loud sounds and cognitive stress**, believed to result in sudden changes in sympathetic discharge.
    - The characteristic T wave of LQT2 is **flat and bifid**.
  - **LQT3** occurs in 5-10% of genotyped patients with LQTS.[18]
    - Associated with **gain-of-function** mutation in *SCN5A*, encoding the α-subunit of the ion channel responsible for the sodium current I_{Na}, resulting in prolongation of the plateau of the cardiac action potential.

- Clinically, events leading to sudden cardiac arrest occur during **rest, especially at night**.
- Characteristic ECG changes in LQT3 include a **long isoelectric ST segment, followed by a narrow-peaked T wave**.
- The **risk of subsequent event** (syncope or sudden cardiac arrest) following the diagnosis of LQTS is variable, and high-risk features have been reported (Table 31-1).
  ○ **Length of QT interval is a powerful predictor of events**, with risk of arrhythmia increasing exponentially with QT prolongation.
  ○ When QT interval measurement is combined with genetic mutation, risk stratification is greatly enhanced and is valuable in guiding therapy (Table 31-2).[10]

TABLE 31-1	HIGH-RISK FACTORS PREDICTING VENTRICULAR ARRHYTHMIA OR EXCESSIVE QT PROLONGATION

ECG changes

- Long QT interval
- Increased QT variance (QTc >500 ms)
- Increased interval from peak to end of T wave
- T-wave alternans
- T-U waves

Electrolyte abnormalities

- Hypokalemia
- Hypomagnesemia

Female gender
Older age
HIV disease
LV systolic dysfunction
Previous history of drug-induced long QT or torsades de pointes
Relatives with history of drug-induced long QT

HIV, human immunodeficiency syndrome; LV, left ventricular; QTc, corrected QT.

TABLE 31-2	RISK STRATIFICATION FOR EVENTS BEFORE AGE 40, USING GENETIC AND ECG DATA

High risk (≥50%)	QTc >500 ms and LQT1 or LQT2, and LQT3 (males)
Intermediate risk (30–49%)	QTc <500 ms and LQT2 (females) and LQT3 (male or females) QTc ≥500 ms and LQT3 (females)
Low risk (<30%)	QTc <500 ms and LQT1 (males) and LQT2 (males)

QTc, corrected QT.
Data from Priori SG, Schwartz PJ, Napolitano C, et al. Risk stratification in the long-QT syndrome. *N Engl J Med.* 2003;348:1866–74.

TREATMENT

- In all patients with prolongation of the QT interval, **electrolyte abnormalities** should be evaluated and corrected, especially low serum **potassium** and **magnesium**. Patients with chronically low levels of serum potassium and magnesium should be prescribed oral supplements.
- In patients with congenital LQTS, **strict avoidance of any medications with known QT-prolonging effects** should be endorsed. Patients should be educated and given access to resources in this regard, such as the website www.crediblemeds.org, created and maintained by a nonprofit organization. It provides a search tool for drug names and identifies drugs classified as having a known, possible, or conditional risk of TdP.
- **Exercise restriction** has been historically recommended in congenital LQTS (particularly given adrenergic trigger in LQT1 and, to some degree, in LQT2 patients). However, there is debate as to whether patients who are deemed low risk can participate in competitive sports. A large recent registry demonstrates that certain patients with LQTS and appropriate therapy can safely participate in exercise and sports.[19]

Medications

- **Pharmacologic arrhythmia suppression** is the pillar of therapy for patients with congenital LQTS.
- **β-Adrenergic blockade** is recommended in patients with congenital LQTS, regardless of QTc interval, unless there is prohibitive comorbid asthma.[2] β-Blockers offer more protection in certain genetic variants than others (LQT1 > LQT2 > LQT3).[20]
  - β-Blockers may be **particularly useful in preventing symptoms in LQT1.**
  - β-Blockers have mixed results in the prevention of events in LQT2, producing the competing effects of adrenergic suppression (antiarrhythmic) and bradycardia (proarrhythmic).
  - β-Adrenergic blockade is less effective in LQT3.
  - Propranolol and nadolol, titrated to tolerated doses, are the β-blockers of choice.
  - Avoid abrupt discontinuation of β-blockers.
- **Mexiletine**, a Vaughan-Williams class IB Na^+ channel-blocking antiarrhythmic drug, may have clinical efficacy in LQT3.[21] Other sodium channel blockers such as flecainide and ranolazine may also be beneficial.

Nonpharmacologic Therapies

- **Implantable cardioverter-defibrillators** (ICDs) provide an effective means of terminating arrhythmias and are potentially lifesaving in patients with LQTS.
- ICD therapy is not recommended in low-risk asymptomatic patients.
- Defibrillator implantation should be considered in patients who are at **high risk for subsequent events** (such as syncope) or who have experienced **resuscitated cardiac arrest**.
- Patients with **events despite optimal treatment with medications** (namely β-blockers, which provide the most therapeutic benefit in LQT1 as noted previously) should be considered for defibrillator implantation.

Surgical Management

- **Left cardiac sympathetic denervation** (LCSD) is a treatment option in patients who are not candidates for ICD placement, or for those who have breakthrough despite β-blockade.
- LCSD interrupts the sympathetic/adrenergic input to the heart that can serve as a trigger for arrhythmias in this population. Given the proposed mechanism, it is expected that LQT1 patients would derive the most benefit from this therapy.[22]

Acquired Prolongation of the QT Interval

GENERAL PRINCIPLES

Definition

- Acquired LQTS implicates a secondary cause for QT interval prolongation, such as drugs or electrolyte derangements.
- Other medical conditions that may be accompanied by a prolonged QT interval include **postmyocardial infarction, hypertrophic cardiomyopathy, dilated cardiomyopathy, myocarditis, hypothyroidism, pheochromocytoma, subarachnoid hemorrhage,** and **Takotsubo cardiomyopathy**.

Epidemiology

- Medications with QT-prolonging effects are exceedingly common, and clinicians should familiarize themselves with some of the most prescribed medications (Table 31-3).
  - Websites like www.crediblemeds.org maintain a comprehensive list of QT-prolonging agents.
  - A total of 2-3% of all medications have known QT-prolonging effects.
- **TdP is more common with antiarrhythmic drugs**, occurring in 1-5%. With other QT-prolonging medications, TdP is very rare, occurring in <0.1% of patients.
- Several clinical characteristics that predict drug-induced TdP have been described, including **female gender, hypokalemia, bradycardia, recent conversion from atrial fibrillation (especially with a QT-prolonging antiarrhythmic drug), heart failure, digitalis use, baseline QT prolongation, subclinical congenital LQTS,** and **hypomagnesemia**.[23]

Pathophysiology

- As with inherited channelopathies, secondary factors such as medications and electrolyte abnormalities can lead to prolonged action potential duration and heterogeneous repolarization, predisposing to ventricular arrhythmias such as TdP.

TABLE 31-3	COMMON MEDICATIONS KNOWN TO PROLONG THE QT INTERVAL

Antiarrhythmic drugs
Dofetilide, amiodarone, sotalol, quinidine, disopyramide, ibutilide

Antipsychotics
Chlorpromazine, haloperidol, thioridazine, clozapine, risperidone

Anti-infective agents
Clarithromycin, erythromycin, amantadine, azithromycin, levofloxacin, ciprofloxacin

Antiemetics
Droperidol, ondansetron, granisetron

Antidepressants
Some serotonin reuptake inhibitors

Other
Cisapride, methadone, arsenic

- In the case of drug-associated QT prolongation, **inhibition of hERG** (responsible for the rapidly activating delayed rectifier potassium current I_{Kr}, and affected LQT2) has been implicated as a common cause.[24]
- The variable risk of QT prolongation has been explained by the concept of **repolarization reserve** (see section on Pathophysiology in Long QT Syndrome). One of the extensions of this concept is the existence of different levels of susceptibility to excessive QT prolongation and TdP.

TREATMENT

- In patients with acquired prolonged QT, suspected medications should be **discontinued** as soon as they are recognized and electrolytes (potassium, magnesium, calcium) should be normalized.
- Often, patients with acquired QT prolongation require no further therapy beyond avoidance of triggers, if the QT interval normalizes after discontinuation of the medication or correction of electrolyte abnormalities.

PREVENTION

- When prescribing QT-prolonging medications, it is important to review a baseline ECG to assess if QT interval is normal.
- Patients should be given guidance regarding risk and asked to promptly report any symptoms of palpitations, dizziness, syncope, or presyncope. In addition, changes in condition that predispose to electrolyte abnormalities such as new medications (especially diuretics), nausea, vomiting, and diarrhea need to be reported.
- Patients with acquired LQTS are often taking multiple medications with QT-prolonging effects. Prompt recognition of common QT-prolonging agents is critical in preventing arrhythmia in patients with **polypharmacy**.

Short QT Syndrome

GENERAL PRINCIPLES

- SQTS is a very rare inherited condition characterized by abnormally short QT interval (Figure 31-5) and an increased risk of atrial and ventricular arrhythmias.[25]
- It was originally described in 2000.[26] Of the total 144 families described in the literature as of 2018, 37 presented clinically with sudden cardiac death or aborted sudden cardiac death, and 15 presented with atrial fibrillation in infancy/childhood.[27]

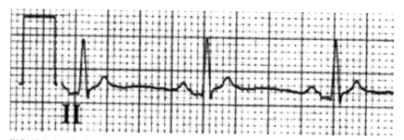

FIGURE 31-6. Lead II in the first patient described with SQTS; heart rate is 60, and QT interval is 230 ms.

Definitions

- Like LQTS, SQTS is suspected primarily by the ECG measurement of the QT interval on the 12-lead surface ECG (Figure 31-1).
- **Lower limit of normal for the QTc interval is 360 ms in males and 370 ms in females.**
- **Because the QT interval in SQTS is minimally affected by heart rate, Bazett formula will overcorrect the QT interval at heart rates >60 beats per minute (bpm), which, in some cases (especially in children with faster heart rates), may lead to missing a diagnosis of SQTS.** The best way to make the ECG diagnosis of a short QT is, therefore, to measure the QT interval at a heart rate as close to 60 bpm as possible.

Pathophysiology

- SQTS has variable inheritance pattern just like LQTS, though, unlike LQTS, most patients have not been genetically categorized. Mutations implicated in SQTS include:
  - **Gain-of-function** mutations in the **KCNH2, KCNQ2,** and **KCNJ2** genes encoding proteins responsible for I_{Kr}, I_{Ks}, and I_{K1}, respectively.
  - **Loss-of-function** mutations in the **CACNA1C** and **CACNB2B** genes encoding proteins responsible for I_{CaL}. Patients with these mutations often have type 1 Brugada pattern ECG at rest or with drug challenge.
  - Both types of mutations result in shortening of the action potential duration.
- Shortening of the action potentials duration leads to a shortened refractory periods and increased dispersion of refractoriness, which, in turn, create a substrate for reentry and tachyarrhythmias, such as atrial and ventricular fibrillation.
- QTc intervals between 345 and 360 ms have been observed in some patients with **early repolarization**, **idiopathic ventricular fibrillation**, and **Brugada syndrome**, all of which convey an increased risk of sudden cardiac arrest.

Epidemiology

- SQTS is a very rare autosomal dominant inherited channelopathy with heterogeneous genetic basis. Variable penetrance has been invoked to explain why there appears to be a male predominance in the cohorts described to date.
- While a short QT interval measured on ECG should lead to the further evaluation of symptoms and family history, it does not automatically imply SQTS. A study of over 18,000 apparently healthy people aged 14 to 35 years found a prevalence of QTc <320 ms of 0.1% (26 individuals) without any increase in cardiac outcomes in the group.[28] In the Framingham Study, 2 standard deviations below the mean QTc was 332 ms in males and 344 ms in females.[29] A strict cutoff defining a pathologically short QT interval does not exist.

Etiology

- SQTS is primarily an inherited condition; however, the causes of acquired shortening of the QT interval are known.
- **Hypercalcemia** is a common cause of shortened QT intervals, often as an effect of **hyperparathyroidism**, **malignancy**, **renal disease**, and **medications**.
- Short QT intervals have also been reported secondary to **hyperkalemia**, **acidosis**, effect of **digoxin**, effect of **catecholamines**, **androgen use**, **enhanced vagal tone**, and **hyperthermia**.

DIAGNOSIS

Clinical Presentation

- In the absence of a family history and ECG, historical information compatible with a diagnosis of SQTS is often nonspecific and is more likely to represent other processes.

- If the patient is **known to have a short QT interval**, complaints consistent with **atrial fibrillation** or **ventricular tachyarrhythmia** strongly favor a diagnosis of SQTS.
- Patients may complain of **palpitations** and unheralded **syncope**.
- **Sudden cardiac arrest** is a possible presentation.

Diagnostic Testing

- No specific QTc on ECG differentiates affected from healthy individuals.
- A short QTc on ECG should prompt further clinical evaluation regarding personal history of syncope and family history of sudden/unexplained death or ICD placement.
- Expert consensus statements recommend using QTc ≤330 ms for diagnosis, or QTc ≤360 ms in the presence of pathogenic mutation, family history of SQTS or sudden death in a family member younger than 40 years of age, or aborted cardiac arrest.[2]
- Other features suggestive of SQTS include:
  ○ **Tall, peaked T waves** especially in left precordial leads are characteristic for some forms of SQTS.
  ○ Lack of changes in QT interval with changes in heart rate is characteristic of SQTS.
  ○ Effective refractory periods are very short in both the atria and the ventricles.
  ○ Ventricular fibrillation is usually inducible during electrophysiologic (EP) study; however, sensitivity is low and thus EPS is not generally used for risk stratification.[30]
- There are no clear guidelines on the evaluation of patients with suspected SQTS.
  ○ It is important to identify and treat secondary causes of QT shortening when possible.
  ○ **Genetic testing** for known mutations can confirm the diagnosis of SQTS.
  ○ The utility of additional studies, including ambulatory monitoring and stress testing for assessment of QT/RR slope and invasive EP testing for assessment of refractory periods, and inducibility of tachyarrhythmias are not well defined.

TREATMENT

- Currently, the only established treatment for patients diagnosed with SQTS is ICD implantation for the prevention of sudden cardiac death.
- There are no independent individual risk factors to guide risk stratification, and there are no data to support ICD placement in asymptomatic patients. ICD is recommended as a secondary prevention strategy (in the case of aborted sudden cardiac death and sustained VT). It can be considered in patients with SQTS and family history of sudden cardiac death.[2]
- The tall peaked T waves found in SQTS have, in some cases, been problematic for sensing of the intracardiac electrogram, causing double counting and inappropriate shocks.
- QT-prolonging drugs have been proposed as treatment options in patients who have an indication but refuse ICD implantation or have recurrent ICD therapies.
  ○ **Quinidine** has been used in the setting of SQT1. It is thought to be effective through blockade of I_{Kr} producing channels, thus prolonging the action potential.
  ○ **Hydroquinidine** has been used to normalize the QT interval and reduce clinical events in small studies of patients with SQT1.[31]

REFERENCES

1. Morita H, Wu J, Zipes DP. The QT syndromes: long and short. *Lancet.* 2008;372:750-63.
2. Priori SG, Wilde AA, Horie M, et al. HRS/EHRA/APHRS expert consensus statement on the diagnosis and management of patients with inherited primary arrhythmia syndromes: document endorsed by HRS, EHRA, and APHRS in May 2013 and by ACCF, AHA, PACES, and AEPC in June 2013. *Heart Rhythm.* 2013;10:1932-63.
3. Drew BJ, Ackerman MJ, Funk M, et al. Prevention of torsade de pointes in hospital settings. *Circulation.* 2010;121:1047-60.

4. Phoon CKL. Mathematic validation of a shorthand rule for calculating QTc. *Am J Cardiol.* 1998;82:400-402.
5. Splawski I, Shen J, Timothy KW, et al. Spectrum of mutations in long-QT syndrome genes. *Circulation.* 2000;102:1178-85.
6. Adler A, Novelli V, Amin AS, et al. An international, multicentered, evidence-based reappraisal of genes reported to cause congenital long QT syndrome. *Circulation.* 2020;141:418-28.
7. Zimetbaum P, Buxton A, Josephson M. Practical clinical electrophysiology. In: *Practical Clinical Electrophysiology.* 2nd ed. Wolters Kluwer; 2018:229.
8. Schwartz PJ, Stramba-Badiale M, Crotti L, et al. Prevalence of the congenital long-QT syndrome. *Circulation.* 2009;120:1761-7.
9. Zareba W, Moss AJ, Schwartz PJ, et al. Influence of the genotype on the clinical course of the long-QT syndrome. *N Engl J Med.* 1998;339:960-5.
10. Priori SG, Schwartz PJ, Napolitano C, et al. Risk stratification in the long-QT syndrome. *N Engl J Med.* 2003;348:1866-74.
11. Viskin S, Alla SR, Barron HV, et al. Mode of onset of torsade de pointes in congenital long QT syndrome. *J Am Coll Cardiol.* 1996;28:1262-8.
12. Bigatello LM, Alam H, Allain RM, et al. *Critical Care Handbook of the Massachusetts General Hospital.* Wolters Kluwer; 2009.
13. Roden DM. Taking the "idio" out of "idiosyncratic": predicting torsades de pointes. *Pacing Clin Electrophysiol.* 1998;21:1029-34.
14. Arnestad M, Crotti L, Rognum TO, et al. Prevalence of long-QT syndrome gene variants in sudden infant death syndrome. *Circulation.* 2007;115:361-7.
15. Schwartz PJ, Moss AJ, Vincent GM, Crampton RS. Diagnostic criteria for the long QT syndrome. An update. *Circulation.* 1993;88:782-4.
16. Al-Khatib SM, Stevenson WG, Ackerman MJ, et al. 2017 AHA/ACC/HRS guideline for management of patients with ventricular arrhythmias and the prevention of sudden cardiac death. *Circulation.* 2018;138:e272–e391.
17. Vyas H, Hejlik J, Ackerman MJ. Epinephrine QT stress testing in the evaluation of congenital long-QT syndrome. *Circulation.* 2006;113:1385-92.
18. Schwartz PJ, Crotti L, Insolia R. Long-QT syndrome. *Circ Arrhythm Electrophysiol.* 2012;5:868-77.
19. Tobert KE, Bos JM, Garmany R, Ackerman MJ. Return-to-play for athletes with long QT syndrome or genetic heart diseases predisposing to sudden death. *J Am Coll Cardiol.* 2021;78:594-604.
20. Priori SG. Association of long QT syndrome loci and cardiac events among patients treated with β-blockers. *JAMA.* 2004;292:1341-4.
21. Mazzanti A, Maragna R, Faragli A, et al. Gene-specific therapy with mexiletine reduces arrhythmic events in patients with long QT syndrome type 3. *J Am Coll Cardiol.* 2016;67:1053-8.
22. Moss AJ, Goldenberg I. Importance of knowing the genotype and the specific mutation when managing patients with long-QT syndrome. *Circ Arrhythm Electrophysiol.* 2008;1:219-26.
23. Roden DM. Drug-induced prolongation of the QT interval. *N Engl J Med.* 2004;350:1013-22.
24. Finlayson K, Witchel HJ, McCulloch J, Sharkey J. Acquired QT interval prolongation and HERG: implications for drug discovery and development. *Eur J Pharmacol.* 2004;500:129-42.
25. Bjerregaard P, Nallapaneni H, Gussak I. Short QT interval in clinical practice. *J Electrocardiol.* 2010;43:390-5.
26. Gussak I, Brugada P, Brugada J, et al. Idiopathic short QT interval: a new clinical syndrome? *Cardiology.* 2000;94:99-102.
27. Bjerregaard P. Diagnosis and management of short QT syndrome. *Heart Rhythm.* 2018;15:1261-7.
28. Dhutia H, Malhotra A, Parpia S, et al. The prevalence and significance of a short QT interval in 18,825 low-risk individuals including athletes. *Br J Sports Med.* 2016;50:124-9.
29. Sagie A, Larson MG, Goldberg RJ, et al. An improved method for adjusting the QT interval for heart rate (the Framingham Heart Study). *J Am Coll Cardiol.* 1992;70:797-801.
30. Giustetto C, Di Monte F, Wolpert C, et al. Short QT syndrome: clinical findings and diagnostic-therapeutic implications. *Eur Heart J.* 2006;27:2440-7.
31. Mazzanti A, Maragna R, Vacanti G, et al. Hydroquinidine prevents life-threatening arrhythmic events in patients with short QT syndrome. *J Am Coll Cardiol.* 2017;70:3010-15.

Adult Congenital Heart Disease

32

Natasha K. Wolfe and Kathryn J. Lindley

Introduction

GENERAL PRINCIPLES

- Congenital heart diseases (CHDs) are malformations of the heart or great vessels that have been present since birth.
- Three factors require particular consideration when caring for an adult patient with CHD:
  - The original congenital cardiac lesion
  - The specific surgical repair(s) that the patient has undergone
  - The anticipated natural history associated with both the condition and the repair

Classification

The recent 2018 American College of Cardiology/American Heart Association (ACC/AHA) guidelines recommend classification of CHD by both anatomic and physiologic complexity.[1] This classification system is presented in Table 32-1. Select conditions are described in more detail later in this chapter.

Epidemiology

- 90% of patients with CHD survive into adulthood.[1]
- An estimated 1.4 million adults live with CHD in the US.[2]
- Gender prevalence varies by cardiac lesion.

Etiology

- Genetic:
  - Chromosomal abnormalities and congenital syndromes are present in almost 20% of patients with congenital heart defects.
  - 40-50% of patients with trisomy 21 have CHD.
  - 15% of patients with tetralogy of Fallot (ToF) or conotruncal defects have 22q11.2 deletion.
  - ~60% of CHD cases are unexplained, suggesting complex, non-Mendelian inheritance patterns.
- Environmental:
  - Maternal infections (e.g., rubella)
  - Medications/drugs (e.g., lithium, thalidomide, alcohol)
  - Maternal conditions (e.g., diabetes, lupus)

Atrial Septal Defect

GENERAL PRINCIPLES

- The most common type of congenital defect found in adults, with an estimated prevalence in adulthood of 0.88 per 1000 patients[3]
- Often asymptomatic until the second to fourth decades of life

TABLE 32-1	CLASSIFICATION OF ADULT CONGENITAL HEART DISEASE (ANATOMY + PHYSIOLOGIC STAGE = ACHD AP CLASSIFICATION)[1]	

ACHD anatomy

I: Simple
- Isolated small ASD, VSD, or mild native PS
- Repaired PDA, ASD, VSD

II: Moderate (repaired or unrepaired)
- Anomalous pulmonary venous connection
- AV canal defect
- Coarctation of the aorta
- Congenital aortic valve disease including subvalvular and supravalvular AS
- Tetralogy of Fallot
- Moderate-to-large unrepaired ASD, PDA, VSD
- Ebstein anomaly

III: Complex
- Fontan
- TGA
- Truncus arteriosus
- Double-outlet RV

Physiologic stage

A:
- NYHA class I symptoms
- No hemodynamic or anatomic sequelae
- No arrhythmias
- No end-organ dysfunction

B:
- NYHA class II symptoms
- Mild hemodynamic sequelae (mild aortic or ventricular enlargement or dysfunction)
- Mild valvular disease
- Arrhythmia not requiring treatment
- Trivial or small shunt

C:
- NYHA class III symptoms
- Significant valvular disease
- ≥ moderate ventricular dysfunction
- Mild-to-moderate hypoxemia
- Arrhythmias controlled with treatment
- < severe PAH
- End-organ dysfunction responsive to therapy

D:
- NYHA class IV symptoms
- Severe aortic enlargement
- Arrhythmias refractory to treatment
- Severe PAH
- Eisenmenger syndrome
- Refractory end-organ dysfunction
- Severe hypoxemia

- Simple anatomic lesion, but complex physiologic changes related to pulmonary vascular remodeling and shunt direction often complicate the presentation and management

Classification
- The types of atrial septal defects (ASDs) are illustrated in Figure 32-1.
- **Secundum ASD:**
  - Defect of the true fossa ovalis due to either enlarged ostium secundum or insufficient septum secundum tissue
  - Most common form of ASD, about 80%

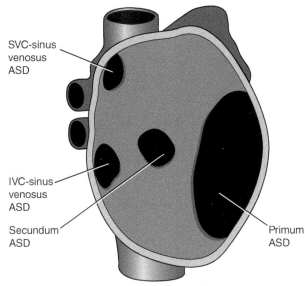

FIGURE 32-1. Anatomic location of common atrial septal defects (ASDs). IVC, inferior vena cava; SVC, superior vena cava.

- ○ Occurs more frequently in women
- ○ Can be associated with mitral valve prolapse
- **Primum ASD**:
  - ○ Defect in lower atrial septum due to defective fusion of septum primum with the endocardial cushions
  - ○ Accounts for 10% of ASDs
  - ○ Associated with trisomy 21, atrioventricular (AV) canal defects, and cleft mitral valve
- **Sinus venosus ASD**:
  - ○ Defect where the superior vena cava (SVC) or inferior vena cava (IVC) meets the right atrium (RA) at the intra-atrial septum; superior defect is more common than inferior.
  - ○ Associated with partially anomalous pulmonary venous return (PAPVR), particularly of the right upper pulmonary vein (PV)
- Unroofed coronary sinus (least common type) is associated with persistent left SVC. It is often missed by traditional imaging modalities. It can be detected by injecting agitated saline contrast bubbles in the left upper extremity and seeing bubbles enter the left atrium (LA) before the RA.
- Other associated defects are valvular pulmonic stenosis (PS) and coronary artery abnormalities.

Pathophysiology

- Under normal conditions, there is left-to-right (L-to-R) shunting from the higher pressure LA to the lower pressure RA.
- Over time, the right-sided chambers can dilate secondary to volume overload, which can lead to atrial arrhythmias.
- In a small percentage of patients (~15%), continued volume overload to the right heart can lead to pulmonary hypertension, and sometimes, pulmonary pressures eventually exceed systemic pressures, causing shunt reversal.

DIAGNOSIS

Clinical Presentation

History
- Majority of patients are asymptomatic, but gradual onset of symptoms often leads to a late diagnosis.[3]
- Early symptoms: dyspnea on exertion and/or fatigue
- Late symptoms: atrial arrhythmias, signs of right-sided heart failure (third to fourth decades)
- End-stage symptoms: In a small percentage of patients, there is the development of **pulmonary hypertension, Eisenmenger syndrome,** and right-sided heart failure.
- Increased risk of paradoxical embolism and stroke

Physical Examination
- **Fixed split S$_2$**
- Loud P$_2$ present in setting of pulmonary hypertension
- Soft systolic murmur at the left upper sternal border secondary to increased flow across the right ventricular outflow tract (RVOT) and pulmonary valve (PV)
- Right ventricle (RV) heave or pulmonary artery (PA) tap with large shunts or the development of pulmonary hypertension
- Large shunts may result in a diastolic rumble at the left lower sternal border.

Diagnostic Testing
- ECG:
  - All types of ASD commonly have an incomplete right bundle branch block (RBBB) pattern (rSR′) and may have some degree of AV block.
  - Secundum ASD may have right-axis deviation with right atrial enlargement (RAE) and right ventricular hypertrophy (RVH).
  - Primum ASD may have left-axis deviation (or extreme right axis).
  - Sinus venosus ASD may have an abnormal P-wave axis (leftward).
- CXR:
  - Typically normal
  - If pulmonary arterial hypertension (PAH) is present, enlarged cardiac silhouette with RA and RV enlargement and increased pulmonary vascular markings may be seen.
- Transthoracic echocardiogram (TTE):
  - Two-dimensional imaging of the atrial septum (parasternal, apical, subcostal views) employing color Doppler to display shunting
  - Contrast echo with agitated saline (bubble study) to confirm an R-to-L shunt if color Doppler is negative/inconclusive
  - Tricuspid regurgitation (TR) jet should be used to estimate PA pressure.
- Transesophageal echocardiogram (TEE) improves lesion definition particularly in the case of sinus venosus and coronary sinus defects.
- MRI and cardiac CT: useful with unclear or inconclusive echocardiography findings and to identify abnormal PV connections
- Cardiac catheterization: used for the measurement of pulmonary pressures, pulmonary vascular resistance (PVR), pulmonary-to-systemic flow ratio (Qp:Qs), and for coronary artery evaluation in patients being evaluated for closure

TREATMENT

Medications
- Anticoagulation is warranted in the presence of atrial fibrillation.
- Rate and rhythm control strategies are used for atrial fibrillation management. Rhythm control should be pursued based on individual patient characteristics with

particular consideration of the congenital defect, not solely on the basis of patient symptoms.
- Pulmonary vasodilators are recommended in those with significant PAH.[3,4]

Surgical Management

- Indications for closure[1,3]:
  - Class I indication for transcatheter or surgical closure in patients with symptoms (impaired functional capacity), enlarged RA and/or RV, and physiologically significant net L-to-R shunt (Qp:Qs ratio ≥1.5:1)
    - Patients should not have cyanosis at rest or with exertion or have PA pressures ≥50% systemic or PVR ≥1/3 SVR (systemic vascular resistance).
    - Transcatheter closure is indicated for uncomplicated secundum ASDs as defect size permits.
    - Primum ASD, sinus venosus ASD, and coronary sinus ASD require surgical closure.
  - Class IIa indication for closure if patients meet the abovementioned criteria but are asymptomatic
  - Class IIb indication for closure in patients with PA pressures ≥50% systemic or PVR ≥1/3 SVR
  - Class III (HARM) for closure in patients with pulmonary pressures and PVR ≥2/3 systemic and/or a net R-to-L shunt. Recent studies demonstrate that pulmonary vasodilators can be used for patients with significant PAH, but still have a net L-to-R shunt, in a "treat-to-close" approach. Approximately 30% of patients treated with pulmonary vasodilators have improvement in pulmonary pressures, allowing for eventual ASD closure and leading to improved RV size, 6-minute walk test (6MWT), and a trend toward improved survival.[4]

Lifestyle/Risk Modification

- Endocarditis prophylaxis: indicated the first 6 months after closure, in patients with net R-to-L shunting (cyanotic), and residual shunt at the site of or adjacent to repair with prosthetic material[1]
- Pregnancy: generally well tolerated, should be avoided if there is presence of significant PAH and/or Eisenmenger syndrome (World Health Organization [WHO] class I if repaired with no residual sequelae, WHO II if unrepaired in the absence of PAH)[1,5]
- Activity[6]:
  - Small defect, normal right heart volume, no PAH: no limitations
  - Large defect with normal pulmonary pressures: no limitations
  - Presence of mild pulmonary hypertension: low-intensity competitive sports
  - Cyanosis or large R-to-L shunt: no participation in competitive sports
  - Symptomatic arrhythmias: preparticipation screening
  - Postclosure: no limitations as long as pulmonary pressures are normal, and there is no evidence of arrhythmia, no second- or third-degree AV block, and no myocardial dysfunction
- Thromboembolic prophylaxis:
  - Dual-antiplatelet therapy for the first 3 to 6 months after surgical or device closure
  - Warfarin or direct oral anticoagulants (DOACs) after documented thromboembolic cerebrovascular event and/or with concomitant atrial fibrillation

Ventricular Septal Defect

GENERAL PRINCIPLES

- Ventricular septal defects (VSDs) are the most common congenital heart defect in infants (0.5-5%).[7]
- The majority of VSDs close spontaneously (~80%).

Classification[7]

- **Type 1** (so-called conal, subpulmonary, infundibular, or supracristal):
  - Accounts for 6% of VSDs in non-Asians, but up to 33% in Asians
  - It is located near the outflow portion of the RV.
  - Frequently associated with aortic insufficiency (AI)
- **Type 2** (so-called perimembranous, membranous, or conoventricular):
  - Overall, the most common type of VSD, about 80%
  - Located in the membranous septum adjacent to tricuspid septal leaflet
  - May be associated with AI
  - May be closed by septal leaflet of the tricuspid valve (TV), leading to a "septal aneurysm"
  - Rarely may be a Gerbode defect (shunting between the LV and the RA)
  - May be associated with subvalvular PS
- **Type 3** (so-called inlet, AV canal type):
  - Accounts for 5-8% of VSDs
  - Common in patients with trisomy 21
  - In the lower RV adjacent to the TV
- **Type 4** (muscular):
  - Accounts for 20% of VSDs in infants but less in adults
  - Central, apical, or at the margin of the septum and free wall of the RV
  - Spontaneous closure is common in childhood.
  - Often seen without other defects
  - Can occur as part of a multilesion syndrome (i.e., ToF, transposition of the great arteries [TGA])

Pathophysiology

- Blood flows preferentially from the high-pressure LV into the RV.
- A sufficiently large Qp:Qs can result in LV volume overload and heart failure.
- Over time, an uncorrected VSD with an L-to-R shunt may cause pulmonary vascular remodeling and eventual reversal of the shunt (Eisenmenger syndrome).
- Small (restrictive): <1/3 size of aortic annulus with a hemodynamically insignificant L-to-R shunt (Qp:Qs <1.5), no LV volume overload, and no PAH
- Moderate: 1/3 to 2/3 size of aortic diameter with a small-to-moderate L-to-R shunt, mild-to-moderate LV volume overload, and mild/no PAH. Qp:Qs is ~1.5:1.9.
- Large: 2/3 size of aortic diameter, a large L-to-R shunt, LV volume overload and RV pressure overload, and PAH is typical. Qp:Qs >2.0.

DIAGNOSIS

Clinical Presentation

- The presentation varies from an asymptomatic murmur to fulminant heart failure.
- When symptomatic, history is significant for dyspnea on exertion and fatigue.
- Physical examination is characterized by a **loud, harsh holosystolic murmur** (as long as the RV pressure is low). As RV pressure rises, the murmur becomes softer.

Diagnostic Testing

- ECG: LA and LV enlargement/hypertrophy with isolated LV volume overload; RVH with progressive pulmonary hypertension
- CXR: cardiomegaly and increased pulmonary vascular markings with a moderate-to-large defect and Qp:Qs >1.5
- TTE:
  - Diagnostic study of choice to confirm diagnosis, location, size, and shunting present at VSD

○ Assess pulmonary pressures, signs of RV pressure overload, and LV volume overload
○ Identification of associated lesions (i.e., AI)
• MRI: assess anatomy and the presence of other lesions
• Cardiac catheterization:
    ○ Higher accuracy for assessment of Qp:Qs and pulmonary vascular pressures and resistance than other imaging modalities
    ○ Confirm VSD anatomy and number, to define coronary anatomy and the presence of valvular lesions preoperatively

TREATMENT

Surgical Management[1]

• Class I indication for surgical or transcatheter closure if there is evidence of LV volume overload and a hemodynamically significant shunt (Qp:Qs ≥1.5:1):
    ○ PA systolic pressure should be <50% systemic and PVR <1/3 systemic.
    ○ Transcatheter closure of muscular and perimembranous VSDs is feasible with good safety and efficacy profile.
• Surgical closure of perimembranous or supracristal VSD is reasonable in adults when there is worsening aortic valve regurgitation caused by the VSD (class IIa).
• Surgical closure of a VSD may be reasonable in adults with a history of infective endocarditis caused by VSD if not otherwise contraindicated (class IIb).
• Class IIb for closure if there is a net L-to-R shunt with PA systolic pressure ≥50% systemic and/or PVR ≥1/3 systemic.
• Class III (HARM) for closure in patients with severe PAH with PA systolic pressure and PVR ≥2/3 systemic and/or a net R-to-L shunt.
• In absence of the previous findings, the VSD is termed "restrictive" and can be observed.

Lifestyle/Risk Modification

• Endocarditis prophylaxis: indicated 6 months following closure, residual shunt at the site of or adjacent to repair with prosthetic material, and R-to-L shunting as with Eisenmenger syndrome (cyanotic)[1]
• Pregnancy: generally well tolerated, should be avoided if there is presence of significant PAH and/or Eisenmenger syndrome (WHO class I if repaired without sequelae, WHO II if unrepaired)[1,5]
• Activity[6]:
    ○ No restrictions with normal PA pressures
    ○ Postrepair:
        ▪ Asymptomatic patients with small residual defect and no PAH, arrhythmia, or myocardial dysfunction can resume normal activity 3 to 6 months after repair.
        ▪ Avoid competitive sports if persistent severe PAH.

Atrioventricular Septal Defect

GENERAL PRINCIPLES

Definition

Atrioventricular septal defect (AVSD) is also known as an AV canal defect, endocardial cushion defect, or common AV canal.

Etiology

• Due to defective fusion of septum primum with endocardial cushions:
    ○ Complete: primum ASD, type 3 VSD, and common AV valve

- ○ Partial: primum ASD and typically a cleft anterior mitral valve leaflet
- ○ Transitional or intermediate: incomplete atrial and VSDs and/or incomplete abnormalities of the common AV valve
- Often seen with trisomy 21 (one-third of AVSDs)[1]
- Partial AVSD is not associated with trisomy 21.
- Associated defects: ToF, conotruncal anomalies, heterotaxy syndromes, and subaortic stenosis (SubAS).[1]

Pathophysiology

- The abnormal connection between the atria and the ventricles causes blood from the right and left heart to mix. This can lead to low systemic oxygen saturation and cyanosis.
- The common AV valve is often incompetent, leading to regurgitant flow returning to the atria, increasing pulmonary congestion and pressures.
- Initially low PVR leads to increased Qp:Qs, volume overload, and LV failure.
- A nonrestrictive VSD leads to RV pressure overload and failure.

DIAGNOSIS

Clinical Presentation

- Most AVSDs are repaired in childhood. If not, those with complete AVSDs will present with Eisenmenger syndrome and symptoms of heart failure, cyanosis, and/or atrial arrhythmias.
- In patients who underwent surgical repair in infancy, most common long-term complications include the development of left AV valve regurgitation and stenosis, left ventricular outflow tract (LVOT) obstruction attributable to the abnormal ("gooseneck deformity") shape of the LVOT, and tachyarrhythmias and bradyarrhythmias.

Diagnostic Testing

- ECG: left-axis deviation, with or without first-degree AV block; signs of any chamber enlargement
- TTE: diagnostic study of choice to confirm the location, size, and severity. Typically sufficient for complete characterization
- MRI: evaluate for associated lesions
- Cardiac catheterization: evaluate PA pressures when considering operation/reoperation

TREATMENT

Surgical Management[1]

- Often done in infancy, but reoperation may be required
- Reoperation recommended (all class I indications):
  - ○ Presence of severe left AV valve regurgitation/stenosis, resulting in symptoms, arrhythmias, increase in LV dimensions, or reduction in LV function
  - ○ LVOT obstruction with peak gradient >50 mm Hg or peak or lower gradient if associated with heart failure symptoms or moderate-to-severe mitral regurgitation (MR) or AI
  - ○ Residual ASD or VSD with a significant L-to-R shunt (as mentioned earlier)
- Regular evaluation of AV conduction system (ECG and Holter monitor) is necessary in repaired patients as surgical repair can lead to AV node and conduction system disease.

Lifestyle/Risk Modification

- Endocarditis prophylaxis: indicated with concomitant prosthetic valve, cyanosis, residual defect near prosthetic patch (thus inhibiting endothelialization of graft), within 6 months of repair[1]

- Pregnancy: usually well tolerated in repaired patient with no residual PAH; in the patient with trisomy 21, there is a 50% risk of transmission to offspring.[1,5]
- Activity: no restrictions in repaired patient if there is no valvular regurgitation, arrhythmia, or LVOT obstruction

Patent Ductus Arteriosus

GENERAL PRINCIPLES

Definition

- Persistent connection between the proximal descending aorta and the roof of the PA.
- Associated defects: ASD and VSD, maternal rubella infection, fetal valproate syndrome, and chromosomal abnormalities

Pathophysiology

- Allows L-to-R blood flow across the patent ductus arteriosus (PDA)
- Patent shunt can lead to left chamber volume overload and increased pulmonary flow.
- May cause remodeling and subsequent pulmonary hypertension/Eisenmenger physiology

DIAGNOSIS

Clinical Presentation

- The presentation largely depends on the size of the PDA, ranging from asymptomatic to dyspnea and fatigue to cyanosis/clubbing with Eisenmenger physiology.[8]
- Physical examination is characterized by a **continuous machinery-type murmur** heard best at left infraclavicular area.
- The pulse is increased, and there is a wide pulse pressure if the PDA is large with a large L-to-R shunt.
- There may be differential cyanosis with clubbing/cyanosis of the feet due to an R-to-L shunt, allowing deoxygenated blood to preferentially be sent to the lower extremities. This occurs when pulmonary pressures meet or exceed systemic pressures.

Diagnostic Testing

- ECG: normal or with left atrial enlargement (LAE) and left ventricular hypertrophy (LVH) if significant L-to-R shunt; RVH with pulmonary hypertension.
- TTE: used to diagnose PDA, evaluate net shunt direction, and estimate PA pressure
- CXR: typically demonstrates left heart enlargement and increased pulmonary vascularity until the development of Eisenmenger syndrome

TREATMENT

Surgical Management[1,8]

- Class I indications for closure:
  - LA or LV enlargement
  - Net L-to-R shunt
  - PA systolic pressure <50% systemic and PVR <1/3 systemic
  - **Catheter-based closure is preferred** unless deemed impossible after consultation with an adult congenital interventional cardiologist.
- Class IIb indications for closure: Patient with PAH (PA systolic pressure ≥50% or PVR ≥1/3 systemic) and net L-to-R shunt
- Class III indication for closure: not indicated in severe PAH (PA systolic pressure or PVR ≥2/3 systemic) with net R-to-L shunt

Lifestyle/Risk Modification

- Endocarditis prophylaxis: not recommended unless the patient is cyanotic[1,8]
- Pregnancy: generally well tolerated, exceptions include large degree of shunting and in the presence of PAH (WHO class I unless left ventricular volume overload (LVVO)/PAH)[5]
- Activity: generally, no restrictions with a small defect or postclosure; larger defects warrant a restriction in activity.[6]

Partial Anomalous Pulmonary Venous Return

GENERAL PRINCIPLES

Definition

- PAPVR occurs when some portion of the PV drainage is to systemic venous structures or to the RA.
- Typical sites of connection include:
  - Left upper PV to the innominate vein
  - Right upper PV to the SVC (most common)
  - Right PV to the IVC, so-called "Scimitar syndrome"
  - Associated with pulmonary sequestration, aortopulmonary collaterals to the right lung, and right branch PA stenosis

Pathophysiology

- The pathophysiology is similar to ASD, predominantly due to L-to-R shunting of blood and volume overload on right heart. However, unlike ASDs, there is no potential for R-to-L shunting.
- This is a frequently isolated congenital defect but may be associated with many other congenital heart abnormalities such as polysplenia-type heterotaxy.

DIAGNOSIS

Clinical Presentation

History
- PAPVR is typically asymptomatic if the shunt is small.
- Exercise intolerance and edema occur with larger shunts.
- Symptoms compatible with RV failure, severe TR, and/or PAH can also occur.

Physical Examination
- RV heave with a large shunt
- Right-sided S_3 in cases of RV failure
- Palpable PA pulsation with a PV opening snap
- Right-sided S_4 in cases of pulmonary hypertension
- Edema may be present in cases of RV failure or severe TR.
- Systolic TR murmur in cases of TR
- Diastolic tricuspid flow murmur in cases of a large shunt

Diagnostic Testing

- ECG: typically normal; RA and RV enlargement and RVH in patients with PAH
- CXR: typically normal; RA and RV enlargement and increased pulmonary vascular markings in patients with PAH

- TTE: typically normal; RA/RV enlargement, TR, high estimated PA systolic pressure in patients with PAH
- CT/MRI will identify anatomy of anomalous PV return.
- Catheterization will quantify degree of shunt and identify location of shunt and presence and the degree of pulmonary hypertension.

TREATMENT

Surgical Management

- Criteria similar to those for secundum ASD repair.
- After surgical repair, 10% of patients will develop PV stenosis at the site of re-anastomosis, which may require stenting or repeat surgery if physiologically significant.

Lifestyle/Risk Modification

- Endocarditis prophylaxis: indicated only for other associated lesions[1]
- Pregnancy: well tolerated unless there is significant PAH (WHO classes I and II)
- Activity: no restrictions

Total Anomalous Pulmonary Venous Return

GENERAL PRINCIPLES

Definition

- Total anomalous pulmonary venous return (TAPVR) is due to failure of fusion of the PV confluence with the posterior wall of the LA.
- Confluence occurs behind RA with a decompressing vein draining to a systemic venous structure, such as the IVC, SVC, innominate vein, coronary sinus, or subdiaphragmatic veins.
- Cor triatriatum: partial fusion with a residual perforated membrane between the PV confluence and the LA

Epidemiology

- 80-90% of patients with asplenia-type heterotaxy have TAPVR.
- TAPVR is also associated with other congenital heart lesions.

Pathophysiology

- All PV return passes to systemic veins and then to the RA and RV.
- Patients depend on atrial, ventricular, or PDA-level R-to-L shunts to survive.
- Must be repaired or palliated in childhood or death will ensue unless there is sufficient mixing at the level of the R-to-L shunt
- There may be stenosis at the site of anastomosis between the PVs and systemic veins.

DIAGNOSIS

Clinical Presentation

- Almost universally recognized in childhood due to cyanosis or cardiogenic shock in infancy
- Adult patients will almost all have had repair or palliation.
- May be no physical findings if the patient has had prior repair
- Signs and symptoms of pulmonary hypertension and RV pressure overload may occur if there is PV obstruction after repair.

- With palliated patients (those who have an ASD or VSD without complete repair), there will be signs and symptoms of RV volume overload and failure. Severe functional TR may occur with progressive RV dysfunction and enlargement.

Diagnostic Testing
- CXR: RA and RV enlargement, pulmonary hypervascularity in unrepaired or palliated patient; repaired patient may be normal.
- ECG: RA and RV enlargement, RVH in unrepaired or palliated patient; repaired patient may be normal.
- TTE:
  ○ RA and RV volume overload
  ○ There will be an evidence of R-to-L shunting at the atrial, ventricular, or PDA level if palliated or unrepaired.
  ○ May be normal in repaired patients
- CT/MRI: useful to identify anastomosis between the PVs and systemic veins before surgical repair
- Catheterization: useful to identify PV stenosis in repaired patients

TREATMENT

Lifestyle/Risk Modification
- Endocarditis prophylaxis: indicated only for other associated lesions if repair is complete; indicated if repair is palliative due to cyanosis[1]
- Pregnancy: well tolerated in the absence of PV stenosis if repaired; contraindicated if palliated due to high risk of maternal morbidity and mortality (WHO classes III and IV)
- Activity: normal if repaired

Surgical Management
- TAPVR is typically repaired in childhood.
- Postoperative monitoring for evidence of PV stenosis should be regularly performed, particularly in patients with poor exercise tolerance or pulmonary hypertension.
- Surgery or stenting is indicated to relieve PV stenosis in repaired patients.
- Complete repair should be considered in patients who are palliated.

Bicuspid Aortic Valve

GENERAL PRINCIPLES

Epidemiology
- Bicuspid aortic valve (BAV) is the most common congenital cardiac malformation, present in 1 in 80 adults.[9]
- Men are affected more than women (3:1).[10]

Etiology
Most cases are spontaneous, but it can be inherited in an autosomal dominant with reduced penetrance manner within families. Echocardiographic screening is recommended for all first-degree relatives of patients with BAV.[1,10]

Pathophysiology
A BAV is made of two unequal sized leaflets, with the larger leaflet having a central raphe that results from fusion of the commissures. Morphologic patterns of the bileaflet valve vary according to which commissures have fused:

- Most common is fusion of the left and right coronary cusps; this is associated with coarctation of the aorta (CoA).
- Fusion of the right and noncoronary cusps has higher rates of developing AS and/or AI.

Associated Conditions

- Nonvalvular findings occur in up to 50% of adults with BAV, the most common being dilation of the thoracic aorta. Dilation thought to occur due to changes in flow dynamics but also structural abnormalities at the cellular level of the aorta, similar to cystic medial necrosis of Marfan syndrome.
- Coexists with other congenital defects, the most common of which is CoA, along with VSDs, PDA, and ASDs[10]
- Many genetic syndromes with cardiac involvement include BAV and left-sided obstructive lesions: Shone complex, Williams syndrome, and Turner syndrome.
- Increased risk of cerebral aneurysms (up to 10%)[11]

DIAGNOSIS

Clinical Presentation

- Two-thirds of patients develop symptoms of AS by the fifth decade.
- Systolic ejection sound due to valve opening (usually disappears by the fourth decade due to calcification)
- **Crescendo–decrescendo mid-systolic murmur at the upper sternal border with radiation to the neck** (in the presence of AS)
- With more significant AS, the murmur becomes more late peaking, and peripheral pulses are diminished and delayed (pulsus parvus et tardus).

Diagnostic Testing

- ECG: may or may not have LVH, LAE, or ST-T repolarization
- TTE:
  - Qualify the lesion (anatomy of cusp fusion)
  - Quantify the degree of AS and/or AI
  - Assess the aortic root
  - May require TEE if difficult to visualize on transthoracic echo
  - Should be done yearly for AS when mean gradient >30 mm Hg or peak gradient >50 mm Hg, every 2 years if gradients are less
  - Screening TTE: first-degree relatives of patients with BAV, fetus of all pregnant women with BAV in the second trimester
- MRI:
  - Noncontrast chest MR angiography (MRA) can be used to intermittently assess the size of the entire thoracic aorta.
  - Serial imaging for aorta should be done every year if >50 mm and less frequently if <45 mm.
  - Noncontrast brain MRA should be done approximately every 10 years in patients with known aortopathy to screen for the development of cerebral aneurysms.

TREATMENT

Medications

At a minimum, high blood pressure (BP) should be aggressively treated in patients with BAV. β-Blockers and angiotensin-receptor blockers (ARBs) have been demonstrated to slow progression of aortic dilatation in Marfan syndrome; however, there are not significant data on the effectiveness of these medications in adults with CHD.[12]

Surgical Management

- **Balloon valvuloplasty** is the procedure of choice in children, adolescents, and young adults if there is severe AS with no valve calcification and no aortic regurgitation (AR).[9,10]
- **Surgical repair/replacement** indications are similar to those for AS or AI with a normal valve (see Chapter 19).[1,13]
- **Transcatheter aortic valve replacement (TAVR)** has been shown to have good safety and efficacy for AS in those with a bicuspid valve, but it is not currently Food and Drug Administration (FDA) approved for use in those with BAV.[14]
- Class I indication for replacement of the aorta when maximum diameter ≥5.5 cm[13]

Lifestyle Modifications

- Endocarditis prophylaxis: not required unless previous valve replacement[1]
- Pregnancy: generally well tolerated unless there is significant AS or aortic root dilatation. Severe AS is a high-risk lesion (WHO class IV)[5]
- Activity: Limitations are based on the degree of AS; avoidance of competitive sports and isometric exercises with severe AS and/or dilated aorta are indicated.[6]

Subaortic Stenosis

GENERAL PRINCIPLES

- SubAS favors males 2:1 and is usually a solitary lesion.
- Other associated abnormalities include VSD (37%), BAV (23%), and AVSD.[1,9]
- SubAS is due to a fibrous ridge or fibromuscular ring in the LVOT.
- Subvalvular accelerated turbulent flow causes aortic valvular damage in the form of obstruction or AI.
- Physiology may be similar to valvular AS if severe.

DIAGNOSIS

Clinical Presentation

- Patients are asymptomatic early, but as the disease progresses, symptoms of AS (valvular or subvalvular) or AI may be present.
- SubAS often presents with a crescendo–decrescendo murmur at left parasternal apical border.
- Murmur of AI may also be appreciated.

Diagnostic Testing

- TTE: the diagnostic study of choice to illustrate the anatomy, gradient, and associated findings (i.e., AI, mitral involvement, systolic function, etc.)
- Stress test: may be reasonable in adults with equivocal indications for intervention to determine exercise capacity, symptoms, ECG changes, or arrythmias[1]

TREATMENT

Surgical Management[1]

- Class I indication for surgery if patient is symptomatic with peak gradient ≥50 mm Hg or if peak gradient ≤50 mm Hg with ischemic symptoms and/or LV dysfunction
- Class IIb indication for surgery to prevent progression of AR if patients are asymptomatic but peak gradient ≥50 mm Hg and at least mild AR
- There is recurrence of the fibromuscular band after surgery in at least one-third of the patients.

Lifestyle Modifications

Pregnancy generally well tolerated if peak gradient is <50 mm Hg, and engagement in competitive sports should be planned and discussed with the treating physician (depends on the severity of gradient).

Supravalvular Aortic Stenosis

GENERAL PRINCIPLES

- Supravalvular AS is a fixed obstruction immediately distal to the sinus of Valsalva.
- The coronary arteries arise proximal to the obstruction (thus they receive high systolic pressure and low diastolic flow).
- Typically seen in **Williams syndrome** (autosomal dominant mutation on chromosome 7 elastin gene): elfin facies, cognitive disorders, joint abnormalities, and behavioral problems[1,9]
- All first-degree relatives should have screening for this heritable condition.
- Aortic valve abnormalities are found in 50% of the patients.
- PA abnormalities (peripheral PA stenoses) are also seen.
- The pathophysiology is similar to AS, except that there is sometimes coronary artery involvement.

DIAGNOSIS

Clinical Presentation

- The clinic presentation may include symptoms of outflow obstruction (dyspnea, angina, and syncope), hypertension, and coronary ischemia.
- Coandă effect: Preferential flow up the right portion of the ascending aorta can lead to discordant amplitude of carotid and upper extremity arterial pulses. There may also be differential BPs in the upper extremities.
- Suprasternal notch thrill may be heard.
- Crescendo–decrescendo murmur at the left upper sterna border with radiation to the right neck

Diagnostic Testing

- TTE: used to characterize the anatomy of the proximal aorta, obstruction, and associated defects
- MRI/CT: may be required to define the anatomy and associated defects
- Proximal renal artery and main and branch PA flow should be evaluated.
- Myocardial perfusion imaging can be used if there is suspicion for coronary ischemia. Periodic screening may be indicated.

TREATMENT

Surgical Management[1,9]

Class I indications for surgery:
- Symptoms or decreased LV systolic function secondary to aortic obstruction
- Coronary artery revascularization is recommended in symptomatic adults with supravalvular AS and coronary ostial stenosis.

Lifestyle/Risk Modifications

- Pregnancy: not advised if unrepaired
- Activity: should avoid competitive sports and isometric exercises if unrepaired

Coarctation of the Aorta

GENERAL PRINCIPLES

- CoA is due to a narrowing near the level of the ligamentum arteriosum.
- These patients also have an intrinsic aortic wall abnormality similar to the aorta of BAV. This predisposes to aortic dilatation and rupture.
- Associated defects:
  - BAV (nearly three-fourths of coarctation patients), brachiocephalic vessel anomalies, SubAS, VSD, arch hypoplasia, circle of Willis cerebral artery aneurysm (10%)[9]
  - One-third of the patients with Turner syndrome have CoA.
- Evidence of hypoperfusion distal to the site of obstruction depends on the degree of narrowing.
- Hypertension is the most common sequela of CoA, whether repaired or unrepaired.

DIAGNOSIS

Clinical Presentation

- Unoperated CoA is typified by systemic arterial hypertension in the upper extremities with a difference in the upper extremity and lower extremity systolic BP by ≥20 mm Hg.
- Other symptoms include headache, epistaxis, and claudication.
- Assess for brachial–femoral pulse delay in all hypertensive patients (class I).[1]
  - Assess the brachial and femoral pulses for timing and amplitude.
  - Measure the brachial and popliteal BPs as well.
- A left infrascapular murmur is classical.

Diagnostic Testing

- CXR: "Figure 3" sign due to indentation at the CoA and postobstructive dilation; rib notching (present on the inferior rib borders)
- TTE: Suprasternal notch window with color flow and continuous wave may show turbulence in the descending aorta with a peak gradient >20 mm Hg and continuous forward diastolic flow.
- Systemic hypertension may not consistently be identifiable at rest; therefore, guidelines recommend ambulatory BP monitoring or stress testing to identify hypertension with exertion.

TREATMENT

Hypertension should be treated with guideline-directed medical therapy. Low-dose antihypertensive for exercise-induced hypertension (but normotensive at rest) should be considered.

Surgical Management[1,9]

- Catheter-based stenting (preferred) or surgical repair for adults with hypertension and significant native or recurrent CoA
- Balloon angioplasty for adults with native and recurrent CoA may be considered if stent placement is not feasible and surgical intervention is not an option.
- Recurrence rate after balloon angioplasty is 7%.

Lifestyle/Risk Modification

- Endocarditis prophylaxis: indicated for patients in whom repair or stenting has been performed in the past 6 months[1]

- Pregnancy: Risk varies according to associated lesions and the presence/absence of aortic root dilatation.[5] It is generally well tolerated if no recurrent coarctation or aortic root dilatation.
- Activity[1,6]:
  - Unrepaired CoA should avoid contact sports, isometric exercises, and most competitive sports.
  - Stress testing can be used before allowing low- to moderate-intensity sports if no associated lesions and low gradients.

MONITORING/FOLLOW-UP

- CoA repair site should be evaluated at least every 5 years (irrespective of repair status) by MRI or CT to evaluate for recurrence and development of aneurysm.
- Brain MRA or CT angiography (CTA) should be done every 10 years to screen for intracranial aneurysms.

Pulmonary Hypertension/Eisenmenger Physiology

GENERAL PRINCIPLES

- Pulmonary hypertension: CHD-related PAH occurs due to one or a combination of:
  - Pulmonary overcirculation
  - Exposure of the pulmonary vasculature to systemic pressures
- Eisenmenger physiology[15]:
  - This is an end-stage complication for many congenital heart defects.
  - **Reversal of blood flow across a defect** at the level of the pulmonary and systemic ventricles or arteries resulting in **pulmonary-to-systemic shunting** of blood that occurs when **pulmonary BPs meet or exceed systemic**.
- PAH can be caused by many forms of CHD: L-to-R shunts (ASD, VSD, AVSD, PDA), TAPVR, PAPVR, truncus arteriosus, TGA, and single ventricle disorders

DIAGNOSIS

Clinical Presentation

- Symptoms may include dyspnea on exertion (most common), palpitations, edema, and progressive cyanosis.
- Physical findings may include central cyanosis, clubbing, and signs of right heart failure (prominent jugular venous pulsations, increased A waves, ascites, RV impulse, PA impulse, palpable P_2, cessation of previous shunt murmur).
- Patients can develop hyperviscosity syndrome due to polycythemia (driven by chronic cyanosis).
- Increased risk of both bleeding and clotting complications including stroke, intrapulmonary thrombosis, pulmonary hemorrhage, hemoptysis, cerebral bleeding, menorrhagia, and epistaxis
- Increased risk of infections such as bacterial endocarditis, cerebral abscess, and pneumonia

Diagnostic Testing

- The initial workup should include additional testing for other causes of PAH (e.g., pulmonary function tests, CT of the chest for identification of pulmonary emboli).
- ECG: RAE, RVH, and right-axis deviation

- TTE demonstrates defect with bidirectional or pulmonary-to-systemic shunting and increased PA pressure. Agitated saline bubble study is contraindicated, as it can result in air embolism.
- Cardiac catheterization is the gold standard for the diagnosis of PAH and to assess the severity of pulmonary vascular disease and shunt direction and magnitude.
- Yearly blood counts, iron level, creatinine, and uric acid are recommended.[1]
- Yearly digital oximetry and treatment with oxygen if responsive[1]

TREATMENT

- Pulmonary vasodilators may improve 6MWT, hemodynamics, and subjective functional ability.[1]
  - Class I indication for use of bosentan in symptomatic patients with Eisenmenger due to ASD or VSD
  - Class IIa indication for use of combination therapy with bosentan and phosphodiesterase inhibitors if symptoms do not improve with either medication alone
  - Class IIa indication for use of bosentan for symptomatic patients with Eisenmenger due to shunts other than ASD/VSD
- The use of anticoagulation in this population remains controversial as patients are at increased risk of bleeding and clotting.
- Iron deficiency should be treated.
- Therapeutic phlebotomy for erythrocytosis is generally not recommended as it can impair oxygen transport capacity, reduce exercise tolerance, induce iron deficiency, and increase the risk of stroke.
- Endocarditis prophylaxis is indicated due cyanotic nature of this lesion.[1]
- Pregnancy should be avoided due to high risk of maternal and fetal morbidity and mortality, and early termination is recommended.[5]
- Activity: avoid strenuous exercise, acute exposure to excessive heat (i.e., a hot tub), high altitudes, and dehydration.[6]

Tetralogy of Fallot

GENERAL PRINCIPLES

Definition

- The primary defect of ToF is anterior deviation of the infundibular septum.
- Consists of four major defects (Figure 32-2):
  - Subpulmonary infundibular stenosis
  - VSD
  - Aorta overriding (posterior malalignment) VSD
  - RVH
- 5% of patients also have an associated ASD (pentalogy of Fallot).[16]
- 25% will have a right-sided aortic arch, and coronary artery anomalies can also occur.[1]

Epidemiology

- ToF represents 5-10% of all CHD and is the most common cyanotic heart disease.[16]
- Sudden death occurs in 1.5% per decade of follow-up in repaired patients (thought to be mediated by ventricular arrhythmia).
- Associated syndromes are 22q11 deletion and trisomy 21.

Pathophysiology

- Narrowed RVOT restricts systemic venous blood flow to the pulmonary vasculature.

Unrepaired Tetrology of Fallot

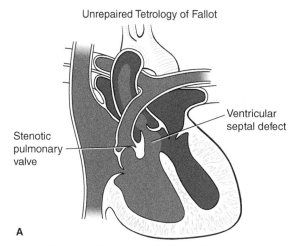

Stenotic
pulmonary
valve

Ventricular
septal defect

A

Surgically Repaired Tetrology of Fallot

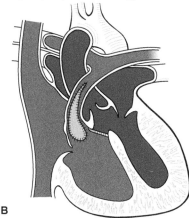

B

FIGURE 32-2. Tetralogy of Fallot with (1) stenotic pulmonic valve (PV), (2) ventral septal defect, (3) right ventricular hypertrophy, and (4) overriding aorta with mixing of oxygenated and deoxygenated blood. (Reprinted with permission from https://www.heart.org/en/health-topics/congenital-heart-defects/about-congenital-heart-defects/tetralogy-of-fallot. Copyright ©American Heart Association, Inc.)

- Dynamic infundibular subpulmonic stenosis is exacerbated during periods of increased myocardial contractility.
- Leads to further increases in resistance to pulmonary blood flow and to preferential shunting of blood from the RV to the LV, producing cyanotic so-called Tet spells

DIAGNOSIS

Clinical Presentation

- Most patients undergo primary surgery in the first year of life.
- Palliative repair varies based on when this was completed.

- Repair typically includes patching of VSD and ASD (if present) with enlargement of the RVOT. The extent of which will depend on the degree and extent of obstruction.
- Patients with prior repair are typically left with significant pulmonary insufficiency (PI). Chronic PI portends significant volume overload on the RV, which, over decades, leads to adverse RV remodeling and eventually RV systolic dysfunction.
- About 20% of patients will develop LV systolic dysfunction later in life.
- Higher risk of ventricular arrhythmias. Typically, due a reentrant rhythm that can form around the surgical ventriculotomy site in the RVOT

History
- Severe PI or residual PS may lead to exertional dyspnea, edema, or other symptoms of RV failure.
- Unrepaired adult patients typically present similar to a nonrestrictive VSD without pulmonary hypertension. This is due to protection of the pulmonary vasculature by subpulmonic stenosis.

Physical Examination
- Postrepair:
  - Systolic murmur from RVOT
  - May or may not have diastolic murmur of PI or residual PS
  - Pansystolic murmur may indicate a VSD patch leak.
- Some patients may have had an arterial-to-pulmonary shunt (i.e., Blalock–Taussig–Thomas [BTT] shunt) before their complete ToF repair, and this may lead to reduced/absent pulses on the ipsilateral side.

Diagnostic Testing

- CXR: Boot-shaped horizontal heart is classic in unrepaired ToF; right-sided aortic arch may be seen; RA and RV enlargement in repaired ToF.
- ECG: RVH and RBBB common in repairs done before 1990s; there is an increased risk of sustained ventricular arrhythmias and sudden death if the QRS is >180 ms.
- TTE: useful for routine follow-up of PI, RVH/RV enlargement, and systolic function; assess for degeneration of repair
- Cardiac MRI: useful for evaluation of severe PI, RV volumes, and RV systolic function

TREATMENT

Surgical Management[1]

- Class I indication for pulmonary valve replacement (surgical or percutaneous) for patients with repaired ToF, moderate or greater pulmonary regurgitation (PR), and cardiovascular symptoms not otherwise explained
- Class IIa indication for pulmonary valve replacement to preserve RV size and function in asymptomatic patients with repaired ToF, moderate or greater PR, and RV enlargement or dysfunction
  - Cardiac MRI should be obtained to get accurate ventricular volumes and function.
  - If patients have two of the following criteria, pulmonary valve replacement is indicated:
    - Mild or moderate RV or LV systolic dysfunction
    - RV end-diastolic volume index $\geq$160 mL/m^2 or RV end-systolic volume index $\geq$80 mL/m^2 or RV end-diastolic volume $\geq$2$\times$ LV end-diastolic volume
    - RVSP due to RVOT obstruction $\geq$2/3 systemic pressure
    - Progressive reduction in objective exercise tolerance
- Class IIb indication for pulmonary valve replacement, in addition to arrhythmia management, for patients with repaired ToF, moderate or greater PR, and ventricular arrhythmias
- Primary prevention implantable cardioverter-defibrillator (ICD) should be considered in adults with ToF and multiple risk factors for sudden cardiac death SCD (see section on Sudden Cardiac Death).[17]

Lifestyle/Risk Modification

- Endocarditis prophylaxis: not indicated in the repaired patient unless within 6 months of repair or there is an evidence of degeneration of prior repair[1]
- Pregnancy[5]:
  - Moderately increased risk of maternal morbidity such as heart failure and arrhythmias; however, pregnancy is generally well tolerated in women postrepair with normal ventricular function.
  - Genetic prenatal counseling is recommended. 4-6% of fetuses born to women with ToF will have a congenital heart defect (in the absence of 22q11 deletion syndrome).
- Activity: In patients with repaired ToF without significant ventricular dysfunction, arrhythmias, or outflow tract obstruction, participation in moderate- to high-intensity sports may be considered, but an exercise test and clinic assessment should be done before clearing.[6]

MONITORING/FOLLOW-UP

- Yearly cardiology follow-up with TTE or MRI (class I indication)
- Annual ECG to assess rhythm and QRS duration
- Intermittent ambulatory ECG monitoring to evaluate for arrhythmias may be indicated.

Transposition of the Great Arteries

GENERAL PRINCIPLES

Classification

- There are two types of TGA:
  - Dextro-TGA (d-TGA)
  - Levo-TGA (l-TGA), also known as congenitally corrected TGA (CCTGA) or double switch
- Associated defects:
  - d-TGA: coronary anomalies, PDA, VSD (45%), LVOT obstruction (25%), and CoA (5%)[1,15]
  - CCTGA: VSD (70%, perimembranous), subvalvular/valvular PS (40%), AI (90% of the systemic semilunar valve), AV block (2% yearly rate), ventricular dysfunction (near universal by adulthood), and Ebstein-like anomaly of TV[18]

Pathophysiology

- d-TGA:
  - Ventriculoarterial discordance where the aorta and main PA are switched in position
  - Path of blood: RA to RV to aorta; LA to LV to PA two parallel circuits where deoxygenated blood circulates through body and oxygenated blood circulates through lungs
  - Septal defect or PDA allows for mixing of deoxygenated/oxygenated blood and thus survival.
  - Presents with cyanosis in infancy. One-third die in the first week without intervention (90% die at 1 year without intervention).
- CCTGA:
  - Ventricular inversion where the RV and LV switch positions
  - Path of blood: RA to LV (first switch) to PA (second switch) to LA to RV to aorta
  - RV functions as the systemic ventricle.

DIAGNOSIS

Clinical Presentation

d-TGA

- Clinical presentation in adulthood is often based on complications associated with the type of repair (Table 32-2).
- Atrial switch operations (i.e., Mustard and Senning procedures) (Figure 32-3)[18]:
  - An intra-atrial baffle is used to redirect blood across the atrium from the SVC and IVC to the mitral valve and out the main PA. PV blood return gets directed to the TV and out the aorta. Results in a systemic RV.
    - Dacron graft or pericardium (Mustard procedure)
    - Atrial septum (Senning procedure)
  - Common problems:
    - Systemic pressure results in RV failure and severe TR.
    - Baffle obstruction or leak occurs in 25% of patients, which may cause paradoxical embolus. Obstruction is more common in the SVC limb.
    - Arrhythmia: 50% develop sinus node dysfunction and 30% develop intra-atrial reentry tachycardia (IART) by age 20.
    - Pulmonary hypertension
  - Atrial switch procedures result in a loud A_2. If there is RV failure, there may be TR and RV heave.
- Arterial switch operation (ASO or Jatene procedure) (Figure 32-3)[18]:
  - PA and aorta trunks are transected and sewn to the contralateral root with transposition of the coronary arteries to the neoaorta. This is preferable as the LV remains the systemic ventricle.
  - Common problems: dilation of the neoaortic root leading to AI, stenosis near anastomosis sites (leads to PS or AS physiology), coronary artery ostial stenosis, supravalvular AS or PS
  - Arterial switch procedure usually results in a normal physical examination.
  - This has become the standard for d-TGA repair since the 1980s.

CCTGA

- >50% are diagnosed in adulthood.
- Presentation varies from asymptomatic to advanced (heart failure, arrhythmias).
- Often, these patients present with systemic AV valve regurgitation and subsequent systemic ventricular dysfunction.
- Physical findings include medial point of maximal impulse (PMI) indicating a rotated heart, single S_2, and possible murmur of VSD, AI, or PS.

Diagnostic Testing

- ECG:
  - Atrial switch: RVH, sinus bradycardia, or junctional escape
  - Arterial switch: normal
  - CCTGA:
    - First-degree AV block (50%) and reversal of precordial Q-wave pattern due to reversed septal activation
    - Complete heart block may be evident (2% per year).[18]
- CXR: "egg on its side" in uncorrected d-TGA patients; cardiomegaly in CCTGA due to left-sided RV enlargement
- TTE:
  - d-TGA: parallel great arteries, aorta anterior and to the right
  - CCTGA: parallel great arteries, aorta is located anterior and to the left

TABLE 32-2 COMMON SURGICAL PROCEDURES PERFORMED IN ADULTS WITH TGA

Name	Description	Advantage	Disadvantage	Consequences
Mustard procedure (atrial switch)	Intra-atrial baffle (pericardium or PTFE)	Low mortality	Arrhythmia, sinus node dysfunction Baffle leak or obstruction Ventricular failure	Most common TGA seen in adults, although supplanted by ASO
Senning procedure (atrial switch)	Intra-atrial baffle (atrial septum)	Low mortality	Arrhythmia, sinus node dysfunction Baffle leak or obstruction Ventricular failure	Supplanted by ASO
Jatene procedure (ASO)	Arterial switch operation, PA and aortic root	Establishes LV as systemic ventricle Less arrhythmia than atrial switch	Coronary artery closure Neoaortic root dilatation	Surgery of choice for TGA repair
Rastelli procedure	Ventricular switch (RV to PA conduit and LV to aorta baffle)	Establishes LV as systemic ventricle	High risk	Used when a VSD and pulmonary stenosis are present with d-TGA
Rashkind procedure	Balloon atrial septostomy	Rapidly creates an ASD to allow for mixing of arterial and venous blood	Palliative	Used in first few days of life to allow for mixing of blood in d-TGA
Blalock–Hanlon procedure	Off-pump surgical atrial septostomy	Off-pump procedure, allows mixing of arterial and venous blood	Palliative	Used before the advent of Rashkind to allow for early mixing of blood in d-TGA

ASO, arterial switch operation; LV, left ventricle; PA, pulmonary artery; PTFE, polytetrafluoroethylene; RV, right ventricle; TGA, transposition of the great arteries; VSD, ventricular septal defect.

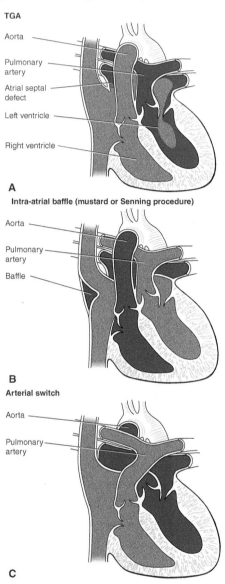

FIGURE 32-3. (**A**) Dextro-transposition of the great arteries (d-TGA). Note the systemic and venous systems in parallel, with mixing only through an atrial septal defect. (**B**) Atrial switch procedure, bringing venous blood to the morphologic left ventricle and out to the lungs. The right ventricle is the systemic ventricle, which is the cause of many of the long-term sequelae in this repair. (**C**) Arterial switch procedure, maintaining the left ventricle as the systemic ventricle.

- May be difficult to identify the morphologic ventricle; these are some clues: RV has a trabeculated apex, RV has moderator band, TV is displaced apically in the RV, LV is attached to a bileaflet AV valve.
- MRI: standard for assessing function and structure
- Diagnostic catheterization:
  - Further assess baffle leaks, presumed stenosis in conduits/baffles/great vessels, or unanticipated sources for ventricular dysfunction
  - Assess coronary anatomy after Jatene operation

TREATMENT

Medications

There are limited data on the use of guideline-directed medical therapy for heart failure, such as angiotensin-converting enzyme inhibitor (ACE-I), ARBs, β-blockers, and aldosterone antagonists in patients with systemic RVs; however, it is reasonable to use such medications in symptomatic patients or those with significant systolic dysfunction.[1,19]

Surgical Management[1,18]

- d-TGA with atrial switch:
  - Interventional catheterization procedures can be done for the treatment of baffle stenosis or leak with placement of stents at sites of obstruction (SVC, IVC, or PVs) or occluder devices at sites of leak.
  - Surgical procedures can be done for moderate-to-severe systemic TR, baffle leak or obstruction not amenable to percutaneous intervention, or symptomatic severe subpulmonary stenosis.
- d-TGA with arterial switch:
  - Interventional catheterization procedure can be done for the treatment of PA stenosis, significant RVOT obstruction (peak gradient >50 mm Hg or RV/LV pressure ration >0.7), coronary artery stenosis via dilation and stenting.
  - Surgical intervention for significant RVOT obstruction, coronary artery stenosis not amenable to percutaneous intervention
  - AVR is indicated for severe neoaortic valve regurgitation with dilated LV, reduced ejection fraction (EF), or symptoms similar to the management for acquired valvular heart disease.[13]
  - Aortic root replacement is indicated for severe neoaortic root dilation. The threshold at which the risk of dissection or rupture exceeds that of operation is not defined, but European guidelines suggest replacement at diameters >55 mm.[20]
- CCTGA: Valve replacement is indicated in severe systemic TR in patients with normal or mildly depressed systemic RV systolic function.

Lifestyle/Risk Modification

- Endocarditis prophylaxis: indicated for prosthetic valve, cyanotic shunt, degeneration of prior repair with prosthetic material and within 6 months of repair[1]
- Pregnancy: significantly increased risk of maternal morbidity such as heart failure and arrhythmias; however, pregnancy can generally be successfully managed with a multidisciplinary team at a tertiary care center.[5]
- Activity[6]:
  - d-TGA:
    - Atrial baffle: can participate in low- to moderate-intensity sports if no history of heart failure, arrhythmia, or syncope
    - Postarterial switch: generally, no restrictions unless there are hemodynamic abnormalities

○ CCTGA: Asymptomatic patients can participate in moderate- to high-intensity sports in the absence of significant chamber enlargement, ventricular dysfunction, or arrhythmia.

MONITORING/FOLLOW-UP[1]

- Patients with TGA should have TTE and/or MRI yearly.
- Intermittent ECG ambulatory monitoring for bradycardia or sinus node dysfunction is recommended in patients with d-TGA after atrial switch.
- It is reasonable to perform a one-time evaluation of coronary artery anatomy (coronary angiography, coronary CTA, or MRA) in asymptomatic patients with d-TGA after arterial switch.

Ebstein Anomaly

GENERAL PRINCIPLES

Classification

- Ebstein anomaly is rare accounting for only 1% of congenital heart defects.[21]
- It has been linked to maternal lithium use.
- It consists of an apically displaced, malformation of the TV with an "atrialized" portion of the RV and is highly variable in severity.
- Ebstein anomaly is surgically classified into four types:
  ○ Type I: anterior TV leaflet large and mobile. Posterior and septal leaflets are apically displaced, dysplastic, or absent. Ventricular chamber size varies.
  ○ Type II: anterior, posterior, and often septal leaflets are present but are small and apically displaced in a spiral pattern. Atrialized ventricle is large.
  ○ Type III: anterior leaflet is restricted, shortened, fused, and chordae are tethered. Frequently, papillary muscles directly insert into the anterior leaflet. Posterior and septal leaflets are displaced, dysplastic, not reconstructable. Large atrialized RV.
  ○ Type IV: anterior leaflet is deformed and displaced into the RVOT. Few to no chordae. Direct insertion of papillary muscle into valve is common. Posterior leaflet is absent or dysplastic. Septal leaflet is a ridge of fibrous material. Small atrialized RV.
- Associated defects include ASD or patent foramen ovale (PFO) (80% of patients), VSD, PS or pulmonary atresia, PDA, and CoA, and 20% have accessory pathways (Wolff–Parkinson–White) and arrhythmias.[1,21]
- Pathophysiologic consequences depend on the severity of malformation, degree of TR or obstruction of the RVOT, and size of the RV cavity/amount of atrialized RV.

DIAGNOSIS

Clinical Presentation

- In children, earlier presentation is associated with worse outcome.
- Adults can present at any age and most commonly present with arrhythmia, exercise intolerance, or right heart failure.
- Sudden death can occur and has been attributed to atrial fibrillation with conduction through an accessory pathway or ventricular arrhythmias.
- Paradoxical embolism may occur and suggests the presence of a concomitant ASD.
- Systolic murmur of TR may be heard (holosystolic at the left lower sternal border that increases with inspiration).

Diagnostic Testing
- CXR: may or may not show cardiomegaly
- ECG: RAE as evidenced by tall Himalayan P waves, QR in V1 up to lead V4, RBBB, splintered QRS complex; accessory pathway is present in one-third of patients.
- TTE:
  - Diagnosis made with echo (apical displacement of septal tricuspid leaflet >8 mm/m^2 and the presence of redundant, elongated anterior leaflet and a septal leaflet tethered to the ventricular septum)
  - Also used to determine the degree of RAE, TR, and presence of associated defects
- Cardiac MRI and/or TEE can be done to better define valve structure and assess RV size and function.

TREATMENT
Surgical Management[1]
- Repair or replacement of TV is indicated in patients with Ebstein anomaly and significant TR when one or more of the following are present (class I):
  - Heart failure symptoms
  - Objective evidence of worsening exercise capacity
  - Progressive RV systolic dysfunction by echo or MRI
- Catheter ablation is recommended in those with a high-risk pathway conduction or multiple accessory pathways (class I).
- Repair or replacement of TV is reasonable in patients with significant TR with (class IIa):
  - Progressive RV enlargement
  - Systemic desaturation from R-to-L atrial shunt
  - Paradoxical embolism
  - Atrial tachyarrhythmias

Lifestyle/Risk Modification
- Endocarditis prophylaxis: warranted in cyanotic patients or those with a prosthetic valve[1]
- Pregnancy: generally well tolerated, requires evaluation before pregnancy, risk of CHD in fetus is about 6%.[5]
- Activity[6]:
  - Patients without cyanosis, mild-to-moderate TR, normal RV size, and no tachyarrhythmias have no restrictions.
  - Severe TR and no arrhythmia can participate in low-intensity sports.

Single Ventricle Disorders and Fontan Palliation

GENERAL PRINCIPLES
Definition
- Includes multiple disorders characterized by one physiologically sized and functional ventricle: tricuspid atresia, hypoplastic left heart syndrome, doublet-inlet left ventricle, double-outlet RV, pulmonary atresia with intact ventricular septum, unbalanced AVSDs, and others[22]
- Typically, these patients undergo a series of three separate cardiac operations in the first 3 to 5 years of life: BTT shunt bidirectional Glenn Fontan. See Table 32-3 and Figure 32-4.[23]

TABLE 32-3	COMMON SURGICAL PROCEDURES IN PATIENTS WITH UNIVENTRICULAR HEART		
Type of repair	Anatomy	Outcome	Complications
Systemic-to-pulmonary artery shunt (i.e., modified Blalock–Taussig–Thomas)	Subclavian or carotid artery connection to right or main PA (now often a graft is used)	Allows for deoxygenated systemic blood to enter pulmonary circulation and palliate cyanosis before Glenn and Fontan completion	Atrial arrhythmias secondary to systemic ventricular dilatation Falsely low blood pressure in the extremity near previous repair
Bidirectional Glenn	SVC is connected to the right and left pulmonary arteries in infancy/early childhood.	Venous return from upper extremities and head bypass the RV and go directly to the lungs. Blood from the IVC continues to enter the RV. This works to improve oxygen saturation.	Pulmonary arteriovenous fistulas develop and can cause cyanosis due to relatively more IVC than SVC flow.
Bidirectional Glenn plus additional pulmonary flow	Includes a concomitant systemic-to-pulmonary shunt	Used to further increase systemic oxygenation (albeit with more load on the ventricle and SVC pressure)	Volume overload to the ventricle
Atriopulmonary Fontan	RA appendage is connected to the main PA shunting both SVC and IVC blood to the lungs.	Completes full systemic flow redirection to the pulmonary arteries Most patients of current adult age had this type of repair.	Atrial arrhythmias due to scarring of the atrium Protein-losing enteropathy Plastic bronchitis Thromboembolic events Chronic congestive hepatopathy Ventricular failure Systemic AV valve regurgitation

Modified Fontan	Extracardiac conduit: IVC → R PA/main PA via synthetic graft outside the RA	Creates a right-to-left shunt to reduce pressure in the systemic system, but results in hypoxia.
	Intra-atrial (lateral) tunnel: IVC → R PA/main PA via partition in the RA	Used once protein-losing enteropathy has developed
	Intracardiac lateral tunnel Fenestration between systemic venous path and LA	Same as with traditional Fontan, except that arrhythmias and thromboembolic events less common
1.5 Ventricle repair	Bidirectional Glenn + IVC flow directed to small pulmonary ventricle	Reduces systemic blood return to a small pulmonary ventricle
2 Ventricle repair	Intraventricular or VSD patch placed to septate a common ventricle (or large VSD)	Separates systemic and pulmonic circulation

AV, arteriovenous; IVC, inferior vena cava; PA, pulmonary artery; R, right; RA, right atrium; SVC, superior vena cava; VSD, ventricular septal defect.

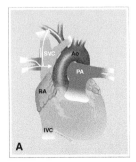
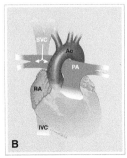
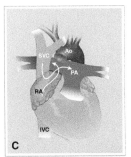
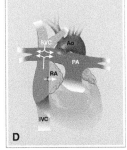
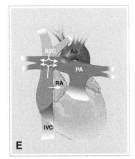

FIGURE 32-4. (A) Blalock–Taussig–Thomas shunt (subclavian artery to PA). **(B)** Bidirectional Glenn shunt (SVC to PA). **(C)** Classic atriopulmonary Fontan with the RA appendage connected to PA. **(D)** Intra-atrial lateral tunnel Fontan connecting IVC to RPA via a partition in the RA with fenestration. **(E)** Extracardiac Fontan connecting IVC to RPA via a synthetic graft conduit outside the heart with fenestration. *Arrows represent blood flow.* IVC, inferior vena cava; PA, pulmonary artery; RA, right atrium; RPA, right pulmonary artery; SVC, superior vena cava. (Reprinted from Wolfe NK, Sabol BA, Kelly JC, et al. Management of Fontan circulation in pregnancy: a multidisciplinary approach to care. *Am J Obstet Gynecol MFM.* 2021;3(1):100257. Copyright © 2020 Elsevier. With permission.)

Pathophysiology

- Fontan procedure remediates cyanosis but poses exceptional challenges for the cardiovascular system.
- Fontan circulation results in complete separation of the pulmonary and systemic circulations and lack of a pumping ventricle into the pulmonary circulation.
  - Body becomes dependent on high systemic venous pressure and low PA resistance to propel nonpulsatile blood flow through the pulmonary circulation.
  - Hallmark of Fontan circulation is sustained elevated ventral venous pressure and decreased cardiac output; highly preload dependent.

DIAGNOSIS

Clinical Presentation

Due to the abnormal hemodynamics of Fontan circulation, there are many long-term sequelae that patients can develop:

- Heart failure and arrhythmias
- Thromboembolism
- Fontan-associated liver disease and increased risk of hepatocellular carcinoma
- Development of chest and mediastinal arteriovenous and venovenous collaterals
- Protein-losing enteropathy
- Plastic bronchitis
- Progressive renal dysfunction

TREATMENT

Medications

- Aspirin should be given to all patients with Fontan; warfarin is indicated for those with an atrial shunt or thrombus, atrial arrhythmias, or a history of thromboembolic event.[1]
- Pulmonary vasodilators have been shown to have some improvement in symptoms and functional capacity in those with Fontan circulation and heart failure symptoms.[1,24]

Surgical Management[1]

- Fontan revision surgery for those with the classic AP type Fontan is reasonable in those with atrial tachyarrhythmias refractory to pharmacologic therapy and catheter ablation who have preserved systolic ventricular function.
- Survival is estimated to be ~85% 30 years after Fontan, and the majority of patients will develop end-stage heart failure or significant end-organ dysfunction by middle age. Thus, most patients will require referral to a heart failure specialist for evaluation of heart transplantation.

Lifestyle/Risk Modification

- Endocarditis prophylaxis: warranted if prosthetic valve, recent repair (within 6 months), previous endocarditis[1]
- Pregnancy[23]:
  - High risk of maternal morbidity, including heart failure, arrhythmias, thromboembolism, and postpartum hemorrhage
  - High risk of miscarriage, stillbirth, intrauterine growth restriction, and prematurity for fetus
  - Patients should have a full cardiovascular evaluation before conception and be managed by a multidisciplinary team at a tertiary care center during pregnancy.
- Activity: Asymptomatic patients can participate in low-intensity activity; participation in higher intensity activity may be considered on an individual basis if patient can complete an exercise test without arrhythmias, hypotension, or concerning clinical symptoms.[5]

MONITORING/FOLLOW-UP

- Patients should have annual echo, ECG, liver imaging (ultrasound or MRI), 6MWT to identify possible desaturation with exertion, and bloodwork (renal function panel, liver functional panel, iron studies, international normalized ratio [INR]).
- Holter monitor and exercise test should be done every 1 to 2 years.
- Cardiac catheterization to assess hemodynamics should be done every 10 years.

Sudden Cardiac Death and Congenital Heart Disease

GENERAL PRINCIPLES

- SCD is a frequent long-term complication in the CHD population, estimated to be the cause of 20-25% of deaths.[25]
- Current guideline indications for ICD in CHD patients have been found to only be moderately predictive of SCD, and many patients with adult CHD (ACHD) still die of SCD.[26]
- Due to the lack of randomized trials and accurate risk prediction algorithms as well as known higher rates of device complications and inappropriate shocks in the ACHD population, the use of ICDs for SCD prevention lags behind use in acquired heart disease.

Risk Factors[25]

- Impaired systemic ventricular function
- Heart failure symptoms
- Prolonged QRS duration
- Atrial arrhythmias

DIAGNOSIS

- Current guidelines on identification of those at high risk of SCD in the ACHD are largely extrapolated from data and guidelines used in patients with acquired cardiomyopathies.
- The need for SCD risk prediction in patients with ACHD is vital as these patients have different anatomy, surgical history, and risk factors for SCD.
- Electrophysiologic (EP) study to identify inducible ventricular arrhythmias can be considered to help risk stratify ACHD patients for SCD and has typically been used in patients with a history of repaired ToF and risk factors for SCD.

TREATMENT

- ICD placement should be considered in those felt to be at high risk of SCD for primary prevention.
- Current Heart Rhythm Society Guidelines published in 2014 identify the following cohorts of ACHD patients as potentially benefitting from ICD therapy for primary prevention[25]:
  - Class I indication in those with systemic LVEF ≤35%, biventricular physiology with the New York Heart Association (NYHA) class II or III symptoms
  - Class IIa indication in those with ToF and multiple risk factors for SCD including LV systolic or diastolic dysfunction, nonsustained ventricular tachycardia (VT), QRS ≥180 ms, extensive RV scarring, or inducible sustained VT on EP study
  - Class IIb indication in those with single ventricle EF <35%, biventricular physiology with systemic RVEF <35%, or syncope with high clinical suspicion (or proven by EP study) of ventricular arrhythmias
- Other SCD risk predictions tools specific to the ACHD population have been developed and validated.
  - In ToF patients, the Khairy risk score stratifies patients into low, intermediate, and high risk of SCD, with points being given for those with prior palliative shunt (i.e., BTT shunt), inducible sustained VT on EP study, QRS duration ≥180 ms, ventriculotomy incision, nonsustained VT, and LV end-diastolic pressure (LVEDP) ≥12 mm Hg.[17] Those in the high-risk category had an annualized rate of appropriate ICD shocks of

TABLE 32-4	PREVENTION-ACHD RISK SCORE MODEL—ANNUAL RISK OF SCD (%)[27]						
Number of risk factors[a]	**1**	**2**	**3**	**4**	**5**	**6**	**7**
Diagnosis							
Eisenmenger syndrome[b]	4	8	16	>25	>25	>25	>25
Cyanotic non-Eisenmenger	3	7	15	>25	>25	>25	>25
Ebstein anomaly	1	2	5	11	23	>25	>25
Fontan circulation	<1	2	5	10	20	>25	NA[c]
TGA atrial switch	<1	2	4	8	17	>25	>25
CCTGA	<1	<1	2	4	9	18	>25
Left-sided lesions	<1	<1	2	3	7	15	>25
Tetralogy of fallot	<1	<1	1	3	6	14	>25
Closed ASD	<1	<1	1	2	5	10	22

Shaded boxes indicate those at high risk of SCD in whom primary prevention ICD should be considered.

TGA, transposition of the great arteries: ASD, atrial septal defect; ICD, implantable cardioverter-defibrillator.

[a]Risk factors are as follows: (1) coronary artery disease, (2) heart failure symptoms (NYHA class II/III), (3) supraventricular tachycardia, (4) impaired systemic ventricular function <40% on echo, (5) impaired subpulmonary ventricular function <40% on echo, (6) QRS duration ≥120 ms, (7) QT dispersion ≥70 ms.

[b]Those with Eisenmenger syndrome are not recognized as ICD candidates by the Heart Rhythm Society guidelines (class III Harm).[25]

[c]Seven risk factors not possible for patients with Fontan circulation as these patients do not have a subpulmonary ventricle.

Modified from Vehmeijer JT, Koyak Z, Leerink JM, et al. Identification of patients at risk of sudden cardiac death in congenital heart disease: the PRospEctiVE study on implaNTable cardIOverter defibrillator therapy and suddeN cardiac death in Adults with Congenital Heart Disease (PREVENTION-ACHD). *Heart Rhythm.* 2021;18(5):785-92. https://creativecommons.org/licenses/by/4.0/

17.5%, compared to <4% in the low- and intermediate-risk groups; thus, high-risk individuals should be referred for a primary prevention ICD.

○ The PREVENTION—ACHD risk score[27] was recently developed in 2021 and can be used to calculate individualized annual risk of SCD based on risk factors and baseline hazard of risk due to underlying anatomy. Those with an estimated ≥3% annual risk of SCD are considered high risk, and primary prevention ICD is recommended. See Table 32-4.

REFERENCES

1. Stout KK, Daniels CJ, Aboulhosn JA, et al. 2018 AHA/ACC guideline for the management of adults with congenital heart disease: a report of the American College of Cardiology/American Heart Association Task Force on Clinical Practice Guidelines. *J Am Coll Cardiol.* 2019;73:e81-192.
2. Gilboa SM, Devine OJ, Kucik JE, et al. Congenital heart defects in the United States. *Circulation.* 2016;134:101-9.
3. Bradley EA, Zaidi AN. Atrial septal defect. *Cardiol Clin.* 2020;38:317-24.

4. Bradley EA, Ammash N, Martinez SC, et al. "Treat-to-close": non-repairable ASD-PAH in the adult: results from the North American ASD-PAH (NAAP) Multicenter Registry. *Int J Cardiol.* 2019;291:127-33.

5. Lindley KJ, Bairey Merz CN, Asgar AW, et al. Management of women with congenital or inherited cardiovascular disease from pre-conception through pregnancy and postpartum: JACC focus seminar 2/5. *J Am Coll Cardiol.* 2021;77:1778-98.

6. Hare GFV, Ackerman MJ, Evangelista JK, et al. Eligibility and disqualification recommendations for competitive athletes with cardiovascular abnormalities: task force 4: congenital heart disease. *Circulation.* 2015;132:e281-91.

7. Minette MS, Sahn DA. Ventricular septal defects. *Circulation.* 2006;114:2190-7.

8. Schneider DJ, Moore JW. Patent ductus arteriosus. *Circulation.* 2006;114:1873-82.

9. Aboulhosn J, Child JS. Left ventricular outflow obstruction: subaortic stenosis, bicuspid aortic valve, supravalvular aortic stenosis, and coarctation of the aorta. *Circulation.* 2006;114:2412-22.

10. Siu SC, Silversides CK. Bicuspid aortic valve disease. *J Am Coll Cardiol.* 2010;55:2789-800.

11. Schievink WI, Raissi SS, Maya MM, Velebir A. Screening for intracranial aneurysms in patients with bicuspid aortic valve. *Neurology.* 2010;74:1430-3.

12. Niwa K. Aortic dilatation in complex congenital heart disease. *Cardiovasc Diagn Ther.* 2018;8:725-38.

13. Otto CM, Nishimura RA, Bonow RO, et al. 2020 ACC/AHA guideline for the management of patients with valvular heart disease: a report of the American College of Cardiology/American Heart Association Joint Committee on Clinical Practice Guidelines. *Circulation.* 2021;143:e72-227.

14. Xie X, Shi X, Xun X, Rao L. Efficacy and safety of transcatheter aortic valve implantation for bicuspid aortic valves: a systematic review and meta-analysis. *Ann Thorac Cardiovasc Surg.* 2016;22:203-15.

15. Dillar GP, Gatzoulis MA. Pulmonary vascular disease in adults with congenital heart disease. *Circulation.* 2007;115:1039-50.

16. Bashore TM. Adult congenital heart disease: right ventricular outflow tract lesions. *Circulation.* 2007;115:1933-47.

17. Khairy P, Harris L, Landzberg MJ, et al. Implantable cardioverter-defibrillators in tetralogy of Fallot. *Circulation.* 2008;117:363-70.

18. Warnes CA. Transposition of the great arteries. *Circulation.* 2006;114:2699-709.

19. Zaragoza-Macias E, Zaidi AN, Dendukuri N, Marelli A. Medical therapy for systemic right ventricles: a systematic review (part 1) for the 2018 AHA/ACC Guideline for the management of adults with congenital heart disease: a report of the American College of Cardiology/American Heart Association task force on clinical practice guidelines. *J Am Coll Cardiol.* 2019;73:1564-78.

20. Baumgartner H, De Backer J, Babu-Narayan SV, et al. 2020 ESC guidelines for the management of adult congenital heart disease. *Eur Heart J.* 2021;42:563-645.

21. Attenhofer Jost CH, Connolly HM, Dearani JA, et al. Ebstein's anomaly. *Circulation.* 2007;115:277-85.

22. Khairy P, Poirier N, Mercier LA. Univentricular heart. *Circulation.* 2007;115:800-12.

23. Wolfe NK, Sabol BA, Kelly JC, et al. Management of Fontan circulation in pregnancy: a multidisciplinary approach to care. *Am J Obstet Gynecol MFM.* 2021;3:100257.

24. Rychik J, Atz AM, Celermajer DS, et al. Evaluation and management of the child and adult with Fontan circulation: a scientific statement from the American Heart Association. *Circulation.* 2019;CIR0000000000000696.

25. Khairy P, Van Hare GF, Balaji S, et al. PACES/HRS Expert Consensus Statement on the Recognition and Management of Arrhythmias in Adult Congenital Heart Disease: developed in partnership between the Pediatric and Congenital Electrophysiology Society (PACES) and the Heart Rhythm Society (HRS). Endorsed by the governing bodies of PACES, HRS, the American College of Cardiology (ACC), the American Heart Association (AHA), the European Heart Rhythm Association (EHRA), the Canadian Heart Rhythm Society (CHRS), and the International Society for Adult Congenital Heart Disease (ISACHD). *Heart Rhythm.* 2014;11:e102-65.

26. Vehmeijer JT, Koyak Z, Budts W, et al. Prevention of sudden cardiac death in adults with congenital heart disease: do the guidelines fall short? *Circ Arrhythm Electrophysiol.* 2017;10:e005093.

27. Vehmeijer JT, Koyak Z, Leerink JM, et al. Identification of patients at risk of sudden cardiac death in congenital heart disease: the PRospEctiVE study on implaNTable cardIOverter defibrillator therapy and suddeN cardiac death in Adults with Congenital Heart Disease (PREVENTION-ACHD). *Heart Rhythm.* 2021;18(5):785-92.

Cardiovascular Disease in Women

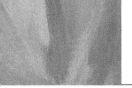

33

Dominique S. Williams, Sonakshi Manjunath, and Zainab Mahmoud

Cardiovascular Disease

GENERAL PRINCIPLES

Epidemiology

- Cardiovascular disease (CVD), including coronary artery disease (CAD), stroke, and heart failure (HF), is the leading cause of death in women, accounting for one-third of all deaths in the US. Approximately 42 million women in the US (34%) have CVD.[1,2]
- The incidence of CVD rises sharply after menopause to nearly equal that of men. Women present ~10 years later in life than men.
- Women are more likely to present with atypical symptoms leading to a delay in diagnosis or missed diagnosis. Women and physicians frequently attribute their chest pain to anxiety, stress, and other psychological problems, which further delays time to diagnosis. Psychological stress is associated with acute cardiac events in women (e.g., stress-induced cardiomyopathy).
- Compared to men, women have a higher incidence of spontaneous coronary artery dissection (SCAD), defined as a spontaneous tear in the coronary arterial wall,[3] myocardial ischemia with no obstructive coronary artery (MINOCA) disease, and coronary vasomotion disorders, defined as a supply–demand mismatch between nutrients delivered from blood flow and myocardial requirements, resulting in a transient ischemia.[4]

Risk Factors

- Women and men have similar risk factors for CVD. Specific risk factors only seen in women are due to adverse events of pregnancy, including preeclampsia, gestational diabetes, and preterm labor.[1]
- Certain risk factors—including diabetes, decreased high-density lipoprotein cholesterol (HDL-C), elevated triglycerides, and depression—are associated with worse outcomes in women.[5]

Prevention

- Preventive measures for CVD in women are similar to those for men.[3]
- The use of low-dose aspirin (75 to 100 mg PO daily) for primary prevention can be considered for men with a 10-year atherosclerotic cardiovascular disease (ASCVD) risk of >10% and for women with an ASCVD risk of >20%, but this decision must be individualized. Rates of serious vascular events are reduced, but cardiovascular mortality does not appear to be significantly lessened.[6-8]
- As ASCVD risk increases, so does the higher benefit of low-dose aspirin in primary prevention. The risk of aspirin use (gastrointestinal or intracranial bleeding) also increases with increasing global risk scores.

DIAGNOSIS

Clinical Presentation

- Chest pain is more predictive of CAD in men than women. A 60-year-old man with typical angina has a 90% chance of having obstructive CAD, whereas a woman presenting with the typical angina chest pain has a 60% chance of CAD.[9,10]
- Women are more likely to present with atypical symptoms, including back, jaw, and neck pain; nausea and/or vomiting; dyspnea; palpitations; indigestion; dizziness; fatigue; loss of appetite; and syncope.[11]
- Women present more often as stable angina rather than an acute ST-segment elevation myocardial infarction (STEMI) and have higher postrevascularization complication rates and higher in-hospital mortality with STEMI.[12]

Diagnostic Testing

- Fewer women are referred for diagnostic testing for CVD.[12]
- Compared to men, treadmill ECG exercise testing has a higher false-positive and lower false-negative rate in women.
- Nuclear stress imaging is associated with breast tissue anterior attenuation artifacts, which may be mistaken for perfusion defects suggestive of ischemia.

TREATMENT

Medications

- Women are underrepresented in randomized controlled trials new therapies for CAD.
- Medical management for secondary prevention of CVD is equally efficacious in women compared to men.
- Women have a higher risk of bleeding from antiplatelet agents, anticoagulants, and thrombolytics. This is most likely due to failure to adjust dosage for smaller body size and advanced age.
- Hormone replacement therapy (HRT) should not be used for the sole purpose of reducing CVD risk in women. Early observational studies and initial data from the Heart and Estrogen/Progestin Replacement study (HERS) suggested a protective effect of HRT on coronary heart disease (CHD) risk in postmenopausal women with established CAD.[13] This protective effect did not persist over an additional 2.7 years of follow-up.[14] In a randomized trial of 27,347 women, women treated with either estrogen alone or combined estrogen and progestin had increased risk of CHD events.[15]

Revascularization

- Success rates of coronary stenting and atherectomy are similar in both men and women.
- Women are less likely than men to undergo coronary artery bypass grafting (CABG) and more likely to undergo percutaneous revascularization (percutaneous coronary intervention [PCI]). This may be due to the higher prevalence of comorbidities and advanced age in the women presenting with CAD and, with this, the perception of higher perioperative risk.

OUTCOME/PROGNOSIS

- **Prognosis of CAD is worse in women**, with higher mortality in the year following myocardial infarction (MI) compared with men.
- Women have a greater likelihood of developing chronic HF, having diabetes and/or hypertension, and being older at disease onset.
- HF in women:
  - Men and women have similar lifetime risk of HF, but women have a higher prevalence of HF with preserved ejection fraction.
  - Risk factors for HF unique to women include premature menopause and adverse pregnancy outcomes, including hypertensive disorders of pregnancy, fetal growth restriction, preterm delivery, and gestational diabetes.[1]
  - See Chapters 11 and 12.

Pregnancy

GENERAL PRINCIPLES

Physiologic Changes in Pregnancy[16]

- In general, pregnancy leads to an increase in cardiac output, plasma volume, stroke volume, and heart rate, while the systemic and pulmonary vascular resistance decreases.
- In the fifth to sixth weeks of pregnancy, cardiac output increases by 40-50% due to increase stroke volume and heart rate. This is associated with an increase in left ventricular (LV) end-diastolic volume and atrial stretch. Arterial blood pressure may fall due to lower systemic vascular resistance.
- During the third trimester, cardiac output is ~7 L per minute and increases further to 10 to 11 L per minute during delivery.
- There is an increase in plasma catecholamines and adrenergic receptor sensitivity.
- The pharmacokinetics of drugs administered during pregnancy are affected by a decrease in serum protein concentration, altered protein-binding affinity, as well as increased renal perfusion and liver metabolism.
- Healthy women are able to meet these increased demands without difficulty.

ARRHYTHMIAS IN PREGNANCY

General Principles

- Arrhythmias may occur during pregnancy in women with and without heart disease. Benign arrhythmias such as sinus tachycardia, premature atrial contractions (PACs), and premature ventricular contractions (PVCs) are common in pregnancy; however, pathologic arrhythmias, both supraventricular and ventricular, are also increasing in prevalence.[17]
- Factors that may exacerbate previously identified arrhythmias or initiate new arrhythmias include:
  - Endogenous risk factors: congenital or acquired structure heart disease, a previous history of cardiac arrhythmia, anemia, hyperthyroidism, and electrolyte imbalances, increasing maternal age
  - Exogenous risk factors: tobacco; caffeine; medication side effects, such as tocolytics and oxytocin; supplements; and illicit drug use

Diagnosis

- Presenting symptoms include palpitations, fatigue, dyspnea, diaphoresis, chest pressure, dizziness, presyncope, syncope, or unexplained seizure.
- Onset, severity, frequency, and duration of symptoms, as well as a comprehensive physical examination and baseline ECG are essential to making the correct diagnosis.
- For symptoms occurring on a daily basis, a 24- or 48-hour continuous Holter monitor can be placed. For less frequent symptoms, a 30-day event monitor can be worn.
- Differential diagnosis:
  - Sinus tachycardia is often physiologic and does not require treatment during pregnancy. Causes include anemia, hyperthyroidism, pulmonary embolism, and HF. Inappropriate sinus tachycardia and postural orthostatic tachycardia syndrome (POTS) should be considered if no physiologic cause is identified. POTS often improves with adequate hydration, sodium intake, and donning of compression stockings.[18]
  - PAC and PVC are common and often benign. Frequent PVCs can be associated with structural heart disease or lead to a cardiomyopathy; thus, evaluation of structural heart disease should be considered. Triggers include excess caffeine, electrolyte disturbances, thyroid disorders, anemia, or lack of sleep.

- Paroxysmal supraventricular tachycardia (SVT) is common and usually has a favorable outcome. In the setting of hemodynamic instability, synchronized electrical cardioversion must be immediately performed. If hemodynamically stable, vagal maneuvers and/or adenosine should be trialed before cardioversion.[18-20]
- Atrial fibrillation/atrial flutter (AF/AFl) is uncommon. A rhythm control strategy is generally preferred for recurrent AF/AFl during pregnancy. Medications such as sotalol, flecainide, and dofetilide have sufficient safety profiles. Women with valvular AF/AFl and a CHA_2DS_2-VASc score of ≥ 2 should be considered for full-dose anticoagulation to prevent systemic thromboembolism. For women who do not have these criteria, low-dose aspirin (<162 mg PO daily) is often recommended. The decision for full-dose anticoagulation is made on an individual basis.[18-20]
- Ventricular tachycardia (VT) and ventricular fibrillation (VF) are rare and predominantly seen in women with structurally abnormal hearts or genetic predisposition to arrhythmias. Treatment should be immediate synchronized cardioversion if VT or defibrillation for VF.
- Bradyarrhythmias are rare. Sinus bradycardia may be due to supine hypotensive syndrome of pregnancy due to uterine compression of the inferior vena cava, leading to paradoxical slowing of the sinus node. Other etiologies of bradycardia include treatment with β-blockers or calcium channel blockers (CCBs), untreated sleep apnea, and hypothyroidism.
- Complete heart block is uncommon, and temporary pacing may be required during delivery.

Treatment

Medications
- Antiarrhythmic agents cross the placenta and can be safely used during pregnancy. Risks versus benefits of any medication must be considered for the underlying condition.
- Treatment should be reserved for those with hemodynamic compromises, severe symptoms, or sustained arrhythmias.
- For long-term management of ventricular arrhythmias, antiarrhythmic medications and β-blocking agents are typically indicated during pregnancy and postpartum.

Nonpharmacologic Therapy
- Vagal maneuvers, carotid massage, and Valsalva maneuver should be attempted in SVT before medical therapy.
- SVT ablation can be performed if recurrent and refractory to medical therapy; however, it is usually deferred until after delivery.[20]
- Permanent pacemakers and internal defibrillators can be implanted during pregnancy if necessary. To minimize radiation exposure, this should be done with echocardiographic guidance or with fluoroscopy, using a shield to protect the fetus.[20]
- Algorithms for the management of narrow- and wide-complex tachyarrhythmias are shown in Figure 33-1.

HYPERTENSION IN PREGNANCY

General Principles

Definition[21]
- Hypertension may occur in pregnancy in women without preexisting hypertension.
- Preexisting hypertension, that is, chronic hypertension, is defined as systolic blood pressure ≥ 140 mm Hg and/or diastolic blood pressure ≥ 90 mm Hg before 20 weeks' gestation.
- **Gestational hypertension** is hypertension diagnosed after 20 weeks' gestation and resolves within 6 weeks postpartum.

- **Preeclampsia** is defined as systolic blood pressure ≥140 mm Hg and/or diastolic blood pressure ≥90 mm Hg after 20 weeks' gestation with proteinuria. In the absence of proteinuria, other criteria include renal insufficiency, elevated liver function test, thrombocytopenia, pulmonary edema, and cerebral involvement.
- Preeclampsia with severe features is defined as systolic blood pressure >160 mm Hg and/or diastolic blood pressure >110 mm Hg with features of preeclampsia.
- Women with chronic hypertension may develop chronic hypertension with superimposed preeclampsia.
- **Eclampsia** is defined as hypertension in pregnancy with seizures, severe headaches, visual disturbance, abdominal pain, nausea, vomiting, and low urinary output and requires emergent medical therapy with delivery.

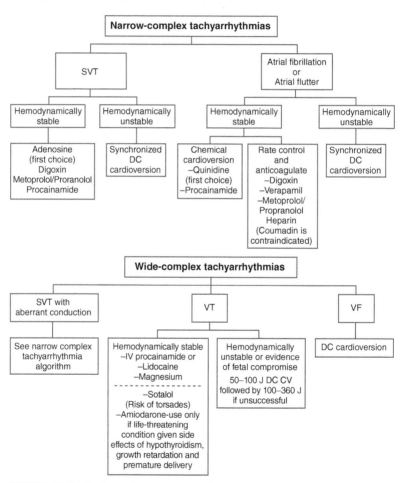

FIGURE 33-1. Tachycardia management in pregnancy. DC, direct current; J, joules; SVT, supraventricular tachycardia; VF, ventricular fibrillation; VT, ventricular tachycardia.

- HELLP (hemolysis, elevated liver enzymes, low platelets) syndrome requires immediate treatment and delivery.
- Hypertension that persists after 6 weeks postpartum is considered chronic hypertension.

Pathophysiology
- The pathophysiology of preeclampsia is not fully understood; however, a leading hypothesis is abnormal placental implantation.
- Remodeling of uterine spinal arteries leads to abnormal placental implantation, causing placental ischemia, which results in an imbalance in circulating levels of soluble Fms-like tyrosine kinase receptor 1 (sFlt-1), vascular endothelial growth factor (VGEF), and placental growth factor (PIGF). This imbalance leads to endothelial dysfunction, oxidative stress, and a vasoconstrictive state in multiple organ systems.[22,23]
- Genetic predisposition, altered sensitivity of the renin–angiotensin system, abnormal placental vasculature development, pro-inflammatory state during pregnancy, dietary changes, and cytokine and immune modulations play a role in the process.[22,23]
- Presentation:
  ○ Chronic hypertension: hypertension before 20 weeks' gestation, often asymptomatic
  ○ Preeclampsia: hypertension after 20 weeks' gestation, new-onset headache not relieved by medication, visual changes, right upper quadrant abdominal pain, pulmonary edema, and seizures
- Diagnostic criteria:
  ○ Preeclampsia is diagnosed in the setting of hypertension with a blood pressure ≥ 140/90 on two occasions at least 4 hours apart after 20 weeks' gestation or blood pressure ≥ 160/110 on one occasion after 20 weeks' gestation with concomitant presence of proteinuria defined as 300 mg or more protein per 24-hour urine collection, protein/creatinine ratio of ≥0.3, or dipstick reading of 2+.
  ○ In the absence of proteinuria, diagnostic criteria include a platelet count <100,000, renal insufficiency defined as serum creatinine >1.1 or doubling of serum creatinine in absence of other renal disease, impaired liver function defined as transaminases elevated to twice normal concentration, pulmonary edema, or new-onset headache unresponsive to medication and not accounted for by alternative diagnoses or visual symptoms.[24]
  ○ Echocardiographic findings in preeclampsia include increased LV wall thickness, reduced LV global longitudinal strain, increased peripheral vascular resistance, decreased cardiac output, and diastolic dysfunction. Markers of diastolic dysfunction include a reduced early diastole/atrial contraction (E/A), lateral e′ of <14 cm per second, and increased pulmonary artery systolic pressure. Right ventricular (RV) dysfunction and reduced RV global longitudinal strain may also be seen.[24,25]

Treatment

- Multiple classes of antihypertensive medications have been shown to be reasonably safe for use during pregnancy.
- The first-line agents include β-blockers and CCBs. Labetalol is commonly used, but other once-daily β-blockers such as carvedilol and metoprolol are also safe to use. Atenolol is contraindicated due to increased growth of intrauterine growth retardation (IUGR).[25,26]
- Methyldopa is safe for pregnancy, although it has fallen out of favor.
- IV β-blockers (labetalol, metoprolol, or esmolol) or hydralazine and immediate-release nifedipine may be safely used for immediate reduction of blood pressure.
- **Drugs to avoid include angiotensin-converting enzyme inhibitors (ACEIs), angiotensin-receptor blockers (ARBs), direct rennin inhibitors, aldosterone antagonist, and nitroprusside** (possible fetal cyanide poisoning).

PERIPARTUM CARDIOMYOPATHY

General Principles

Definitions

Peripartum cardiomyopathy (PPCM) is defined as LV systolic dysfunction, LV ejection fraction (LVEF) ≤45%, presenting in the last month of pregnancy or the first 5 months postpartum, and no preexisting LV dysfunction or alternative etiology for the patient with HF.[27,28]

Etiology

- Likely multifactorial etiology with potential contributions from genetic predisposition, nutritional deficiencies, autoimmune processes, viral myocarditis, and angiogenic imbalance
- Elevated levels of sFlt-1, commonly found in preeclampsia, have also been noted in PPCM. This may partially explain why preeclampsia is a strong risk factor for PPCM.[28-31]

Risk Factors[27,28,31]

- Risk factors include advanced maternal age, African ancestry, multiparity, multiple pregnancy, chronic pregnancy, and hypertensive disorders of pregnancy, including preeclampsia and eclampsia.
- Occurs in 1 in 3000 to 4000 pregnancies in the US
- African American women have higher risk compared to non-African American women. There are reports as high as 1 in 100 deliveries in Nigeria and 1 in 300 deliveries in Haiti.

Diagnosis

Clinical Presentation

- PPCM may be difficult to recognize as dyspnea on exertion and lower extremity edema are common in late pregnancy.
- Patients frequently present with signs and symptoms of HF but can range from mild symptoms to sudden cardiac death as the initial presentation.
- Thromboembolic events (systemic and pulmonary emboli) may occur.

Diagnostic Testing

- Elevated brain natriuretic peptide (BNP) and N-terminal proBNP can be seen in preeclampsia and PPCM.[27,28,31]
- Echocardiography:
  - LV systolic dysfunction, with an LVEF <45%
  - Fractional shortening <30%
  - LV dilatation, although all four chambers may be dilated
  - Functional MR is relatively common.
  - LV thrombus is common in patients with LVEF <35%.
- ECG: LV hypertrophy (LVH) and ST–T-wave abnormalities

Treatment

- Treatment includes standard guideline-directed medical therapy for HF.
- Hydralazine and nitrates are used in pregnancy in place of ACEI/ARBs. Angiotensin receptor-neprilysin inhibitors (ARNIs) are not recommended in pregnancy or breast-feeding women.
- β-Blockers reduce the catecholaminergic tone, heart rate, the incidence of arrhythmia, and risk of sudden cardiac death. Metoprolol succinate, carvedilol, and bisoprolol are recommended.

- Digoxin is safe during pregnancy and is used to augment contractility and rate control. Levels must be closely monitored.
- Diuretics are used for preload reduction and symptom relief.
- Anticoagulation in those with thromboembolism and LVEF ≤30% due to the increased risk of LV thrombus. Low-molecular-weight heparin (LMWH) or warfarin is recommended in pregnancy and breastfeeding women. Direct oral anticoagulants can be considered in nonbreastfeeding women.

Outcome/Prognosis

- PPCM carries a better prognosis than other nonischemic cardiomyopathies. Complete recovery approaches 72%.[27-32]
- Extent of ventricular recovery at 6 months postdelivery predicts overall recovery; however, continued improvement has been seen 2 to 3 years after diagnosis. African American women have poorer outcomes and longer times to recovery of LV function despite similar rates of medical therapy.[32]
- Prepregnancy LVEF is the strongest predictor of outcomes in subsequent pregnancies for women with PPCM. Subsequent pregnancies can be associated with significant deterioration in LV function and death in women with a prepregnancy LVEF <50%. In women with a prepregnancy LVEF >50%, mortality is unlikely; however, significant LV deterioration may occur.[27-32]
- Mortality rates differ significantly based on racial groups, geographical region, and duration of follow-up. At 1-year follow-up in the US, mortality rates have differed from 4% in the IPAC study to 11% in a population, with 96% being African American women.[27-32]
- Contraception, counseling, and family planning are essential in women with PPCM, regardless of the extent of recovery. In women who do not recover LV to an LVEF >50%, subsequent pregnancies should be highly discouraged.[20,27,28,30-32]

PREGNANT WOMEN WITH CARDIOVASCULAR DISEASE

General Principles

- Women with CVD are at increased risk of adverse cardiovascular events with pregnancy. Severity of risk depends on the severity of cardiac disease and prepregnancy state. There are risks to both the mother and the fetus.
- Risk scores have been created to assist with risk prediction and patient management.[33-35]
  - ZAHARA risk score (in Dutch, Zwangerschap bij vrouwen met een Aangeboren HARtAfwijking) is limited to women with a history of congenital heart disease.
  - The Cardiac Disease in Pregnancy (CARPREG) risk score determines pregnancy complications by assessing the composite risk of impaired systolic function, stroke, left heart obstruction (mitral/aortic stenosis), and New York Heart Association >II.
  - The modified World Health Organization (mWHO) score categorizes cardiac lesions as low risk (I), medium risk (II), high risk (III), or contraindicated for pregnancy (IV). The mWHO risk score is widely used and has proven to be the most reliable score in multiple studies.
- High-risk lesions include pulmonary arterial hypertension, PPCM with residual LV dysfunction, and aortopathy with high risk of aortic dissection (Marfan syndrome > 45 mm or Loeys–Dietz > 45 mm, severe left-sided obstructive lesions, and HF). Pregnancy is highly discouraged, and termination may be considered.[33-35]
- Low-risk lesions include simple congenital lesions that have been repaired (i.e., septal defects, patent ductus arteriosus).
- A multidisciplinary approach with cardiology, obstetrics, and anesthesiology is needed to ensure a safe and successful pregnancy and delivery.

- Maternal cardiovascular risks include arrhythmia, stroke, HF, pulmonary edema, and death.
  - The risk is determined by a woman's ability to adapt to the physiologic stresses placed on their cardiovascular system during pregnancy.
  - The risks associated with different congenital conditions (Table 33-1)[36] are determined by the patient's anatomy, previous operations, and hemodynamic status.
- The risk of fetal adverse events is higher than that in the general population:[37]
  - Includes IUGR, preterm birth, intracranial hemorrhage, and fetal loss
  - Risks are higher in women with poor functional class, cyanotic heart disease, and LV outflow tract (LVOT) obstruction.
  - Offspring of adults with congenital heart disease have an increased risk of congenital heart disease. There is an ~3-7% risk of congenital heart disease in the fetus, with risk varying by the specific condition, compared with a baseline risk of 0.8% in the general population.[36-39]

Treatment

- Low-risk patients can receive care locally, while moderate- to high-risk patients should be followed at a tertiary care facility.
- Highest risk pregnancies require serial monitoring with additional BNP measurements, echocardiogram, or other imaging as needed.
- Highest risk patients should have a delivery plan established before the third trimester. Some women may require scheduled hospitalization near delivery for close monitoring, oxygen, and medication optimization, such as β-blockers, pulmonary vasodilators, or antiarrhythmics. In some cases, surgeries such as balloon valvuloplasty or surgical valve replacement may be indicated.

CARDIAC DRUGS COMMONLY USED DURING PREGNANCY[20,26,31,40]

- Adenosine:
  - Rapid action and short half-life; rapid metabolism reduces amount crossing the placenta.
  - First choice for acute SVT presentation
- β-Blockers:
  - Widely used in pregnancy to treat hypertension, arrhythmias, cardiomyopathy, hypertrophic cardiomyopathy, thyrotoxicosis, mitral stenosis, and fetal tachycardia
  - Use leads to reduce umbilical blood flow and increase uterine contractility
  - β-1 selective agents may be preferable for peripheral vasodilation and uterine relaxation.
  - Atenolol is contraindicated.
- CCBs:
  - Widely used to treat maternal arrhythmias, fetal SVT, and hypertension
  - Verapamil preferred for maternal and fetal SVT (acute and chronic).
  - Amlodipine and nifedipine are often used for maternal hypertension.
  - No teratogenicity, but maternal/fetal hypotension, bradycardia, atrioventricular (AV) nodal blockade, and decreased LV contractility reported.
  - IV verapamil has been associated with maternal hypotension and decreased uterine blood flow.
  - Excreted in breast milk
- Digoxin:
  - Widely used for maternal/fetal arrhythmias
  - Freely crosses the placenta
  - Digoxin levels decrease by up to 50% due to increase in renal excretion.
  - Digoxin toxicity is associated with fetal loss.

TABLE 33-1 CONGENITAL HEART DISEASE IN PREGNANCY

Low-Risk Lesions	Potential Maternal and Fetal Risks	Preconception and Pregnancy Diagnostic and Treatment Recommendations
Uncomplicated septal defects (e.g. atrial septal defects (ASD), ventricular septal defects (VSD)	Arrhythmias Increased risk of endocarditis if unoperated or residual VSD Thromboembolism in unoperated or residual ASD	Assess for pulmonary hypertension and valvular disease Consider thromboprophylaxis with low dose aspirin or low molecular weight heparin
Repaired coarctation	Independently associated with increased risk of preeclampsia Aortic dissection Heart Failure	Associated with aortopathy and bicuspid aortic valve Assess for re-coarctation and aneurysm formation Close monitoring of blood pressure during pregnancy and postpartum B-blockers recommended if medical therapy is necessary to control hypertension
Repaired Tetralogy of Fallot without residual valvular disease and normal ventricular function	Arrythmias, including ventricular arrhythmias Heart failure Endocarditis Aortic dissection	Assess for left and right ventricular dysfunction, pulmonary regurgitation and stenosis, aortic aneurysm Associated with DiGeorge Syndrome
Bioprosthetic valves with normal function, annuloplasty rings without regurgitation or stenosis	Arrythmias Heart failure Endocarditis	Assess for valvular dysfunction and ventricular dysfunction Low dose aspirin recommended in bioprosthetic valves

Moderate-Risk Lesions	Potential Maternal and Fetal Risks	Preconception and Pregnancy Diagnostic and Treatment Recommendations
Moderate mitral stenosis	Atrial arrythmias Thromboembolism Heart failure, pulmonary edema Pulmonary hypertension Hemorrhage in anticoagulated patients Preterm Labor, small for gestational age, intrauterine growth restriction	Assess for pulmonary hypertension and ventricular dysfunction Assess for additional left sided obstructive lesions (Shone's Complex) Therapeutic anticoagulation for atrial fibrillation and flutter Consider low dose aspirin or thromboprophylaxis in selected patients B – blockers recommended for hypertension and tachycardia
Moderate aortic valve stenosis	Atrial arrythmias Heart failure, pulmonary edema Pulmonary hypertension Angina Endocarditis Aortic dissection Preterm Labor, small for gestational age, intrauterine growth restriction	Bicuspid aortic valves associated with aortopathy and coarctation of the aorta Assess for additional left sided obstructive lesions (Shone's Complex) Assess ventricular dysfunction
Systemic right ventricle, mild ventricular dysfunction	Arrhythmias (atrial, ventricular, and bradyarrhythmias) Thromboembolism Heart failure, pulmonary edema Hemorrhage in anticoagulated patients Preterm Labor, small for gestational age, intrauterine growth restriction	Serial assessment of for ventricular dysfunction Women with moderate and severe ventricular dysfunction at higher risk of complications Therapeutic anticoagulation for atrial fibrillation and flutter Consider low dose aspirin or thromboprophylaxis in selected patients B – blockers recommended for hypertension and tachycardia

(continued)

TABLE 33-1 CONGENITAL HEART DISEASE IN PREGNANCY *(continued)*

Moderate-Risk Lesions	Potential Maternal and Fetal Risks	Preconception and Pregnancy Diagnostic and Treatment Recommendations
Fontan Circulation	Atrial and ventricular arrythmias Heart failure Thromboembolism Hemorrhage High risk of preterm labor Small for gestational age, intrauterine growth restriction, stillbirth	Assess for ventricular dysfunction and valvular disease Consider low dose aspirin or low molecular weight heparin throughout pregnancy and peripartum period Preload dependent, maintain filling pressures, avoid dehydration
Tetralogy of Fallot with ventricular dysfunction and/or severe pulmonary regurgitation or stenosis	Arrhythmias (atrial and ventricular) Thromboembolism Heart failure, pulmonary edema Endocarditis Aortic dissection Preterm Labor, small for gestational age, intrauterine growth restriction	Serial assessment of left and right ventricular dysfunction, aortic aneurysm Associated with DiGeorge Syndrome

High-Risk Lesions Pregnancy not recommended, consider therapeutic termination	Potential Maternal and Fetal Risks	Preconception and Pregnancy Diagnostic and Treatment Recommendations
Marfan Syndrome or aortopathy with higher risk of aortic dissections (Loeys-Dietz, Bicuspid aortic valve, Turner's syndrome, vascular Ehlers-Danlos)	Aortic dissection, including type B Heart Failure Myocardial infarction Small for gestational age, intrauterine growth restriction Maternal and fetal death	Consider aortic root intervention prior to pregnancy: – Marfan Syndrome and Loeys – Dietz and aortic root >4 cm – Bicuspid valve and aortic root > 5 cm – Turner's syndrome and aortic root > 2-2.5 cm/m2 Vascular Ehlers- Danlos associated with visceral organ rupture Aggressive blood pressure and heart rate control B- blockers recommended if medical therapy is necessary for blood pressure and/or heart rate control Serial assessments of aorta in pregnancy Elective cesarean section Extended postpartum hospital monitoring

Condition	Complications	Management
Eisenmenger's Syndrome	Atrial and ventricular arrythmias Heart failure Thromboembolism Hemorrhage High risk of preterm labor Small for gestational age, intrauterine growth restriction, stillbirth Maternal death	Serial assessment of ventricular function Pulmonary vasodilator therapy Supplemental oxygen Consider low dose aspirin or thromboprophylaxis in selected patients Extended postpartum hospital monitoring
Severe left sided obstructive lesions (severe mitral stenosis, severe symptomatic aortic stenosis, severe coarctation of the aorta)	Arrythmias Heart failure, pulmonary edema Pulmonary hypertension Small for gestational age, intrauterine growth restriction, stillbirth Maternal death	Therapeutic anticoagulation for atrial fibrillation and flutter Coarctation of the aorta and aortic stenosis may be associated with aortopathy and risk of aortic dissection Increased risk of thromboembolism in severe mitral stenosis Serial assessments of ventricular dysfunction in pregnancy B- blockers recommended if medical therapy is necessary for blood pressure and/or heart rate control Balloon valvuloplasty for severe aortic stenosis, surgical AV replacement may be considered in patients who are not candidates for balloon valvoplasty Extended postpartum monitoring

Adapted from Uebing A, Steer PJ, Yentis SM, Gatzoulis MA. Pregnancy and congenital heart disease. BMJ. 2006 Feb 18;332(7538):401-6.

- Flecainide:
  - Used in maternal and fetal SVT
  - No evidence of teratogenicity or fetal adverse effects
  - Crosses placenta, but effectively excreted by fetal renal function
  - Excreted in breast milk
- Anticoagulation and antiplatelet therapy:
  - LMWH does not cross the placenta. Anti-Xa monitoring is recommended.
  - LMWH or warfarin can be used for mechanical valves or thromboembolism. Women should be admitted before induction or scheduled cesarean and changed to unfractionated heparin.
  - Warfarin is associated with teratogenicity and may lead to skeletal and central nervous system (CNS) malformations and intracranial hemorrhage. During the first 6 to 12 weeks' gestation, warfarin embryopathy and miscarriage may occur. Risks of adverse fetal effects of warfarin are dose dependent. Guidelines suggest continuation of warfarin during the first trimester if the daily dose is ≤5 mg.
  - Therapeutic anticoagulation with warfarin at the time of delivery mandates delivery by cesarean section due to increased risk of fetal intracranial hemorrhage during vaginal delivery.[20,37,40]
- Low-dose aspirin (75 to 100 mg daily): High-dose aspirin is associated with premature closure of the ductus arteriosus.
- Clopidogrel: No adverse effects noted in animal studies; limited data in humans. Insufficient data on other platelet inhibitors such as ticagrelor and prasugrel.
- Statins: associated with low risk of congenital malformations; avoidance recommended
- Sotalol:
  - Used in fetal and maternal SVT
  - Increased risk of prolonged QT and torsade de pointes, fetal bradycardia, hypoglycemia, and fetal growth restriction
- Lidocaine:
  - Crosses placenta, but not known to increase fetal malformations
  - Causes increase in myometrial tone, decrease in placental blood flow, and fetal bradycardia
  - If fetus is acidotic, it can result in neonatal cardiac and CNS toxicity.
  - Small amounts are excreted in breast milk.
- Mexiletine: limited data, used in ventricular arrhythmias
- Procainamide: limited data, no reports of teratogenicity in the first trimester

CARDIAC DRUGS NOT SAFE FOR USE IN PREGNANCY[20,40]

- **ACEIs and ARBs:** risk of neonatal renal failure, hypotension, renal tubular dysgenesis, IUGR, and decreased skull ossification
- **Amiodarone:** may be used in life-threatening conditions but carries the risk of fetal hypothyroidism and potential brain damage
- **Spironolactone:** amiloride preferred if a potassium-sparing diuretic is needed
- **Direct oral anticoagulants (apixaban, rivaroxaban, edoxaban):** limited data, not recommended in pregnancy or breastfeeding

DELIVERY PLANNING[20,40]

- Delivery in tertiary care centers should be prioritized for intermediate- to high-risk women with CVD.
- Vaginal delivery is preferred in most women unless the patient is unstable due to refractory life-threatening arrhythmias, severe valvular disease, HF, pulmonary arterial hypertension, acute aortic dissection or high risk for an aortic dissection (i.e., Marfan syndrome with an aorta >4.5 cm), and acute coronary syndrome.

- An assisted second stage should be considered to minimize duration of Valsalva.
- Patients on anticoagulation should be switched to unfractionated heparin before scheduled delivery to minimize bleeding risk. For such patients, vaginal delivery is associated with less blood loss.
- Anesthesia is recommended for pain, heart rate, and blood pressure reduction. Anesthesia decreases catecholamine secretion. Hypotension may occur in some women with anesthesia and may lead to adverse effects depending on the cardiac lesion (i.e., hypertrophic cardiomyopathy). Predelivery anesthesia consultation is recommended in intermediate- to high-risk women. High-risk women may benefit from delivery in the operating room or intensive care unit (ICU) with invasive blood pressure monitoring.

Contraception[20]

- Discussion of safe and effective contraception must be had early on in women with a history of heart disease. Family planning counseling with a cardiologist is recommended in women with known heart disease before discontinuation of birth control.
- Estrogen-containing contraceptives have the highest risk of thromboembolic events and are generally not recommended in women with CVD. Estrogen-containing contraceptives are contraindicated in women with a history of hypertension.
- Progestin-only contraceptives given as an implant or depot are preferred. This includes the levonorgestrel intrauterine device (IUD), etonogestrel implant, and medroxyprogesterone depot.
- A copper IUD and tubal ligation are also safe and effective options for contraception.

REFERENCES

1. Parikh NI, Gonzales JM, Anderson AM, et al. Adverse pregnancy outcomes and cardiovascular disease risk: unique opportunities for cardiovascular disease prevention in women: a scientific statement from the American Heart Association. *Circulation.* 2021;143:e902-16.
2. Go AS, Mozaffarian D, Roger VL, et al. Heart disease and stroke statistics—2013 update: a report from the American Heart Association. *Circulation.* 2013;127:e6-245.
3. Saw J, Humphries K, Aymong E, et al. Spontaneous coronary artery dissection: clinical outcomes and risk of recurrence. *J Am Coll Cardiol.* 2017;70:1148-58.
4. Ford TJ, Ong P, Sechtem U, et al. Assessment of vascular dysfunction in patients without obstructive coronary artery disease: why, how, and when. *JACC Cardiovasc Interv.* 2020;13:1847-64.
5. Huxley R, Barzi F, Woodward M. Excess risk of fatal coronary heart disease associated with diabetes in men and women: meta-analysis of 37 prospective cohort studies. *BMJ.* 2006;332:73-8.
6. Mosca L, Banka CL, Benjamin EJ, et al. Evidence-based guidelines for cardiovascular disease prevention in women: 2007 update. *Circulation.* 2007;115:1481-501.
7. Antithrombotic Trialists' (ATT) Collaboration. Aspirin in the primary and secondary prevention of vascular disease: collaborative meta-analysis of individual participant data from randomised trials. *Lancet.* 2009;373:1849-60.
8. Seshasai SR, Wijesuriva S, Sivakumaran R, et al. Effect of aspirin on vascular and nonvascular outcomes: meta-analysis of randomized controlled trials. *Arch Intern Med.* 2012;172:209-16.
9. Pryor DB, Harrell FE Jr, Lee KL, et al. Estimating the likelihood of significant coronary artery disease. *Am J Med.* 1983;75:771-80.
10. Castelli WP. Epidemiology of coronary heart disease: the Framingham study. *Am J Med.* 1984;76:4-12.
11. Patel H, Rosengren A, Ekman I. Symptoms in acute coronary syndromes, does sex make a difference? *Am Heart J.* 2004;148:27-33.
12. Daly C, Clemens F, Lopez Sendon JL, et al. Gender differences in the management and clinical outcome of stable angina. *Circulation.* 2006;113:490-8.
13. Hulley S, Grady D, Bush T, et al. Randomized trial of estrogen plus progestin for secondary prevention of coronary heart disease in postmenopausal women. Heart and Estrogen/progestin Replacement Study (HERS) Research Group. *JAMA.* 1998;280:605-13.

14. Grady D, Herrington D, Bittner V, et al. Cardiovascular disease outcomes during 6.8 years of hormone therapy. Heart and Estrogen/Progestin Replacement Study Follow-up (HERS II). *JAMA*. 2002;288:49-57.

15. Manson LE, Hsia J, Johnson KC, et al. Women's Health Initiative Investigators: estrogen plus progestin and risk of coronary heart disease. *N Engl J Med*. 2003;349:523-34.

16. Sanghavi M, Rutherford JD. Cardiovascular physiology of pregnancy. *Circulation*. 2014;130:1003-8.

17. Vaidya VR, Arora S, Patel N, et al. Burden of arrhythmia in pregnancy. *Circulation*. 2017;135:619-21.

18. Lindley KJ, Judge N. Arrhythmias in pregnancy. *Clin Obstet Gynecol*. 2020;63:878-92.

19. Lip GYH, Banerjee A, Boriani G, et al. Antithrombotic therapy for atrial fibrillation: CHEST guideline and expert panel report. *Chest*. 2018;154:1121-201.

20. Regitz-Zagrosek V, Roos-Hesselink JW, Bauersachs J, et al. 2018 ESC guidelines for the management of cardiovascular diseases during pregnancy. *Eur Heart J*. 2018;39:3165-241.

21. Unger T, Borghi C, Charchar F, et al. 2020 International Society of hypertension global hypertension practice guidelines. *Hypertension*. 2020;75:1334-57.

22. Ives CW, Sinkey R, Rajapreyar I, Tita ATN, Oparil S. Preeclampsia-pathophysiology and clinical presentations: JACC state-of-the-art review. *J Am Coll Cardiol*. 2020;76:1690-702.

23. Thilaganathan B, Kalafat E. Cardiovascular system in preeclampsia and beyond. *Hypertension*. 2019;73:522-31.

24. Vaught AJ, Kovell LC, Szymanski LM, et al. Acute cardiac effects of severe pre-eclampsia. *J Am Coll Cardiol*. 2018;72:1-11.

25. Gestational hypertension and preeclampsia: ACOG Practice Bulletin, Number 222. *Obstet Gynecol*. 2020;135:e237-60.

26. Bateman BT, Heide-Jørgensen U, Einarsdóttir K, et al. β-Blocker use in pregnancy and the risk for congenital malformations: an international cohort study. *Ann Intern Med*. 2018;169:665-73.

27. Davis MB, Arany Z, McNamara DM, Goland S, Elkayam U. Peripartum cardiomyopathy: JACC state-of-the-art review. *J Am Coll Cardiol*. 2020;75:207-21.

28. Bauersachs J, König T, van der Meer P, et al. Pathophysiology, diagnosis and management of peripartum cardiomyopathy: a position statement from the Heart Failure Association of the European Society of Cardiology Study Group on peripartum cardiomyopathy. *Eur J Heart Fail*. 2019;21:827-43.

29. Parikh P, Blauwet L. Peripartum cardiomyopathy and preeclampsia: overlapping diseases of pregnancy. *Curr Hypertens Rep*. 2018;20:69.

30. Hoes MF, Arany Z, Bauersachs J, et al. Pathophysiology and risk factors of peripartum cardiomyopathy. *Nat Rev Cardiol*. 2022. doi:10.1038/s41569-021-00664-8

31. Elkayam U, Goland S, Pieper PG, Silverside CK. High-risk cardiac disease in pregnancy: part I. *J Am Coll Cardiol*. 2016;68:396-410.

32. McNamara DM, Elkayam U, Alharethi R, et al. Clinical outcomes for peripartum cardiomyopathy in North America: results of the IPAC Study (Investigations of Pregnancy-Associated Cardiomyopathy). *J Am Coll Cardiol*. 2015;66:905-14.

33. Siu SC, Sermer M, Colman JM, et al. Prospective multicenter study of pregnancy outcomes in women with heart disease. *Circulation*. 2001;104:515-21.

34. van Hagen IM, Roos-Hesselink JW. Pregnancy in congenital heart disease: risk prediction and counselling. *Heart*. 2020;106:1853-61.

35. Kim YY, Goldberg LA, Awh K. Accuracy of risk prediction scores in pregnant women with congenital heart disease. *Congenit Heart Dis*. 2019;14:470-8.

36. Uebing A, Steer PJ, Yentis SM, Gatzoulis MA. Pregnancy and congenital heart disease. *BMJ*. 2006;332:401-6.

37. Hayward RM, Foster E, Tseng ZH. Maternal and fetal outcomes of admission for delivery in women with congenital heart disease. *JAMA Cardiol*. 2017;2:664-71.

38. Burn J, Brennan P, Little J, et al. Recurrence risks in offspring of adults with major heart defects: results from first cohort of British collaborative study. *Lancet*. 1998;351:311-6.

39. Gill HK, Splitt M, Sharland GK, Simpson JM. Patterns of recurrence of congenital heart disease: an analysis of 6,640 consecutive pregnancies evaluated by detailed fetal echocardiography. *J Am Coll Cardiol*. 2003;42:923-9.

40. Halpern DG, Weinberg CR, Pinnelas R, Mehta-Lee S, Economy KE, Valente AM. Use of medication for cardiovascular disease during pregnancy: JACC state-of-the-art review. *J Am Coll Cardiol*. 2019;73:457-76.

Cardiovascular Disease in Older Patients

34

Mustafa Husaini and Michael W. Rich

Introduction

GENERAL PRINCIPLES

Epidemiology[1]

- The number of Americans aged 65 years or older will increase from ~49.2 million in 2016 to ~73.1 million in 2030. The most rapidly growing segment of the US population comprises individuals aged 75 years or older.
- The prevalence of cardiovascular disease (CVD) increases progressively with age and exceeds 80% in men and women aged 80 years or older.[1] See Figure 34-1.[2]
- People aged 65 years or older account for 63% of all CVD hospitalizations in the US, including[1]:
  - Over 50% of percutaneous and surgical revascularization procedures
  - 55% of implantable cardioverter-defibrillator (ICD) implantations
  - 75% of arterial endarterectomies
  - 80% of permanent pacemaker (PM) insertions
- Older patients have been markedly underrepresented in clinical trials.

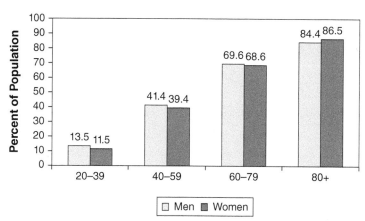

FIGURE 34-1. Prevalence of cardiovascular disease in adults aged 20 years or older by age and sex (National Health and Nutrition Examination Survey: 2011-2014). Data include coronary heart disease, heart failure, stroke, and hypertension. (Reprinted with permission from Benjamin EJ, Virani SS, Callaway CW, et al. Heart disease and stroke statistics—2018 update: a report from the American Heart Association. *Circulation.* 2018;137(12):e67-492. Copyright © 2018 American Heart Association, Inc.)

Pathophysiology

Effects of Aging on the Cardiovascular System[3,4]

- Aging is associated with diffuse changes throughout the cardiovascular system (Table 34-1).
- Resting cardiac performance (i.e., contractility and cardiac output) is generally preserved in healthy older individuals, but there is a progressive decline in cardiovascular reserve.
- As a result, the heart is less able to compensate in response to stress, both physiologic (e.g., exercise) and pathologic (e.g., acute coronary syndrome [ACS], pneumonia, or surgery).
- Older patients are at increased risk for complications, including ischemia, heart failure (HF), arrhythmias, and death, in the setting of both cardiac and noncardiac illnesses and procedures.

Geriatric Syndromes and Key Effects of Aging on Other Organ Systems[5-10]

- **Geriatric syndromes**
  - *Frailty*: a state of increased vulnerability resulting from aging-associated declines in reserve and function across multiple physiologic systems, leading to impaired ability to cope with acute stressors. Frailty is associated with increased risk for procedural complications, disability, hospitalization, institutionalization, and death.[9]
  - *Multimorbidity*: the presence of two or more chronic conditions. Multimorbidity is associated with increased risk for health care utilization, disability, and death.
  - *Polypharmacy and hyperpolypharmacy*: use of ≥5 and ≥10 medications, respectively. They are associated with increased risk for drug–drug and drug–disease interactions, medication side effects and costs, and nonadherence.
  - *Cognitive impairment*: decline in executive function and memory that manifests as difficulty with activities of daily living (ADLs), including management of medications and adherence to other health care recommendations

TABLE 34-1	PRINCIPAL EFFECTS OF AGING ON THE CARDIOVASCULAR SYSTEM
Effect	**Clinical implications**
Increased arterial stiffness	Increased afterload, systolic blood pressure, and pulse pressure
Impaired myocardial relaxation and increased myocardial stiffness	Impaired diastolic filling and increased risk for diastolic heart failure and atrial fibrillation
Impaired sinus node function and decreased conduction velocity in the AV node and infranodal conduction system	Increased prevalence of sick sinus syndrome, bundle branch block, and supraventricular and ventricular arrhythmias
Impaired responsiveness to β-adrenergic stimulation	Decreased maximum heart rate and cardiac output Impaired thermoregulation
Impaired endothelium-mediated vasodilation	Reduced maximum coronary blood flow, increased risk for demand ischemia and atherosclerosis
Decreased baroreceptor responsiveness	Increased risk for orthostatic—hypotension, falls, and syncope

- *Functional decline*: decreased functional capacity and mobility related to loss of muscle mass and strength (sarcopenia) and the cumulative effects of medical illnesses, often exacerbated by hospitalization and associated with delayed recovery and increased decline after hospital discharge
- *Delirium*: an acute state of disorientation and confusion, usually waxing and waning, characterized by disorganized thinking and altered level of consciousness, often due to illness, medications, and unfamiliar surroundings, commonly precipitated or exacerbated by hospitalization, especially surgery and/or intensive care unit (ICU) care
- *Falls*: markedly increased risk for falls and injurious falls during and after hospitalization
- *Pressure ulcers*: associated with immobility; increased risk during hospitalization
- *Urinary incontinence*: underdiagnosed and undertreated syndrome associated with significant psychological and physical challenges, increased risk for pressure ulcers, and nonadherence to diuretics
- **Effects of aging on other organ systems**
  - Renal:
    - Decline in glomerular filtration rate (GFR) (~8 mL/min/decade)
    - Decreased concentrating and diluting capacity
  - Pulmonary:
    - Decreased vital capacity
    - Increased ventilation/perfusion mismatching
  - Gastrointestinal:
    - Altered absorption and elimination of drugs
    - Altered hepatic metabolism of drugs
  - Hematologic:
    - Altered balance between thrombosis and fibrinolysis in favor of thrombosis
    - Increased risk of arterial (stroke, myocardial infarction [MI]) and venous thrombosis (deep vein thrombosis [DVT] and pulmonary embolism [PE])
    - Increased risk of hemorrhage, particularly with antiplatelet, anticoagulant, or fibrinolytic therapy
  - Musculoskeletal:
    - Osteopenia: loss of bone (increased risk for falls and fractures)
    - Sarcopenia: loss of muscle mass and strength (increased risk for falls and functional decline)
  - Neurologic:
    - Decreased central nervous system (CNS) autoregulatory capacity (increased susceptibility to hypoperfusion)
    - Altered reflex responsiveness (increased risk of orthostatic hypotension and falls)
    - Impaired thirst mechanism (increased risk for dehydration)

Cardiovascular Risk Factors

- Age itself is a potent risk factor for the development of CVD.
- Hypertension:
  - Prevalence exceeds 70% in men and women older than 70 years.
  - Isolated systolic hypertension accounts for >90% of all hypertension after 75 years of age.
  - **Systolic blood pressure is the strongest independent risk factor for CVD after age 65.**
  - In a subgroup analysis of ambulatory patients aged 75 years or older in SPRINT, aggressive blood pressure reduction led to a reduction of cardiovascular morbidity and mortality.[11]
  - The 2017 American College of Cardiology/American Heart Association (ACC/AHA) Hypertension guidelines recommend that select elderly patients be treated to a goal blood pressure <130/80 mm Hg if this can be achieved without undue side effects.[12]

- Diabetes mellitus (DM):
  - Prevalence increases up to age 80.
  - ~50% of all individuals with diabetes in the US are aged 65 years or older.
  - **The attributable risk of diabetes to CVD is greater in patients aged 65 years or older than in younger individuals, and higher in women than in men.**
  - Hemoglobin A1C treatment targets in older adults should be individualized based on health status and life expectancy:
    - <7.5% for relatively healthy older adults with life expectancy of at least 10 years
    - <8.0% for moderately complex older adults with good life expectancy, for example, 5 to 10 years
    - <8.5% for older adults with advanced chronic illness, dementia, frailty, and/or limited life expectancy
- Dyslipidemia:
  - In men, total cholesterol levels increase until about age 70.
  - In women:
    - Total cholesterol levels rise rapidly after menopause and average 15 to 20 mg/dL higher than in men after age 60.
    - High-density lipoprotein (HDL) cholesterol levels average about 10 mg/dL higher than in men throughout adult life.
  - High total cholesterol to HDL-cholesterol ratios remain independently associated with coronary events among individuals aged 80 years or older.
  - Strength of association of dyslipidemia with CVD declines with age.
  - Management of dyslipidemia in older adults should be individualized, taking into consideration risk profile, comorbidities and polypharmacy, life expectancy, and personal preferences.
- Tobacco:
  - Smoking prevalence declines with age, in part due to premature smoking-related deaths.
  - Smoking cessation is associated with a marked reduction in CVD risk in all individuals.
  - Tobacco users of all ages should be strongly advised to quit, and those interested in quitting should be provided access to counseling and appropriate pharmacotherapy.
- Other risk factors:
  - The association between obesity and CVD risk in older adults is unclear and likely confounded by collider bias. Mild-to-moderate obesity (body mass index [BMI] 30 to 40 kg/m^2) may confer a more favorable prognosis in older patients with coronary artery disease (CAD) or HF, the so-called obesity paradox.
  - Physical inactivity is associated with increased CVD risk and worse prognosis in individuals of all ages.
  - Clonal hematopoiesis of indeterminate potential (CHIP), an age-related disorder due to somatic mutations in hematopoietic stem cells, is associated with a higher rate of death from CVD and other noncancer causes.[13]
  - The clinical utility of C-reactive protein, B-type natriuretic protein, coronary artery calcium scores, ankle–brachial index, and carotid artery intima–media thickness in the routine assessment of CVD risk in older adults remains undefined.[14]

DIAGNOSIS

- Diagnosis and management of older adults with CVD should be undertaken in the context of their overall health status, goals of care, and treatment preferences utilizing a process of shared decision-making.[15]
- Assessment of overall health status should include consideration of:
  - Cognitive and physical function
  - Living environment and social support

- ○ Prevalent comorbidities, polypharmacy, and geriatric syndromes
- ○ Level of independence in ADLs and instrumental ADLs (IADLs)
- ○ Patient perception of overall health (excellent, very good, good, fair, poor)
- Older patients often present with nonspecific and vague symptoms, as well as atypical or nondiagnostic physical findings.
- The diagnosis of specific CVDs is discussed in the following sections relevant to those conditions.

TREATMENT

- The evidence base for managing older patients with CVD is severely limited, as **this population has been markedly underrepresented in randomized clinical trials and observational studies**.
- Management is further complicated by the **high prevalence of comorbid conditions** that impact the benefit-to-risk ratio of diagnostic procedures and therapeutic interventions.
- **Management must be individualized**, with consideration given to the nature and severity of the patient's cardiac and noncardiac conditions, psychosocial factors, and personal preferences, including the patient's perception of the importance of quality of life versus length of life.
- **Age alone is rarely a contraindication** to implementation of interventions that have a reasonable likelihood of improving quality and/or quantity of life.

Chronic Coronary Artery Disease[7]

GENERAL PRINCIPLES

- A general discussion regarding chronic CAD can be found in Chapter 7.
- Autopsy studies indicate that up to 70% of adults aged 70 years or older have significant CAD, defined as ≥50% obstruction of one or more major coronary arteries.
- The prevalence of clinically manifest CAD is ~22% in men and 13% in women aged 75 years or older.
- People aged 65 years or older account for approximately two-thirds of MIs in the US, with 40-45% occurring in people aged 75 years or older.
- Women account for 26% of MIs in the 45- to 64-year age group, 35% of MIs in the 65- to 74-year age group, and 55% of MIs in the ≥75-year age group.
- Over 80% of deaths from MI occur in patients aged 65 years or older, and ~60% occur in patients aged 75 years or older.

DIAGNOSIS

- Older patients are more likely to report nonspecific symptoms (fatigue, dyspnea, nausea, epigastric discomfort) rather than classic angina pectoris. In addition, sedentary lifestyle and limited exercise capacity due to noncardiac conditions (e.g., arthritis, frailty) may obfuscate symptoms of ischemia.
- Older patients have more extensive CAD at the time of diagnosis, and there is a higher prevalence of left main CAD, multivessel CAD, and left ventricular (LV) dysfunction.
- **Exercise or pharmacologic stress test is the initial diagnostic procedure of choice in older patients with stable symptoms**. An exercise test is preferred in patients who are able to exercise.
- Coronary CT angiography may be limited in older adults by high coronary calcium burden, comorbid atrial fibrillation (AF), or renal dysfunction.
- The risk of invasive coronary angiography increases slightly with age, but the risk of major complications in experienced centers is <2%, even in nonagenarians.

TREATMENT

Medications and Lifestyle Interventions

- Hypertension, dyslipidemia, and DM should be treated in accordance with published guidelines.
- Aspirin 81 mg daily is indicated in all patients with CAD and without contraindications.
- β-Blockers, calcium channel antagonists, long-acting nitrates, and ranolazine are effective, either alone or in combination, to control symptoms of ischemia.
- β-Blockers (carvedilol, metoprolol succinate, and bisoprolol) are indicated in most patients with prior MI and in patients with a left ventricular ejection fraction (LVEF) ≤40%.
- Angiotensin-converting enzyme (ACE) inhibitors, or angiotensin-receptor blockers (ARBs) in ACE inhibitor–intolerant patients, are indicated in patients up to age 85 with established CAD and an estimated GFR ≥30 mL/min, as well as in patients with an LVEF ≤40%.
- Smoking cessation with behavioral and/or pharmacologic support should be provided as needed.
- Regular exercise is recommended, and cardiac rehabilitation is effective in improving exercise tolerance and in supporting behavioral modifications in patients with stable CAD.

Revascularization

- Indications for percutaneous coronary intervention (PCI) and coronary artery bypass graft (CABG) surgery are similar in older and younger patients.
  - Revascularization improves quality of life in older patients whose symptoms fail to respond to aggressive medical therapy.
  - Risk of procedure-related complications increases with age.
- Up to 50% of older patients undergoing CABG experience postoperative cognitive decline that may persist for 3 to 6 months following surgery. Although a small percentage experience persistent cognitive impairment, this may reflect progression of preexisting cognitive dysfunction.
- Cardiac rehabilitation should be initiated before hospital discharge with subsequent referral to a structured rehabilitation program.

Acute Coronary Syndromes[7,16,17]

GENERAL PRINCIPLES

- General principles for the care of older patients with CAD are presented in the preceding section.
- A detailed discussion regarding ACS and acute MI can be found in Chapters 8 and 9.

DIAGNOSIS

- The likelihood of chest pain as a presenting symptom of ACS declines with age.
  - Shortness of breath is the most common presenting symptom in patients older than >80 years.
  - ~20% of patients aged 85 years or older present with altered mental status, confusion, dizziness, or syncope.
  - Silent infarcts may account for one-third of MIs in older patients.
  - For these reasons, a high index of suspicion for ACS is appropriate in older patients.

- The initial ECG is more likely to be nondiagnostic due to higher prevalence of conduction abnormalities, LV hypertrophy, prior MI, or paced rhythm.
- The proportion of patients with non–ST-segment elevation MI (NSTEMI) increases with age.
- Delays in presentation and diagnosis contribute to worse outcomes.
- Elevated cardiac biomarkers due to noncoronary myocardial injury can be caused by infection, anemia, arrhythmias, hypotension, hypertension, respiratory failure, renal failure, HF, or other causes.
  ○ Clinical judgment is essential in determining whether elevated cardiac biomarkers are due to coronary-mediated myocardial injury or other causes.
  ○ In patients with elevated cardiac biomarkers due to reasons other than ACS, urgent coronary angiography and PCI are unlikely to be beneficial.

TREATMENT

- In general, treatment for ACS is similar to that in younger patients.
- Age-related cardiovascular changes and comorbid conditions alter the benefit-to-risk analysis for virtually all interventions.

Medications

- Aspirin and β-blocker therapy unless there are contraindications.
- Addition of an ACE inhibitor or ARB is reasonable in elderly patients with adequate renal function (GFR ≥30 mL/min) and HF or LV systolic dysfunction.
- Early initiation of a statin is reasonable.
- Indications for the use of adjunctive antithrombotic agents (i.e., heparin, low molecular heparin, bivalirudin, clopidogrel, ticagrelor, and other antithrombotic drugs) are similar to younger patients, with the exception of prasugrel, which is not recommended for patients aged 75 years or older due to an increased risk of bleeding.
  ○ Adjustment for weight and renal function is essential to minimize the risk of hemorrhage.
  ○ Bleeding risk increases progressively with the number of antithrombotic agents administered.

Nonpharmacologic Therapies

- **Early reperfusion** (i.e., within 6 to 12 hours) in patients with ST-segment elevation MI (STEMI) is desirable.
- **Primary PCI is associated with more favorable outcomes** than fibrinolytic therapy (at least up to age 85).
- **Early invasive strategy in patients with NSTEMI/unstable angina is associated with lower mortality and reinfarction rates** than an initial strategy of optimal medical therapy. However, few patients aged 80 years or older with significant comorbidities have been enrolled in these trials.
- Referral to a cardiac rehabilitation program following hospital discharge is recommended.

Valvular Heart Disease[9]

GENERAL PRINCIPLES

- A general discussion of valvular heart disease is found in Chapters 21 to 23.
- The incidence and prevalence of valvular heart disease increase with age.
  ○ Mitral regurgitation (MR) and aortic stenosis (AS) are the most prevalent valvular conditions in the elderly.

- ◦ The prevalence of tricuspid regurgitation (TR) also increases with age and is often due to left-sided heart disease.
- ◦ Aortic valve replacements (AVRs) and mitral valve repair or replacements are the second and third most common indications for open-heart surgery in older adults, respectively.
- AS is most commonly due to fibrosis and calcification of a previously normal trileaflet aortic valve, but congenital bicuspid aortic valve accounts for 10-20% of AS in older patients.
- **Aortic regurgitation** (AR) may be either acute or chronic. The most common etiologies include primary valve disease (e.g., coexisting AS or infective endocarditis) and diseases of the ascending aorta (e.g., aortic aneurysm or dissection).
- **Mitral stenosis** (MS) in older patients is most commonly due to nonrheumatic calcification of the mitral valve annulus and subvalvular apparatus.
- MR may be either acute or chronic. The most common etiologies of clinically significant MR include myxomatous degeneration of the valve, ischemic papillary muscle dysfunction, and annular dilatation due to ischemic or nonischemic dilated cardiomyopathy.

DIAGNOSIS

- Older patients with valvular disease present similarly to younger patients, but older patients often present at a more advanced stage.
- In contrast to younger patients, older patients with severe AS often have preserved carotid upstrokes due to age-associated increased stiffness of the great vessels.

TREATMENT

- Older patients being considered for a valve procedure are optimally managed by a multidisciplinary "heart team" that considers available options in the context of the patient's comorbidities, functional status, and preferences via a shared decision-making process.
- Indications for AVR and mitral valve repair or replacement are similar to younger patients.
- Bioprosthetic valves are recommended in patients aged ≥65 years or older.
- Mitral valve repair is preferable to mitral valve replacement when feasible.
- Operative mortality for patients aged 80 years or older:
  - ◦ 3-10% for elective aortic valve procedures
  - ◦ 5-15% for elective mitral valve procedures
- There is an increased risk of perioperative complications, and length of hospital stay and recovery time tend to be longer.
- Long-term outcomes are generally favorable, especially following AVR for severe AS.
- Transcatheter aortic valve replacement (TAVR)[18]:
  - ◦ TAVR is associated with superior outcomes compared to medical therapy in patients with very high or prohibitive operative risk.
  - ◦ TAVR is associated with equivalent or superior outcomes compared to surgical AVR in patients with intermediate to high operative risk.
  - ◦ TAVR compared to surgical AVR is associated with equivalent and/or superior outcomes in low-risk patients with severe AS. In the PARTNER 3 trial (The Safety and Effectiveness of the SAPIEN 3 Transcatheter Heart Valve in Low Risk Patients with Aortic Stenosis), TAVR was associated with superior outcomes to surgical AVR at 1 year. In the Evolut Low Risk trial (Medtronic Evolut Transcatheter Aortic Valve Replacement in Low Risk Patients), TAVR was noninferior to surgical AVR outcomes at 2 years. In 2019, the Food and Drug Administration (FDA) extended the indication of several transcatheter valves for use in low-risk patients.

○ Potential complications of TAVR include valve thrombosis, complete heart block requiring a permanent PM, and significant residual AR.
○ For reasons that have not been elucidated, some older patients undergoing TAVR do not derive significant survival or quality of life benefit.

Heart Failure[19]

GENERAL PRINCIPLES

See Chapters 10 to 12 for a full discussion of HF.

Epidemiology

• The incidence and prevalence of HF increase progressively with age and are projected to double over the next two decades.
• **HF is the leading cause of hospitalization and rehospitalization in older adults**.
• HF is a major cause of chronic disability and impaired quality of life in older individuals.
• The median age of patients hospitalized with HF in the US is ~75 years.
• Two-thirds of deaths attributable to HF occur in individuals aged 75 years or older.
• Ten percent of people aged 80 years or older, half of whom are women, have HF.
• One-year mortality is 25-30% among patients with newly diagnosed HF.
• Median survival is 2 to 3 years, and 5-year survival is ~20-25%.

Etiology

• The etiology of HF in older patients is most often **multifactorial**.
• The most common antecedent condition is hypertension:
  ○ Principal cause of HF in 60-70% of older women
  ○ Principal cause of HF in 30-40% of older men with a similar percentage attributable to CAD
• Other common causes include valvular heart disease, amyloidosis, and nonischemic dilated cardiomyopathy.
• Less common causes include hypertrophic cardiomyopathy, other forms of restrictive cardiomyopathy, and pericardial diseases.
• The prevalence of HF with preserved ejection fraction (HFpEF) increases with age:
  ○ ~50% of all HF cases in patients aged 70 years or older.
  ○ More common in women than in men.

DIAGNOSIS

• HF in older patients is **more likely to present with atypical symptoms**, such as confusion, lethargy, irritability, anorexia, or gastrointestinal irregularities.
• Classic signs and CXR findings of HF are both less sensitive and less specific.
• B-type natriuretic peptide (BNP) and N-terminal pro-BNP (NT-proBNP) levels increase with age; therefore, their specificity for diagnosing HF is reduced in older patients.
• Transthoracic echocardiography with color and spectral Doppler is indicated for newly diagnosed HF or an unexplained deterioration in clinical status.
• Stress testing followed by coronary angiography, if indicated, is appropriate for those with suspected CAD who are suitable candidates for revascularization.

TREATMENT

• Older patients are more likely to have multiple comorbidities that may complicate therapy.

- Patients with advanced HF and anticipated life expectancy <6 months should be offered palliative care services and hospice.[20] Palliative care services have been shown to improve quality of life in patients with HF.[21]
- Completion of an advance directive and assignment of durable power of attorney for health care decisions should be encouraged due to the poor prognosis associated with HF in older patients.

Medications

- Pharmacotherapy of HF with reduced ejection fraction (HFrEF) is similar in older and younger patients.
- Older patients are at increased risk for adverse drug effects and interactions—slower dose titration and cautious addition of new medications are warranted.
- No pharmacologic agents have been shown to reduce mortality in patients with HFpEF.
- Treatment of HFpEF should focus on controlling hypertension, reducing ischemic burden (if applicable), optimizing rhythm or rate control for AF, and normalizing volume status with judicious diuretic use.
- Spironolactone for improving symptoms and reducing hospitalizations in patients with HFpEF is reasonable.
- Avoid NSAIDs in all HF patients due to adverse effects on renal function and tendency to promote sodium and water retention, as well as drug interactions with renin–angiotensin system antagonists.

Nonpharmacologic Therapies

- Moderate dietary sodium restriction (2000 to 2500 mg/day)
- Avoid excess fluid intake (>48 to 64 oz per day)
- Regular exercise as tolerated (including flexibility, strengthening, and aerobic exercises), as exercise has been associated with improved exercise capacity in patients with either HFpEF or HFrEF.
- HF self-care education (e.g., daily weights, adherence to medications, and other recommended behaviors)
- Referral to an HF disease management program if available for patients with advanced HF (New York Heart Association classes III to IV)
- ICD therapy in appropriately selected patients with systolic HF up to 80 years of age. The utility of ICDs in patients older than 80 years is uncertain.
- Cardiac resynchronization therapy (CRT) is a reasonable option in appropriately selected patients of advanced age (including 80 years or older) with prolonged QRS duration, especially with a left bundle branch block pattern, and persistent limiting symptoms despite optimal medical therapy.

Atrial Fibrillation[8,22]

GENERAL PRINCIPLES

- AF is reviewed in Chapter 28.
- The incidence and prevalence of AF increase markedly with age:
  - Median age of patients with AF in the US is 75 years.
  - Prevalence of about 10% in Americans aged 80 years or older, somewhat higher in men than women
- The incidence of stroke attributable to AF also increases with age, accounting for 25-30% of strokes in those aged 80 years or older.

- The risk of stroke in older patients with AF is higher in women than in men by a factor of about 1.8.
- AF is also an independent risk factor for all-cause mortality.

DIAGNOSIS

- The most common symptoms of AF in older patients include palpitations, shortness of breath, fatigue, and exercise intolerance.
- Many patients are asymptomatic, while others develop acute HF and pulmonary edema, often associated with elevated troponin levels.
- Stroke, transient ischemic attack, or other thromboembolic event may be the presenting symptom.
- Diagnostic evaluation should include ECG, serum electrolytes, thyroid function tests, and transthoracic echocardiography.

TREATMENT

- Principal goals of therapy are to **alleviate symptoms** and **minimize the risk of thromboembolic events**.
- **Compared to rate control and anticoagulation, restoring sinus rhythm has not been shown to reduce stroke or mortality in older AF patients with mild symptoms.**[23]
- Lenient rate control with resting heart rate up to 110 bpm is as effective in controlling symptoms and reducing the risk of adverse events compared to more stringent rate control with resting heart rate <80 bpm over medium-term follow-up.[24]
  - Lenient rate control is also associated with fewer side effects and symptomatic bradycardia in elderly patients, who have a higher prevalence of intrinsic conduction system disease.
  - However, the effect of resting heart rates up to 110 bpm over many years is unknown.
- In the CHA_2DS_2-VASc score, age >65 (1 point) and age >75 (2 points) exemplify the impact of age on risk of stroke.
  - Similarly, age >65 years is a risk factor for major bleeding in the HAS-BLED score.
  - Thus, the decision to start oral anticoagulation should be individualized based on stroke risk, bleeding risk, renal function, comorbidity burden, and patient preferences.

Medications

Rhythm Control

- Rhythm control is appropriate for persistent moderate or marked symptoms despite measures to control heart rate.
- Amiodarone is the most effective agent for maintaining sinus rhythm but is associated with multiple limiting side effects in older patients.
- Additional pharmacologic agents for rhythm control include sotalol, dofetilide, flecainide, propafenone, and dronedarone.

Anticoagulation[25,26]

- As noted earlier, older age is an independent risk factor for stroke.
- **Anticoagulation is indicated in all patients aged 75 years or older and in almost all patients aged 65 to 74 years with paroxysmal or persistent AF in the absence of contraindications**.
- Warfarin reduces stroke risk by 60-70% in patients with nonvalvular AF.
- In nonvalvular AF, the direct oral anticoagulants (DOAC) have similar efficacy to warfarin in preventing ischemic strokes.

- Compared to warfarin, DOACs are associated with a lower risk of intracranial bleeding, more predictable pharmacokinetics with less CYP enzyme drug interactions, and no need for dietary alterations or routine monitoring. DOACs are not recommended for creatinine clearance (CrCL) < 15 mL/min.
  - Dabigatran is a direct thrombin inhibitor that requires dose reduction for CrCL 15 to 30 mL/min.
  - The factor Xa inhibitors include rivaroxaban, apixaban, and edoxaban.
    - Rivaroxaban should be taken with the largest meal to improve bioavailability; reduce dose for CrCL 15 to 50 mL/min.
    - Apixaban dose should be reduced if two out of three criteria are met (age >80 years, weight <60 kg, and serum creatinine >1.5 mg/dL).
    - Edoxaban is not indicated if CrCL >95 mL/min as warfarin shown to be superior in that population; reduce dose for CrCL 15 to 50 mL/min.
    - Aspirin may be considered in patients with a CHADS-VASc score of 0 (males) or 1 (females). A prior studied showed a 20-25% risk reduction in stroke in AF patients younger than 75 years. Aspirin is **ineffective in patients aged 75 years or older.**
- Risk of falls is the most common reason for withholding oral anticoagulation therapy in older adults.
  - The benefit of anticoagulation on stroke risk outweighs the potential bleeding risk associated with falls in the majority of cases.
  - In patients with a CHA_2DS_2-VASc score ≥2 and history of falls or high fall risk, anticoagulation is associated with a net clinical benefit.

Nonpharmacologic Therapies

- Catheter ablation of the left atrial myocardium, pulmonary vein isolation, is effective for maintaining sinus rhythm in selected older patients, especially those with paroxysmal AF and small left atrial size.
- Atrioventricular (AV) junction ablation with permanent ventricular pacing is effective in preventing rapid ventricular rates in symptomatic patients resistant to (or ineligible for) other therapies, but does not obviate the need for anticoagulation.
- The surgical Maze procedure is a reasonable option for treating symptomatic AF in older patients who require open-heart surgery for another indication (e.g., CABG, mitral valve surgery).
- Left atrial appendage occlusion devices were approved by the FDA in 2015 as a nonpharmacologic approach to reduce thromboembolic risk in highly selected patients.

Ventricular Arrhythmias[8]

- Frequent ventricular premature beats are associated with increased mortality in older patients with structural heart disease, but treatment should be directed at the underlying cardiac condition.
- The diagnosis and management of ventricular arrhythmias is similar in older and younger adults.
  - The indications for an ICD are similar in younger and older patients up to age 80 years.
  - The value of ICDs in patients aged 80 years or older has not been established.

Bradyarrhythmias[8]

- The incidence and prevalence of bradyarrhythmias and conduction disorders increases with age due to age-related changes in the sinus node, AV node, and infranodal conduction system.

- ~75% of PM recipients in the US are aged 65 years or older and ~50% are aged 75 years or older. Most common indications for PM are sinus node dysfunction (42%) and AV block (39%).[8]
- **Sick sinus syndrome** is manifested by resting sinus bradycardia, chronotropic incompetence (failure to increase heart rate commensurate with increased demands), sinus pauses, and/or sinus arrest.
  - Accounts for up to 50% of PM insertions in older adults
- In general, the diagnosis and management of bradyarrhythmias and conduction disorders is similar in older and younger patients (see Chapter 27).
- Sick sinus syndrome is often associated with paroxysmal supraventricular tachyarrhythmias (tachy-brady syndrome), and treatment of the tachyarrhythmias may exacerbate the bradyarrhythmias and necessitate PM implantation.
- Dual-chamber pacing is associated with reduced incidence of AF and HF compared to single chamber ventricular pacemakers (VVI), but beneficial effects on mortality and stroke have not been demonstrated.

REFERENCES

1. Benjamin EJ, Virani SS, Callaway CW, et al. Heart disease and stroke statistics—2018 update: a report from the American Heart Association. *Circulation.* 2018;137:e1-e427.
2. Go AS, Mozaffarian D, Roger VL, et al. Heart disease and stroke statistics—2018 update: a report from the American Heart Association. *Circulation.* 2018;137:e67-e493.
3. Lakatta EG, Levy D. Arterial and cardiac aging: major shareholders in cardiovascular disease enterprises: part I: aging arteries: a "set up" for vascular disease. *Circulation.* 2003;107:139-46.
4. Lakatta EG, Levy D. Arterial and cardiac aging: major shareholders in cardiovascular disease enterprises: part II: the aging heart in health: links to heart disease. *Circulation.* 2003;107:346-54.
5. Stolker JM, Kim DH, Rich MW. Cardiovascular disease in the elderly: pathophysiology and clinical implications. In: Fuster V, Harrington RA, Narula J, Eapen ZJ, eds. *Hurst's the Heart.* 14th ed. McGraw Hill Education; 2017:1571-93.
6. Forman DE, Rich MW, Alexander KP, et al. Cardiac care for older adults: time for a new paradigm. *J Am Coll Cardiol.* 2011;57(18):1801-10.
7. Madhavan MV, Gersh BJ, Alexander KP, et al. Coronary artery disease in patients ≥80 years of age. *J Am Coll Cardiol.* 2018;71(18):2015-40.
8. Curtis AB, Karki R, Hattoum A, et al. Arrhythmias in patients ≥80 years of age: pathophysiology, management, and outcomes. *J Am Coll Cardiol.* 2018;71:2041-57.
9. Kodali SK, Velagapudi, Hahn RT, et al. Valvular heart disease in patients ≥80 years of age. *J Am Coll Cardiol.* 2018;71:2058-72.
10. Xue QL. The frailty syndrome: definition and natural history. *Clin Geriatr Med.* 2011;27:1-15.
11. Williamson JD, Supiano MA, Applegate WB, et al. Intensive vs standard blood pressure control and cardiovascular disease outcomes in adults aged ≥75 years: a randomized clinical trial. *JAMA.* 2016;315:2673-82.
12. Whelton PK, Carey RM, Aronow WS, et al. 2017 ACC/AHA/AAPA/ABC/ACPM/AGS/APhA/ASH/ASPC/NMA/PCNA guideline for the prevention, detection, evaluation, and management of high blood pressure in adults. *Hypertension.* 2018;71:1269-324.
13. Jaiswal S, Natarajan P, Silver AJ, et al. Clonal hematopoiesis and risk of atherosclerotic cardiovascular disease. *N Engl J Med.* 2017;377:111-21.
14. US Preventive Services Task Force. Risk assessment for cardiovascular disease with nontraditional risk factors: US Preventive Services Task Force recommendation statement. *JAMA.* 2018;320:272-80.
15. Merchant FM, Dickert NW, Howard DH. Mandatory shared decision making by the Centers for Medicare & Medicaid Services for cardiovascular procedures and other tests. *JAMA.* 2018;320:641-42.
16. Alexander KP, Newby LK, Cannon CP, et al. Acute coronary care in the elderly, part I: non-ST-segment-elevation acute coronary syndromes. *Circulation.* 2007;115:2549-69.
17. Alexander KP, Newby LK, Armstrong PW, et al. Acute coronary care in the elderly, part II: ST-segment-elevation myocardial infarction. *Circulation.* 2007;115:2570-89.

18. Braghiroli J, Kapoor K, Thielhelm TP, Ferreira T, Cohen MG. Transcatheter aortic valve replacement in low risk patients: a review of PARTNER 3 and Evolut low risk trials. *Cardiovasc Diagn Ther.* 2020;10:59-71.
19. Jugdutt BI. Heart failure in the elderly: advances and challenges. *Expert Rev Cardiovasc Ther.* 2010;8:695-715.
20. Goodlin SJ. Palliative care in congestive heart failure. *J Am Coll Cardiol.* 2009;54:386-96.
21. Rogers JG, Patel CB, Mentz RJ, et al. Palliative care in heart failure: the PAL-HF randomized, controlled clinical trial. *J Am Coll Cardiol.* 2017;70(3):331-41.
22. Fang MC, Chen J, Rich MW. Atrial fibrillation in the elderly. *Am J Med.* 2007;120:481-7.
23. Wyse DG, Waldo AL, DiMarco JP, et al. A comparison of rate control and rhythm control in patients with atrial fibrillation. The atrial fibrillation follow-up investigation of rhythm management (AF-FIRM) investigators. *N Engl J Med.* 2002;347:1825.
24. Van Gelder IC, Groenveld HT, Crijns HJGM, et al. Lenient versus strict rate control in patients with atrial fibrillation. *N Engl J Med.* 2010;362:1363-73.
25. Ruff CT, Giugliano RP, Braunwald E, et al. Comparison of the efficacy and safety of new oral anticoagulants with warfarin in patients with atrial fibrillation: a meta-analysis of randomised trials. *Lancet.* 2014;383:955-62.
26. Sardar P, Chatterjee S, Chaudhari S, et al. New oral anticoagulants in elderly adults: evidence from a meta-analysis of randomized trials. *J Am Geriatr Soc.* 2014;62(5):857-64.

Echocardiography

Manoj Thangam and Majesh Makan

GENERAL PRINCIPLES

Definition

- Echocardiography is ultrasound imaging of the heart.
- Images are acquired by placing the ultrasound probe on the chest with transthoracic echocardiography (TTE) or by intubating the esophagus using a modified probe with transesophageal echocardiography (TEE).[1]
- Diagrams of TTE and TEE along with common views of the heart obtained from these two modalities can be seen in Figures 35-1[2] through 35-8.[2]

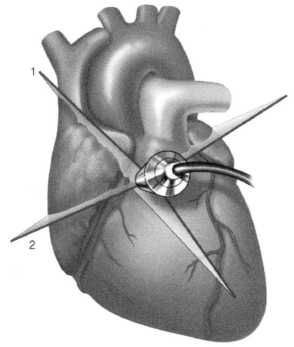

FIGURE 35-1. Transducer orientation used for acquiring parasternal views. Plane 1 represents a parasternal long-axis view. Scanning plane 2 is obtained by rotating the transducer 90 degrees and can be used to obtain a family of short-axis views of the heart. (Reprinted with permission from Feigenbaum H. *Echocardiography*. 4th ed. Lea & Febiger; 1986.)

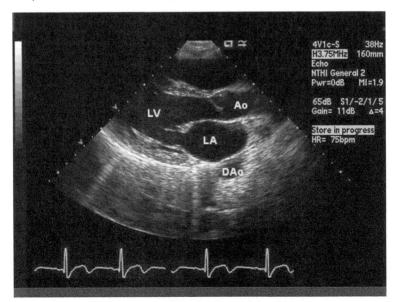

FIGURE 35-2. Parasternal long-axis view. Ao, aortic root; DAo, descending aorta; LA, left atrium; LV, left ventricle.

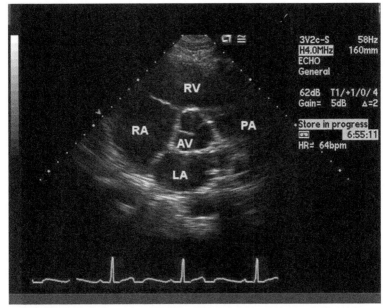

FIGURE 35-3. Short-axis 2D echocardiogram at the level of the aortic valve (AV). LA, left atrium; PA, pulmonary artery; RA, right atrium; RV, right ventricle.

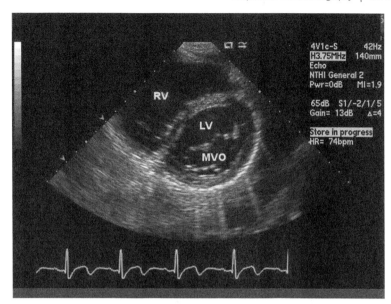

FIGURE 35-4. Short-axis 2D echocardiogram at the level of the mitral valve. LV, left ventricle; MVO, mitral valve orifice; RV, right ventricle.

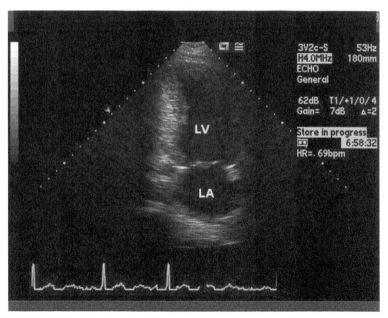

FIGURE 35-5. Apical two-chamber view of the left ventricle (LV). LA, left atrium.

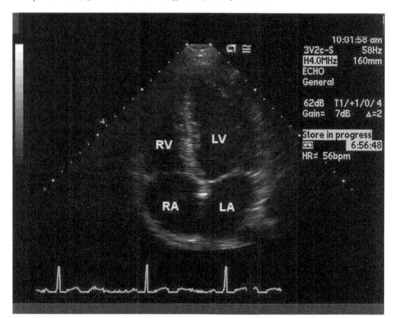

FIGURE 35-6. Apical four-chamber view of the heart. LA, left atrium; LV, left ventricle; RA, right atrium; RV, right ventricle.

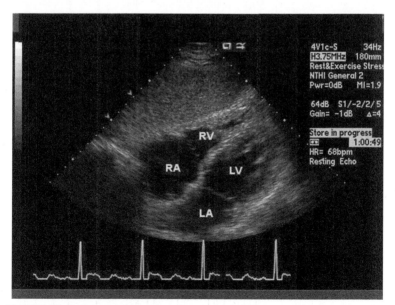

FIGURE 35-7. Subcostal four-chamber view. LA, left atrium; LV, left ventricle; RA, right atrium; RV, right ventricle.

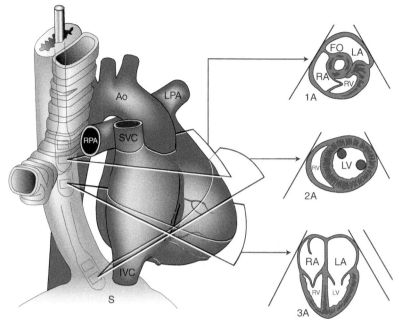

FIGURE 35-8. Transesophageal echocardiography views obtained in the horizontal transducer position. 1A from the upper esophagus, 2A from the midesophagus, and 3A is recorded in the gastric position. Ao, aorta; IVC, inferior vena cava; LA, left atrium; LAA, left atrial appendage; LUPV, left upper pulmonary vein; LV, left ventricle; RA, right atrium; RPA, right pulmonary artery; RV, right ventricle; S, stomach; SVC, superior vena cava. (Reprinted with permission from Feigenbaum H. *Echocardiography*. 4th ed. Lea & Febiger; 1986.)

Physics

- High-frequency sound waves (20,000 Hz) are emitted by a transducer, which are modified by the body and reflected back to the transducer.
- Ultrasound can pass easily through fluids but poorly through bones and air. Rib shadows can limit the available windows for visualizing the heart when using TTE.
- Hyperechoic structures
  - Black regions on ultrasound where waves are attenuated
  - Blood, pleural effusions, and pericardial effusions all appear black.
- Hypoechoic structures
  - Appear as gray areas of varying brightness
  - Often depend on how well the structure reflects ultrasound waves
  - Myocardium, valves, vessel walls, masses, thrombi, and vegetations all appear gray.

Modalities

- Color Doppler[1]:
  - Pixelated display showing the direction and velocity of blood flow
  - Flow toward the transducer is displayed in red.
  - Flow away is displayed in blue.

- Pulse-wave Doppler[1]:
  - Displays, over time, a selected range of velocities and flows within a gated (localized) area
  - Useful in assessing the severity of valvular lesions and pressure gradients
- Continuous-wave Doppler[1]
  - Displays real-time velocities and flows along a single trajectory from the transducer, allowing detection and measurement of the highest velocity
  - Differs from pulse-wave because it is not gated, thus limiting the ability to localize the highest velocity observed
- Continuous- and pulse-wave Doppler are complementary in hemodynamic assessment.
- Tissue Doppler[1]:
  - Assesses myocardial velocity and displacement instead of blood velocity
  - Useful for assessing diastolic function, right ventricular (RV) function, differentiating between constriction/restriction, and efficacy of cardiac resynchronization therapy
- Strain imaging[1,3]:
  - Measures myocardial deformation within a cardiac cycle
  - Useful for quantifying regional myocardial function about multiple axes
  - Strain imaging is used in the assessment of left ventricular (LV) and RV function. It can also be used in assessing atrial function.
  - Used as an additive marker to assess LV and RV function
  - Strain imaging is sensitive for detecting subclinical LV dysfunction and can be used for risk stratification and prognosis.
  - Strain imaging is used in dilated cardiomyopathy, hypertensive heart disease, cardiotoxicity, diabetes, valvular heart disease, infiltrative cardiomyopathy, and hypertrophic cardiomyopathy. Specific patterns of strain imaging can be seen in amyloidosis and apical hypertrophic cardiomyopathy, assisting with diagnosis.
- Contrast echocardiography[1]:
  - Contrast is composed of lipid microspheres filled with perfluorocarbon gas that permits for improved delineation of the endocardial border.
  - Uses
    - Difficult image acquisition
    - Assessment of wall motion abnormalities
    - Detection of LV thrombus
- Agitated saline echocardiography[4]:
  - Created by mixing normal saline with a small volume of air to create a microbubble suspension
  - Resultant microbubbles injected IV and well visualized in the right-sided cardiac chambers.
  - Bubbles have a larger diameter than red blood cells and cannot cross the pulmonary microvasculature. Therefore, they are absorbed into the lungs unless a shunt exists, which would then allow the microbubbles to cross into the left side of the heart.
  - Appearance of saline bubbles in the left-sided cardiac chambers within three heartbeats of visualization in the right chambers consistent with intracardiac shunt
  - Visualization after three heartbeats may suggest intrapulmonary shunt.
- Three-dimensional echocardiography[5]:
  - Technological improvements now allow for real-time 3D volumetric acquisition and display.

Detailed measurements of LV volume and mass, RV volume and function, congenital malformations, and valvular pathology (particularly involving the mitral valve)

APPLICATIONS

The American Society of Echocardiography has developed **appropriateness criteria**.[6]

Transthoracic Echocardiogram

- Common indications for TTE:
  - Coronary artery disease
  - Acute myocardial infarction
  - Cardiomyopathy
  - Heart failure with reduced and preserved ejection fraction
  - Respiratory failure
  - Valvular heart disease
  - Pericardial effusion
  - Arrhythmias
  - Candidacy for primary prevention implantable cardioverter-defibrillator (ICD) placement
  - Endocarditis
  - Congenital heart disease
  - Pulmonary hypertension
  - Pulmonary embolus
  - Ascending aortic aneurysm
  - Stroke
  - Assessment of change in LV function with regard to heart failure, chemotherapy, and cardiac resynchronization therapy
- TTE advantages:
  - Portable, noninvasive, affordable, and able to answer most cardiac clinical questions
  - Provides accurate assessment of structure, hemodynamics, and physiology
- TTE disadvantages:
  - Can be limited by body habitus
  - Obesity and chronic obstructive pulmonary disease can limit image quality.

Transesophageal Echocardiogram[7]

- Common indications for TEE (similar to TTE with the following):
  - Assessment of aortic pathology
  - Evaluation of left atrium (LA) appendage for thrombus
  - Assessment of valvular pathology
  - Inability to visualize the heart with TTE due to poor windows
- TEE advantages:
  - Better at visualizing posterior structures such as the atria, atrial appendage, aortic valve, and mitral valve
  - Effective in evaluation of the aorta
  - Higher frequency transducer can give better visualization of the valves and nonbiologic structures (i.e., pacemaker leads).
- TEE disadvantages:
  - Semi-invasive procedure
  - Poor visualization of distal structures, such as the LV apex

Comparision of TEE & TTE

- TTE is very good with hemodynamics and function, whereas TEE is very good with structure and anatomy.
- TEE will give excellent pictures of a stenotic aortic valve, whereas TTE will provide more accurate valvular gradients.

Stress Echocardiography[8]

TTE that is performed at rest and immediately after cardiovascular stress used to assess abnormalities in LV/RV contractility, diastolic function, and development of new or worsening regional myocardial wall motion abnormalities.

- Exercise or chemical agents, such as dobutamine, are used to stress the heart.

- More specific but less sensitive than myocardial perfusion imaging (see Chapter 37). A greater degree of myocardial ischemia is needed to see a wall motion defect compared to a perfusion defect.
- Dobutamine stress testing with low- and high-dose dobutamine can be used to assess for myocardial viability and LV contractile reserve.
- Exercise stress echocardiography can be used in the assessment of valvular disease (i.e., asymptomatic mitral regurgitation, asymptomatic severe aortic stenosis).

REFERENCES

1. Mitchell C, Rahko PS, Blauwet LA, et al. Guidelines for performing a comprehensive transthoracic echocardiographic examination in adults: recommendations from the American Society of Echocardiography. *J Am Soc Echocardiogr*. 2019;32:1-64.
2. Feigenbaum H. *Echocardiography*. 4th ed. Lea & Febiger; 1986.
3. Potter E, Marwick TH. Assessment of left ventricular function by echocardiography: the case for routinely adding global longitudinal strain to ejection fraction. *JACC Cardiovasc Imaging*. 2018;11(2 Pt 1):260-74.
4. Bernard S, Churchill TW, Namasivayam M, Bertrand PB. Agitated saline contrast echocardiography in the identification of intra- and extracardiac shunts: connecting the dots. *J Am Soc Echocardiogr*. 2020 Oct 23;S0894-7317(20)30615-5.
5. Lang RM, Addetia K, Narang A, et al. 3-Dimensional echocardiography. Latest developments and future directions. *JACC Cardiovasc Imaging*. 2018;11:1854-78.
6. Doherty JU, Kort S, Mehran R, et al. ACC/AATS/AHA/ASE/ASNC/HRS/SCAI/SCCT/SCMR/STS 2019 appropriate use criteria for multimodality imaging in the assessment of cardiac structure and function in nonvalvular heart disease: a report of the American College of Cardiology Appropriate Use Criteria Task Force, American Association for Thoracic Surgery, American Heart Association, American Society of Echocardiography, American Society of Nuclear Cardiology, Heart Rhythm Society, Society for Cardiovascular Angiography and Interventions, Society of Cardiovascular Computed Tomography, Society for Cardiovascular Magnetic Resonance, and the Society of Thoracic Surgeons. *J Am Soc Echocardiogr*. 2019;32:553-79.
7. Hahn RT, Abraham T, Adams MS, et al. Guidelines for performing a comprehensive transesophageal echocardiographic examination: recommendations from the American Society of Echocardiography and the Society of Cardiovascular Anesthesiologists. *J Am Soc Echocardiogr*. 2013;26(9):921-64.
8. Pellikka PA, Arruda-Olson A, Chaudhry FA, et al. Guidelines for performance, interpretation, and application of stress echocardiography in ischemic heart disease: from the American Society of Echocardiography. *J Am Soc Echocardiogr*. 2020;33:1-41.e8.

Cardiac Computed Tomography and Magnetic Resonance Imaging

36

Manoj Thangam and Anita R. Bhandiwad

Cardiac Computed Tomography

GENERAL PRINCIPLES

Definitions

- Coronary CT angiography (CCTA) involves imaging the coronary arteries. It also allows the evaluation of cardiac chambers and surrounding structures.
- Coronary calcium scoring has a role in risk stratification for primary prevention of coronary artery disease.
- Fractional flow reserve (FFR) may be derived from CCTA and assist in revascularization planning.

Physics

- Multidetector technology (MDCT) allows for multiple CT slices to be taken per rotation of the CT tube, allowing for finer spatial resolution.
- The thinnest image that can be reconstructed from the data collected is determined by the slice thickness of the scanner.
- The 64-slice scanner's ability to obtain thinner slice thickness makes it superior to the traditional scanners (4- or 16-slice detector technology). Imaging of sub-millimeter coronary vasculature requires very high spatial resolution. Scanners with 128-, 512-, and 640-slice capacities are being utilized in research centers and may eventually be incorporated into widespread clinical practice.
- As the source of ionizing radiation in a CT rotates around the body, CT radiation differs from that of a standard plain radiograph.
- Potential radiation effects and magnitude of dose are dependent on many factors.
- The effective dose or dose equivalent, defined in Sievert (Sv), is the weighted sum of the radiation dose to a number of body tissues (Table 36-1).[1,2]

Interpretation and Image Analysis

- Image acquisition must be timed with the cardiac cycle.
- Image acquisition is coupled with ECG triggering.
- Retrospective gating:
  - Plain radiographs applied throughout the cardiac cycle
  - Desired images are selected postacquisition.
  - Results in increased radiation exposure
- Prospective gating:
  - Application of plain radiographs only at specific times in the cardiac cycle
  - Preferred as it minimizes radiation exposure
  - Gating is often timed with mid diastole and end systole when the heart is relatively still to minimize motion artifacts
- Imaging of the heart during a complete cardiac cycle allows cine imaging and is useful for measuring ejection fraction, wall motion, and valvular orifice area.

TABLE 36-1	COMPARISON OF AVERAGE EFFECTIVE RADIATION DOSES IN CARDIAC IMAGING
Yearly background radiation	3 mSv
Posteroanterior and lateral CXR	0.1 mSv
Diagnostic cardiac catheterization	7 mSv
Nuclear myocardial perfusion stress test	9–40 mSv
Nongated chest CT	7 mSv
Coronary calcium CT scan	1–3 mSv
Retrospective gated coronary CT angiography (64-slice)	18–22 mSv
Prospective dose modulation-gated coronary CT angiography (64-slice)	2–5 mSv

Based on data from Mettler FA, Huda W, Yoshizumi TT, Mahesh M. Effective doses in radiology and diagnostic nuclear medicine: a catalog. *Radiology.* 2008;248:254–63; Halliburton SS, Abbara S, Chen MY, et al. SCCT guidelines on radiation dose and dose-optimization strategies in cardiovascular CT. *J Cardiovasc Comput Tomogr.* 2011;5:198–224.

APPLICATIONS

Coronary Computed Tomography Angiography

- Define cardiac anatomy:
  - Congenital anomalies
  - Pulmonary vein configuration
  - Bypass graft location and patency
  - Tumors/thrombi
  - Coronary anomalies
  - Vein or arterial mapping
  - Pericardial anatomy
- Chest pain syndrome in the intermediate-risk patient with either indeterminate ECG or inability to exercise:
  - Ability of CCTA to assess severity and extent of atherosclerosis in comparison to conventional angiography has been validated in multiple studies with both 16- and 64-slice scanners.[3-10] Limited data suggest that 128-slice scanners may also have similar efficacy in evaluating coronary disease.[5,11,12]
  - Strong negative predictive value to exclude significant coronary stenosis[3,5,6,13,14]
- Assessment of both the lumen and the arterial wall for positive remodeling and plaque vulnerability
  - Positive remodeling
    - In response to increasing plaque burden, there is expansion of the arterial cross-sectional area in an attempt to preserve the luminal area.
    - Not well appreciated on conventional angiography (Figure 36-1)
  - Plaque vulnerability
    - Most plaques associated with myocardial infarction are nonobstructive in nature.
    - Often, noncalcified plaques are more prone to rupture than their obstructive, more calcified counterparts.
  - Acute chest pain in the intermediate-risk patient with normal ECG and negative serial enzymes. Excellent negative predictive value in ruling out acute coronary syndrome (ACS) among patients when no coronary lesions were seen.[3,5,6,13,14]
  - Appropriate use criteria have been developed regarding the use of CCTA.[16]

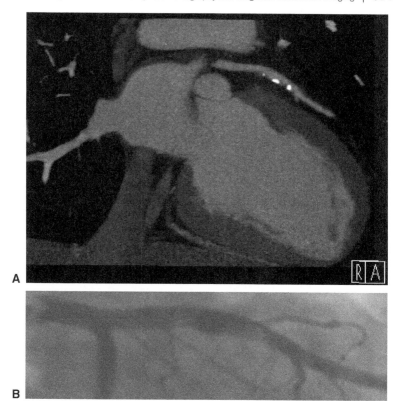

FIGURE 36-1. Atherosclerosis of the proximal left axis deviation with positive remodeling. **(A)** Coronary CT angiography. **(B)** Conventional angiography.

Coronary Artery Calcification

- Coronary artery calcification (CAC) imaging can be applied to a specific area of stenosis or calculated as an overall calcium score.
- There is a strong correlation of atherosclerotic burden with CAC.[17-21]
  - Predictive of long-term cardiovascular events. The results of one such study of over 6000 persons followed for a median of 3.8 years are presented in Table 36-2.[18]
  - Overall atherosclerotic burden, rather than a specific stenosis, can be important in the prediction of long-term cardiovascular events.
- Quantification of CAC is performed as a CAC score or Agatston score.[22]
  - Computer generated by multiplying the calcium plaque area (in square millimeters) by the calcium plaque density (Hounsfield number)
  - A high CAC score does not equate to a severely stenotic lesion but rather to a high atherosclerotic burden and an increased risk of cardiovascular events.[17-21]
- CAC may have a role in the risk stratification of asymptomatic individuals at an intermediate risk for cardiovascular event by the Framingham criteria.[19,23]
- CAC scores of ≥300 Agatston units or higher than the 75th percentile may support an upward revision of risk assessment for individuals in whom pharmacologic therapy initiation is uncertain.[24]

TABLE 36-2	CORONARY CALCIUM SCORE AND CARDIOVASCULAR RISK[a]	
Coronary calcium score	Major coronary event[b] (HR)	Any coronary event (HR)
0	1.00	1.00
0–100	3.89	3.61
101–300	7.08	7.73
>300	6.84	9.67

HR, hazard ratio.

[a]After adjustment for standard coronary risk factors.

[b]Myocardial infarction or death from coronary artery disease.

Data from Detrano R, Guerci AD, Carr JJ, et al. Coronary calcium as a predictor of coronary events in four racial or ethnic groups. *N Engl J Med.* 2008;358:1336-45.

- Disadvantages of CAC include relatively moderate specificity for predicting significant coronary artery lesions, limited quantification of noncalcified plaque, and radiation exposure.

Fractional Flow Reserve

- Invasive FFR
  - FFR is the ratio of maximal myocardial flow in the presence of a coronary stenosis to a theoretical normal maximal flow in the absence of stenosis.
  - Traditionally, FFR is measured using a pressure wire during coronary angiography to assess mean pressure distal to a stenosis compared to mean pressure proximal to the stenosis during hyperemia induced by adenosine administration.
  - A threshold of ≤0.80 is used as a guide for revascularization and has been shown to improve cardiovascular outcomes.[25-27]
- CT fractional flow reserve (FFR$_{CT}$)
  - Calculated using a process termed computational fluid dynamics[28-30]
  - CCTA images are used to generate a three-dimensional model of coronary arteries.
  - A physiologic model of microcirculation is then derived using patient-specific data, including myocardial mass, microvascular resistance, vessel size, and physical laws of fluid dynamics.
  - This generates an FFR$_{CT}$ value for any area of the coronary circulation.
  - FFR$_{CT}$ values of ≤0.80 in vessels ≥2 mm in size are considered positive.
  - FFR$_{CT}$ may be a useful tool in determining hemodynamically significant coronary artery disease and has been shown to influence the management of patients compared to CCTA alone.[28-31]
  - Disadvantages of FFR$_{CT}$ include variability of image quality, limited data on long-term outcomes, and ongoing development of technology and algorithms.

Other Applications

- Transcatheter aortic valve replacement (TAVR) planning: assessment of the aortic valve apparatus, ascending aorta, and iliac arteries[32]
- Peripheral angiography
- Valve fluoroscopy

LIMITATIONS

- Contraindications:
  - High risk for contrast nephropathy (e.g., increased serum creatinine, cutoff varies with institution at >1.5 or 2 mg/dL)
  - Pregnancy
  - Breastfeeding may need to be postponed for 24 hours after contrast.
  - History of severe allergy to IV contrast
- Image quality will be reduced in patients with the following conditions:
  - Irregular heart rhythms (atrial fibrillation/flutter, frequent premature atrial/ventricular contractions) with improper ECG triggering. Can result in slice misregistration and/or errors in radiation dose modulation
  - High regular heart rate (>70 bpm) refractory to rate-lowering agents causes motion artifact.
  - Extreme obesity (body mass index [BMI] >40 kg/m^2) leads to excessive radiation attenuation with a subsequent reduction in the signal-to-noise ratio.
- Metallic objects (e.g., surgical clips, mechanical heart valves, or the wires of a pacemaker/implanted cardiac defibrillator) are prone to radiation scatter, producing streaking artifacts. Coronary stent patency assessment is possible, but not always reliable.
- Severe coronary calcification can obscure the coronary artery lumen.
- Small vessels (<1.5 mm), typically affecting distal coronary segments and some side branch vessels, are not well evaluated.

Cardiac Magnetic Resonance Imaging

GENERAL PRINCIPLES

Definitions

- The high spatial and temporal resolutions of cardiovascular MR (CMR) allow the detailed examination and measurement of cardiac structure and function.
- A strong magnetic field and radiofrequency waves provide detailed tomographic images of internal organs and tissues.
- Assessment of ventricular size, regional and global systolic function, and ventricular wall thickness/mass does not require IV contrast.
- Steady-state–free precession (SSFP): used for functional imaging, ventricular size, volumes, and mass. Blood is bright and heart is dark.
- Spin echo: used for anatomic imaging. Blood is dark, and heart is bright.
- Phase contrast (flow velocity encoding): used for measuring blood flow, quantification of valve regurgitation, stenosis, and intracardiac shunt
- T1 mapping: newer technique calculating a value for the T1 relaxation of the myocardium and used to assess etiology of cardiomyopathy

Physics

- Hydrogen nuclei align their magnetic moments when exposed to an electromagnetic field.
- Application of a radiofrequency pulse stimulates the protons to spin out of equilibrium.
- When the pulse is discontinued, protons release energy as they realign with the magnetic field that is received and converted into an image.
- MR provides markedly detailed images by exploiting the difference in water content in soft tissue. The relation between applied field strength, detected frequency, and the time for proton realignment allows for imaging and differentiation of tissues.

- Lack of radiation exposure is particularly important in cases where serial studies are needed.
- Simple breath-holding techniques, cardiac gating, and respiratory gating improve image quality and reduce motion artifact during imaging of the heart and coronary arteries.

APPLICATIONS

Cardiomyopathy[33]

- CMR is well established in the evaluation of left ventricular (LV) and right ventricular (RV) mass and function due to its accuracy and reproducibility.
- Can distinguish between ischemic and nonischemic cardiomyopathy with gadolinium enhancement including:
  - Hypertrophic cardiomyopathy: location and extent of hypertrophy (Figure 36-2), extent of late gadolinium enhancement (LGE) is associated with progressive ventricular dilation and sudden death[34,35]
  - Arrhythmogenic RV cardiomyopathy
  - Infiltrative cardiomyopathies such as
    - Amyloid heart disease
    - Iron overload (hemochromatosis, transfusional iron overload)
    - Sarcoidosis
    - Fabry disease
  - Focal inflammatory changes in myocarditis: first-line imaging technique to diagnose myocarditis
  - Serial assessment of rejection episodes following heart transplantation
  - Identification of fibrotic areas linked to the risk of sudden cardiac death and development of heart failure
  - Quantification of infarcted myocardium and determination of viability in ischemic cardiomyopathy
  - LV noncompaction, the failure of loosely arranged muscle fibers to form mature compacted myocardium during embryonic development, is increasingly recognized during high-resolution CMR studies. Diagnosis of LV noncompaction cardiomyopathy often requires clinical correlation as increased sensitivity of CMR can lead to overdiagnosis.
- High sensitivity and specificity for LV thrombus detection (Figure 36-3)[36,37]

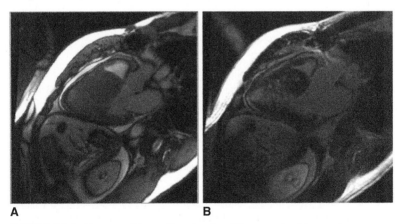

A   B

FIGURE 36-2. Hypertrophic cardiomyopathy. **(A)** noncontrast image demonstrating marked anteroseptal hypertrophy. **(B)** Patchy late gadolinium enhancement (bright areas) seen in hypertrophied septum.

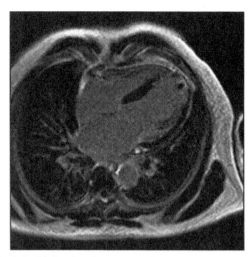

FIGURE 36-3. Apical infarction demonstrated as white scarring by late gadolinium enhancement and left ventricular thrombus in apex (dark).

Pericardial Disease

- Pericardial effusion
- Pericardial thickening in the evaluation of constrictive pericarditis (Figure 36-4)
- Real-time visualization of septal interdependence during respiration
- Pericardial enhancement can be seen after gadolinium administration and can suggest an inflammatory process.
- Tumor infiltration into the pericardium with differentiation of cystic tumors, fatty tumors, melanoma metastasis, hemorrhage, and vascular tumors

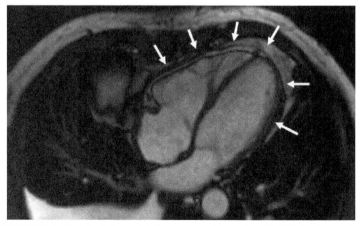

FIGURE 36-4. Pericardial constriction: concentric pericardial thickening and constriction around the left ventricle and right ventricle (white arrows).

Congenital Heart Disease[33,38,39]

- The ability to delineate complex cardiac anatomy without radiation exposure is advantageous in young patients who need sequential studies.
- Can quantify cardiac shunt to assist in treatment and prognosis
- Particularly helpful for postoperative follow-up where RV assessment and complex postoperative anatomy can pose difficulties for 2D echocardiography

Vascular Disease: Aorta and Peripheral Arterial Disease[40]

- CMR can image many aspects of the vessel wall, including the assessment of dissection, thrombus, inflammation, and atherosclerotic plaque.
- MR angiography (MRA) may be done without contrast injection using "time-of-flight" techniques or with IV gadolinium. This is useful in patients with contraindications to CT contrast.
- A rare but significant side effect of gadolinium contrast agents, nephrogenic systemic fibrosis (NSF), has been described in patients with severe renal insufficiency; therefore, caution is warranted in these patients (see later).[33,40]
- MRA combined with vascular wall imaging is valuable in the detection and serial monitoring of thoracic and abdominal aortic aneurysms.
- Location and extent of aortic aneurysm and dissection flap with assessment of true and false lumen flow

Coronary Artery Disease

- Easily assesses proximal coronary artery course for delineation of anomalous coronary arteries. The lack of radiation exposure makes CMR a first-line choice for imaging in a child or young adult (Figure 36-5).

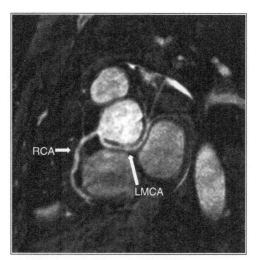

FIGURE 36-5. Anomalous left main coronary artery (LMCA). Anomalous LMCA originates from the right coronary cusp with right coronary artery (RCA) and takes a retroaortic course on coronary MR angiography. (Image courtesy of Warren Manning, MD, Beth Israel Deaconess Medical Center, Boston, MA.)

- The direct visualization of coronary arteries with coronary MRA has improved in recent years but still faces technical challenges, mainly due to motion artifacts. CT or cardiac catheterization is preferable for assessing the degree of coronary stenosis.
- Ischemia[41-43]
  - Gadolinium-enhanced CMR incorporated with a pharmacologic agent such as dobutamine, regadenoson, adenosine, or dipyridamole
  - Dobutamine stress CMR: visualizes segmental wall motion abnormalities during incremental dose increases of dobutamine
  - Vasodilator perfusion CMR (regadenoson, adenosine, or dipyridamole): visualize ischemia as areas of myocardial hypoperfusion as the contrast washes through the myocardium (first-pass perfusion study) during administration of medication that induces vasodilation
- Infarction: delayed imaging of LGE is highly sensitive for the detection of myocardial fibrosis. Acute and chronic infarctions can be imaged. CMR can be used to assess viability. Negative predictive value of ~90% of no functional recovery in segments with >50% transmural infarction detected by LGE. 78% positive predictive value for recovery in segments without LGE after revascularization.[44]
- The combination of stress and infarction imaging techniques allows the determination of myocardial ischemia, infarction, and prediction of myocardial recovery following revascularization.

Valvular Heart Disease

- Allows for morphologic and functional assessment of cardiac valves[33,45-48]
- Not prone to poor acoustic windows that may be encountered in transthoracic echocardiography
- Valuable alternative when transesophageal echocardiography is not desired
- Measure peak velocity; estimate the pressure gradient to evaluate the severity of stenosis
- Direct valve orifice planimetry
- Volume quantification permits accurate assessment of valvular regurgitation.
- Most prosthetic valves are safe for imaging, but focal artifacts may obscure the images.
- Vegetations are not always visualized due to erratic motion.
- Quantification of LV dimensions, volume, and systolic function can assist in determining the timing for valve surgery.
- Usually second-line technique when echocardiography is inadequate

CONTRAST ENHANCEMENT

- MRI benefits from the use of contrast agents.
- These agents generate effects by altering the local magnetic field and relaxation parameters within the imaged tissue.
- The most used contrast agents are gadolinium chelates.
- Gadolinium is an extracellular contrast agent that is normally not retained in myocardium.
- It is retained in areas of infarction and fibrosis where it is seen as a bright signal on imaging.
- Anaphylactoid reactions with these agents have been observed in <0.1% of cases.[33,40]
- NSF
  - A rare but serious complication
  - Described with administration of certain gadolinium chelates
  - Gadolinium-based contrast agents should be avoided unless the diagnostic information is essential and not available with non–contrast-enhanced MRI in the following patients:
    - Acute or chronic severe renal insufficiency
    - Renal dysfunction of any severity due to hepatorenal syndrome

- In the perioperative liver transplantation period
- Dialysis patients should receive gadolinium agents only when this is essential, and if so, dialysis should be performed as soon as possible after scan.

CONTRAINDICATIONS

- Absolute
  - Metallic fragments in the eye are not held in place by scar tissue. An orbital plain radiography should be performed before MRI if a metal fragment is suspected to be in the eye.
  - Aneurysm clips in the brain are not protected by scar tissue.
- Relative
  - Cardiac implantable electronic devices (CIEDs): Potential interactions can result in atrial and ventricular arrhythmias, changes in sensing or capture thresholds, asynchronous pacing and inhibition of tachycardia therapies, electrical reset, inappropriate function and therapies, and imaging artifacts. Devices that are MRI conditional can safely undergo required imaging.[49-51] Recent data suggest that thoracic and nonthoracic MRI examinations may be safely performed even in devices that are not MRI conditional.[52]
  - Insufficient safety data for abandoned, epicardial, or fractured leads[51]
  - Cochlear implants, insulin pumps, and nerve stimulators
  - Mechanical cardiac valves if dehiscence is suspected[33,50]
  - Orthopedic implants are usually stable if embedded for several weeks but cause artifacts when adjacent to the area of interest.
- Acoustic noise is due to the currents in the wires of the gradient magnets:
  - In 3T scanners, depending on the imaging techniques, the noise can reach more than 130 dB.
  - Appropriate ear protection is mandatory.
- Pregnancy
  - Limited data exist on the effects of MR on the developing fetus.
  - Current guidelines recommend that a pregnant woman should undergo MRI only when essential and ideally after the first trimester after organogenesis is complete.[53,54]
  - No direct harm to a fetus has been demonstrated with the use of non–contrast-enhanced MRI.[53,54]
  - The use of gadolinium enhancement may be associated with adverse outcomes extending into childhood.[54]
  - Due to unclear risk related to gadolinium compounds and known placental crossing of the chemical compound, they are not recommended for use in pregnancy.

REFERENCES

1. Mettler FA, Huda W, Yoshizumi TT, Mahesh M. Effective doses in radiology and diagnostic nuclear medicine: a catalog. *Radiology.* 2008;248:254-63.
2. Halliburton SS, Abbara S, Chen MY, et al. SCCT guidelines on radiation dose and dose-optimization strategies in cardiovascular CT. *J Cardiovasc Comput Tomogr.* 2011;5:198-224.
3. Budoff MJ, Dowe D, Jollis JG, et al. Diagnostic performance of 64-multidetector row coronary computed tomographic angiography for evaluation of coronary artery stenosis in individuals without known coronary artery disease: results from the prospective multicenter ACCURACY (Assessment by Coronary Computed Tomographic Angiography of Individuals Undergoing Invasive Coronary Angiography) trial. *J Am Coll Cardiol.* 2008;52:1724-32.
4. Garcia MJ, Lessick J, Hoffmann MH, et al. Accuracy of 16-row multidetector computed tomography for the assessment of coronary artery stenosis. *JAMA.* 2006;296:403-11.
5. Hoffmann U, Truong QA, Schoenfeld DA, et al. Coronary CT angiography versus standard evaluation in acute chest pain. *N Engl J Med.* 2012;367:299-308.
6. Meijboom WB, Meijs MF, Schuijf JD, et al. Diagnostic accuracy of 64-slice computed tomography coronary angiography: a prospective, multicenter, multivendor study. *J Am Coll Cardiol.* 2008;52:2135-44.

7. Miller JM, Rochitte CE, Dewey M, et al. Diagnostic performance of coronary angiography by 64-row CT. *N Engl J Med.* 2008;359:2324-36.

8. Ollendorf DA, Kuba M, Pearson SD. The diagnostic performance of multi-slice coronary computed tomographic angiography: a systematic review. *J Gen Intern Med.* 2011;26:307-16.

9. Paech DC, Weston AR. A systematic review of the clinical effectiveness of 64-slice or higher computed tomography angiography as an alternative to invasive coronary angiography in the investigation of suspected coronary artery disease. *BMC Cardiovasc Disord.* 2011;11:32.

10. Stein PD, Yaekoub AY, Matta F, Sostman HD. 64-slice CT for diagnosis of coronary artery disease: a systematic review. *Am J Med.* 2008;121:715-25.

11. Chae MK, Kim EK, Jung KY, et al. Triple rule-out computed tomography for risk stratification of patients with acute chest pain. *J Cardiovasc Comput Tomogr.* 2016;10:291-300.

12. Ayad SW, ElSharkawy EM, ElTahan SM, et al. The role of 64/128-slice multidetector computed tomography to assess the progression of coronary atherosclerosis. *Clin Med Insights Cardiol.* 2015;9:47-52.

13. The SCOT-HEART Investigators. CT coronary angiography in patients with suspected angina due to coronary heart disease (SCOT-HEART): an open-label, parallel-group, multicenter trial. *Lancet.* 2015;385:2383-91.

14. Litt HI, Gatsonis C, Snyder B, et al. CT angiography for safe discharge of patients with possible acute coronary syndromes. *N Engl J Med.* 2012;366:1393-403.

15. Wolk MJ, Bailey SR, Doherty JU, et al. ACCF/AHA/ASE/ASNC/HFSA/HRS/SCAI/SCCT/SCMR/STS 2013 multimodality appropriate use criteria for the detection and risk assessment of stable ischemic heart disease: a report of the American College of Cardiology Foundation Appropriate Use Criteria Task Force, American Heart Association, American Society of Echocardiography, American Society of Nuclear Cardiology, Heart Failure Society of America, Heart Rhythm Society, Society for Cardiovascular Angiography and Interventions, Society of Cardiovascular Computed Tomography, Society for Cardiovascular Magnetic Resonance, and Society of Thoracic Surgeons. *J Am Coll Cardiol.* 2014;63:380-406.

16. Budoff MJ, Hokanson JE, Nasir K, et al. Progression of coronary artery calcium predicts all-cause mortality. *JACC Cardiovasc Imaging.* 2010;3:1229-36.

17. Detrano R, Guerci AD, Carr JJ, et al. Coronary calcium as a predictor of coronary events in four racial or ethnic groups. *N Engl J Med.* 2008;358:1336-45.

18. Greenland P, LaBree L, Azen SP, et al. Coronary artery calcium score combined with Framingham score for risk prediction in asymptomatic individuals. *JAMA.* 2004;291:210-15.

19. O'Rourke RA, Brundage BH, Froelicher VF, et al. American College of Cardiology/American Heart Association Expert Consensus document on electron-beam computed tomography for the diagnosis and prognosis of coronary artery disease. *Circulation.* 2000;102:126-40.

20. Taylor AJ, Bindeman J, Feuerstein I, et al. Coronary calcium independently predicts incident premature coronary heart disease over measured cardiovascular risk factors: mean three-year outcomes in the Prospective Army Coronary Calcium (PACC) project. *J Am Coll Cardiol.* 2005;46:807-14.

21. Agatston AS, Janowitz WR, Hildner FJ, et al. Quantification of coronary artery calcium using ultrafast computed tomography. *J Am Coll Cardiol.* 1990;15:827-32.

22. Greenland P, Alpert JS, Beller GA, et al. 2010 ACCF/AHA guideline for assessment of cardiovascular risk in asymptomatic adults: executive summary. *Circulation.* 2010;122:2748-64.

23. Goff DC Jr, Lloyd-Jones DM, Bennett G, et al. 2013 ACC/AHA guideline on the assessment of cardiovascular risk: a report of the American College of Cardiology/American Heart Association task force on practice guidelines. *J Am Coll Cardiol.* 2014;63:2935-59.

24. Tonino PA, De Bruyne B, Pijls NHJ, et al. Fractional flow reserve versus angiography for guiding percutaneous coronary intervention. *N Engl J Med.* 2009;360:213-24.

25. De Bruyne B, Pijls NJH, Kalesan B, et al. Fractional flow reserve-guided PCI versus medical therapy in stable coronary disease. *N Engl J Med.* 2012;367:991-1001.

26. Xaplanteris P, Fournier S, Pijls NHJ, et al. Five-year outcomes with PCI guided by fractional flow reserve. *N Engl J Med.* 2018;e1-10.

27. Koo BK, Erglis A, Doh JH, et al. Diagnosis of ischemia-causing coronary stenosis by noninvasive fractional flow reserve computed from coronary computed tomographic angiograms. *J Am Coll Cardiol.* 2011;58:1989-97.

28. Min JK, Leipsic J, Pencina MJ, et al. Diagnostic accuracy of fractional flow reserve from anatomic CT angiography. *JAMA.* 2012;308:1237-45.

29. Norgaard BL, Leipsic J, Gaur S, et al. Diagnostic performance of noninvasive fractional flow reserve derived from coronary computed tomography angiography in suspected coronary artery disease. *J Am Coll Cardiol.* 2014;63:1145-55.

30. Curzen NP, Nolan J, Zaman AG, et al. Does the routine availability of CT-derived FFR influence management of patients with stable chest pain compared to CT angiography alone?: the FFR$_{CT}$ RIPCORD study. *JACC Cardiovasc Imaging.* 2016;9:1188-94.

31. Schoenhagen P, Kapadia SR, Halliburton SS, et al. Computed tomography evaluation for transcatheter aortic valve implantation (TAVI): imaging of the aortic root and iliac arteries. *J Cardiovasc Comput Tomogr.* 2011;5:293-300.

32. Hundley WG, Bluemke DA, Finn JP, et al. ACCF/ACR/AHA/NASCI/SCMR 2010 expert consensus document on cardiovascular magnetic resonance. *Circulation.* 2010;121:2462-508.

33. Moon JC, McKenna WJ, McCrohon JA, et al. Toward clinical risk assessment in hypertrophic cardiomyopathy with gadolinium cardiovascular magnetic resonance. *J Am Coll Cardiol.* 2003;41:1561-7.

34. Chan RH, Maron BJ, Olivotto I, et al. Prognostic value of quantitative contrast-enhanced cardiovascular magnetic resonance for the evaluation of sudden death risk in patients with hypertrophic cardiomyopathy. *Circulation.* 2014;130:484-95.

35. Srichai MB, Junor C, Rodriguez LL, et al. Clinical, imaging, and pathological characteristics of left ventricular thrombus: a comparison of contrast-enhanced magnetic resonance imaging, transthoracic echocardiography, and transesophageal echocardiography with surgical or pathological validation. *Am Heart J.* 2006;152:75-84.

36. Weinsaft JW, Kim RJ, Ross M, et al. Contrast-enhanced anatomic imaging as compared to contrast-enhanced tissue characterization for detection of left ventricular thrombus. *JACC Cardiovasc Imaging.* 2009;2(8):969-79.

37. Weber OM, Higgins CB. MR evaluation of cardiovascular physiology in congenital heart disease: flow and function. *J Cardiovasc Magnet Res.* 2006;8:607-17.

38. Wood JC. Anatomical assessment of congenital heart disease. *J Cardiovasc Magnet Res.* 2006;8:595-606.

39. Kramer CM, Budoff MJ, Fayad ZA, et al. ACCF/AHA clinical competence statement on vascular imaging with computed tomography and magnetic resonance. A report of the American College of Cardiology Foundation/American Heart Association/American College of Physicians task force on clinical competence and training. *J Am Coll Cardiol.* 2007;50:1097-114.

40. Lee DC, Johnson NP. Quantification of absolute myocardial blood flow by magnetic resonance perfusion imaging. *JACC Cardiovasc Imaging.* 2009;2:761-70.

41. Nandalur KR, Dwamena BA, Choudhri AF, et al. Diagnostic performance of stress cardiac magnetic resonance imaging in the detection of coronary artery disease. *J Am Coll Cardiol.* 2007;50:1343-53.

42. Pennell DJ. Contemporary reviews in cardiovascular medicine: cardiovascular magnetic resonance. *Circulation.* 2010;121:692-705.

43. Kim RJ, Wu E, Rafael A, et al. The use of contrast-enhanced magnetic resonance imaging to identify reversible myocardial dysfunction. *N Engl J Med.* 2000;343:1445-53.

44. Djavidani B, Debl K, Lenhart M, et al. Planimetry of mitral valve stenosis by magnetic resonance imaging. *J Am Coll Cardiol.* 2005;45:2048-53.

45. McVeigh ER, Guttman MA, Lederman RJ, et al. Real-time interactive MRI-guided cardiac surgery: aortic valve replacement using a direct apical approach. *Magn Reson Med.* 2006;56:958-64.

46. Rent P, Lederlin M, Lafitte S, et al. Absolute assessment of aortic valve stenosis by planimetry using cardiovascular magnetic resonance imaging: comparison with transesophageal echocardiography, transthoracic echocardiography, and cardiac catheterization. *Eur J Radiol.* 2006;59:276-83.

47. Suzuki J, Caputo GR, Kondo C, Higgins CB. Cine MR imaging of valvular heart disease: display and imaging parameters affect the size of the signal void caused by valvular regurgitation. *Am J Roentgenol.* 1990;155:723-7.

48. Williamson BD, Gohn DC, Ramza BM, et al. Real-world evaluation of magnetic resonance imaging in patients with a magnetic resonance imaging conditional pacemaker system. *JACC Clin Electrophysiol.* 2017;3:1231-9.

49. Levine GN, Gomes AS, Arai AE, et al. Safety of magnetic resonance imaging in patients with cardiovascular devices. *Circulation.* 2007;116:2878-91.

50. Indik JH, Gimbel, JR, Abe H, et al. 2017 HRS expert consensus statement on magnetic resonance imaging and radiation exposure in patients with cardiovascular implantable electronic devices. *Heart Rhythm.* 2017;14:e97-153.

51. Nazarian S, Hansford R, Rahsepar AA, et al. Safety of magnetic resonance imaging in patients with cardiac devices. *N Engl J Med.* 2017;377:2555-64.

52. ACOG Committee. Guidelines for diagnostic imaging during pregnancy and lactation. *Obstet Gynecol.* 2017;130:e210-16.

53. Ray JG, Vermeulen MJ, Bharatha A, et al. Association between MRI exposure during pregnancy and fetal and childhood outcomes. *JAMA.* 2016;316:952-61.

Nuclear Cardiology

37

Rahul A. Chhana, Thomas H. Schindler, Chirayu Gor, and Sudhir K. Jain

GENERAL PRINCIPLES

Definitions

- **Single-photon emission computed tomography** (SPECT) is a modality utilized for the assessment of myocardial perfusion and viability.
- Clinical application includes the following:
  - Myocardial perfusion imaging (MPI)
    - This is the most common clinical application of SPECT.
    - Useful for stress imaging where images at rest are compared to those at stress (pharmacologic or exercise)
    - For patients with active anginal symptoms, only resting images are performed for detection of ongoing ischemia or infarction.
  - Assessment of myocardial viability if positron emission tomography (PET) imaging is not available, which is the preferred modality
  - Measurement of left ventricular (LV) volume and function

Physics

- After the radiotracer is administered IV, it is extracted from the blood by viable myocytes and retained for a given time period.
- As the isotope decays, a γ-camera (Figure 37-1) captures the emitted photons and produces a digital image by rotating in an orbital path around the patient.[1]
  - As the camera rotates, multiple images are obtained with 20 to 25 seconds of emission data, giving different angles of the myocardium.
  - Imaging information from each view is back projected onto an imaging matrix, creating a reconstruction of the heart (Figure 37-2).[1]
  - After the images are acquired, various software applications are applied to improve image quality, such as attenuation correction.
- The tomographic images are displayed in three standard planes (Figure 37-3).[1]
  - **Short-axis images** are obtained by cutting perpendicular to the long axis of the heart.
    - This produces doughnut-like slices.
    - These images are similar to the parasternal short-axis view on two-dimensional echocardiography.
  - **Vertical long-axis images** are obtained by cutting parallel to the long axis of the heart. This allows for easy evaluation of the anterior and inferior walls.
  - **Horizontal long-axis images** are also cut parallel to the long axis of the heart; however, they are orthogonal to the vertical long-axis image. This allows for easy evaluation of the septal and lateral walls.
- Representative images are presented in Figures 37-4, 37-5, and 37-6.[2]

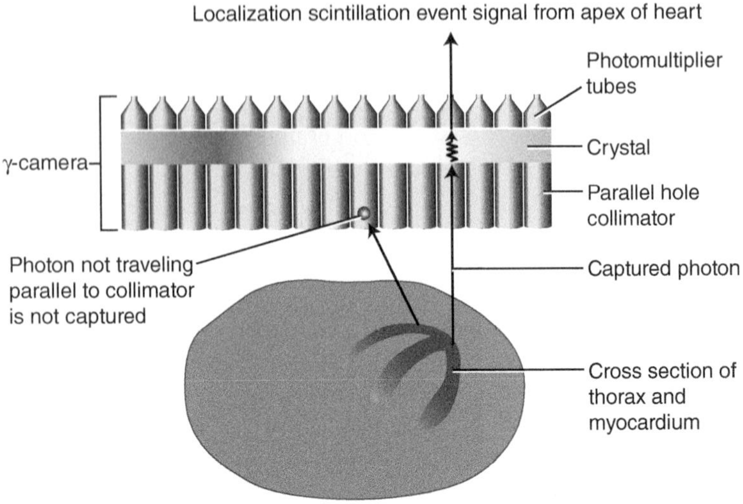

Localization scintillation event signal from apex of heart

Photomultiplier tubes

γ-camera

Crystal

Parallel hole collimator

Photon not traveling parallel to collimator is not captured

Captured photon

Cross section of thorax and myocardium

FIGURE 37-1. Transmission of photons emitted from myocardium to a γ-camera. (Reprinted from Udelson JE, Dilsizian V, Bonow RO. Nuclear cardiology. In: Libby P, Bonow RO, Mann DL, et al, eds. *Braunwald's Heart Disease: A Textbook of Cardiovascular Medicine.* 8th ed. Elsevier; 2008:345-91. Copyright © 2008 Elsevier. With permission.)

Radiotracers

- Most SPECT studies use agents based on either **technetium-99m** (^{99m}Tc) (^{99m}Tc-sestamibi, ^{99m}Tc-tetrofosmin, and ^{99m}Tc-teboroxime) or **thallium-201** (^{201}Tl).
- Understanding SPECT MPI requires understanding the properties of these tracers.[3]
- **^{99m}Tc**
  - This is a relatively newer agent with a half-life of 6 hours.
  - Emits 140 keV of photon energy. Higher energy photons allow for higher counts and less noise.
  - First-pass absorption is only 60%, and there is very little redistribution. Perfusion is fixed at the time of injection, allowing for quicker imaging and functional assessment.
  - Given these qualities of the isotope, various protocols can be used in the appropriate clinical scenario:
    - **Stress/rest protocol**
      - Inject 10 to 12 mCi for stress images, followed by 30 mCi for rest if needed.
      - Stress images are performed first; if stress first imaging has normal perfusion and normal wall motion, then there is no need for rest imaging.
      - This is most commonly performed with SPECT-CT, which allows for attenuation correction for the inferior wall (liver, diaphragm) and the anterior wall (breast-induced attenuation in women). Attenuation correction helps avoid false-positive findings and thus improves study quality, sensitivity, and, in particular, specificity.
      - Advantages of stress/rest protocol include lower radiation dose (3 to 4 mSv), improved patient comfort, and less time (60- to 90-minute examination vs. 2 to 3 hours for standard rest/stress protocol).
      - Disadvantages of stress/rest protocol include reduced image quality in obese patients and women with large breasts due to the lower injection dose (10 to 12 mCi).

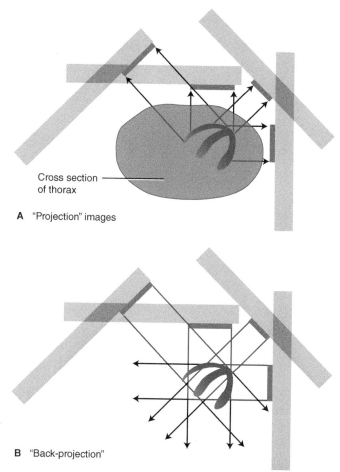

Cross section of thorax

A "Projection" images

B "Back-projection"

FIGURE 37-2. A) Detection of photons by a γ-camera. The camera is rotated to different angles to enable image acquisition from multiple views. B) Imaging information from each view is back-projected onto an imaging matrix, creating a reconstruction of the heart. (Republished with permission of Elsevier Science &Technology Journals from Udelson JE, Dilsizian V, Bonow RO. Nuclear cardiology. In: Zipes DP, Libby P, Bonow RO, et al, eds. *Braunwald's Heart Disease: A Textbook of Cardiovascular Medicine.* 7th ed. Elsevier; 2005:287-335; permission conveyed through Copyright Clearance Center, Inc.)

- **Rest/stress protocol**
  - This is the standard protocol utilized at most institutions.
  - 10 to 12 mCi of isotope is injected for rest images, followed by 30 to 35 mCi for stress imaging.
  - To overcome any residual isotope activity from the rest injection, a two to three times higher dose is needed for stress imaging.
  - Advantages of rest/stress protocol: Stress perfusion images are of better quality due to the higher stress injection dose (30 to 35 mCi) compared to stress/rest protocol

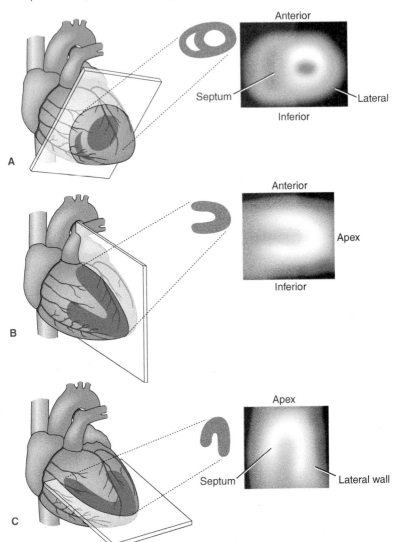

FIGURE 37-3. Tomographic views of the left ventricle. Short-axis view, vertical long-axis view, and horizontal long-axis view (top to bottom). (Reprinted from Udelson JE, Dilsizian V, Bonow RO. Nuclear cardiology. In: Libby P, Bonow RO, Mann DL, et al, eds. *Braunwald's Heart Disease: A Textbook of Cardiovascular Medicine.* 8th ed. Elsevier; 2008:345-91. Copyright © 2008 Elsevier. With permission.)

(10 to 12 mCi). The higher stress injection dose reduces attenuation artifacts and improves detection of wall motion abnormalities. In addition, images are easier to read due to optimal image quality of stress perfusion imaging, specifically in obese patients or women with large breasts. Finally, this is the best protocol for SPECT-only cameras (when CT is not available for attenuation correction).

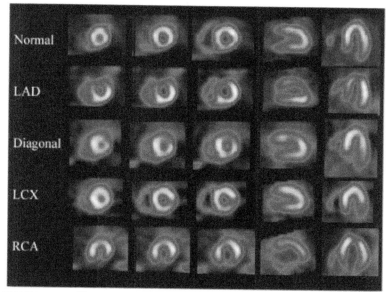

FIGURE 37-4. ^{99m}Tc stress images showing perfusion defects in each of the respective coronary distributions. LAD, left anterior descending; LCX, left circumflex artery; RCA, right coronary artery. (Republished with permission of McGraw Hill LLC from Berman DS, Hayes SW, Hachamovitch R, et al. Nuclear cardiology. In: Fuster V, Walsh RA, Harrington RA, eds. *Hurst's The Heart.* 13th ed. McGraw-Hill, 2011:570; permission conveyed through Copyright Clearance Center, Inc.)

- □ Disadvantages of rest/stress protocol include a longer study protocol time of 3 to 4 hours with less patient throughput due to longer times. In addition, radiation exposure is about 7 to 12 mSv compared to 3 to 4 mSv in stress/rest protocol.
- **^{201}Tl**
  - ○ This radiotracer has a half-life of ~73 hours and emits 80 keV of photon energy.
  - ○ Less commonly used for ischemia. Most commonly used for viability when MRI or PET is not available.
  - ○ Uptake
    - ■ Early myocardial uptake of ^{201}Tl is primarily related to regional blood flow.
    - ■ Poorly perfused myocardium will take up a small amount of ^{201}Tl during the initial 5 to 10 minutes.
    - ■ After this initial phase of myocardial uptake, any subsequent perfusion is primarily due to redistribution across a concentration gradient. This contrasts with ^{99m}Tc that has very little redistribution.
    - ■ Since blood vessels with atherosclerosis do not perfuse myocardium as well as blood vessels of normal caliber, the initial uptake under peak stress will be low.
  - ○ Stress/rest protocol
    - ■ Technetium is preferred for stress/rest protocol perfusion imaging (two injections); however, it is possible to perform stress/rest protocols with thallium (one injection only).
    - ■ Single imaging with peak stress-only injection, followed by stress imaging and subsequent rest imaging.
    - ■ If there is a fixed defect on the stress/rest images, then repeat injection of thallium and reimaging after 1 hour would allow for determination of viability. Alternatively, one

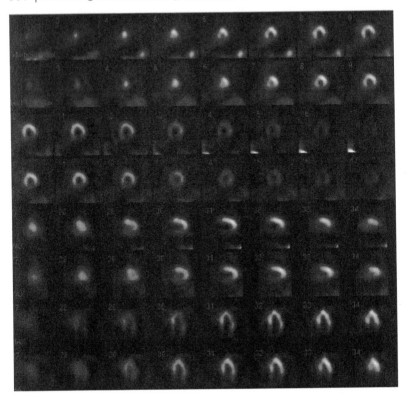

FIGURE 37-5. Rest and SPECT MPI images. Upper row represents stress images; lower row represents rest images. There is a large transmural infarction of the inferior wall and large, moderately severe ischemia of the inferolateral and lateral walls. SPECT MPI, single-photon emission computed tomography-myocardial perfusion imaging.

could reimage again after 8 hours without reinjection as this time lag allows thallium to redistribute to the viable myocardium.

- **18-Fluorodeoxyglucose (FDG)**
  - FDG is generally considered a PET radiotracer.
  - Two studies have demonstrated similar sensitivity to reinjection or redistribution of ^{201}Tl SPECT at detecting viable myocardium but increased specificity with FDG-SPECT.[3]
  - Although the image quality and resolution of PET are clearly superior to those of SPECT, several studies have shown good correlations of viability between FDG-PET and FDG-SPECT (Figure 37-7).[4-6]
  - The magnitude of tracer uptake is proportional to the magnitude of preserved tissue viability.
  - FDG-PET in conjunction with rest perfusion assessment is commonly seen as a reference in the assessment of myocardial viability. It is commonly applied for specific viability assessment when there is a fixed defect and ≥4 segments (within the 17-segment model) on stress/rest images on SPECT. In about 20-40% of patients with fixed perfusion defects, FDG-PET still identifies significant amount of viable but ischemic compromised myocardium.

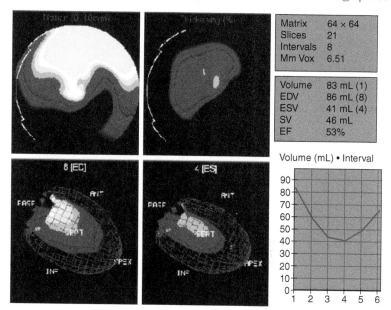

Matrix	64 × 64
Slices	21
Intervals	8
Mm Vox	6.51

Volume	83 mL (1)
EDV	86 mL (8)
ESV	41 mL (4)
SV	46 mL
EF	53%

FIGURE 37-6. ECG-gated SPECT images used to measure left ventricular ejection fraction, wall motion, and volume. EDV, end-diastolic volume; EF, ejection fraction; ESV, end-systolic volume; SPECT, single-photon emission computed tomography; SV, stroke volume.

Interpretation and Image Analysis

- SPECT myocardial scan analysis involves describing the following:
  - The presence and location of perfusion defects
  - The size and severity of the perfusion abnormality
  - The reversibility of defects seen on stress images
  - The presence of infarction (size and severity)
- Similar regions of myocardium are compared at rest and at stress.
  - A defect seen in at least two tomographic planes is more likely to represent a true abnormality compared with a defect seen on one plane.
  - An ischemic region will show a normal perfusion pattern at rest, but reduced uptake of scintillation counts during stress.
  - An infarcted area will demonstrate reduced perfusion at rest and at stress.
  - If a persistent defect is present (suggesting infarction), it is important to pay attention to the adjacent myocardium. One may see a fixed defect on both stress and rest images, but the stress images may show peri-infarct ischemia that is not demonstrated on resting images.
  - Abnormalities seen on rest images, but not stress, are suspicious for artifact.
- ECG gating allows assessment of wall motion abnormalities.
- The extent (size) and the severity of the perfusion abnormality are independently associated with the risk of adverse events over time.[7]
- **Transient ischemic dilation** (TID) refers to the appearance of LV cavity enlargement on stress images when compared to resting pictures.
  - It is suggestive of diffuse subendocardial ischemia and is a marker for severe and extensive coronary artery disease (CAD).
  - TID is also suggestive that the patient may have multivessel disease.
- Detection of lung uptake of radiotracer also suggests multivessel disease on ^{201}Tl stress images.

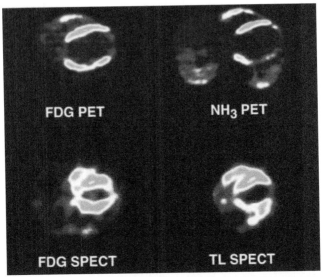

FIGURE 37-7. Comparison of myocardial viability by both PET and SPECT. Both modalities demonstrate apical infarction with metabolically active myocardium in the other walls. Note the improved spatial resolution of PET over SPECT. FDG, fluorodeoxyglucose; PET, positron emission tomography; SPECT, single-photon emission computed tomography; Tl, thallium. (This research was originally published in JNM. Bax JJ, Visser FC, Blanksma PK, et al. Comparison of myocardial uptake of fluorine-18-fluorodeoxyglucose imaged with PET and SPECT in dyssynergic myocardium. *J Nucl Med.* 1996;37(10):1631-36. © SNMMI.)

Artifacts

- Breast tissue can reduce the scintillation counts registered on the γ-camera.
  - This may cause a mild-to-moderate severe fixed defect of the anterior or anterolateral wall.
  - Fixed defects more likely represent breast attenuation artifacts rather than true infarct when associated with preserved wall motion.
- Attenuation artifacts of the inferior wall can be caused by extracardiac structures that interfere with scintillation count measurements.
  - The diaphragm overlaps the inferior wall and can lead to the interpretation of a fixed defect in that region.
  - Placing the patient in a prone position can shift the diaphragm off the inferior wall.

APPLICATIONS

Stable Chest Pain Syndromes

- The goal of MPI is to identify normally perfused, ischemic, and infarcted myocardium.
- The most common way of performing SPECT MPI is as a stress test.
- Initial studies have demonstrated a strong relationship between the extent of ischemia and the risk of cardiac death or myocardial infarction (MI)—the greater the extent of ischemia, the higher the event risk.[8,9]

- SPECT MPI gives incremental prognostic information regarding the risk of cardiac death or nonfatal MI.[10]
- The likelihood of cardiac death or nonfatal MI is very low with normal MPI, $\leq 1\%$ per year over extended follow-up (13 to 89 months).[11]

Suspected Acute Coronary Syndromes

- Patients presenting to the emergency department with symptoms suggestive of an acute coronary syndrome (ACS) but nondiagnostic ECG and cardiac biomarkers can undergo ^{99m}Tc-based MPI.
  - The patient is injected with ^{99m}Tc at rest and then scanned in 45 to 60 minutes.
  - As there is little redistribution of radiotracer, the images obtained in a patient with symptoms due to active ischemia reflect myocardial blood flow at the time of injection (during the ischemic state).
  - Stress imaging is not necessary (and should not be performed) in patients with ongoing symptoms.
- The presence of perfusion defects by ^{99m}Tc imaging suggests either active ischemia or infarction. This provides appropriate risk stratification for the patient based on the pretest probability of ACS.

Assessment after Acute Myocardial Infarction

- In stable patients following ST-segment elevation MI (STEMI), SPECT MPI can help risk-stratify patients for future cardiac events.
- An MPI study that does not demonstrate reversible defects has been associated with lower risk of cardiac death and nonfatal MI.

Assessment of Myocardial Viability

- Myocardial viability can be assessed by using either ^{201}Tl or FDG.
- ^{201}Tl is an excellent agent for viability due to its long half-life and ability to redistribute.
  - Myocardial viability assessment should ideally be performed 24 hours after ^{201}Tl injection, as this can detect additional viable segments that may be missed by 1-day rest/stress SPECT MPI alone.
  - The presence of ^{201}Tl after redistribution implies preserved myocyte activity.
- Using SPECT-CT in conjunction with PET viability imaging

INDICATIONS

Exercise Stress Testing

- Exercise stress testing is discussed in detail in Chapter 7.
- In patients who are able to exercise to an adequate workload (at least 85% of age-adjusted maximal predicted heart rate and 5 metabolic equivalents), this is the preferred modality.

Pharmacologic Stress Testing

- Pharmacologic stress testing is discussed in detail in Chapter 7.
- Indications for the use of pharmacologic stress testing include:
  - Inability to perform adequate exercise (e.g., pulmonary disease, peripheral vascular disease, musculoskeletal limitations, or cognitive concerns)
  - Baseline ECG abnormalities including left bundle branch block (LBBB), ventricular preexcitation, and permanent ventricular pacing
  - Risk stratification of clinically stable patients into low- and high-risk groups very early after acute MI (>1 day) or presentation to the emergency department with presumptive ACS

- There are three vasodilator agents currently used: **dipyridamole, adenosine,** and **regadenoson.**[3]
  - Adenosine
    - Causes coronary vasodilation through A2A receptors. There is greater vasodilation in normal coronary blood vessels compared to those with atherosclerotic lesions.
    - Undesirable effects of adenosine are mediated through its activation of the A1 (atrioventricular [AV] block), A2B (peripheral vasodilation), and A3 (bronchospasm) receptors.
    - Adenosine can cause hypotension, severe bronchospasm, and AV dissociation.
    - It should not be used in patients with AV block, active bronchospasm, or hypotension.
  - Dipyridamole
    - An adenosine deaminase inhibitor
    - Less commonly used and has a side-effect profile similar to adenosine
  - Regadenoson (commonly known as Lexiscan)
    - Similar to adenosine in that it causes coronary vasodilation but has **a higher avidity for the A2A receptor** and less for the A1, A2B, and A3 receptors. Thus, **its side-effect profile is more favorable** than for adenosine.
    - Unlike adenosine, patients with mild asthma or chronic obstructive lung disease can receive regadenoson with close monitoring.
    - Common side effects including flushing, headache, and shortness of breath. These are self-limiting and generally resolve quickly.
- Methylxanthines (e.g., caffeine, theophylline, theobromine)
  - These drugs must be held before testing as they are competitive inhibitors of both adenosine and regadenoson.
  - Aminophylline 50 to 250 mg IV is used to reverse the bronchospastic effect of the vasodilator agents.

Limitations

- MPI is unable to quantify absolute myocardial blood flow.
  - May underestimate the severity of CAD in patients with so-called balanced ischemia[11]
  - Potential for false-negative stress test with triple-vessel CAD where myocardial perfusion will appear identical in all three coronary distributions
- Prone to attenuation artifact
  - Emitted photons scatter in different directions as they travel through tissue in the body rather than moving directly in their initial trajectory.
  - This decreases the spatial resolution of MPI.

Radiation Safety

- The most important determinant of appropriate use criteria for cardiac radionuclide imaging is often radiation exposure.
- Physicians should be **guided by the principle of "as low as reasonably achievable" (ALARA) to reduce lifetime biologic risk from radiation exposure.**
- Table 37-1 outlines the relative radiation exposures with various cardiac imaging modalities.[12,13]

REFERENCES

1. Bonow RO, Mann DL, Zipes DP, Libby P. *Braunwald's Heart Disease: A Textbook of Cardiovascular Medicine.* 9th ed. Saunders; 2011.
2. Fuster V, Walsh RA, Harrington RA. *Hurst's The Heart.* 13th ed. McGraw-Hill; 2011.

TABLE 37-1	RADIATION EXPOSURE OF CARDIAC IMAGING MODALITIES

Imaging	Estimates of effective doses (in mSV)
Pacemaker insertion	1.5
Background level of radiation absorbed from natural sources in the US	≤3.0
Cardiac CT (without contrast, for assessment of coronary calcium)	3.0
Myocardial perfusion imaging study with ejection fraction (stress only)	3–4
Comprehensive electrophysiologic evaluation	5.7
Diagnostic coronary angiography	7
Cardiac blood pool imaging, gated equilibrium (MUGA); planar single study at rest or at stress	7.8
Myocardial perfusion imaging study with ejection fraction (stress/rest protocol)	7–10
Myocardial perfusion imaging study with ejection fraction (rest/stress protocol)	8–12
Percutaneous coronary intervention	15
Cardiac CT (with contrast, for assessment of coronary arteries, without assessment for coronary calcium)	16

MUGA, multigated acquisition scan; US, ultrasound.

Adapted from Mettler FA Jr, Huda W, Yoshizumi TT, Hahesh H. Effective doses in radiology and diagnostic nuclear medicine: a catalog. *Radiology.* 2008;248:254–63; Gerber TC, Carr JJ, Arai AE, et al. Ionizing radiation in cardiac imaging: a science advisory from the American Heart Association Committee on Cardiac Imaging of the Council on Clinical Cardiology and Committee on Cardiovascular Imaging and Intervention of the Council on Cardiovascular Radiology and Intervention. *Circulation.* 2009;119:1056–65.

3. Henzlova MJ, Cerqueira MD, Hansen CL, et al. ASNC imaging guidelines for nuclear cardiology procedures: stress protocols and tracers. *J Nucl Cardiol.* 2009. Accessed 6/10/22. https://www.asnc.org/files/Stress%20Protocols%20and%20Tracers%202009.pdf
4. Schiepers C. *Diagnostic Nuclear Medicine.* 2nd ed. Springer; 2005.
5. Bax JJ, Visser FC, Blanksma PK, et al. Comparison of myocardial uptake of fluorine-18-fluorodeoxyglucose imaged with PET and SPECT in dyssynergic myocardium. *J Nucl Med* 1996;37:1631-6.
6. Martin WH, Delbeke D, Patton JA, et al. FDG-SPECT: correlation with FDG-PET. *J Nucl Med.* 1995;36:988-95.
7. Berman DS, Hachamovitch R, Kiat H, et al. Incremental value of prognostic testing in patients with known or suspected ischemic heart disease: a basis for optimal utilization of exercise technetium-99m sestamibi myocardial perfusion single-photon emission computed tomography. *J Am Coll Cardiol.* 1995;26:639-47.

8. Hachamovitch R, Berman DS, Kiat H, et al. Exercise myocardial perfusion SPECT in patients without known coronary artery disease: incremental prognostic value and use in risk stratification. *Circulation.* 1996;93:905-14.

9. Vanzetto G, Ormezzano O, Fagret D, et al. Long-term additive prognostic value of thallium-201 myocardial perfusion imaging over clinical and exercise stress test in low to intermediate risk patients: study in 1137 patients with 6-year follow-up. *Circulation.* 1999;100:1521-7.

10. Bourque JM, Beller GA. Stress myocardial perfusion imaging for assessing prognosis: an update. *JACC Cardiovasc Imaging.* 2011;4:1315-9.

11. Metz LD, Beattie M, Hom R, et al. The prognostic value of normal exercise myocardial perfusion imaging and exercise echocardiography: a meta-analysis. *J Am Coll Cardiol.* 2007;49:227-37.

12. Mettler FA Jr, Huda W, Yoshizumi TT, Hahesh H. Effective doses in radiology and diagnostic nuclear medicine: a catalog. *Radiology.* 2008;248:254-63.

13. Gerber TC, Carr JJ, Arai AE, et al. Ionizing radiation in cardiac imaging: a science advisory from the American Heart Association Committee on Cardiac Imaging of the Council on Clinical Cardiology and Committee on Cardiovascular Imaging and Intervention of the Council on Cardiovascular Radiology and Intervention. *Circulation.* 2009;119:1056-65.

Cardiovascular Positron Emission Tomography

38

Adefolakemi Babatunde, Jiafu Ou, Robert J. Gropler, and Thomas H. Schindler

GENERAL PRINCIPLES

Definitions

While single-photon emission computed tomography (SPECT) has been the dominant nuclear modality in clinical practice, positron emission tomography (PET) has transitioned from a valuable research technique to an important clinical modality.[1]

Physics

- Positron emission is a type of β-decay of an unstable radionuclide.
- In this unstable radionuclide, a proton undergoes spontaneous decay into a neutron, a neutrino, and a β⁺-particle (positron).
- After a high-energy positron is emitted from a nucleus, it travels a few millimeters in the tissue losing kinetic energy until it ultimately collides with an electron (a negatively charged β-particle).
- This collision results in complete annihilation of both the positron and the electron, with conversion to energy in the form of electromagnetic radiation composed of two high-energy γ-rays, each with an energy of 511 keV.
- The discharged γ-rays travel in opposite directions (180 degrees from each other).
- These γ-rays can be simultaneously detected by a PET scanner, which is referred to as coincidence detection.
- The PET scanner consists of multiple stationary detectors that encircle the thorax and can be programmed to register only events with temporal coincidence of photons that strike at directly opposing detectors using electronic collimation (Figure 38-1).[1]
- By determining where these γ-rays originated, the PET scanner can create an image showing where in the body the annihilation occurred.
- Coincidence detection offers greater sensitivity and spatial resolution compared with SPECT scans.
- Three Food and Drug Administration (FDA)-approved PET tracers are available for cardiovascular (CV) applications: **rubidium-82 (^{82}Rb) and ^{13}N-ammonia for perfusion and fluorine-18 radiolabeled fluorodeoxyglucose (^{18}F-FDG) for metabolism**.
- ^{82}Rb
  - Rubidium is a potassium analog with kinetics similar to thallium-201; thus, uptake correlates with blood flow.
  - It has a high myocardial extraction fraction over a wide range of coronary blood flow.
  - With a short half-life of 75 seconds, any trapped ^{82}Rb quickly disappears from the myocardium by physical decay.
  - ^{82}Rb is produced from strontium-82 via a commercially available generator that can be purchased and kept on-site.
  - The generator costs ~$30,000 per unit and due to the half-life of the strontium-82 requires 13 units per year.

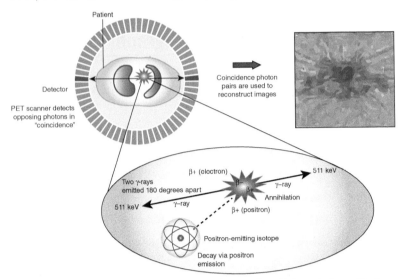

FIGURE 38-1. Schematic of positron and electron β-particle emission, with detection by a coincidence camera, as the basis of positron emission tomography (PET) imaging. (Reprinted from Udelson JE, Dilsizian V, Bonow RO. Nuclear cardiology. In: Libby P, Bonow RO, Mann DL, et al, eds. *Braunwald's Heart Disease: A Textbook of Cardiovascular Medicine.* 8th ed. Elsevier; 2008:345-91. Copyright © 2008 Elsevier. With permission.)

- ^{13}N-ammonia
  - Nitrogen-13 is cyclotron produced and used to radiolabel ammonia to yield ^{13}N-ammonia.
  - ^{13}N-ammonia is a partially extractable perfusion tracer whose uptake is proportion to myocardial perfusion.
  - It has a 9.9-minute half-life and favorable myocardial kinetics.
  - Its image quality is generally superior to that obtained with the shorter half-life of ^{82}Rb.
  - The main limitation with ^{13}N-ammonia is the requirement of an on-site cyclotron.
- ^{18}F-FDG
  - ^{18}F is cyclotron produced and used to radiolabel fluorodeoxyglucose to yield ^{18}F-FDG.
  - ^{18}F has a half-life of about 110 minutes.
  - Following injection of 5 to 10 mCi, ^{18}F-FDG rapidly exchanges across the capillary and cellular membranes.
  - It is then phosphorylated by hexokinase to FDG-6-phosphate and is not metabolized further or used in glycogen synthesis.
  - Because the dephosphorylation rate of ^{18}F-FDG is slow, it becomes trapped in the myocardium, permitting PET or SPECT imaging of regional glucose metabolism.

Interpretation and Image Analysis

- Similar to SPECT, emission data are displayed as tomograms in the horizontal and vertical long- and short-axis views.

- If the data are acquired in dynamic mode, with appropriate mathematical modeling, myocardial perfusion and metabolic data can be displayed in absolute terms:
  - Milliliters per gram per minute (mL/g/minute) for blood flow
  - Moles per gram per minute for metabolism

APPLICATIONS

Clinically available cardiac PET radiotracers fall within two broad categories: myocardial perfusion imaging (MPI) and myocardial metabolism.

Myocardial Perfusion Imaging

- MPI requires radiotracer injection both at rest and after stress. Images are obtained after each injection.
- Stress is usually pharmacologically induced vasodilatation with adenosine, dipyridamole, or regadenoson.
- Exercise stress test is typically not performed due to the short half-life of ^{82}Rb of 75 seconds.
  - Conceptually, exercise stress test can be performed with ^{13}N-ammonia due to a relatively long half-life of 9.9 minutes.
  - Such exercise stress test with IV injection of ^{13}N-ammonia outside the PET scanner would not allow quantification of myocardial blood flow (MBF) in mL/g/minute as the dynamic image acquisition would miss the arterial input function and early radiotracer uptake on initial dynamic frames.
- Clinical uses:
  - Detects myocardial ischemia and infarction
  - Assesses left ventricular (LV) systolic function
  - Relative regional differences of radiotracer uptake can be detected and quantified by PET to identify the regions of ischemia or infarction (similar to SPECT).
  - Detection and evaluation of extensive multivessel coronary artery disease (CAD) with balanced ischemia on qualitative images
  - Absolute regional MBF at rest and during stress (in mL/g/minute) can be obtained and myocardial flow reserve (MFR = MBF peak stress/MBF rest) can be calculated.
    - Reduced MFR in all three major coronary artery territories of the left anterior descending (LAD), left circumflex artery (LCx), and right coronary artery (RCA) in conjunction with drop in left ventricular ejection fraction (LVEF) from rest to stress likely signifies diffuse ischemia due to significant left main and/or advanced three-vessel CAD disease that otherwise could be missed by conventional perfusion imaging.
    - Regional hyperemic MBF and MFR may afford the evaluation of the significance of a given lesion in multivessel disease.
    - Normal LV perfusion images, diffuse reductions in hyperemic MBFs and MFR, and normal wall motion at peak stress and at rest signify coronary microvascular dysfunction that may account for chest pain syndromes in patients without obstructive CAD.
  - Monitoring of therapeutic strategies
  - Diagnostic test of choice in patients who may be prone to artifacts that could lead to an indeterminate SPECT test, such as severely obese patients.
- Advantages[2-4]
  - Better sensitivity and specificity compared with SPECT[5-7]
  - Provides ischemic burden data and higher diagnostic accuracy
  - Increased procedure efficiencies and patient throughput as stress and rest perfusion protocols completed in less time than with SPECT
  - Lower radiation exposure compared with SPECT

- Limitations
  - The expense of both scanners and the radiopharmaceuticals. Some studies, however, suggest that it can be cost-saving in specific patient populations.[8,9]
  - Inability to routinely perform treadmill stress test

Myocardial Viability

- ^{18}F-FDG is most commonly used for assessing myocardial viability.
- Ischemic myocardium that is viable remains metabolically active (utilizes glucose).
- Assessed either by administering ^{18}F-FDG with ^{13}N-ammonia or [82]Rb or by utilizing a SPECT MPI study.

Myocardial Metabolism

- Myocardium requires a continuous supply of oxygen and metabolic substrates to meet its energy demands.
  - Fatty acids are the preferred energy source for overall oxidative metabolism under normal conditions.
  - Fatty acids cannot be oxidized in ischemic myocardium, and glucose becomes the preferred energy source.[10]
  - This metabolic phenomenon is useful for the identification of myocardium that is under perfused but still viable.
    - Such tissue is often hypokinetic or akinetic but will exhibit improved function if blood flow is restored.
    - MPI with either PET or SPECT should accompany ^{18}F-FDG cardiac PET imaging so that the areas of hypoperfusion are identified.
  - Stress MPI may be performed to identify the presence and amount of reversible perfusion defects unless there is a contraindication for stress testing.
  - **[18]F-FDG PET imaging should be performed following a 6- to 12-hour fast followed by a glucose load** and supplemental insulin administered PRN **to favor metabolism of glucose over fatty acids by the heart**.
  - ^{18}F-FDG images are typically compared with resting MPI.
- Clinical implications
  - Cardiac ^{18}F-FDG PET imaging has been considered the gold standard for the assessment of myocardial viability.[10-15]
  - Useful in patients with LV dysfunction due to CAD who are eligible for coronary revascularization and have resting myocardial perfusion defects in order to differentiate viable (i.e., hibernation or stunning) from nonviable myocardium (i.e., scar).
  - Four major patterns of perfusion metabolism comparisons can be seen and quantified (Figure 38-2)[14]:
    - "Match" findings between perfusion and FDG uptake:
      - Myocardial perfusion defect and no FDG uptake: transmural infarction
      - Similar degree of reduced myocardial perfusion and reduced FDG uptake: nontransmural infarction
    - "Mismatch" findings between perfusion and FDG uptake:
      - Reduced myocardial perfusion with diminished but still maintained FDG uptake, $\geq 50\%$: corresponding to nontransmural necrosis with viable but ischemic/compromised myocardium
      - Reduced myocardial perfusion and near-normal FDG uptake: corresponding near-complete viable and ischemic/compromised myocardium
- Potential for improved heart failure symptoms following revascularization correlates with the magnitude of the PET mismatch pattern.
- The presence of ischemic viable myocardium is a marker of an increased CV risk.
- Patients with preserved myocardial viability who undergo revascularization have reduction in the risk of cardiac death.[10-12]

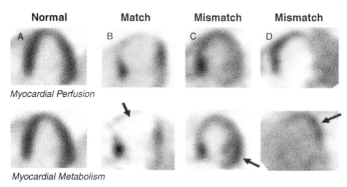

| Normal | Match | Mismatch | Mismatch |

Myocardial Perfusion

Myocardial Metabolism

FIGURE 38-2. Patterns of myocardial perfusion (upper panel) and metabolism (with ^{18}F-FDG lower panel). (Republished with permission of McGraw Hill LLC from Schelbert HR. PET for the noninvasive study and quantitation of myocardial blood flow and metabolism. In: Fuster V, O'Rourke R, Walsh R, et al, eds. *Hurst's the Heart.* 12th ed. McGraw Hill; 2007; permission conveyed through Copyright Clearance Center, Inc.)

- Revascularization conferred no natural history advantage in patients without substantial myocardial viability.
- Advantages
  - Detection scheme yields higher image quality in obese patients.
  - More accurate than thallium-201 SPECT and more sensitive than dobutamine echocardiography
  - Can use when contraindications to cardiac MRI
  - Most experience in patients with severe ischemic cardiomyopathy
- Disadvantages
  - Glucose preloading with adequate insulin availability is required for successful results.
  - Relatively expensive

Cardiac Sarcoidosis[16-18]

- Sarcoidosis is the accumulation of noncaseating granulomas in various organs.
- Cardiac involvement is only diagnosed in 5% of patients; however, it is thought to be underdiagnosed due to the difficulty in diagnosis. Autopsies estimate that as many as 20-25% of patients with systemic sarcoidosis have cardiac involvement.
- Cardiac manifestations include conduction abnormalities, arrhythmias, LV dysfunction, and sudden death.
- Diagnosis is based on the 2006 Japanese Ministry of Health and Welfare Diagnostic Guidelines for Cardiac Sarcoidosis (Table 38-1).
- Perfusion and FDG-PET are performed for detection and characterization of cardiac sarcoidosis.
  - Patient preparation: high-fat/no-carbohydrate diet for 2 to 3 meals followed by a prolonged fast of at least 12 hours, plus unfractionated heparin intravenously (10 to 50 IU/kg) 15 minutes before ^{18}F-FDG injection. Scan obtained 60 to 90 minutes after ^{18}F-FDG injection
  - Unfractionated heparin activates lipoprotein and hepatic lipase, which increase plasma free fatty acid levels and reduce glucose consumption by normal myocytes. Patients should be evaluated for heparin-induced thrombocytopenia (HIT) and bleeding risk before administration.

TABLE 38-1	DIAGNOSIS OF CARDIAC SARCOIDOSIS
Histologic diagnosis	Cardiac sarcoidosis is confirmed when endomyocardial biopsy specimens demonstrate noncaseating epithelioid cell granulomas with histologic or clinical diagnosis of extracardiac sarcoidosis.
Clinical diagnosis	**Major criteria** • Advanced AV block • Basal thinning of the interventricular septum • Positive ^{67}Ga uptake in the heart • Depressed ejection fraction of the left ventricle (<50%) **Minor criteria** • Abnormal ECG: ventricular arrhythmias, complete RBBB, abnormal axis, abnormal Q wave • Abnormal echocardiogram: regional wall motion or morphologic abnormality • Nuclear medicine: perfusion defect by ^{201}Tl or ^{99m}Tc myocardial scintigraphy • Gadolinium-enhanced CMR: delayed enhancement of the mid-myocardium or subepicardium • Endomyocardial biopsy: interstitial fibrosis or monocyte infiltration over moderate grade

Diagnosis of cardiac sarcoidosis is made when ≥2 of 4 major criteria or 1 major and ≥5 minor criteria are present.

AV, atrioventricular; CMR, cardiac magnetic resonance; ^{67}Ga, Gallium-67; RBBB, right bundle branch block; ^{99m}Tc, technetium-99m; ^{201}Tl, thallium-201.

Adapted with permission of Nancy International Ltd Subsidiary AME Publishing Company from Hulten E, Aslam S, Osborne M, et al. Cardiac sarcoidosis—state of the art review. *Cardiovasc Diagn Ther.* 2016;6(1):50-63; permission conveyed through Copyright Clearance Center, Inc.

- ○ Rest perfusion study should be obtained before ^{18}F-FDG PET/CT. Perfusion study will allow for comparison to ^{18}F-FDG PET/CT for evaluation of scar, normal myocardium, or active sarcoid.
- ○ There should be no myocardial FDG uptake in the normal setting, given an optimal suppression of physiologic glucose uptake of the myocardium (fatty-rich and no-carbohydrate meals the day before), fasting state of at least 12 hours, and adjunct subcutaneous heparin application before the PET scan.
- ○ In the setting of immune cell-mediated inflammation and macrophage infiltration, FDG may be taken up avidly by the macrophages, signifying myocardial inflammation.
- Myocardial perfusion may signify nonischemic perfusion deficits predominantly in the basal segments or with patchy pattern to signify fibrosis and/or scar tissue.
- A so-called "mismatch" between reduced perfusion and FDG uptake at the same and typical location (basal segments) enhances the diagnosis for active inflammatory cardiac sarcoidosis.
- Clinical indications for cardiac sarcoidosis detection with PET
  - ○ Patients <55 years of age presenting with second- or third-degree atrioventricular block of unknown etiology
  - ○ Unexplained monomorphic ventricular tachycardia
  - ○ Patients with extracardiac sarcoidosis *and* abnormal ECG, Holter, or echocardiogram in whom cardiac sarcoidosis is suspected
  - ○ Patients with established cardiac sarcoidosis for evaluation of treatment response
- Limitations include difficulties in optimal suppression of myocardial glucose suppression.
- Advantages
  - ○ Highest sensitivity for detection of cardiac sarcoidosis

- Application also in patients having contraindication to cardiac magnetic resonance (CMR) such as implantable devices or renal dysfunction
- Assessment of extracardiac sarcoid activity by adding thoracic or whole-body FDG-PET
- Best imaging method for assessing treatment response in sarcoidosis

Infective Endocarditis

- Infective endocarditis is usually diagnosed using the Modified Duke Criteria. The imaging modality of choice in the Duke criteria is echocardiogram. Transesophageal echocardiogram has higher sensitivity and specificity for endocarditis than transthoracic, especially in the case of prosthetic valve endocarditis.[19,20]
  - Despite echocardiography and blood cultures, there are 20% of prosthetic valve endocarditis cases that remain inconclusive.
  - FDG-PET/CT can aid as an "additional" tool in the workup of patients with prosthetic valve endocarditis.
- Allows for imaging of the entire body, which provides the opportunity to evaluate infective emboli
- Aids in determining the extent of infection in prosthetic valves including perivalvular involvement, suggesting the need for surgical intervention

Identification of Other Vascular Infections

- Cardiac implantable electronic device (CIED)
  - As the indications for CIEDs increase, there has been a corresponding increase in their use.
  - Infection is not an uncommon adverse event. Most infections are seen in the first year after implantation.
  - As the clinical signs and symptoms for CIED infections can be nonspecific, there is a need to differentiate between pocket infections (superficial) and deep infections (involving the device).
  - FDG-PET/CT can help identify the site of infection, which can direct management. This can include antibiotic use alone or removal of the device in addition to antibiotics.
- Left ventricular assist device (LVAD)[21]
  - LVADs are used for patients with advanced heart failure.
  - Complications with LVADs include bleeding, thrombosis, and infection. It is estimated that as many as 20-40% of patients with an LVAD will develop sepsis 1 to 2 years after implantation. The clinical determination of the extent of LVAD infection can be difficult. Management and prognosis differ between superficial and deep infections.
  - FDG-PET/CT can be applied in the early detection of LVAD infections and to localize the site of infection.
- Prosthetic vascular graft infection
  - The incidence of graft infection is reported to be relatively low at 1-5%, but the associated morbidity with limb loss or mortality has been estimated to be quite high.
  - FDG-PET/CT can help distinguish soft-tissue infection from graft infection, which will help determine whether the graft needs to be removed or if the patient can be treated with antibiotics alone.
  - Limitations
    - False positive. Postsurgical inflammation within <3 months after surgery
    - Low-grade infection or prior antibiotic use may reduce sensitivity of study.
    - Can be difficult to determine whether there has been eradication of infection or suppression by antibiotics. There can still be residual FDG-PET activity from inflammation after completion of treatment and no active infection.

Vasculitis

- Vasculitis is defined as inflammation within the blood vessel walls.
- Inflammation of the aorta (aortitis) and its major branches can occur in various conditions, including Takayasu arteritis and giant cell arteritis.

- Takayasu arteritis is more common in women compared to men, and onset is usually in patients aged <50 years. It can affect the carotids and subclavian arteries.
- Giant cell arteritis is more common in older persons. It may affect the aorta, with a predilection for the carotids and vertebral arteries.

REFERENCES

1. Udelson JE, Dilsizian V, Bonow RO. Nuclear cardiology. In: Libby P, Bonow RO, Mann DL, Zipes DP, eds. *Braunwald's Heart Disease: A Textbook of Cardiovascular Medicine.* 8th ed. Elsevier; 2008:345-91.
2. Heller GV, Calnon D, Dorbala S. Recent advances in cardiac PET and PET/CT myocardial perfusion imaging. *J Nucl Cardiol.* 2009;16:962-9.
3. Schindler TH, Schelbert HR, Quercioli A, et al. Cardiac PET imaging for the detection and monitoring of coronary artery disease and microvascular health. *J Am Coll Cardiol.* 2010;3:623-40.
4. Bengel FM, Higuchi T, Javadi MS, Lautamäki R. Cardiac positron emission tomography. *J Am Coll Cardiol.* 2009;54:1-15.
5. Nandalur KR, Dwamena BA, Choudhri AF, et al. Diagnostic performance of positron emission tomography in the detection of coronary artery disease: a meta-analysis. *Acad Radiol.* 2008;15:444-51.
6. Di Carli MF, Hachamovitch R. New technology for noninvasive evaluation of coronary artery disease. *Circulation.* 2007;115:1464-80.
7. Schindler TH. Myocardial blood flow: putting it into clinical perspective. *J Nucl Cardiol.* 2016;23:1056-71.
8. Merhige ME, Breen WJ, Shelton V, et al. Impact of myocardial perfusion imaging with PET and (82) Rb on downstream invasive procedure utilization, costs, and outcomes in coronary disease management. *J Nucl Med.* 2007;48:1069-76.
9. Patterson RE, Eisner RL, Horowitz SF. Comparison of cost-effectiveness and utility of exercise ECG, single photon emission computed tomography, positron emission tomography, and coronary angiography for diagnosis of coronary artery disease. *Circulation.* 1995;91:54-65.
10. Peterson LR, Gropler RJ. Radionuclide imaging of myocardial metabolism. *Circ Cardiovasc Imaging.* 2010;3:211-22.
11. Schinkel AF, Bax JJ, Poldermans D, et al. Hibernating myocardium: diagnosis and patient outcomes. *Curr Probl Cardiol.* 2007;32:375-410.
12. Allman K, Shaw L, Hachamovitch R, Udelson JE. Myocardial viability testing and impact of revascularization on prognosis in patients with coronary artery disease and left ventricular dysfunction: a meta-analysis. *J Am Coll Cardiol.* 2002;39:1151-8.
13. Boehm J, Haas F, Bauernschmitt R, et al. Impact of preoperative positron emission tomography in patients with severely impaired LV-function undergoing surgical revascularization. *Int J Cardiovasc Imaging.* 2010;26:423-32.
14. Dilsizian V, Bacharach SL, Beanlands RS, et al. PET myocardial perfusion and metabolism clinical imaging. *J Nucl Cardiol.* 2009;16:651-80.
15. Schelbert HR. Positron emission tomography for the noninvasive study and quantitation of myocardial blood flow and metabolism in cardiovascular disease. In: Fuster V, O'Rourke R, Walsh R, Poole-Wilson R, eds. *Hurst's The Heart.* 12th ed. McGraw Hill; 2007.
16. Hulten E, Aslam S, Osborne M, et al. Cardiac sarcoidosis—state of the art review. *Cardiovasc Diagn Ther.* 2016;6(1):50-63.
17. Chareonthaitawee P, Beanlands RS, Chen W, et al. Joint SNMMI-ASNC expert consensus document on the role of 18F-FDG PET/CT in cardiac sarcoid detection and therapy monitoring. *J Nucl Med.* 2017;58:1341-53.
18. McArdle BA, Leung E, Ohira H, et al. The role of F(18)-fluorodeoxyglucose positron emission tomography in guiding diagnosis and management in patients with known or suspected cardiac sarcoidosis. *J Nucl Cardiol.* 2013;20:297-306.
19. Lawal I, Sathekge M. F-18 FDG PET/CT imaging of cardiac and vascular inflammation and infection. *Br Med Bull.* 2016;120:55-74.
20. Swart L, Scholtens AM, Tanis W, et al. ^{18}F-fluorodeoxyglucose positron emission/computed tomography and computed tomography angiography in prosthetic heart valve endocarditis: from guidelines to clinical practice. *Eur Heart J.* 2018;39:3739-49.
21. Kim J, Feller E, Chen W, et al. FDG PET/CT for early detection and localization of left ventricular assist device infection. *JACC Cardiovasc Imaging.* 2019;12(4):722-9.

Coronary Angiography and Intravascular Imaging

39

Manuel Rivera Maza, Prashanth D. Thakker, and John Lasala

Coronary Angiography

GENERAL PRINCIPLES

- Coronary angiography permits the direct visualization of the coronary vasculature and enables the diagnosis and treatment of coronary artery disease (CAD).
- Cardiac catheterization uses fluoroscopy to obtain real-time images.
  - Plain radiography signals are emitted by the plain radiography tube located under the patient's table.
  - The signals are captured by an image intensifier (II), located directly above the patient, and are subsequently processed to obtain a live image.
  - Both the plain radiography source and the II move in opposite directions: cranial-caudal and right anterior oblique (RAO)–left anterior oblique (LAO) to obtain the necessary images.
- Coronary angiography provides a two-dimensional representation of the three-dimensional coronary vessel lumen.
  - Image accuracy is dependent on vessel orientation with respect to the image plane since, if foreshortening occurs, the degree of vessel stenosis can be underestimated.
  - This limitation is addressed by interrogating the coronary tree in multiple angiographic projections. Further discussion on angiographic projections is highlighted later in this chapter.

Indications

- The decision to perform coronary angiography should balance the risk of the procedure with the anticipated benefit from angiography and possible intervention.
- Appropriate use of diagnostic catheterization is outlined in the multisociety appropriate use criteria document. The reader should be familiar with appropriate indications for diagnostic coronary angiography.[1]
- A list of indications for coronary angiography include:
  - Acute coronary syndromes
  - Suspected CAD if high pretest probability and no prior noninvasive stress imaging
  - Suspected CAD if high-risk findings on prior stress test with imaging
  - Known CAD on medical therapy and with worsening symptoms and intermediate- or high-risk noninvasive findings
  - Newly recognized left ventricular (LV) systolic dysfunction or new wall motion abnormality found on echocardiogram
  - Suspected significant ischemic complication related to CAD (e.g., ischemic mitral regurgitation or ventricular septal defect)
  - Resuscitated cardiac arrest with return of spontaneous circulation, unclear etiology after initial evaluation
  - Ventricular fibrillation (VF) or sustained ventricular tachycardia (VT) with or without symptoms, unclear etiology after initial evaluation
  - Preoperative assessment before valvular surgery (especially with risk factors for CAD)

Patient Evaluation and Preparation

- In nonemergent cases, patients should be NPO for >6 hours. Patients who are intubated should have their feedings stopped for this same period.
- A history focused on the reason for the study, medication, allergies, known history of peripheral vascular disease/interventions, and anticoagulation therapy should be reviewed.
- Prior cardiac imaging studies (transthoracic echocardiogram, transesophageal echocardiogram, CT scans, stress tests, and prior cardiac catheterization films) should be comprehensively reviewed.
- History of cardiovascular surgeries should be reviewed.
- Laboratory work including complete blood count (CBC), basic metabolic panel (BMP), and international normalized ratio (INR) should be obtained before procedure.
- Patients should be screened for absolute and relative contraindications for cardiac catheterization.
  - **Relative contraindications to diagnostic cardiac catheterization**:
    - Acute major bleeding/severe anemia hemoglobin (Hgb) <7.0 g/dL
    - Coagulopathy, thrombocytopenia
    - Electrolyte imbalance
    - Infection and fever
    - Pregnancy
    - Decompensated heart failure
    - Recent stroke
    - Acute kidney failure
  - Absolute contraindication: patient refusal
- Physical examination and history should also evaluate the current hemodynamic status of the patient. Carotid and peripheral pulses should be examined.
  - Radial and ulnar pulses should be checked.
  - Despite historical data, Allen and Barbeau tests are not a useful triage strategy for transradial access.[2]
- 12-lead ECG should be obtained and reviewed.
- The patients American Society of Anesthesiologist (ASA) physical status classification should be identified to determine eligibility for conscious sedation.
- **A description of the procedure and the following procedure-related risks should be explained to the patient before consenting for diagnostic catheterization**[3]:
  - Risk of death ~0.1%
  - Risk of myocardial infarction ~0.05%
  - Risk of stroke ~0.17%
  - Risk of serious ventricular arrhythmia ~0.5%
  - Bleeding events within 72 hours of the procedure ~0.5%
  - New requirement for dialysis ~0.14%. Well-validated risk prediction models are available and should be used before cardiac catheterization.[4]

PROCEDURE

- At least one functional IV (20 gauge or higher) should be present.
- Conscious sedation is favored. First-line agents for this include fentanyl (25 μg) and midazolam (0.5 to 1 mg) pushes.
  - Careful attention must be paid to the patient's mental status and should be reassessed periodically.
  - The patient should be able to respond appropriately to verbal instructions.
- Vital signs (oxygenation, capnography, blood pressure, heart rate) should be closely monitored.

Vascular access

- There has been much debate comparing radial access to femoral access. Advantages and limitations of both approaches are listed in Table 39-1.[5,6]
- Given the constraints each approach poses, operators should be familiar and trained in both transradial and transfemoral procedures.

Radial access

- Following administration of local anesthesia, arterial access is obtained by using the modified Seldinger technique. Ultrasound guidance is recommended as it reduces complications, number of attempts, and risk of spasm.
- Prevention of radial artery spasm[7]:
  - Following radial sheath insertion and before advancing catheter, administer nitroglycerin 100 to 200 µg and verapamil 2.5 to 5 mg (or nicardipine) through sheath.
  - Dose can be repeated if radial spasm develops during procedure.
- Intra-arterial or IV heparin at 50 U/kg should always be administered to prevent radial artery occlusion.

Femoral access

- Access should be obtained at the common femoral artery—defined as the segment proximal to the femoral bifurcation and distal to the superficial epigastric artery—over the midportion of the femoral head.
- Following administration of local anesthesia, arterial access is obtained by using the modified Seldinger technique.
  - Ultrasound guidance reduces complications.[8]
  - Use of micropuncture technique reduces vascular complications as it allows for direct contrast injection through a 4F micropuncture catheter to ensure appropriate landing zone.[9]

TABLE 39-1	COMPARISON OF FEMORAL AND RADIAL ACCESS	
Feature	**Femoral**	**Radial**
Access site bleeding Arterial complications	3–4% pseudoaneurysm, retroperitoneal bleed, AV fistula, painful hematoma	Rare local irritation, pulse loss 3–9%
Ambulation	2–4 hours	Immediate
Extra costs	Closure device	Band
Procedure time	Perceived shorter	Perceived longer
Fluoroscopy time	Perceived shorter	Perceived longer
Access to LIMA	Easy	Hard from RRA
Learning curve	Short	Longer
Bigger guide catheters	No problem	Maximum 7F in men Up to 6F in women
PVD, obese	Problematic	Not a limitation

AV, arteriovenous; LIMA, left internal mammary artery; PVD, peripheral vascular disease; RRA, right radial artery.

Adapted from Kern MJ, Sorajja P, Lim MJ. *The Interventional Cardiac Catheterization Handbook.* 4th ed. Elsevier; 2018.

Diagnostic Catheter Selection

- Diagnostic catheters can be divided into universal catheters (same catheter used to engage right and left coronary arteries) and dedicated left and right coronary catheters.
- The most commonly used catheters include (Figure 39-1):
  - Dedicated catheters:
    - Judkins left (JL) and Judkins right (JR)
    - Amplatz left (AL) and Amplatz right (AR) or AR modified
    - Internal mammary artery catheter
  - Universal catheters:
    - Jacky catheter (radial)
    - Tiger catheter (radial)
    - Multipurpose catheter
- Preformed JLs have a 90-degree primary curvature and a 180-degree secondary curvature. JRs have a 90-degree primary curvature and a 30-degree secondary curvature.
  - The distance between the primary and secondary curvature is variable (JL4—4 cm, JL5—5 cm, JR4—4 cm, etc.).
  - It is adapted based on approach (radial or femoral), patient height, and aortic root diameter.
- Amplatz catheters are an alternative to Judkins catheters. Catheter size indicates the diameter of the tip of the catheter curve. Available sizes are the same as for Judkins catheters.
- Catheter selection for femoral approach:
  - For the left coronary, the JL4, AL1, or AL2 fit most normal-sized adults.
  - For the right coronary, the JR4, AL0.75, and AR1 (modified) are adequate for most adults.
- Catheter selection for radial approach:
  - Typically, universal radial catheters are selected (Jacky, Sarah, Tiger).
  - If using Judkins catheters from the right radial approach:

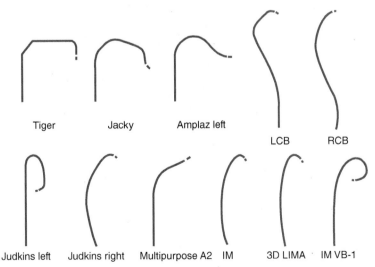

Tiger   Jacky   Amplaz left

LCB   RCB

Judkins left   Judkins right   Multipurpose A2   IM   3D LIMA   IM VB-1

FIGURE 39-1. Coronary angiography catheter shapes.

- For JL catheters, 0.5 cm smaller curve than that used for femoral approach should be chosen.
- For JR catheters, 1 cm larger curve than that used for femoral approach should be chosen.
  ○ In contrast, when selecting left radial approach, same standard femoral catheter sizes can be used.

BASIC ANGIOGRAPHIC PROJECTIONS

- Angulations (cranial, caudal, RAO, LAO, anteroposterior [AP]) indicate the position of the II relative to the patient.
- The standard views for the left coronary system include the "four corners"[7]:
  ○ RAO 15 to 30 degrees, cranial 10- to 30 degrees view (Figure 39-2)
  ○ LAO 20 to 45 degrees, cranial 30 to 60 degrees view (Figure 39-3)
  ○ LAO 20 to 45 degrees, caudal 20 to 45 degrees view, the "spider" view (Figure 39-4)
  ○ RAO 15 to 30 degrees, caudal 10 to 30 degrees view (Figure 39-5)
- Examples of views for the right coronary artery are given in Figures 39-6 and 39-7.
- In general, cranial views are used to address overlapping coronary segments that are obscured in regular views. Cranial views typically are best for the left anterior descending (LAD) and diagonal branches. Caudal views are best for the circumflex and left main.
- Suggested views for coronary angiography are described in Table 39-2[10] and shown in Figures 39-1 through 39-6.

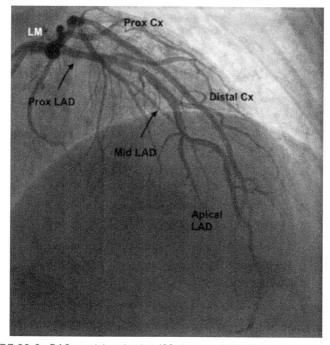

FIGURE 39-2. RAO cranial projection (29 degrees RAO, 25 degrees cranial). LAD, left anterior descending; RAO, right anterior oblique. (Photo courtesy of Sudhir Jain, MD, Washington University School of Medicine, St. Louis, MO.)

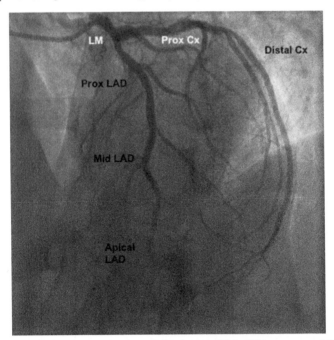

FIGURE 39-3. LAO cranial projection (20 degrees LAO, 35 degrees cranial). LAD, left anterior descending; LAO, left anterior oblique. (Photo courtesy of Sudhir Jain, MD, Washington University School of Medicine, St. Louis, MO.)

Diagnostic Criteria

- Angiographic classification of lesion severity. Stenosis severity is visually estimated ($\pm 20\%$ interobserver variability) and reported as percent narrowing of the most stenotic segment compared to a normal vessel segment.
  - Mild CAD <50% stenosis
  - Moderate CAD 50-75% stenosis
  - Severe CAD >75% stenosis
  - Total occlusion (100% stenosis)
- Angiographically determined stenosis severity should not be assumed to result in abnormal physiology and ischemia.
- Significant coronary artery stenosis is defined as:
  - 70% luminal diameter narrowing by visual assessment of epicardial stenosis in angiogram
  - 50% luminal diameter narrowing by visual assessment of a left main stenosis in angiogram
  - 40-70% luminal diameter narrowing by visual assessment of epicardial stenosis in angiogram with an abnormal functional assessment study, such as fractional flow reserve (FFR) or instantaneous wave-free ratio (iFR)

Classification of Angiographic Blood Flow

Angiographic blood flow is qualitatively assessed by using the Thrombolysis in Myocardial Infarction (TIMI) flow grading.
- TIMI 3 flow: normal flow, fills the distal coronary bed completely within 3 to 4 beats
- TIMI 2 flow: delayed of sluggish antegrade flow with complete filling to the distal territory after 4 beats

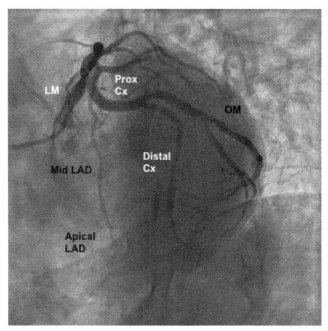

FIGURE 39-4. LAO caudal projection (31 degrees LAO, 20 degrees caudal). LAD, left anterior descending; LAO, left anterior oblique. (Photo courtesy of Sudhir Jain, MD, Washington University School of Medicine, St. Louis, MO.)

- TIMI 1 flow: faint antegrade coronary flow beyond the occlusion, although filling of the distal coronary bed is incomplete
- TIMI 0 flow: absence of any antegrade flow beyond a coronary occlusion

CATHETER AND SHEATH REMOVAL

- Close monitoring of puncture site is advised, regardless of method for hemostasis.
- Look for expanding hematoma, pseudoaneurysm formation, or persistent pain.

Radial Access

- Several compression devices are available to assist in the hemostasis of radial artery after cardiac catheterization. The device is fitted around the wrist, and patent hemostasis of the radial artery is achieved with an air-titratable compression balloon.
- It is imperative to use a protocol for removal of the hemostatic device.
  - Maintenance of patent hemostasis for 1 hour
  - If activated clotting time (ACT) <180 seconds after 1 hour, then start loosening the device by removing 3 to 4 mL of air every 30 minutes until all air is removed.
  - If bleeding occurs, reinject 4 mL of air until achieving hemostasis.

Femoral Access

- If heparin has been given during procedure, arterial sheath is not removed until ACT falls <180 seconds. Firm, three-finger pressure is held over femoral arteriotomy site while achieving patent hemostasis.

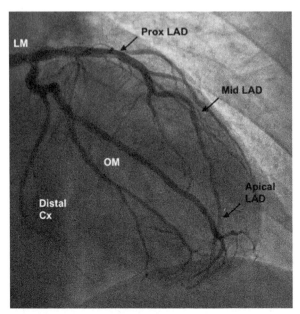

FIGURE 39-5. RAO caudal projection (24 degrees RAO, 15 degrees caudal). LAD, left anterior descending; RAO, right anterior oblique. (Photo courtesy of Sudhir Jain, MD, Washington University School of Medicine, St. Louis, MO.)

- Manual pressure should be held firmly for ~5 minutes per sheath size.[6]
- Multiple arterial closure devices can also be used; these decrease the time to ambulation when compared to manual compression.
  - Femoral mechanical compression devices (Femo-Stop®) are also available.
  - Use of vascular closure devices is cautioned in patients with peripheral vascular disease.
  - Femoral angiogram via micropuncture catheter when getting vascular access is recommended and can determine suitability for closure device.
- When ipsilateral femoral arterial and venous access have been obtained, the arterial sheath should be removed first to reduce the risk of arteriovenous (AV) fistula formation.

COMPLICATIONS

Femoral Access Complications

Pseudoaneurysm
- Results from failure of sealing the initial arterial puncture
- They present in the form of a pulsatile hematoma with or without a bruit.
- Risk factors include:
  - Calcified arteries
  - Hemodialysis
  - Anticoagulation
  - Inadequate compression postprocedure
- If pseudoaneurysm fails to close, active treatment is indicated.
  - Ultrasound-guided compression: External application of pressure using a vascular clamp guided by Doppler ultrasound probe results in obliteration of pseudoaneurysm tract and clotting.

| TABLE 39-2 | SUGGESTED VIEWS FOR CORONARY ANGIOGRAPHY |

Coronary artery	Suggested views
Left main	
Ostial	Shallow RAO; LAO cranial; AP caudal
Body	RAO shallow/caudal/cranial; AP
Distal	LAO caudal/cranial; RAO caudal
Left anterior descending	
Ostial/proximal diagonals	Cranial LAO; RAO shallow/cranial/lateral
Proximal/mid diagonals	LAO cranial; RAO cranial/lateral
Distal/apical	RAO lateral
Left circumflex	
Ostial/proximal	LAO; LAO cranial/caudal
Ostial/ramus	LAO; LAO caudal; RAO caudal
Mid/marginals	RAO shallow/caudal; LAO caudal
Distal (dominant)	LAO shallow/cranial; RAO shallow/caudal
Right coronary	
Ostial/proximal	LAO; LAO cranial; left lateral
Mid	LAO; LAO cranial; RAO shallow; left lateral
Distal/bifurcation of posterior descending	LAO cranial; RAO shallow/lateral; AP caudal
Posterior descending	RAO shallow, LAO cranial; AP caudal
Posterolateral to left ventricle	RAO shallow, LAO cranial; AP caudal

AP, anteroposterior; caudal, toward the feet; cranial, toward the head; LAO, left anterior oblique; lateral, 90° from vertical; RAO, right anterior oblique; shallow, 15° to 30° angulation from vertical with neither caudal or cranial angulation.

Reprinted from Bashore TM, Bates ER, Berger PB, et al. American College of Cardiology/Society for Cardiac Angiography and Interventions Clinical Expert Consensus Document on cardiac catheterization laboratory standards: a report of the American College of Cardiology Task Force on Clinical Expert Consensus Documents. *J Am Coll Cardiol.* 2001;37(8):2170-214. With permission.

○ Thrombin injection: 1000 U of thrombin is diluted in a 1-mL syringe and injected to pseudoaneurysm under ultrasound guidance.
○ Vascular surgery is only required for complex pseudoaneurysms (>3 cm and multi-lobed) that are resistant to thrombin injection.[6]

Arteriovenous fistula
• Palpable thrill or audible continuous bruit
• Most fistulas produce low shunt volumes and are asymptomatic. AV fistulas that exceed 30% of the cardiac output are often symptomatic.
• Conservative management is favored as 90% of AV fistulas will close spontaneously; 10% will ultimately require surgical repair.

Bleeding
• Bleeding is characterized by the Bleeding Academic Research Consortium (BARC) definitions.[11]
• The most common complication of femoral cardiac catheterization is local hematoma formation (BARC type 1).

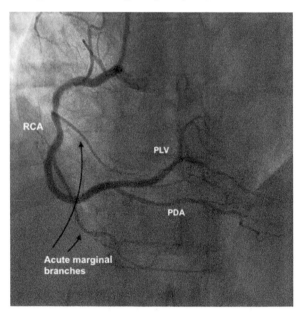

FIGURE 39-6. Straight LAO projection (24 degrees LAO, 10 degrees cranial). LAD, left anterior descending; LAO, left anterior oblique; PDA, posterior descending artery; PLV, posterolateral vessel; RCA, right coronary artery. (Photo courtesy of Sudhir Jain, MD, Washington University School of Medicine, St. Louis, MO.)

- Severe, actionable bleeding includes large femoral hematoma (incidence ~2.5%) and retroperitoneal hematoma (incidence ~0.3%). Signs and symptoms of retroperitoneal hematoma include hypotension, tachycardia, and groin/abdominal/flank pain.
- For the most part, treatment focuses on supportive management with IV fluids and blood products.
- If rapidly expanding hematoma and patient persistently hemodynamically unstable despite fluid resuscitation, early vascular surgery consultation is recommended.

Radial Access Complications

- Radial artery spasm can occur from manipulation with catheters.
  - Spasm tends to improve with intra-arterial vasodilators.
  - Severe spasm can entrap the radial sheath.
    - It is imperative to not to force withdraw catheters or radial sheaths, given risk of radial artery avulsion.
    - Local nerve block or general anesthesia is usually required in these instances.
- Forearm hematoma and compartment syndrome:
  - Results from perforation within the course of the radial artery
  - Should have a high suspicion if increasing pain and hematoma formation during or after the procedure
  - Blood pressure should be controlled, compression is achieved with ACE bandage, and further anticoagulation should be avoided.
  - Pain, paresthesia, and expanding forearm/arm diameters are concerning for compartment syndrome (incidence <0.01%) and warrant evaluation by surgery.

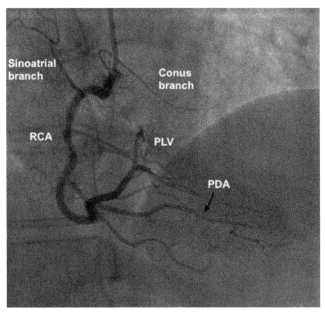

FIGURE 39-7. RAO cranial projection (15 degrees RAO, 20 degrees cranial). LAD, left anterior descending; PDA, posterior descending artery; PLV, posterolateral vessel; RAO, right anterior oblique; RCA, right coronary artery. (Photo courtesy of Sudhir Jain, MD, Washington University School of Medicine, St. Louis, MO.)

- Atheroembolism:
  - Results from plaque dislodgement from scraping of the great vessels by diagnostic or guide catheters
  - This can result in cholesterol embolization syndrome, multiorgan embolization, and stroke.
  - Prevention always includes the following:
    - Advancing catheters over a guidewire along the aorta
    - Blood aspiration from the catheter to clear debris that might have been picked up by the catheter while in transit to the aortic cusps

Anaphylaxis to Radiocontrast Media

- Documentation of prior exposure to IV administered iodinated contrast and type of reaction is important to ascertain validity.
- Shellfish allergy is not cross-reactive with contrast allergy.
- A true contrast allergy is an anaphylactoid reaction characterized by hypotension, hives, and bronchospasm.
- Can minimize risk with use of either low-ionic contrast media and/or premedication before procedure.[12] A typical premedication regimen includes:
  - Prednisone 50 mg PO given 13, 7, and 1 hour before procedure
  - Diphenhydramine 50 mg PO given 1 hour before procedure
  - H_2 blocker may also be given 1 hour before procedure.

Contrast-Induced Nephropathy

- Risk stratification models should be used to identify individuals at high risk for contrast-induced nephropathy (CIN).[4]

- Rise in creatine may continue 72 hours after cardiac catheterization. Appropriate laboratory follow-up should be arranged for those patients at risk.
- Prevention:
  - Prehydration with 1 to 3 mL/kg/h for 2 to 12 hours for a total volume of 3 to 12 mL/kg
  - Posthydration with 1 to 3 mL/kg/h for 2 to 12 hours for a total volume of 3 to 12 mL/kg; although posthydration should ideally be guided by the left ventricular end-diastolic pressure (LVEDP)[13]
  - No proven benefit of IV sodium bicarbonate or oral acetylcysteine over IV isotonic sodium chloride[14]
- Angiotensin converting enzyme inhibitors, angiotensin-receptor blockades (ARBs), NSAIDs, and diuretics should be stopped 24 hours before the procedure and can often be restarted 24 hours after.
- It is important to minimize the dose of contrast media used.
- Contrast media agents have different characteristics (Table 39-3).[15] Iso-osmolar, nonionic agents should be favored in patients considered high risk for CIN.

SPECIAL POPULATIONS

Patients with Diabetes Mellitus

- If contrast-induced renal dysfunction develops, concomitant metformin can result in profound lactic acidosis.
- Metformin should be stopped the morning of the procedure and restarted once the creatinine level is stable, usually 48 hours after cardiac catheterization.

TABLE 39-3	CLASSIFICATION AND PROPERTIES OF CONTRAST AGENTS			
Quality	High osmolar[a]	Low osmolar	Low osmolar	Iso-osmolar
Osmolality	>1500	600	600–1000	280
Ionicity	Ionic	Ionic	Nonionic	Nonionic
Number of benzene rings	Monomer	Dimer	Monomer	Dimer
Name	Iothalamate (Conray) Diatrizoate (Hypaque)	Ioxaglate (Hexabrix)	Iohexol (Omnipaque) Iopamidol (Isovue) Ioversol (Optiray)	Iodixanol (Visipaque)
Viscosity	Low	Low	Intermediate	High
Ratio (iodine/osmotically active particles)	1.5	3	3	6

[a]No longer commercially available in the US due to side effects.

Adapted from Klein LW, Sheldon MW, Brinker J, et al. The use of radiographic contrast media during PCI: a focused review: a position statement of the Society of Cardiovascular Angiography and Interventions. *Catheter Cardiovasc Interv.* 2009;74(5):728-46. Copyright © 2009 Wiley-Liss, Inc. Reprinted by permission of John Wiley & Sons, Inc.

TABLE 39-4	CESSATION OF DOAC BEFORE CARDIAC CATHETERIZATION		
Agent	**eGFR >50 mL/min**	**eGFR 31–50 mL/min**	**eGFR ≤30 mL/min**
Apixaban	48 hours	48 hours	≥72 hours
Rivaroxaban	48 hours	48 hours	≥72 hours
Dabigatran	48–72 hours	96 hours	≥120 hours

DOAC, direct-acting oral anticoagulant; eGFR, estimated glomerular filtration rate.

Adapted from Doherty JU, Gluckman TJ, Hucker WJ, et al. 2017 ACC Expert Consensus Decision Pathway for periprocedural management of anticoagulation in patients with nonvalvular atrial fibrillation: a report of the American College of Cardiology Clinical Expert Consensus Document Task Force. *J Am Coll Cardiol.* 2017;69(7):871-98. Copyright © 2017 by the American College of Cardiology Foundation. With permission.

Antithrombotic Medications

- Patients on warfarin should discontinue three doses before cardiac catheterization.
- An INR of <1.8 is acceptable for elective cardiac catheterization.
- Preprocedural management of direct oral anticoagulants is dependent on creatinine clearance and shown in Table 39-4.[16]
- Cardiac catheterization can be carried out while on heparin without concern.
- Heparin activity can be estimated by the ACT.
  - Can be reversed by protamine if significant bleeding
  - Protamine can lead to allergic reactions in diabetic patients on NPH insulin.

Intravascular Ultrasound

GENERAL PRINCIPLES

- Intravascular ultrasound (IVUS) is a catheter-based imaging modality used for cross-sectional imaging of the coronary vasculature (Table 39-5).[5,6]
  - Coronary stenosis quantified by IVUS has fewer anatomic limitations when compared to angiography.
  - IVUS enables accurate intraluminal vessel measurements and allows to better define plaque morphology and volume.
- There are two different types of IVUS catheters:
  - Mechanical state/rotating transducer catheters: rotating transducer housed in catheter and capturing images with each revolution
  - Solid state/electronic array: multiple phased-array elements around the catheter tip receiving backscattered ultrasound signals, does not require rotation
- IVUS catheters sizes range from 3.2 to 3.5F and are compatible with 5F and 6F guide catheters.

PROCEDURE

- Following administration of heparin or bivalirudin, after coronary guidewire has been positioned in the distal coronary vessel, and after intracoronary vasodilators, IVUS is advanced over a wire and positioned distally to the coronary stenosis.
- The catheter is then pulled back; lesion severity, length, and plaque characteristics can then be assessed.
- All ultrasound measurements should be performed on end-diastolic frames.

TABLE 39-5	CORONARY IMAGING DEVICES IN THE CATHETERIZATION LABORATORY				
Quality	Angiogram	IVUS (20–40 MHz)	HD IVUS ACIST Hdi® (60 MHz)	NIRS	OCT
Axial resolution (μm)	100–200	80–120	<50	[a]	10–15
Probe size (μm)	NA	700	=	1000	140
Contact	No	Yes	Yes	Yes	Yes
Ionizing radiation	Yes	No	No	No	No
Other	Lumen/ flow only	Assessment of plaque characteristics (calcium), dimensions, and adequacy of stent deployment.	2–3× better resolution compared to conventional IVUS; echogenicity of blood increases with higher frequencies	Modality combined with conventional IVUS; identifies vulnerable plaques with large lipid pools	10× better resolution compared to IVUS Drawback: shallow depth of penetration

HD IVUS, high-definition intravascular ultrasound, IVUS, intravascular ultrasound; NIRS, near-infrared spectroscopy; OCT, optical coherence tomography.

[a]Makoto™ imaging system by Infraredx™ with axial resolution <50 μm.

Adapted from Kern MJ, Sorajja P, Lim MJ. *The Interventional Cardiac Catheterization Handbook.* 4th ed. Elsevier; 2018.

CLINICAL APPLICATIONS

- Common clinical applications for IVUS include:
  - Guiding percutaneous coronary intervention (PCI) strategy
    - Establishes reference vessel size
    - Determines lesion length and extent of disease
    - Determines plaque composition
    - Ensures complete stent expansion and apposition with lack of edge dissection or other complications
    - Assesses ischemic potential of left main coronary artery based on minimal lumen area (MLA)[17,18]
      - If MLA >6 mm^2, then not consistent with ischemia.
      - If MLA <4.5 mm^2, then likely resulting in ischemia.

- Equivocal angiographic findings:
  - Angiographically indeterminate left main and ostial lesions
  - Unusual lesion morphology
  - Assessment of plaque vulnerability
- In-stent restenosis mechanisms:
  - Stent underexpansion
  - Neointimal hyperplasia
- Expert consensus recommendations on the use of IVUS are shown in Table 39-6.[19]

ANATOMIC INFORMATION

IVUS enables the anatomic evaluation of coronary vessel wall layers (Figure 39-8).
- Inner layer:
  - Normal coronaries: Usually, the intima is not seen. The internal elastic lamina appears as a very thin echogenic layer.
  - Disease coronaries: Atheromatous intima appears as a thick echogenic layer.
- Middle hypoechoic layer: corresponds to the media and is echolucent. The external elastic lamina (EEL) can be seen as a thin echodense layer.
- Outer echogenic layer: The adventitia is the most echodense structure in normal coronaries and surrounds the hypoechoic media.

PLAQUE MORPHOLOGY

- Based on their visual appearance, atheroma identified with grayscale IVUS have been classified into four categories (Figure 39-9).
  - Soft plaque: >80% of intimal lesion area with lower (but homogenous) echogenicity when compared to surrounding adventitia
  - Fibrous plaque: >80% of intimal lesion area with similar echogenicity to surrounding adventitia

TABLE 39-6	EXPERT CONSENSUS STATEMENT ON THE USE OF IVUS
Beneficial	IVUS is an accurate method to corroborate stent deployment and for sizing vessels before PCI.
Probably beneficial	IVUS can be used to appraise the significance of LMCA stenosis (a cutoff MLA = 6 mm^2, determines need for LMCA PCI).
Possibly beneficial	IVUS can be useful for the assessment of plaque morphology.
No proven value/ should be discouraged	IVUS measurements for determination of non-LMCA lesion severity should not be relied upon if there is no additional functional evidence.

IVUS, intravascular ultrasound; LMCA, left main coronary artery; MLA, minimum luminal area; PCI, percutaneous coronary intervention.

Adapted from Lotfi A, Jeremias A, Fearon WF, et al. Expert consensus statement on the use of fractional flow reserve, intravascular ultrasound, and optical coherence tomography: a consensus statement of the Society of Cardiovascular Angiography and Interventions. *Catheter Cardiovasc Interv.* 2014;83(4):509-18. Copyright © 2013 Wiley Periodicals, Inc. Reprinted by permission of John Wiley & Sons, Inc.

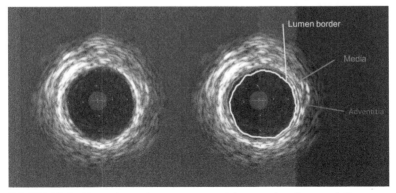

FIGURE 39-8. Normal vessel appearance on intravascular ultrasound. (Images provided courtesy of Philips.)

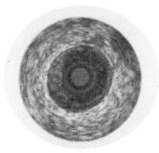

Soft (Fatty) plaque
Echolucent light gray flecks

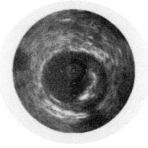

Fibrous plaque
Echogenic, light gray with white surfaces

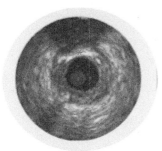

Calcified plaque
Highly echogenic white areas with shade

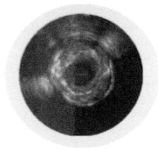

Mixed plaque
Combination of tissues of different echogenicity

FIGURE 39-9. Different plaque morphology by intravascular ultrasound.

○ Calcified plaque: highly echogenic intimal lesion with resulting in acoustic shadowing involving >90% of the vessel wall circumference

○ Mixed plaque: does not meet the criteria listed earlier. Often with a unique acoustical subtype

• "Vulnerable" plaques" appear eccentric on IVUS and are characterized by echolucent zones representing large necrotic lipid pools.

INTRAVASCULAR ULTRASOUND IN PERCUTANEOUS CORONARY INTERVENTION GUIDANCE

• IVUS can determine stent length and assess true vessel size to optimize stent size selection.[20]

○ Proximal and distal stent landing zones should avoid segments with abundant calcification, attenuation, and large plaque burden.

○ Aggressive stent sizing strategy should be avoided in lesions with negative remodeling (Figure 39-10)[21] due to the risk of perforation. Stent sizing strategies from least to most aggressive are as follows:

■ Largest reference lumen, whether proximal or distal

■ Mid-wall (halfway between lumen and EEL)

■ Media to media (0.5 mm subtracted)

• The use of IVUS guidance for PCI is associated with a 23% risk reduction in major adverse cardiac events (cardiac death, myocardial infarction, or stent thrombosis), 60% risk reduction of stent thrombosis, and a 35% risk of target vessel myocardial infarction at 2 years when compared to angiographic guidance alone.[22]

• Optimal stent deployment by IVUS is defined by:

○ Minimal stent area (MSA) >5.5 mm^2 (non-left main) or 90% of distal reference lumen cross-sectional area (CSA)

○ Plaque burden at the 5 mm proximal or distal to stent edge <50%

○ No edge dissection involving media with length >3 mm

Optical Coherence Tomography

GENERAL PRINCIPLES

• Optical coherence tomography (OCT) is a catheter-based modality used to image the coronary arterial wall and lesions.

• Instead of ultrasound, OCT uses near-infrared light and produces high-resolution images out of the backscattering light from the vessel wall and intraluminal structures. The wavelengths

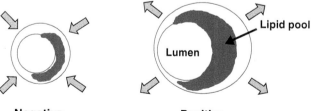

Negative   **Positive**

FIGURE 39-10. Negative and positive remodeling. (Adapted from Schoenhagen P, Ziada KM, Vince DG, et al. Arterial remodeling and coronary artery disease: the concept of "dilated" versus "obstructive" coronary atherosclerosis. *J Am Coll Cardiol.* 2001;38(2):297-306. Copyright © 2001 American College of Cardiology. With permission.)

of near-infrared light used in OCT range 1.25 to 1.35 μm; this limits its penetration to 1 to 3 mm compared to IVUS, which penetrates the vessel wall by about 4 to 8 mm.[23]
- The spatial resolution with OCT is in the order of 10 to 15 μm, making it the imaging modality that best correlates with tissue histology. OCT allows a better understanding of plaque biology with good visualization of fibrous caps and is also useful to verify stent apposition and determine mechanisms of stent failure (stent thrombosis or restenosis).
- Improved resolution comes at the cost of beam penetration into vessel walls.[24]
- Available OCT catheters sizes are 2.6F (Terumo) and 2.7F (Abbott) and are compatible with 5F and 6F guide catheters.

PROCEDURE

- Red blood cells (RBC) result in backscattering (OCT wavelength ~1.3 mm vs. RBC diameter ~8 mm). Thus, image acquisition requires blood clearance with contrast or low-molecular-weight dextran solutions.[25]
- The sequence of steps to follow for OCT imaging is the same as for IVUS imaging.
  ○ Administration of anticoagulants
  ○ Guidewire should be positioned in the distal coronary vessel, and intracoronary vaso-dilators should be delivered.
  ○ OCT is then advanced over the wire and positioned distally to the area of interest.
  ○ The catheter is then pulled back, and lesions are assessed.
  ○ OCT measurements should also be performed on end-diastolic frames.
- Structures and lesions are described based on:
  ○ Attenuation referring to the reduction in intensity of light waves as they pass through tissue
    ▪ High attenuation: Structure or lesion limits light penetration. Deep tissue beyond lesion appears dark and is not well visualized.
    ▪ Low attenuation: Light penetrates structures and allows visualization of deep tissue.
  ○ Backscatter intensity or brightness
    ▪ High backscatter describes a region or lesion that appears bright and "signal rich."
    ▪ Low backscatter describes a region or lesion that appears darker and is "signal poor."

ANATOMIC INFORMATION

All three vascular layers are seen along healthy segments of coronary arteries with OCT. Normal vessel walls have a "bright-dark-bright" trilaminar appearance (Figure 39-11).
- Intima (innermost layer and appears slightly brighter than media)
- Media (appears as a slightly darker band than the intima and adventitia)
- EEL is the outer layer of the media.
- Adventitia (outermost layer, appears slightly brighter than media)

PLAQUE MORPHOLOGY

- Lipidic, fibrous, or calcific lesions can be identified with OCT based on lesion attenuation and backscatter (Figure 39-12).
- Figure 39-13 presents a simplified algorithm to identify plaque type.[26]

OPTICAL COHERENCE TOMOGRAPHY FOR PERCUTANEOUS CORONARY INTERVENTION GUIDANCE

- The use of OCT for PCI guidance improves stent placement strategy (by assessing morphology, lesion length, and diameter) and optimization (by assessing stent apposition, stent expansion, and excluding vessel dissection).

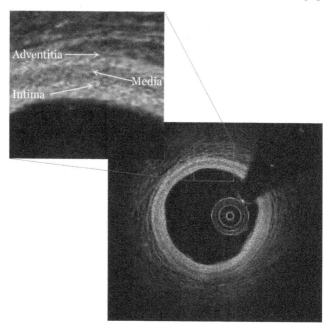

FIGURE 39-11. Vessel wall anatomy by optical coherence tomography. (OPTIS is a trademark of Abbott or its related companies. Reproduced with permission of Abbott, © 2022. All rights reserved.)

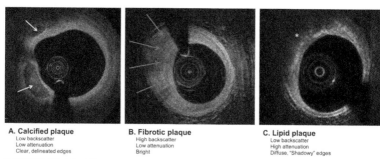

A. Calcified plaque
Low backscatter
Low attenuation
Clear, delineated edges

B. Fibrotic plaque
High backscatter
Low attenuation
Bright

C. Lipid plaque
Low backscatter
High attenuation
Diffuse, "Shadowy" edges

FIGURE 39-12. Plaque characteristics by optical coherence tomography. **(A)** Calcified lesions (arrows). **(B)** Fibrous plaque (arrows). **(C)** Fatty lesion (asterisk). (OPTIS is a trademark of Abbott or its related companies. Reproduced with permission of Abbott, © 2022. All rights reserved.)

- OCT is a tool that is useful in identifying lesions with high calcium burden prone to stent underexpansion and, in this way, at risk for stent restenosis and early thrombosis. The rule of the 5's has been proposed to identify these lesions that can benefit from plaque modification[27]:
  - ○ Calcific lesion >0.5 mm thickness
  - ○ Lesion length >5 mm
  - ○ Lesion involving >50% of the vessel arc

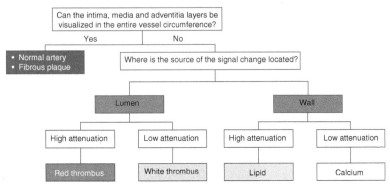

FIGURE 39-13. Simplified algorithm for interpretation of optical coherence tomographic images in the native coronary arteries. (Reprinted from Ali ZA, Karimi Galougahi K, Maehara A, et al. Intracoronary optical coherence tomography 2018: current status and future directions. *JACC Cardiovasc Interv.* 2017;10(24):2473-87. Copyright © 2017 by the American College of Cardiology Foundation. With permission.)

- Stent sizing can be done based on reference vessel EEL sizing strategy (when the EEL is visible) or reference vessel luminal sizing strategy.
  - EEL sizing strategy: Mean EEL to EEL diameter of the reference vessel is measured, and diameter is rounded down to the nearest stent size.
  - Luminal sizing strategy: Mean lumen diameter of the reference vessel is measured, and diameter is rounded up to nearest stent size.
- OCT criteria for optimal stent deployment include[24]:
  - MSA >4.5 mm^2 (non-left main) or $\geq 90\%$ of distal reference lumen CSA
  - No major edge dissection or intramural hematoma is defined as:
    - <60 degree of the vessel circumference
    - <3 mm in length and not involving deep layers (media or adventitia)
  - Good apposition is defined as:
    - Incomplete stent apposition distance <0.3 mm
    - Involving a vessel segment that is <1 mm
- OCT is noninferior to IVUS for PCI guidance for acute procedural result as well as mid-term clinical outcomes. Although long-term outcome studies are currently ongoing, by consensus, IVUS and OCT are considered to be equivalent and superior to angiography in guiding PCI.[24]

REFERENCES

1. Patel MR, Bailey SR, Bonow RO, et al. ACCF/SCAI/AATS/AHA/ASE/ASNC/HFSA/HRS/SCCM/SCCT/SCMR/STS 2012 appropriate use criteria for diagnostic catheterization: American College of Cardiology Foundation Appropriate Use Criteria Task Force Society for Cardiovascular Angiography and Interventions American Association for Thoracic Surgery American Heart Association, American Society of Echocardiography American Society of Nuclear Cardiology Heart Failure Society of America Heart Rhythm Society, Society of Critical Care Medicine Society of Cardiovascular Computed Tomography Society for Cardiovascular Magnetic Resonance Society of Thoracic Surgeons. *Catheter Cardiovasc Interv.* 2012;80(3):E50-81.
2. Valgimigli M, Campo G, Penzo C, Tebaldi M, Biscaglia S, Ferrari R. Transradial coronary catheterization and intervention across the whole spectrum of Allen test results. *J Am Coll Cardiol.* 2014;63:1833-41.

3. Dehmer GJ, Weaver D, Roe MT, et al. A contemporary view of diagnostic cardiac catheterization and percutaneous coronary intervention in the United States: a report from the CathPCI Registry of the National Cardiovascular Data Registry, 2010 through June 2011. *J Am Coll Cardiol* 2012;60:2017-31.

4. Tsai TT, Patel UD, Chang TI, et al. Validated contemporary risk model of acute kidney injury in patients undergoing percutaneous coronary interventions: insights from the National Cardiovascular Data Registry Cath-PCI Registry. *J Am Heart Assoc* 2014;3:e001380.

5. Kern M, Sorajja P, Lim M. *The Interventional Cardiac Catheterization Handbook.* 4th ed. Elsevier; 2018.

6. Kern M, Sorajja P, Lim M. *The Cardiac Catheterization Handbook.* 6th ed. Elsevier; 2016.

7. Zipes D, Libby P, Bonow R., Mann D, Tomaselli G. *Braunwald's Heart Disease: A Textbook of Cardiovascular Medicine.* 11th ed. Elsevier; 2019.

8. Sobolev M, Slovut DP, Lee Chang A, Shiloh AL, Eisen LA. Ultrasound-guided catheterization of the femoral artery: a systematic review and meta-analysis of randomized controlled trials. *J Invasive Cardiol.* 2015;27:318-23.

9. Ben-Dor I, Sharma A, Rogers T, et al. Micropuncture technique for femoral access is associated with lower vascular complications compared to standard needle. *Catheter Cardiovasc Interv.* 2021;97:1379-85.

10. Bashore TM, Bates ER, Berger PB, et al. American College of Cardiology/Society for Cardiac Angiography and Interventions Clinical Expert Consensus Document on cardiac catheterization laboratory standards. A report of the American College of Cardiology Task Force on Clinical Expert Consensus Documents. *J Am Coll Cardiol.* 2001;37:2170-214.

11. Mehran R, Rao SV, Bhatt DL, et al. Standardized bleeding definitions for cardiovascular clinical trials: a consensus report from the Bleeding Academic Research Consortium. *Circulation.* 2011;123:2736-47.

12. Naidu SS, Aronow HD, Box LC, et al. SCAI expert consensus statement: 2016 best practices in the cardiac catheterization laboratory: (Endorsed by the Cardiological Society of India, and sociedad Latino Americana de Cardiologia intervencionista; Affirmation of value by the Canadian Association of Interventional Cardiology-Association canadienne de cardiologie d'intervention). *Catheter Cardiovasc Interv.* 2016;88:407-23.

13. Brar SS, Aharonian V, Mansukhani P, et al. Haemodynamic-guided fluid administration for the prevention of contrast-induced acute kidney injury: the POSEIDON randomised controlled trial. *Lancet.* 2014;383:1814-23.

14. Weisbord SD, Gallagher M, Jneid H, et al. Outcomes after angiography with sodium bicarbonate and acetylcysteine. *N Engl J Med.* 2018;378:603-14.

15. Klein LW, Sheldon MW, Brinker J, et al. The use of radiographic contrast media during PCI: a focused review: a position statement of the Society of Cardiovascular Angiography and Interventions. *Catheter Cardiovasc Interv.* 2009;74:728-46.

16. Doherty JU, Gluckman TJ, Hucker WJ, et al. 2017 ACC expert consensus decision pathway for periprocedural management of anticoagulation in patients with nonvalvular atrial fibrillation: a report of the American College of Cardiology Clinical Expert Consensus Document Task Force. *J Am Coll Cardiol.* 2017;69:871-98.

17. Johnson TW, Räber L, di Mario C, et al. Clinical use of intracoronary imaging. Part 2: acute coronary syndromes, ambiguous coronary angiography findings, and guiding interventional decision-making: an expert consensus document of the European Association of Percutaneous Cardiovascular Interventions. *Eur Heart J.* 2019;40:2566-84.

18. de la Torre Hernandez JM, Hernández Hernandez F, Alfonso F, et al. Prospective application of pre-defined intravascular ultrasound criteria for assessment of intermediate left main coronary artery lesions results from the multicenter LITRO study. *J Am Coll Cardiol.* 2011;58(4):351-8.

19. Lotfi A, Jeremias A, Fearon WF, et al. Expert consensus statement on the use of fractional flow reserve, intravascular ultrasound, and optical coherence tomography: a consensus statement of the Society of Cardiovascular Angiography and Interventions. *Catheter Cardiovasc Interv.* 2014;83:509-18.

20. Mintz GS. IVUS in PCI guidance. American College of Cardiology. Accessed December 21. 2021. https://www.acc.org/latest-in-cardiology/articles/2016/06/13/10/01/ivus-in-pci-guidance

21. Schoenhagen P, Ziada KM, Vince DG, Nissen SE, Tuzcu EM. Arterial remodeling and coronary artery disease: the concept of "dilated" versus "obstructive" coronary atherosclerosis. *J Am Coll Cardiol.* 2001;38:297-306.

22. Maehara A, Mintz GS, Witzenbichler B, et al. Relationship between intravascular ultrasound guidance and clinical outcomes after drug-eluting stents. *Circ Cardiovasc Interv.* 2018;11:e006243.

23. Bezerra HG, Costa MA, Guagliumi G, Rollins AM, Simon DI. Intracoronary optical coherence tomography: a comprehensive review clinical and research applications. *JACC Cardiovasc Interv.* 2009;2:1035-46.

24. Räber L, Mintz GS, Koskinas KC, et al. Clinical use of intracoronary imaging. Part 1: guidance and optimization of coronary interventions. An expert consensus document of the European Association of Percutaneous Cardiovascular Interventions. *Eur Heart J* 2018;39:3281-300.

25. Maehara A, Matsumura M, Ali ZA, Mintz GS, Stone GW. IVUS-guided versus OCT-guided coronary stent implantation: a critical appraisal. *JACC Cardiovasc Imaging.* 2017;10:1487-503.

26. Ali ZA, Karimi Galougahi K, Maehara A, et al. Intracoronary optical coherence tomography 2018: current status and future directions. *JACC Cardiovasc Interven.* 2017;10(24):2473-87.

27. Fujino A, Mintz GS, Matsumura M, et al. A new optical coherence tomography-based calcium scoring system to predict stent underexpansion. *EuroIntervention.* 2018;13:e2182-9.

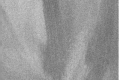

Cardiovascular Emergencies

Hannah Wey, Mustafa Husaini, and Marc Sintek

40

GENERAL PRINCIPLES

- Cardiovascular emergencies require urgent care by a cardiovascular care team and treatment in an intensive care unit (ICU) or emergency department setting after initial stabilization.
- For each situation discussed in this chapter, there is risk of abrupt progression to cardiac arrest. It is imperative to be cognizant of the patient's clinical stability during assessment of any cardiovascular emergency and to ensure adequate means of resuscitation and hemodynamic monitoring. During the initial evaluation, we suggest the following:
  - Ensure adequate IV access.
  - Ensure a reliable form of hemodynamic monitoring, either by frequent cuff measurement or by arterial line.
  - Ensure that the appropriate team members are present. For example, the primary nurse, appropriate medical providers, respiratory therapy, rapid response team members, and the cardiac arrest resuscitation team all have important roles in managing these cardiovascular emergencies.
  - Obtain supplies that you may need for immediate bedside resuscitation. These may include items such as, but not limited to, a crash cart, bedside ultrasound, central line kit, and transcutaneous pacing pads.
  - Obtain a brief, focused history and physical examination, typically facilitated by the primary service physicians.
- Topics presented in this chapter include symptomatic bradycardia, symptomatic tachycardia, ST-segment elevation myocardial infarction (STEMI), cardiac tamponade, hypertensive emergencies, cardiogenic shock, and implantable cardiac device emergencies.
- This chapter is meant as a hands-on, rapid checklist to help manage patients with the abovementioned cardiovascular emergencies. Detailed discussion of each disease can be found elsewhere in this book.

Symptomatic Bradycardia

GENERAL PRINCIPLES

- Assess if the patient is hemodynamically stable or if they are having any symptoms of bradycardia, which can include hypotension, lightheadedness, fatigue, presyncope, or syncope.
- Advanced Cardiac Life Support (ACLS) guidelines for symptomatic bradycardia are provided in Figure 40-1.[1]

DIAGNOSIS

- *Bradycardia* in an adult is defined as a resting heart rate <60 beats per minute (bpm); however, it is rarely symptomatic unless <50 bpm.[2] Correlate a palpated pulse with an ECG. **Asymptomatic bradycardia does not require emergent treatment**.
- Symptomatic bradycardia at rest or with hypotension or syncope requires immediate attention to the circulation, airway, and breathing and initiation of basic life support if appropriate.

Adult bradycardia algorithm

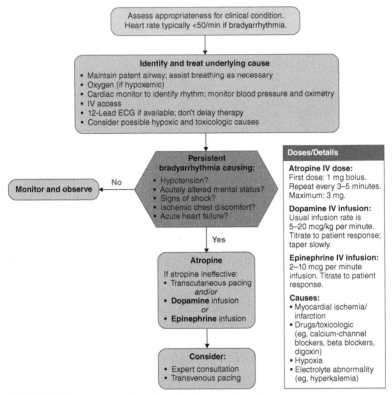

FIGURE 40-1. Advanced Cardiac Life Support algorithm for management of bradycardia. (Reprinted with permission from *Advanced Cardiovascular Life Support Provider Manual.* Copyright ©2020 American Heart Association, Inc.)

- A brief review of the rhythm strip or 12-lead ECG is important to determine whether the bradycardia originates above or below the atrioventricular node (AVN).
  - Bradycardia from above the AVN (sinus bradycardia, sinus node dysfunction, sinus arrest) should respond to treatment with IV atropine.
  - Advanced AV block (type II second- or third-degree AV block) is unlikely to respond to the increased atrial heart rates that atropine provides and will likely need urgent pacing.
  - Ventricular escape bradycardia is unstable and requires preparation for urgent pacing.

TREATMENT

Medications

- **Atropine**: 0.5 to 1.0 mg IV. Doses can be repeated every 3 to 5 minutes. The **exception** to using atropine is type II second-degree AV block, which may be worsened by atropine due to increased AVN refractoriness with increased stimulation leading to complete AV block.

- **Dopamine**: 2.5 to 20 µg/kg per minute IV to keep systolic blood pressure (SBP) >90 mm Hg
- **Epinephrine**: 2 to 10 µg per minute or 0.1 to 0.5 µg/kg per minute IV to keep SBP >90 mm Hg
- **Isoproterenol**: 20 to 60 µg bolus, followed by continuous IV infusion of 1 to 20 µg per minute titrated to heart rate
- **If drug toxicity due to AVN-blocking agents:**
  ○ β-Blockade: IV glucagon 3 to 10 mg bolus followed by infusion of 2 to 5 mg per hour, consider high-dose IV insulin: 1 unit/kg bolus followed by 0.5 unit/kg per hour infusion
  ○ Calcium channel blockade: IV calcium (10% calcium chloride or 10% calcium gluconate) given as IV bolus or as continuous infusion, followed by high-dose IV insulin infusion
  ○ Digoxin: anti-digoxin fab, dose dependent on estimated amount of digoxin ingested or known serum level. Typically, 1 vial binds 0.5 mg of digoxin.
- **Post-heart transplant:**
  ○ Aminophylline: 6 mg/kg in 100 to 200 mL fluid administered over 20 to 30 minutes
  ○ Theophylline: 300 mg IV bolus followed by oral dose 5 to 10 mg/kg per day
- **Spinal cord injury:**
  ○ Aminophylline: 6 mg/kg in 100 to 200 mL fluid administered over 20 to 30 minutes
  ○ Theophylline: oral dose 5 to 10 mg/kg per day

Nonpharmacologic Therapies

Transcutaneous Pacing
- Place pads on the anterior and posterior chest walls. Initially, begin pacing at the highest output and ensure capture with a palpated pulse. **Remember that pacer spikes do not always translate to ventricular capture.** Rapidly reduce the output until ventricular capture is lost and then increase the output until regular capture is seen. If hypotension is not severe, sedate the patient, as transcutaneous pacing can be painful and traumatic for awake patients.
- Prepare for transvenous pacing (see Chapter 27).

SPECIAL CONSIDERATIONS

- In patients with temporary pacemakers, frequently ensure that capture threshold and outputs are stable as pacing wires may migrate.
- Patients who undergo transcatheter aortic valve replacement (TAVR), cardiac surgery, alcohol septal ablation and those with preexisting conduction delay are at high risk for development of conduction abnormalities and complete heart block postprocedurally and are often closely monitored or receive prophylactic temporary pacing strategies.[2]
- Assess for noncardiac (and possible reversible) etiologies of bradycardia, including respiratory failure and hypoxia, acidosis, electrolyte abnormalities, drug toxicities, and evolving neurologic process.

Symptomatic Tachycardia

GENERAL PRINCIPLES

- *Tachycardia* is defined as atrial and/or ventricular rate >100 bpm. However, symptomatic or hemodynamically significant tachycardia typically occurs at heart rate >150 bpm in an adult.[3]
- Similar to the assessment of the patient with bradycardia, the first question to ask yourself is, "Is this person stable?" Check the palpable pulse, blood pressure (BP), and oxygen saturation. If the patient is pulseless or clinically unstable, proceed to defibrillation as described in section Clinically Unstable and ACLS guidelines for tachycardia in Figure 40-2.[1]
- Analysis of the ECG dictates management of the clinically stable patient.

Adult tachycardia with a pulse algorithm

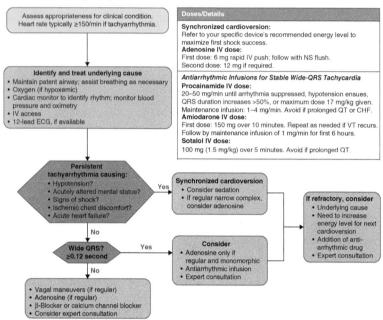

FIGURE 40-2. Advanced Cardiac Life Support algorithm for management of tachycardia. (Reprinted with permission from *Advanced Cardiovascular Life Support Provider Manual.* Copyright ©2020 American Heart Association, Inc.)

DIAGNOSIS

Narrow QRS Complex Tachycardias

- Supraventricular tachycardia (SVT) with a QRS complex <120 milliseconds duration on ECG.
- The most common SVTs in order of frequency are:
  - Sinus tachycardia
  - Atrial fibrillation
  - Atrial flutter
  - AVN reentry tachycardia (AVNRT)
  - AV reentry tachycardia (AVRT, accessory pathway mediated)
  - Atrial tachycardia (ectopic and reentrant)
  - Multifocal atrial tachycardia
  - Junctional tachycardia
- Narrow QRS complex arrhythmias are further diagnosed and often treated by slowing the conduction through the AVN. This can demonstrate the underlying atrial rhythm without large ventricular QRS complexes obscuring the rhythm (atrial fibrillation, flutter, and ectopic atrial tachycardia). In addition, slowing AVN conduction can halt the tachycardia if it is dependent on the AVN as part of the tachycardia circuit (AVNRT and AVRT).

Wide QRS Complex Tachycardia

- QRS duration ≥120 milliseconds:
  - Ventricular tachycardia (VT)
  - SVT with aberrancy
  - Preexcited tachycardias (Wolff–Parkinson–White syndrome)
  - Ventricular pacemaker
- Wide QRS complex tachycardias are more challenging to manage as they require a working diagnosis to aid in the differential diagnosis.
- The treatment for VT can be vastly different from SVT with aberrancy or a preexcited tachycardia.
- There are multiple ECG criteria that are used to differentiate SVT from VT (Brugada criteria, Vereckei criteria, etc.); the following suggest VT as the cause:
  - **Known structural disease:** Patients with coronary disease or ventricular dysfunction are more likely to have VT as the cause of wide-complex tachycardia.
  - **Change in QRS morphology:** a major change in QRS morphology and/or a shift in axis in comparison with QRS morphology in sinus rhythm
  - **AV dissociation**
  - Presence of **fusion/capture beats**
  - Positive or negative concordance of QRS in ECG leads V1 to V6

TREATMENT

Clinically Unstable

- **Patients who are clinically unstable with tachycardia require immediate synchronized cardioversion, or if ventricular fibrillation, with unsynchronized defibrillation by means of high-energy shocks** (200 J, 300 J, 360 J) followed by appropriate ACLS, focusing on high-quality cardiopulmonary resuscitation compressions.
- **Amiodarone** (300 mg IV once, repeat at 150 mg IV once) should be given for continued pulseless VT.
- **Epinephrine** 1 mg IV/IO should be given every 3 to 5 minutes.
- Maximum output defibrillation should continue every 2 minutes for shockable rhythms after pulse and rhythm checks in concordance with the ACLS protocol.
- Therapies aimed at the working diagnosis should also be given if suspected (i.e., magnesium if presumed torsades de pointes, calcium and bicarbonate if hyperkalemia is suspected).

Clinically Stable

Narrow QRS Complex Tachycardia

- AVN slowing can be achieved by **increasing vagal tone** with a carotid sinus massage or bearing down; however, this should be avoided in patients with known carotid artery disease.
- First-line AVN-blocking agent: **Adenosine** can be rapidly pushed (6, 12, or 18 mg) IV with a flush.[3]
  - Ideally, adenosine should be given through a central line if available or a large-bore peripheral IV in the antecubital fossa or proximally.
  - Warn the patient about a flushing/unpleasant sensation.
  - Ensure that there is a continuous 12-lead ECG printing as a "rhythm strip" to document the response.
- Second-line AVN-blocking agent: if can hemodynamically tolerate, can administer IV β-blockade such as esmolol or metoprolol tartrate, IV diltiazem (0.25 mg/kg bolus), IV or verapamil (5 to 10 mg IV bolus).[3] Avoid negative inotropic agents in patients who are decompensated with evidence of volume overloaded and heart failure with reduced ejection fraction as these may precipitate cardiogenic shock.

- Third-line agents: Flecainide and propafenone can be used in the absence of structural or ischemic heart disease. Sotalol, digoxin, dofetilide, and amiodarone are antiarrhythmic agents that can be used to treat SVT in patients with structural heart disease.
- If pharmacologic therapy is contraindicated or ineffective, synchronized cardioversion should be pursued.[3]

Wide QRS Complex Tachycardia

- **Monomorphic VT**: Amiodarone (150 mg IV over 10 minutes, followed by 1 mg per minute continuous infusion for 6 hours and then 0.5 mg per minute continuous infusion for the next 18 hours) should be used. Alternative options include IV lidocaine, IV procainamide, or sotalol. If the patient becomes unstable or the VT persists, synchronized cardioversion should be considered with sedation.
- In the absence of contraindications, the general order of medical treatment for **recurrent VT (VT storm)** is (1) IV amiodarone, (2) IV and oral β-blockers, (3) IV lidocaine, (4) IV and oral benzodiazepine, and (5) general anesthesia and endotracheal intubation.
- Electrophysiologic study with catheter ablation may play a role for treating VT. Selective sympathetic denervation (spinal anesthesia and stellate ganglion surgery) and ventricular support devices (intra-aortic balloon pump [IABP], percutaneous left ventricular assist device [LVAD] [Impella], or extracorporeal membrane oxygenation [ECMO]) can be considered.
- **Polymorphic VT**: This can become unstable quickly. A prolonged QT interval in sinus rhythm should raise the concern of torsades de pointes. Immediate treatment should include administering 4 g IV magnesium, overdrive pacing if temporary pacing wire or permanent pacemaker are available, or isoproterenol at 5 μg per minute infusion. Amiodarone (150 mg IV over 10 minutes) may be helpful, particularly if the QT interval is normal at baseline. Underlying medications or overdoses should be investigated.
- Persistent **torsades de pointes** requires defibrillation.

SPECIAL CONSIDERATIONS

- Patients with a prolonged QT interval at their baseline should have their medications reviewed for QT-prolonging agents.
- Patients who are started on an antiarrhythmic medication should have continuous telemetry monitoring and periodic 12-lead ECGs. Class 3 antiarrhythmics (amiodarone and sotalol) can prolong the QT interval. Class 1 antiarrhythmics can prolong the QRS complex.
- For patients on IV lidocaine, there should be frequent neurologic checks, and serum lidocaine levels should be checked to avoid toxicity.
- In patients with evidence of preexcitation and/or known or suspected accessory pathway, management of SVT depends on mechanism of tachycardia and directionality of the accessory pathway. In patients with orthodromic AVRT, vagal maneuvers and adenosine can be used to terminate AVN-dependent AVRT. Synchronized cardioversion should be performed if hemodynamically unstable or pharmacologic therapy is ineffective. Second-line agents include AVN-blocking agents; however, there exists the risk of conversion from a macro-reentrant SVT to atrial fibrillation and subsequent VF.
- In patients with atrial fibrillation and manifest accessory pathways with evidence of preexcitation on ECG, AVN-blocking agents such as digoxin, amiodarone, β-blockade, and calcium channel blockade are contraindicated due to risk of selective conduction down the accessory pathway, leading to ventricular fibrillation.[3] In hemodynamically stable patients with atrial fibrillation and preexcitation, observational studies support the use of IV procainamide or ibutilide.[4,5]

- Ultimately, patients with accessory pathways and symptomatic arrhythmias should be referred for ablative therapy evaluation.
- Two or more internal cardioverter-defibrillator (ICD) shocks in the span of 24 hours are generally considered concerning. We discuss device failure and inappropriate defibrillation later in this chapter.
- In pregnant patients, treatment of SVT with vagal maneuvers, adenosine, β-blockade (metoprolol tartrate, labetalol, and propranolol), verapamil, procainamide, and synchronized cardioversion are all reasonable options. Amiodarone can be used in life-threatening SVT (but for short courses, due to risk of fetal toxicities) if other therapies have failed.[6]

Cardiac Tamponade

GENERAL PRINCIPLES

- Cardiac tamponade is caused by compression of the cardiac chambers by a pericardial effusion, mechanically inhibiting diastolic filling and, therefore, reducing stroke volume and ultimately cardiac output.
- The presence of a pericardial effusion does not necessarily imply that tamponade physiology is present.
- Detailed discussion on the etiology, pathophysiology, and nonemergent management of pericardial effusion is presented in Chapter 17.

DIAGNOSIS

- Cardiac tamponade is a **clinical diagnosis** associated with relative hemodynamic compromise.
- Characterized by the following parameters:
  ○ Elevation of intrapericardial pressure
  ○ Limitation of right ventricular (RV) diastolic filling
  ○ Reduction of LV stroke volume and cardiac output
- History can reveal a potential cause and rate of fluid accumulation.
- It is important to remember that the size of the effusion is irrelevant in terms of causing tamponade physiology.
  ○ Small effusions that accumulate acutely are as likely to cause tamponade as large effusions that develop over time.
  ○ Large effusions that accumulate slowly will not always lead to tamponade physiology.
- Pertinent physical examination findings include altered mental status, hypotension, tachycardia, jugular venous distension, and pulsus paradoxus (Figure 40-3).[7]
- If the patient is in the ICU and has arterial access, pulsus paradoxus can also be observed and measured on the arterial waveform.
- Supporting diagnostic information can be obtained by evaluating an ECG for low voltage and electrical alternans and a CXR for a water bottle–shaped heart.

Echocardiography

- Confirm the presence of a pericardial effusion by using the descending aorta in the parasternal long-axis view
  ○ If the effusion is anterior to the descending aorta, then pericardial effusion
  ○ If the effusion is posterior to the descending aorta, then pleural effusion

- The most sensitive finding of tamponade physiology is a dilated inferior vena cava that does not demonstrate respiratory variation. Thus, if this is not seen, then there is a low likelihood of cardiac tamponade.
- Distinguishing features on a transthoracic echocardiogram:
  - RV diastolic collapse
  - Right atrial systolic notching
  - Tricuspid and mitral valve inflow variation in Doppler velocities of >40% and >25%, respectively (Figure 40-3)
  - Dilated inferior vena cava
  - Systolic reversal of flow in hepatic veins assessed by pulsed-wave Doppler

TREATMENT

- **Initial medical management:**
  - **Volume expansion:** Initial management consists of increasing preload with IV fluids.

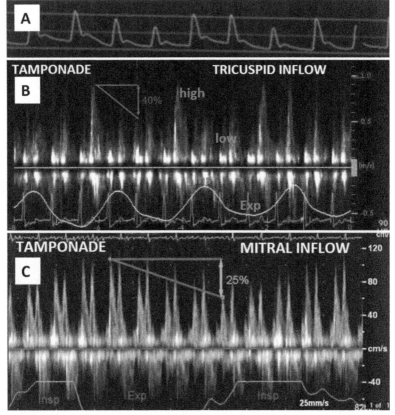

FIGURE 40-3. Cardiac tamponade. **(A)** An arterial line waveform illustrating pulsus paradoxus with a decrease in inspiratory systolic pressure >10 mm Hg. **(B and C)** Tricuspid inflow variation >40% and mitral inflow variation >25%, respectively, in different patients with cardiac tamponade.

- ○ **BP**: Maintain BP with norepinephrine and dobutamine as needed.
- ○ Avoid venodilators, vasodilators, and diuretics.
- The decision to drain the pericardial fluid, as well as the method (surgical or percutaneous) and timing (emergent or elective) of the procedure, should be individualized to each patient considering the acuity of the patient's condition, etiology of the effusion, and availability of trained personnel.
- **Pericardiocentesis**:
  - ○ Pericardiocentesis is a potentially life-threatening procedure, which should be performed by trained personnel with hemodynamic monitoring and echocardiographic guidance whenever possible.
  - ○ Loculated or posterior pericardial effusions are unlikely to be safely reached or relieved with pericardiocentesis alone, and if a patient is symptomatic, may require surgical drainage.
  - ○ Blind percutaneous pericardiocentesis may be needed to stabilize a hemodynamically unstable patient, though emergent pericardiocentesis with ultrasound guidance in the cardiac catheterization lab is preferred. If available, assess nearby structures with ultrasound at the subcostal position to avoid injury to the liver, bowel, and lung.
  - ○ Insert the 8-cm, 19-gauge blunt tipped needle attached to a syringe through the subxiphoid region.
  - ○ Direct the needle tip 30 degrees left of midline and 30 degrees posteriorly toward the patient's left shoulder and slowly advance the needle with gentle aspiration.
  - ○ Confirmation of pericardial cannulation can be performed with ultrasound visualization of agitated saline injection.
  - ○ Aspiration of clear, serous fluid may be from the pericardium or pleural effusion. Aspiration of bloody fluid may be from the pericardium or the RV.
  - ○ Removal of 50 to 100 mL of pericardial fluid should cause a hemodynamic improvement if tamponade is the cause of the hypotension.

Hypertensive Emergency

GENERAL PRINCIPLES

- Severe hypertension affects the renal (elevated serum creatinine and hematuria), cardiovascular (angina, heart failure, and aortic dissection), and neurologic (headache, mental status changes, vision alterations from retinal damage, and papilledema) systems.
- **Hypertensive emergency** is the presence of end-organ damage from elevated BP, necessitating rapid reduction by using IV medications.
- In contrast, **hypertensive urgency** can be treated with oral medications with the goal of BP reduction over the course of days.

DIAGNOSIS

- Elevated BP recordings, often with SBP >180 mm Hg and/or diastolic blood pressure (DBP) >120 mm Hg
- End-organ damage can manifest with an abnormal neurologic examination, acute pulmonary edema, angina, or laboratory markers of acute pathology.

TREATMENT

- In adults with hypertensive emergency and compelling conditions including aortic dissection, severe preeclampsia, eclampsia, or pheochromocytoma crisis, SBP should be decreased to <140 mm Hg in the first hour and <120 mm Hg in the first hour in aortic dissection.[8]

- For patients without a compelling condition, **SBP should be reduced by no >25% within the first hour.** Then, if stable, reduced to <160/100 within the first 6 hours, then cautiously to <130/80 over the following 24 to 48 hours.
- A larger reduction in BP in the first few hours may worsen end-organ damage, particularly in the brain.
- Placement of an arterial line should be strongly considered for the most accurate BP measurement.
- Specific antihypertensive medications should be adjusted for the situation.
- Table 40-1 describes first-line antihypertensive agents and usual doses recommended.[8]

SPECIAL CONSIDERATIONS

- Reversible causes of severe, medical refractory hypertension are warranted for patients who present with hypertensive urgency or emergency. These include blood tests for hyperaldosteronism and a noninvasive scan for renal artery stenosis.
- **Hypertensive encephalopathy:**
  ○ Agents of choice are nitroprusside or labetalol.
  ○ Central nervous system depressants, such as clonidine, should be avoided.
  ○ Antiepileptics may help patients with seizures and lower BP.
- **Cerebrovascular injury:**
  ○ **The need to maintain cerebral perfusion pressure (CPP) outweighs the acute need to lower BP.**
  ○ CPP should be kept >70 mm Hg if intracerebral pressure (ICP) monitoring is available (CPP = MAP − ICP).
  ○ Acute stroke or intracranial hemorrhage:
    ▪ BP >230/140 mm Hg: Nitroprusside is the agent of choice.
    ▪ BP 180–230/140–105 mm Hg: labetalol, esmolol, or other easily titratable IV antihypertensive
    ▪ BP <180/105: Defer hypertensive management.
- **Aortic dissection:**
  ○ Type A dissection: Patients should be referred for emergent surgical correction and aggressively treated with antihypertensives.
  ○ Type B dissection: treated with antihypertensives. Labetalol or esmolol should be started initially to lower heart rate, followed by nitroprusside if necessary. See Chapter 20 for a detailed approach to aortic dissection.
- **LV failure with pulmonary edema:**
  ○ Rapid reduction in BP should be achieved with a nitrate or nitroglycerin.
  ○ Small doses of loop diuretics are often effective.
- **Myocardial ischemia:**
  ○ IV nitroglycerin will improve coronary blood flow, decrease LV preload, and moderately decrease systemic arterial pressure.
  ○ β-Blockers should be added to decrease heart rate and BP.
- **Preeclampsia and eclampsia:**
  ○ Hypertensive emergency in pregnancy is defined as SBP ≥170 mm Hg or DBP ≥110 mm Hg.[6]
  ○ Methyldopa, a centrally acting α-blocker, is the drug of choice for hypertension in pregnancy due to large experience in this setting.
  ○ IV labetalol or nifedipine may also be used with appropriate fetal monitoring.
  ○ Hydralazine is no longer a first-line agent due to elevated risk of perinatal adverse events compared to other antihypertensive agents available. However, if BP remains uncontrolled, it can be used as an additional agent.
  ○ IV sodium nitroprusside can be used as a last-line therapy due to risk of fetal cyanide toxicity with prolonged use.

Class	Drug(s)	Usual Dose Range	Comments
Dihydropyridine calcium channel blockers	Nicardipine	• **Initial 5 mg/h** • Increasing every 5 minute by 2.5 mg/h • **Maximum 15 mg/h**	• Contraindicated in advanced aortic stenosis • No dose adjustment needed for elderly.
	Clevidipine	• **Initial 1–2 mg/h** • Doubling every 90 seconds until BP approaches target, then increasing by less than double every 5–10 minutes • **Maximum dose 32 mg/h** • Maximum duration 72 hours	• Contraindicated in patients with soybean, soy product, egg, and egg product allergy • Contraindicated in patients with defective lipid metabolism (e.g., pathologic hyperlipidemia, lipoid nephrosis, or acute pancreatitis). • Use low-end dose range for elderly patients.
Vasodilators (nitric oxide dependent)	Sodium nitroprusside	• **Initial 0.3–0.5 μg/kg/min** • Increase in increments of 0.5 μg/kg/min to achieve BP target • **Maximum dose 10 μg/kg/min** • Duration of treatment as short as possible.	• Lower dosing adjustment required for elderly. • **Tachyphylaxis common** with extended use. • **Cyanide toxicity with prolonged use** can result in irreversible neurologic changes and cardiac arrest. • For infusion rates ≥4–10 μg/kg/min or duration >30 minutes, thiosulfate can be coadministered to prevent cyanide toxicity.
	Nitroglycerin	• **Initial 5 μg/min** • Increase in increments of 5 μg/min every 3–5 minutes • **Maximum of 20 μg/min**	• Use only in patients with **acute coronary syndrome** and/or **acute pulmonary edema**. • Do not use in volume-depleted patients.

(continued)

TABLE 40-1 IV ANTIHYPERTENSIVE DRUGS FOR TREATMENT OF HYPERTENSIVE EMERGENCIES (*continued*)

Class	Drug(s)	Usual Dose Range	Comments
Direct vasodilators	Hydralazine	• **Initial 10 mg** via slow IV infusion (maximum initial dose 20 mg) • Repeat every 4–6 hours as needed.	• **BP begins to decrease within 10–30 minutes, and the fall lasts 2–4 hours.** • **Unpredictability of response and prolonged duration of action** do not make hydralazine a desirable first-line agent for acute treatment in most patients.
Adrenergic blockers—β₁-receptor selective antagonist	Esmolol	• **Loading dose 500–1000 µg/kg/min** over 1 minute followed by a **50-µg/kg/min infusion.** • For additional dosing, the bolus dose is repeated and the infusion increased in 50-µg/kg/min increments as needed • **Maximum of 200 µg/kg/min.**	• **Contraindicated in patients with concurrent β-blocker therapy, bradycardia, or decompensated HF.** • Monitor for bradycardia. • May worsen HF. • Higher doses may block β₂ receptors and impact lung function in reactive airway disease.
Adrenergic blockers—combined α₁ and nonselective β-receptor antagonist	Labetalol	• **Bolus dosing with initial 0.3–1.0-mg/kg dose** (maximum 20 mg) slow IV injection every 10 minute • **Infusion dose with 0.4–1.0 mg/kg/h** IV infusion up to 3 mg/kg/h. • Adjust rate up to **total cumulative dose of 300 mg.** • This dose can be repeated every 4–6 hour.	• **Contraindicated in reactive airways disease or chronic obstructive pulmonary disease.** • **Especially useful in hyperadrenergic syndromes.** • May worsen HF and should not be given in patients with second- or third-degree heart block or bradycardia.

Adrenergic blockers—nonselective α-receptor antagonist	Phentolamine	• IV bolus dose 5 mg. • Additional bolus doses every 10 minute as needed to lower BP to target.	• Used in hypertensive emergencies induced by catecholamine excess • Pheochromocytoma • Interactions between monoamine oxidase inhibitors and other drugs or food • Cocaine toxicity • Amphetamine overdose • Clonidine withdrawal
Dopamine₁-receptor selective agonist	Fenoldopam	• **Initial 0.1–0.3 µg/kg/min** May be increased in increments of 0.05–0.1 µg/kg/min every 15 minute until target BP is reached. • **Maximum infusion rate 1.6 µg/kg/min.**	• Contraindicated in patients at risk of increased intraocular pressure (glaucoma) or intracranial pressure • Contraindicated in patients with sulfite allergy.
ACE inhibitor	Enalaprilat	• **Initial 1.25 mg** over a 5-minute period. • Doses can be increased up to 5 mg every 6 hour as needed to achieve BP target.	• Contraindicated in pregnancy and should not be used in acute MI or bilateral renal artery stenosis. • Mainly useful in hypertensive emergencies associated with high plasma renin activity. • Dose not easily adjusted. • Relatively slow onset of action (15 minute) and unpredictability of BP response.

BP, blood pressure; CCB, calcium channel blocker; HF, heart failure; MI, myocardial infarction.

Adapted from Whelton PK, Carey RM, Aronow WS, et al. 2017 ACC/AHA/AAPA/ABC/ACPM/ AGS/APhA/ASH/ASPC/NMA/PCNA guideline for the prevention, detection, evaluation, and management of high blood pressure in adults: a report of the American College of Cardiology/American Heart Association Task Force on Clinical Practice Guidelines. *J Am Coll Cardiol.* 2018;71(19):e127-248. Copyright © 2018 by the American College of Cardiology Foundation. With permission.

- IV nitroglycerin is a first-line therapy for preeclampsia associated with pulmonary edema.
- Angiotensin-converting enzyme (ACE) inhibitors, angiotensin II receptor blockers (ARBs), and direct renin inhibitors are contraindicated in pregnancy.[6]
- **Pheochromocytoma crisis:**
  - May present with a markedly elevated BP, labile BP, profound sweating, marked tachycardia, pallor, and numbness/coldness/tingling in the extremities[9]
  - **Phentolamine,** 5 to 10 mg IV, is the drug of choice and should be repeated as needed.
  - Short-acting vasodilators including nitroprusside and nicardipine may be added if necessary.
  - β-Blocker should be added only after phentolamine to avoid unopposed α-adrenergic activity. Of note, labetalol (α-blocker and nonselective β-blocker) and clonidine interfere with catecholamine assays used in the diagnosis of pheochromocytoma, so they should be held before the diagnosis is made.
  - Due to lability, patients often require significant IV fluid resuscitation during periods of subsequent hypotension.
- **Cocaine-related hypertensive emergency** can be treated with **benzodiazepines.**
  - Severe hypertension should be treated with nondihydropyridine calcium channel blockers (e.g., IV diltiazem), nitroglycerin, nitroprusside, or phentolamine.
  - β-Blockers should be theoretically avoided, given the risk of unopposed α-adrenergic activity; however, various studies have not illustrated an association with harm. If given, should use selective β-blockers or those with α-antagonist activity.

ST-Segment Elevation Myocardial Infarction

- Early successful coronary reperfusion strategies lead to improved short- and long-term outcomes.
- IV thrombolytic medication and/or percutaneous coronary intervention may achieve reperfusion in appropriate patients.
- A detailed discussion can be found in Chapter 9.

Cardiogenic Shock

GENERAL PRINCIPLES

- Cardiogenic shock is a spectrum of disease that requires various amounts of therapeutic support and has various outcomes depending on etiology of shock. An algorithm for the assessment and treatment of acute decompensated heart failure (ADHF) is presented in Figure 40-4.
- Even with advances in reperfusion therapy and mechanical circulatory support, inpatient mortality remains high, with nationally reported mortality rates of 27-51%.[10,11]

Definition

- Clinical syndrome of a low cardiac output state with signs and symptoms of organ hypoperfusion and tissue hypoxia[10-14]
- The physiologic definition of cardiogenic shock includes an SBP <90 mm Hg, cardiac index <2.2 L/min/m^2, pulmonary capillary wedge pressure (PCWP) >15 mm Hg, and evidence of end-organ damage, such as elevated serum lactate, oliguria, or altered mental status.

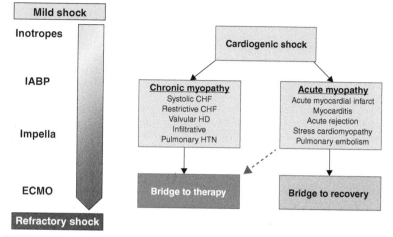

FIGURE 40-4. Cardiogenic shock as a spectrum of disease. Cardiogenic shock can be differentiated by acuity (right side of figure) and (severity left side of figure). CHF, congestive heart failure; ECMO, extracorporeal membrane oxygenation; HD, heart disease; HTN, hypertension; IABP, intra-aortic balloon pump.

Etiology

- **The most common cause is an extensive MI**, which severely and acutely compromises LV function.
- ~6-8% of patients with acute coronary syndrome will develop cardiogenic shock during hospitalization, most often due to an STEMI.[15]
- Other causes include:
  - LV dysfunction
  - Acute valvular failure
  - Electrical instability
  - Pericardial disease
  - RV infarction
  - Mechanical complications such as papillary muscle dysfunction or rupture, ventricular septal rupture, and free wall rupture

Pathophysiology

- Acute LV dysfunction as a result of an acute myocardial infarction (AMI) leads to elevated cardiac filling pressures, decreased cardiac output, and a systemic inflammatory response system (SIRS) response.[11]
- This confluence of events leads to end-organ hypoperfusion, which then leads to further cardiac ischemia, progressive cardiac dysfunction, and, ultimately, death.

Risk Factors

- Risk factors for developing shock include older age, diabetes, anterior infarct, history of previous MI, peripheral vascular disease, decreased LV ejection fraction, underlying cardiomyopathy, and large infarct territory size.
- Predictors of mortality include older age, shock on presentation, clinical evidence of end-organ hypoperfusion, anoxic brain injury, noninferior MI, serum creatine >1.9, prior coronary artery bypass surgery, and SBP.[16]

DIAGNOSIS

Clinical Presentation

- A majority of patients with AMI-induced cardiogenic shock are profoundly hypotensive and peripherally vasoconstricted (cool to touch). However, there is a subset of the population that can present "warm and wet" due to concomitant vasodilatory shock from the SIRS.[11]
- Pulses are diminished and rapid. Cardiac examination may reveal tachycardia with the presence of an S_3 and/or S_4.
- Pay close attention to systolic murmurs indicative of a ventricular septal defect (VSD) or papillary muscle rupture and acute valvular regurgitation.
- Jugular venous distention and pulmonary rales may also be present.

Diagnostic Testing

- May show arterial hypoxemia, elevated creatinine, and lactic acidosis
- CXR may reveal evidence of pulmonary congestion.
- Bedside echocardiography gives rapid information regarding LV systolic function and mechanical complications, including acute VSD, severe mitral regurgitation, free wall rupture, and tamponade.
- Placement of a pulmonary artery catheter (PAC) is appropriate in this setting and allows for differentiation of LV and RV infarction, mechanical complication, and volume depletion.
- In addition, a PAC will guide treatment when starting inotropes, assessing volume status, and titrating afterload reduction.
- In a subanalysis of the SHOCK trial, cardiac power output (CPO) and index were the strongest independent hemodynamic correlates of inpatient mortality.[17] The relationship between CPO and inpatient mortality is shown in Figure 40-5.
  - Cardiac Power Output (CPO) = $\dfrac{\text{Cardiac Output (L/min)} \times \text{MAP (mm Hg)}}{451}$
  - With equal sensitivity and specificity (0.66), CPO <0.53 indicates a 58% positive predictive value of in-hospital mortality.

Classification of Cardiogenic Shock

- **Given the potential for rapid deterioration and high mortality, early recognition and classification of cardiogenic shock is essential. Recognizing the severity of shock can prompt timely initiation of appropriate medical therapies and mechanical support.**
- The Society of Cardiovascular Angiography and Interventions (SCAI) published an expert consensus statement including a schema for stages of cardiogenic shock illustrated in Figure 40-6 and Table 40-2.[18] This statement is also endorsed by the American College of Cardiology (ACC), the American Heart Association (AHA), the Society of Critical Care Medicine (SCCM), and the Society of Thoracic Surgeons (STS).[18]

TREATMENT

Immediate Management

- **Ultimately, identify and treat the underlying cause of shock**: early revascularization for AMI complicated by cardiogenic shock, antiarrhythmic therapy or cardioversion for unstable arrhythmia, transvenous pacing for unstable bradyarrhythmia, pericardiocentesis or pericardial window for tamponade, and emergent surgical consultation for mechanical complications
- **Oxygen**: Maintain O_2 saturation >92% if possible. Intubation may be necessary. Be prepared for the further hypotension that results from the sedation and decreased cardiac filling with positive pressure ventilation.

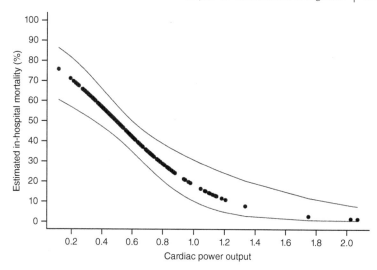

FIGURE 40-5. Analysis of SHOCK trial demonstrated increased in-hospital mortality with lower cardiac power output. Correlation of Cardiac Power Output (x-axis) and in-hospital mortality (y-axis). (Reprinted from Fincke R, Hochman JS, Lowe AM, et al. Cardiac power is the strongest hemodynamic correlate of mortality in cardiogenic shock: a report from the SHOCK trial registry. *J Am Coll Cardiol.* 2004;44(2):340-8. Copyright © 2004 American College of Cardiology Foundation. With permission.)

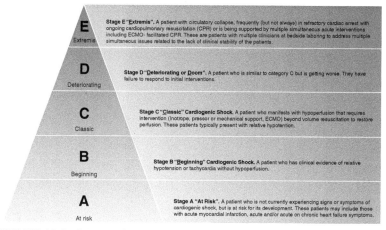

FIGURE 40-6. Schema of cardiogenic shock stages proposed by the Society of Cardiovascular Angiography and Interventions clinical expert consensus statement on classification of cardiogenic shock. (From Baran DA, Grines CL, Bailey S, et al. SCAI clinical expert consensus statement on the classification of cardiogenic shock. *Catheter Cardiovasc Interv.* 2019;94(1):29-37. Copyright © 2019 Wiley Periodicals, Inc. Reprinted by permission of John Wiley & Sons, Inc.)

TABLE 40-2 DESCRIPTIVE FINDINGS OF CARDIOGENIC SHOCK STAGES PROPOSED BY SCAI CLINICAL EXPERT CONSENSUS STATEMENT ON CLASSIFICATION OF CARDIOGENIC SHOCK

Stage	Description	Physical examination/ bedside findings	Biochemical markers	Hemodynamics
A At risk	A patient who is not currently experiencing signs or symptoms of CS, but is at risk for its development. These patients may include those with **large acute myocardial infarction or prior infarction acute or infarction acute and/or acute on chronic heart failure** symptoms.	Normal JVP Lung sounds clear Warm and well perfused Strong distal pulses Normal mentation	Normal renal function Normal lactic acid	Normotensive (SBP ≥100 or normal for the patient) If hemodynamics available: • Cardiac index ≥2.5 • CVP <10 • PA sat ≥65%
B Beginning CS	A patient who has clinical evidence of **relative hypotension** or **tachycardia without hypoperfusion.**	Elevated JVP Rales in lung fields Warm and well perfused Strong distal pulses Normal mentation	**Normal lactate** Minimal renal function impairment Elevated BNP	SBP <90 **OR** MAP 30 mm Hg drop from baseline Pulse ≥100 If hemodynamics available: • Cardiac index ≥2.2 • PA sat ≥65%
C Classic CS	A patient who manifests with hypoperfusion that **requires intervention beyond volume resuscitation** to restore perfusion. Interventions include inotrope, pressor or mechanical circulatory support	Looks unwell Ashen, mottled, dusky Volume overload Killip class 3 or 4 BiPAP or mechanical ventilation Cold, clammy Acute alteration in mental status Urine output <30 mL/h	*May Include Any of:* Lactate ≥2 Creatinine doubling **OR** >50% drop in GFR Increased LFTs Elevated BNP	SBP <90 **OR** MAP 30 mm Hg drop from baseline **AND** drugs/ device used to maintain BP above these targets Hemodynamics: • Cardiac index <2.2 • PCWP >15 • RAP/PCWP ≥0.8 • PAPI <1.85 • Cardiac power output ≤0.6 *May Include Any of:*

			Any of Stage C AND:
D Deteriorating/doom	A patient who is similar to category C but is getting worse. They have **failure to respond to initial interventions.**	**Any of stage C**	**Any of Stage C AND:** Deteriorating	Requiring multiple pressors **OR** addition of mechanical circulatory support devices to maintain perfusion
E Extremis	A patient who is experiencing cardiac arrest with ongoing CPR and/or ECMO, being supported by multiple interventions.	Near pulselessness Cardiac collapse Mechanical ventilation Defibrillator used	"**Trying to die**" CPR (A-modifier) pH ≤7.2 Lactate ≥5	No SBP without resuscitation PEA or refractory VT/VF Hypotension despite maximal support

BiPAP, bilevel positive airway pressure; BNP, brain natriuretic peptide; CPR, cardiopulmonary resuscitation; CS, cardiogenic shock; CVP, central venous pressure; ECMO, extracorporeal membrane oxygenation; GFR, glomerular filtration rate; JVP, jugular venous pressure; LFT, liver function tests; MAP, mean arterial pressure; PA, pulmonary artery; PAPI, pulmonary artery pulsatility index; PEA, pulseless electrical activity; PCWP, pulmonary capillary wedge pressure; RAP, right atrial pressure; SBP, systolic blood pressure; SCAI, Society of Cardiovascular Angiography and Interventions; VF, ventricular fibrillation; VT, ventricular tachycardia.

Adapted from Baran DA, Grines CL, Bailey S, et al. SCAI clinical expert consensus statement on the classification of cardiogenic shock. *Catheter Cardiovasc Interv.* 2019;94(1):29-37. Copyright © 2019 Wiley Periodicals, Inc. Reprinted by permission of John Wiley & Sons, Inc.

- **Medications**: Discontinue negative inotropic agents such as β-blockers and calcium channel blockers immediately. If hypotensive, discontinue vasodilators.
- **IV fluids**: Goal PCWP is ~18 mm Hg. Patients with low PCWP will benefit from gentle hydration. Patients with pulmonary edema or elevated PCWP will often benefit from diuresis with IV loop diuretics.
- **Inotropes and vasopressors**: Inotropic and vasopressor medications can be useful in the management of cardiogenic shock. They should be titrated with PAC guidance as inappropriate use increases the risk of exacerbating ischemia and developing malignant arrhythmias.
  ○ If SBP is <90 mm Hg, start norepinephrine at 2 μg per minute and titrate to 20 μg per minute to achieve a mean arterial pressure of 65 mm Hg.
  ○ With SBP >90 mm Hg, dobutamine is the preferred agent. Dobutamine is started at 2.5 μg/kg per minute and slowly titrated to effect (usual maximum dose is 10 μg/kg per minute). The phosphodiesterase inhibitor milrinone can alternatively be used; it acts as an inotrope and vasodilator.
- Overall, there is a relative paucity of high-quality evidence from randomized controlled trials regarding optimal inotropic and vasodilator strategy to improve patient mortality. A 2020 Cochrane review of inotropes and vasodilators in cardiogenic shock showed poor level of evidence for one strategy over another.[19]
- Studies support the use of norepinephrine as a first-line vasopressor in cardiogenic shock compared with dopamine, vasopressin, and epinephrine due to decreased risk of arrhythmia, improved CPO, and improved short-term mortality.[20-22]

Advanced Support

- Due to the high incidence of morbidity and mortality from irreversible organ damage secondary to pump failure, advanced percutaneous or surgically implanted therapeutic options have been developed for cardiogenic shock.
- It is reasonable to consider transferring the patient to a facility capable of advanced therapies for cardiogenic shock.
- Therapeutic interventions and devices include:
  ○ **Coronary reperfusion**: Several trials have examined the benefit of revascularization (percutaneously or surgically) or medical treatment in patients with cardiogenic shock. The SHOCK trial prospectively examined patients who developed cardiogenic shock within 36 hours of AMI and compared revascularization with aggressive medical management.[13] Although there was no mortality benefit at 30 days, there were significant mortality benefits at 6 months and 1 year with early revascularization. Younger patients (75 years or younger) showed greater benefit with revascularization, whereas older patients had better outcomes with medical management.
  ○ **IABP:** An IABP reduces afterload, increases coronary perfusion, augments DBP, and promotes a slight increase in cardiac output.[14-18] While the IABP-SHOCK II trial did not illustrate a 30-day mortality benefit in patients prospectively randomized to IABP placement after AMI-induced cardiogenic shock, IABPs are still used clinically due to their modest effect on cardiac output and ease of placement.[23]
  ○ Percutaneous LVAD: Devices such as the Impella, TandemHeart, and ECMO serve to unload the LV to decrease cardiac work, which can slow or stop the ischemic "shock spiral."

SPECIAL CONSIDERATIONS

When patients are being considered for mechanical support, their candidacy for advanced heart failure therapies including heart transplant and durable LVAD should also be considered before implantation.

Implantable Cardiac Device Emergencies (Pacemakers and Defibrillators)

GENERAL PRINCIPLES

There are two types of cardiac emergencies for patients with cardiac devices:
- Pacemaker malfunction in a patient who is pacemaker dependent, that is, with underlying symptomatic bradycardia or asystole in the absence of pacing
- Multiple ICD shocks in a patient with a defibrillator

DIAGNOSIS

- Prompt interrogation of the cardiac device and subsequent review of the information can confirm the clinical diagnosis.
- **Identify the device**. Patients with cardiac devices are asked to carry an identification card, which gives the information regarding the type of device and device manufacturer.
- **Identify the rhythm**. A 12-lead ECG can rapidly determine the patient's rhythm and the response of the cardiac device.
- A pacemaker may fail to either sense a beat or capture the heart with a pacing output. This can become an emergency if the patient has underlying symptomatic bradycardia or asystole without effective pacing.
- Two or more ICD shocks in the span of 24 hours are generally considered concerning. This may be due to either appropriate shocks for recurrent ventricular arrhythmia, shocks for an SVT with a fast ventricular rate, or inappropriate ICD sensing, which is most commonly due to a lead fracture or migration.

TREATMENT

- Device interrogation and CXR can often help identify the problematic heart rhythm or device programming/function. Further treatment is tailored toward the arrhythmia or device settings.
- If the patient has symptomatic bradycardia, treatment should focus on maintaining a reasonable heart rate (see section Symptomatic Bradycardia).
- If the patient is receiving inappropriate ICD shocks, a medical magnet may be placed over the pulse generator, which suspends ICD therapy, but not pacing.

SPECIAL CONSIDERATIONS

- Regular cardiac device checkups can monitor for changes in lead performance, which can herald lead failure.
- Wireless home monitoring is available for many newer cardiac devices and has been shown to quickly identify important clinically actionable events.
- Medical treatment and/or catheter ablation of tachyarrhythmias can often prevent future ICD shocks.

REFERENCES

1. Link MS, Berkow LC, Kudenchuk PJ, et al. Part 7: adult advanced cardiovascular life support: 2015 American Heart Association guidelines for cardiopulmonary resuscitation and emergency cardiovascular care. *Circulation.* 2015;132:S444-64.
2. Kusumoto FM, Schoenfeld MH, Barrett, C, et al. 2018 ACC/AHA/HRS guideline on the evaluation and management of patients with bradycardia and cardiac conduction delay: a report of the American College of Cardiology/American Heart Association task force on clinical practice guidelines and the Heart Rhythm Society. *J Am Coll Cardiol.* 2019;74(7):e51-156.

3. Page RL, Joglar JA, Caldwell MA, et al. 2015 ACC/AHA/HRS guideline for the management of adult patients with supraventricular tachycardia: a report of the American College of Cardiology/American Heart Association Task Force on clinical practice guidelines and the Heart Rhythm Society. *J Am Coll Cardiol.* 2016;67(13):e27-115.

4. Wellens HJ, Braat S, Brugada P, et al. Use of procainamide in patients with Wolff–Parkinson–White syndrome to disclose a short refractory period of the accessory pathway. *Am J Cardiol.* 1982;50(5):1087-9.

5. Varriale P, Sedighi A, Mirzaietehrane M. Ibutilide for termination of atrial fibrillation in the Wolff–Parkinson–White syndrome. *Pacing Clin Electrophysiol.* 1999;22(8):1267-9.

6. Regitz-Zagrosek V, Roos-Hesselink JW, Bauersachs J, et al. 2018 ESC guidelines for the management of cardiovascular diseases during pregnancy. *Eur Heart J.* 2018;39(34):3165-241.

7. Roy CL, Minor MA, Brookhart MA, et al. Does this patient with a pericardial effusion have cardiac tamponade? *JAMA.* 2007;297:1810-8.

8. Whelton PK, Carey RM, Aronow WS, et al. 2017 ACC/AHA/AAPA/ABC/ACPM/ AGS/APhA/ASH/ASPC/NMA/PCNA guideline for the prevention, detection, evaluation, and management of high blood pressure in adults: a report of the American College of Cardiology/American Heart Association task force on clinical practice guidelines. *J Am Coll Cardiol.* 2018;71:e127-248.

9. Kizer JR, Koniaris LS, Edelman JD, et al. Pheochromocytoma crisis, cardiomyopathy, and hemodynamic collapse. *Chest.* 2000;118(4):1221-3.

10. Jeger RV, Radovanovic D, Hunziker PR, et al. Ten-year trends in the incidence and treatment of cardiogenic shock. *Ann Intern Med.* 2008;149:618-26.

11. Van Diepen S, Katz JN, Albert NM, et al. Contemporary management of cardiogenic shock: a scientific statement from the American Heart Association. *Circulation.* 2017;136:e232-68.

12. Goldberg RJ, Spencer FA, Gore JM, et al. Thirty-year trends (1975 to 2005) in the magnitude of, management of, and hospital death rates associated with cardiogenic shock in patients with acute myocardial infarction: a population-based perspective. *Circulation.* 2009;119:1211-9.

13. Hochman JS, Sleeper LA, Webb JG, et al. Early revascularization in acute myocardial infarction complicated by cardiogenic shock. SHOCK Investigators. Should we emergently revascularize occluded coronaries for cardiogenic shock. *N Engl J Med.* 1999;341:625-34.

14. Thiele J, Schuler G, Neumann FJ, et al. Intraaortic balloon counterpulsation in acute myocardial infarction complicated by cardiogenic shock: design and rationale of the Intraaortic Balloon Pump in Cardiogenic Shock II (IABP-SHOCK II) trial. *Am Heart J.* 2012;163:938-45.

15. Barron HV, Every NR, Parsons LS, et al. Investigators in the national registry of myocardial infarction 2. *Am Heart J.* 2001;14:933-9.

16. Sleeper LA, Reynolds HR, White HD, et al. A severity scoring system for risk assessment of patients with cardiogenic shock: a report from the SHOCK Trial and Registry. *Am Heart J.* 2010;160(3):443-50.

17. Fincke R, Hochman JS, Lowe AM, et al. Cardiac power is the strongest hemodynamic correlate of mortality in cardiogenic shock: a report from the SHOCK trial registry. *J Am Coll Cardiol.* 2004;44(2):340-8.

18. Baran DA, Grines CL, Bailey S, et al. SCAI clinical expert consensus statement on the classification of cardiogenic shock. *Catheter Cardiovasc Interv.* 2019;94:29-37.

19. Uhlig K, Efremov L, Tongers J, et al. Inotropic agents and vasodilator strategies for the treatment of cardiogenic shock or low cardiac output syndrome. *Cochrane Database Syst Rev.* 2020;11(11):CD009669.

20. De Backer D, Biston P, Devriendt J. et al. Comparison of dopamine and norepinephrine in the treatment of shock. *N Engl J Med.* 2010;362(9):779-89.

21. Levy B, Meziani F, Leone M, et al. Comparison of epinephrine and norepinephrine for the treatment of cardiogenic shock following acute myocardial infarction. OPTIMA CC study. *Ann Intensive Care.* 2008;8(suppl 1):65.

22. Levy B, Perez P, Perny J, et al. Comparison of norepinephrine-dobutamine to epinephrine for hemodynamics, lactate metabolism, and organ function variables in cardiogenic shock. A prospective, randomized pilot study. *Crit Care Med.* 2011;39:450-5.

23. Sjauw KD, Engström AD, Vis MM, et al. A systematic review and meta-analysis of intra-aortic balloon pump therapy in ST-elevation myocardial infarction: should we change the guidelines? *Eur Heart J.* 2009;30:459-68.

Procedures in Critical Care

Manuel Rivera Maza and Alan Zajarias

GENERAL PRINCIPLES

- Planning and organization are essential for all procedures described in this chapter.
- Requisites for good preparation include:
  - An assessment of the physical environment (hospital setting and patient-related factors) to determine the feasibility of using aseptic technique
  - Availability of necessary and standardized equipment
  - Hands-on assistance from colleagues/nursing staff
  - Use of a checklist or protocol for the procedure in question[1]
- Before beginning the procedure, the operator must ensure that:
  - Procedure and procedure-related risks have been explained to the patient and consent has been obtained.
  - A history focused on the reason for the procedure, medication allergies, known history of vascular disease/interventions, and anticoagulation therapy has been documented.
  - Laboratory work including a complete blood count (CBC), basic metabolic panel (BMP), and coagulation parameters has been reviewed.
  - Relevant imaging (when available) should also be reviewed.
  - Patient has been screened for procedural absolute and relative contraindications.
  - Equipment, supplies, lighting, and assistance are readily available.
  - Analgesia and sedation are available.

CENTRAL VENOUS CATHETERIZATION

- Central venous catheterization is used in critical care for both diagnosis (e.g., central venous pressure measurement) and treatment (e.g., IV fluids, pacemaker).[2]
- Patients should be evaluated for the presence of other central venous devices (long-term central venous catheters [CVCs], ports, or leads) and signs of central venous obstruction (distended collateral veins about the shoulder and neck).

Contraindications

- Absolute contraindications
  - Thrombosis of the target vein
  - Infection of the area overlying the target vein
  - Fracture of ipsilateral clavicle (for subclavian approach)
- Relative contraindications
  - Coagulopathy (international normalized ratio [INR] > 2 or activated partial thromboplastin time [aPTT] > 2× upper limit of normal)
  - Thrombocytopenia (platelet count < 50,000/μL)

Types of Catheters

- CVCs are classified based on the following:
  - Number of lumens
  - Location

- ○ Lifespan (short, intermediate, long term)
- ○ Site of insertion
- An important determination for the type and location of the CVC is the intended lifespan based on the clinical need.
  - ○ Short term (≤14 days)
    - Examples include triple lumen and temporary hemodialysis catheters.
    - Most frequently used CVC in critical care given ease and speed of access at bedside.
    - Common sites of insertion include the internal jugular, subclavian, and femoral veins.
    - Optimal catheter length varies depending on access site chosen[3]:
      - □ Right internal jugular vein: 12 to 15 cm
      - □ Left internal jugular vein: 15 to 20 cm
      - □ Femoral veins: 19 to 24 cm
  - ○ Intermediate term (2 to 6 weeks)
    - Example is a peripherally inserted central catheter (PICC).
    - A PICC is inserted into peripheral veins of the upper extremities and advanced to upper portion of the right atrium. Adequate position should be radiographically documented.
    - This allows access to the central circulation without risks associated with direct puncture of internal jugular, subclavian, or femoral veins.[4]
    - Commonly used for inotrope infusion, home parenteral nutrition, or long-term IV antibiotic infusion
  - ○ Long-term (≥31 days)
    - Example is a tunneled catheter.
    - Considered for prolonged infusions (e.g., inotropes, IV pulmonary vasodilators) and long-term hemodialysis
    - These may be cuffed or noncuffed. Cuffed devices have a polyethylene or silicone flange that anchors the catheter within the SC tissue and limits entry of bacteria along the extraluminal surface.

Internal Jugular Access

- The internal jugular vein is easily and rapidly accessible in most patients.
- Advantages of this site include decreased risk of pneumothorax compared with the subclavian approach and ready compressibility of the vessels in case of bleeding.

Anatomic Landmarks

- Both the common carotid artery and internal jugular vein run inside the sternocleidomastoid (SCM) triangle.
- The apex of said triangle is formed by the heads of the SCM muscle, while the clavicle forms its base.
- Ultrasound should be used for confirmation after identifying anatomic landmarks.
- Ultrasound guidance reduces the risk of failed catheter placement, number of attempts, and time to successful catheterization.[5]

Procedure

- The patient should be positioned in the Trendelenburg position. Head should be down and rotated 45 degrees away from the site of cannulation.
- Clean skin with at least 0.5% chlorhexidine preparation with alcohol.
- After both identifying anatomic landmarks and confirming with ultrasound, administer local anesthesia (e.g., 1% lidocaine SC injection).
- Under ultrasound guidance, starting lateral to the carotid pulse, insert an 18-gauge needle at the apex of the SCM triangle at a 45-degree angle toward the ipsilateral nipple.

- Confirm needle placement is in venous blood and not within the carotid artery. This can be done with a manometer, fluoroscopy (if available), blood gas analysis (if available), and characteristics of the color and pulsatility of blood return (least ideal confirmation method).
- Once central venous blood return is achieved, apply **Seldinger technique**:
  ○ While keeping the needle anchored with your hand, decrease the angle of the needle to allow easy passage of the flexible guidewire into the vein through the needle.
  ○ Remove the needle using the wire as a guide.
  ○ Create a small nick on the skin at the puncture site to allow passage of the dilator.
  ○ Dilate tract over the wire.
  ○ Advance CVC over the wire to the cavoatrial junction. Be sure to **maintain control of the guidewire at all times**.
  ○ Remove guidewire.
- Confirm blood return from all blood ports and subsequently flush with saline.
- Secure catheter to the patient's neck at a minimum of two sites.
- Confirm adequate CVC placement with CXR.

Subclavian Vein Approach

- The subclavian approach to the central venous system is generally most comfortable for the patient and easiest to maintain.
- Subclavian vein lines have lower risk of infection compared to internal jugular and femoral lines.[6,7]

Anatomic Landmarks

- The subclavian vein runs just under the middle third of the clavicle. This is where the clavicle angles posteriorly.
- Both subclavian artery and apical pleura lie posterior to the vein.[8]

Procedure

- The patient is placed in 15-degree Trendelenburg position. It is helpful to roll a towel under the spine to prop up the shoulders and make the clavicles more prominent.
- Identify the middle third of the clavicle. The insertion site should be ~2 cm lateral to this point. Orient the needle parallel to and under the clavicle.
- Clean skin with at least 0.5% chlorhexidine preparation with alcohol.
- After identifying anatomic landmarks and following confirmation with ultrasound, administer local anesthesia (e.g., 1% lidocaine) to subcutaneous (SC) tissue and infraclavicular space.
- Under ultrasound guidance, insert catheterization needle at a 30-degree angle toward the sternal notch. Once needle is under skin, decrease the angle so that the needle can run parallel to and under the clavicle; then advance under negative pressure until obtaining central access.
- Apply Seldinger technique to insert CVC.
- Confirm blood return from all blood ports and subsequently flush with saline.
- Secure catheter and apply a sterile dressing.
- Confirm appropriate CVC placement with CXR.

Femoral Vein Approach

- The femoral vein is the easiest site for obtaining central access and is the preferred approach for central venous access during cardiopulmonary resuscitation.
- Limitations to femoral lines include interference with patient mobility and high risk of catheter contamination. Therefore, in elective situations, femoral access should be a last resort when other sites are not a viable option.

Anatomic Landmarks
- The common femoral artery crosses the inguinal ligament approximately midway between the anterosuperior iliac spine and the pubic tubercle.
- The femoral vein runs medial to the artery as they cross the inguinal ligament.

Procedure
- Place patient in supine position and identify the femoral pulse using anatomic landmarks. Confirm vascular structures and patency with ultrasound.
- Clean skin with at least 0.5% chlorhexidine preparation with alcohol.
- Administer local anesthesia (e.g., 1% lidocaine) in the SC tissue medial to the femoral artery and inferior to the inguinal ligament.
- Under ultrasound guidance, insert needle medial to femoral pulse at a 30-degree angle and directing it cephalad with constant negative pressure until obtaining venous return.
- Use Seldinger technique to insert CVC.
- Confirm blood return from all ports are aspirated and flush with saline.
- Secure catheter to patients' groin at a minimum of two sites and apply sterile dressing.

Complications

Some of the risks associated with central venous catheterization include:
- Pneumothorax
  - Internal jugular vein and subclavian vein CVCs carry a nontrivial risk of pneumothorax.
  - Placement of a CVC, or a failed attempt, should be followed by an erect CXR.
- Carotid artery injury
  - Inadvertent carotid artery puncture is usually tolerated in the noncoagulopathic patient and treated by direct pressure over the carotid artery.
  - Although carotid artery puncture is usually benign, inadvertent cannulation can result in stroke or iatrogenic arteriovenous fistula (AVF).
  - A general rule based on size is as follows:
    - If the dilator or catheter is ≤7 French, remove catheter/dilator and apply direct pressure over carotid puncture site and observe patient closely.
    - If the dilator or catheter is >7 French, vascular surgery should be consulted.
- Guidewire-related complications
  - Advancement of the guidewire into the right atrium or ventricle can cause arrhythmias, which usually resolve once the wire is withdrawn.
  - CVC insertion can be performed under fluoroscopy in patients with indwelling devices to minimize the possibility of entanglement of the guidewire with these structures.
- Thrombosis
  - The spectrum of thrombotic complications ranges from fibrin sleeve formation around the catheter to mural or occlusive thrombus.
  - Although only 3-5% of CVCs develop clinically significant thromboses, 33-67% of patients form venous thrombi when the indwelling time of the catheter surpasses 1 week.
- Other potential complications
  - Air embolus
  - Perforation of the right atrium or ventricle with resultant hemopericardium and cardiac tamponade
  - Injury to the trachea, esophagus, thoracic duct, vagus nerve, phrenic nerve, or brachial plexus

Central Line–Associated Bloodstream Infections

Definition
- Catheter colonization is defined as ≥15 CFU on semiquantitative culture.
- The definition of central line–associated bloodstream infections (CLABSI) requires bacteremia or fungemia as well as the following criteria:

○ Clinical signs of infection (fever, chills, tachycardia, hypotension, leukocytosis)
○ No identifiable source for bloodstream infection
○ Isolation of the same organism from semiquantitative culture of the catheter and from the blood

Pathogenesis
Infection occurs by means of three common mechanisms:
- Local insertion site infection. Skin flora at the insertion site migrates along the external surface of the catheter and colonizes the intravascular tip.
- Hub colonization progressing to bloodstream infection via intraluminal colonization
- Hematogenous. The central line is seeded from another focus of infection.

Risk Factors
- Several factors increase the risk of CLABSI, including neutropenia, malignancy, parenteral feeding, intensive care setting, thrombus, and multilumen catheters.
- The risk for infection varies with the catheter insertion site, with the femoral vein associated with a much higher infection rate than jugular and subclavian vein access.
- The likelihood of infection directly correlates with length of time a catheter has been in place.

Management
- Routine catheter replacement after an arbitrary length of time has not been demonstrated to decrease the incidence of CLABSI.[6]
- Catheters inserted during medical emergencies where adherence to aseptic technique cannot be ensured should be replaced as soon as possible.

ARTERIAL LINE PLACEMENT

- Arterial lines allow invasive monitoring of blood pressure as well as access to arterial blood for measurement of arterial oxygenation and frequent blood gas sampling.
- Continuous blood pressure monitoring is indicated in critically ill and hemodynamically unstable patients requiring vasopressors or inotropes.
- Radial artery is the preferred site for catheterization since it is easily accessible and has a low rate of complications.
- See Chapter 39 for a discussion on complications of radial and femoral artery puncture.

Contraindications
- Thrombosis of the target blood vessel
- Infection of the area overlying the target blood vessel
- Traumatic injury proximal to the insertion site
- Severe peripheral vascular disease
- Impaired collateral circulation
- Severe coagulopathy

Preparation
- Physical examination and history should assess hemodynamic status of the patient.
- Imperative that arterial pulses are examined.

Procedure for Radial Access
- Use flexible board or roll to place the patient's hand in moderate dorsiflexion. Use ultrasound to identify vascular structures and confirm patency.
- Clean skin with at least 0.5% chlorhexidine preparation.
- Administer a small amount of local anesthesia (e.g., 1% lidocaine) in the SC tissue.

- Under ultrasound guidance, introduce needle between radial styloid process and flexor carpi radialis tendon at a 30-degree angle from the skin. Advance slowly until obtaining pulsatile blood return.
- Insert catheter using Seldinger technique.
- Once the catheter is successfully placed, secure and connect to a sterile transduction system.

PULMONARY ARTERY CATHETERIZATION

Pulmonary artery catheterization serves as an adjunct in the diagnosis and management of multiple conditions encountered in critical care, including cardiogenic shock, cardiac tamponade, pulmonary hypertension, and mixed shock states.[9]

Contraindications

- Absolute contraindications
  - Thrombosis of the target vein
  - Infection of the area overlying the target blood vessel
  - Fracture of ipsilateral clavicle, if utilizing a subclavian approach
  - Right-sided endocarditis, tumors, or masses that could be dislodged during catheter advancement through right-sided cardiac structures
- Relative contraindications
  - Coagulopathy (INR > 2 or aPTT > 2× upper limit of normal)
  - Thrombocytopenia (platelet count < 50,000/μL)
  - Patients with underlying left bundle branch block are at risk of complete heart block during advancement of pulmonary catheter.

Special Equipment

- Balloon-tipped flow-directed pulmonary artery catheters (PACs) are 110 cm long and 5 to 8 French in diameter. These catheters all have three to four ports and may have a thermistor wire (Figure 41-1).

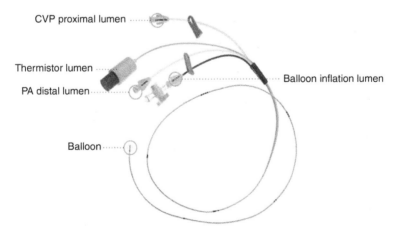

FIGURE 41-1. Pulmonary artery (PA) catheter anatomy. CVP, central venous pressure. (Image courtesy of Teleflex Incorporated. © [2021] Teleflex Incorporated. All rights reserved.)

- Ports are configured as follows:
  - Proximal port (blue)
    - Connects to lumen 30 cm from tip
    - Used to transduce right atrial pressures once catheter in final position
  - Distal port (yellow)
    - Connects to catheter tip
    - Transduces all pressures during insertion
    - Transduces pulmonary and wedge pressures once catheter in final position
  - Infusion port (clear/white and present in larger catheters): connects to a second lumen 30 cm from tip
  - Inflation port (red)
    - Used to inflate the balloon at the catheter tip
    - The syringe packaged with the catheter should be used exclusively.
- A plastic sleeve ("Swandom") should be used to cover the exterior portion of the catheter to maintain sterility and decrease risk of infections.
- A pressure monitor connected to the distal yellow port will transduce intracavitary pressures as the catheter is advanced to the pulmonary circulation.
- The use of fluoroscopy for pulmonary artery catheterization is highly recommended.

Procedure

- Place patient in supine position. After selecting central vein for insertion, the steps to insert the introducer sheath are the same steps described earlier for CVC insertion.
- Attach distal port of the PAC to pressure monitor and calibrate.
- Advance PAC 15 cm through the introducer sheath and inflate balloon tip.
- Progressively advance PAC while tracking pressure waveform tracings (Table 41-1)[9]; catheter position can also be confirmed with fluoroscopy.

TABLE 41-1	HEMODYNAMICS OF PULMONARY ARTERY CATHETER			
Location	**RA**	**RV**	**PA**	**PCWP**
Distance (cm)	~20	~30	~40	~50
Normal pressure (mm Hg)	Mean ≤ 5	Systolic 15–30 Diastolic 1–7	Systolic 15–30 Mean 9–19 Diastolic 4–12	Mean ≤ 12

PA, pulmonary artery; PCWP, pulmonary capillary wedge pressure; RA, right atrium; RV, right ventricle.
Adapted from Kelly CR, Rabbani LE. Videos in clinical medicine. Pulmonary-artery catheterization. *N Engl J Med.* 2013;369(25):e35.

- After obtaining pulmonary capillary wedge pressure, deflate balloon tip. Pulmonary artery pressure waveform should reappear. If this does not occur, slowly withdraw catheter until it does.
- Aspirate blood from the distal port to measure mixed venous oxygen saturation.
- Secure the catheter and deploy plastic sleeve.
- Confirm adequate PAC placement under CXR.

Aftercare

- If a pulmonary capillary wedge pressure waveform is apparent, ensure the balloon tip is deflated and then slowly withdraw the catheter until the pulmonary artery pressure waveform reappears.
- Capillary wedge pressure can be assessed periodically by inflating the balloon tip; the balloon should be deflated right after these assessments.
- Pulmonary catheter allows continuous monitoring of the right atrial pressure and pulmonary pressure.

TRANSVENOUS TEMPORARY PACEMAKER

- Temporary cardiac pacing is used to treat a symptomatic bradyarrhythmia that can lead to hemodynamic instability.
- Transvenous pacing (TVP) is the preferred approach to cardiac pacing. Compared to other forms of temporary pacing, TVP is the most comfortable and durable option.
- Placement of a TVP can usually be performed swiftly and with ease.
- Indications for transvenous temporary pacing include the following:
  - Reversible causes of bradyarrhythmia
  - Emergent situations when permanent pacemaker is not immediately available
  - When the risk of implanting a permanent pacemaker exceeds the benefits

Special Equipment

- Temporary transvenous pacemaker leads are flexible and balloon tipped, allowing flow-directed lead positioning with low risk for cardiac perforation.
- External pulse generator
- Pulse generator connectors
- Fluoroscopy

Procedure

- Place patient in supine position. After selecting central vein for insertion (preferred access sites are the left subclavian and the right internal jugular), the steps to insert the introducer sheath are as for CVC insertion.
- Advance the pacemaker lead 15 cm through the introducer sheath.
- Akin to PAC placement, inflate the balloon located at the tip of the TVP lead.
- The lead is then flow directed to the right ventricle under fluoroscopic guidance.
- Optimal position of transvenous ventricular lead is at or near the right ventricular apex. The pacing lead should be allowed some "slack" to reduce risk of lead dislocation.
- Once the lead is in its final position, connect lead to pulse generator and program.
  - Temporary pacing rate should be titrated to optimize patient's hemodynamics (usually 60 beats per minute in adults).
  - Determine pacing threshold and program the pulse generator output two to three times the pacing threshold.
  - Sensitivity should be adjusted so that the pacemaker senses intrinsic electrical activity (in individuals who are not fully pacemaker dependent).

• Secure the lead and deploy plastic sleeve.
• Confirm adequate pacemaker lead placement with CXR.
• Obtain 12-lead ECG at the end of the procedure.

Aftercare

• Continuous ECG monitoring is necessary.
• Pacing thresholds should be checked daily.
• Daily physical examinations should evaluate for pericardial friction rubs, hypotension with muffled heart sounds and venous distention, and asymmetrical or absent breath sounds.
• CXR should be repeated if there is concern for lead dislodgement.

Complications

• Lead dislodgement and asystole
• Perforation of the myocardium
• Pneumothorax
• Air embolism
• Arrhythmia
• Extracardiac stimulation
• Infection

INTRA-AORTIC BALLOON PUMP

• Intra-aortic balloon counterpulsation is widely used for the management of cardiogenic shock. As it improves afterload reduction, it is often used in chronic heart failure.
• The intra-aortic balloon pump (IABP) is inserted percutaneously and has two lumens.
  ○ A central lumen used for over-the-wire balloon insertion. Once in its final position, this lumen is used for distal aspiration/flushing and to transduce aortic pressures.
  ○ A second lumen used to transfer helium from the console inflating and deflating the intra-aortic balloon.
• Counterpulsation enhances coronary flow by increasing diastolic blood pressure and reduces myocardial workload and oxygen demand by lowering afterload (Figure 41-2).

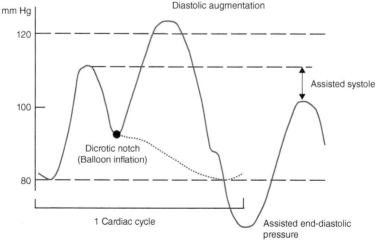

FIGURE 41-2. Optimal counterpulsation timing.

- Optimal timing of inflation/deflation is guided by direct pressure reading or ECG.
  - IABP should inflate at the aortic dicrotic notch that corresponds to the closure of the aortic valve and is correlated with the T wave on the ECG.
  - Deflation should occur during early systole (at or before R wave), thereby reducing aortic end-diastolic pressure.
- Adjustments of balloon timing cycle should be done at 1:2 counterpulsation. Generally, assisted end-diastolic pressure should be lower than unassisted end-diastolic pressure due to the unloading that occurs within the assisted beat.
  - Assisted systolic pressure is lower than unassisted systolic pressure.
  - Peak diastolic augmentation should be greater than unassisted systolic pressure.
- Importantly, IABP augments cardiac output roughly by 0.3 to 0.5 L/minute.
- Femoral approach for IABP insertion is presented in this section.

Indications for Intra-Aortic Balloon Pump Counterpulsation

- Acute myocardial infarction with mechanical complications such as ventricular septal defects or severe mitral regurgitation from ruptured papillary muscles
- Cardiogenic shock
- Refractory unstable angina
- Intractable ventricular tachycardia attributed to myocardial ischemia
- Bridge to another assist device
- High-risk PCI in the setting of severely depressed left ventricular (LV) function
- High-risk PCI involving unprotected left main or last remaining patent vessel

Contraindications

- Absolute contraindications
  - Moderate or severe aortic valve insufficiency
  - Aortic dissection or aneurysm
  - Previous aortic stenting
- Relative contraindications
  - Severe atherosclerosis
  - Blood dyscrasias
  - End-stage cardiomyopathy unless bridging to ventricular assist device (VAD)
  - Severe sepsis

Procedure

- Balloon size is chosen based on patient's height (Table 41-2).[10]
- Follow steps described for femoral CVC insertion for placement of introducer sheath (7 or 8 French depending on the balloon size).
- Connect one-way valve syringe to balloon inflation lumen and aspirate until completely collapsed.
- Under fluoroscopy, advance 0.018″ J-tipped guidewire through introducer sheath to thoracic aorta.
- Load and advance balloon over the 0.018″ wire to proximal descending aorta at ~1 to 2 cm below the origin of the left subclavian artery. This corresponds to the area between the second and third intercostal space.
- Once the catheter is positioned, remove guidewire and flush central lumen.
- Connect to pressure transducer and console.
- Start counterpulsation and optimize on 1:2 counterpulsation mode (Figure 41-2).
- Secure catheter at a minimum of two sites.
- Confirm IABP position with CXR. Low threshold to recheck if patient had major movement (e.g., attempted to get out of bed, transfer to/off bed).

TABLE 41-2 STANDARD INTRA-AORTIC BALLOON SIZING GUIDE

Patient height	Intra-aortic balloon volume (mL)	Body surface area (m²)
147–162 cm (<5'4")	30	<1.8
162–182 cm (5'4"–6'0")	40	>1.8
>182 cm (>6'0")	50	>1.8

Reprinted from Samim A, Berg R. High-risk patients and interventions. In: Kern MJ, Sorajja P, Lim MJ, eds. *The Interventional Cardiac Catheterization Handbook.* 4th ed. Elsevier; 2018:237-60. Copyright © 2018 Elsevier. With permission.

Anticoagulation

- Risks and benefits of systemic anticoagulation should be weighed on a case-by-case basis.
- Omitting anticoagulation for patients considered to be at high risk of bleeding appears to be safe and does not increase the risk of thrombus or limb ischemia when on 1:1 counterpulsation.
- Additional indications and contraindications to anticoagulation should be considered rather than it being an automatic response to IABP use.[11]

REFERENCES

1. ASA Task Force on Central Venous Access. Practice guidelines for central venous access 2020: an updated report by the American Society of Anesthesiologists Task Force on Central Venous Access. *Anesthesiology.* 2020;132(1):8-43.
2. Graham AS, Ozment C, Tegtmeyer K, Lai S, Braner DA. Videos in clinical medicine. Central venous catheterization. *N Engl J Med.* 2007;356(21):e21.
3. KDIGO Acute Kidney Injury Work Group. KDIGO clinical practice guideline for acute kidney injury. *Kidney Int Suppl.* 2012;2(1):1-138.
4. Chopra V, Flanders SA, Saint S, et al. The Michigan Appropriateness Guide for Intravenous Catheters (MAGIC): results from a multispecialty panel using the RAND/UCLA appropriateness method. *Ann Intern Med.* 2015;163(6 suppl):S1-40.
5. Hind D, Calvert N, McWilliams R, et al. Ultrasonic locating devices for central venous cannulation: meta-analysis. *BMJ.* 2003;327(7411):361.
6. O'Grady NP, Alexander M, Burns LA, et al. Summary of recommendations: guidelines for the prevention of intravascular catheter-related infections. *Clin Infect Dis.* 2011;52:1087-99.
7. Institute for Healthcare Improvement. Measures: prevent central line infection—central line bundle compliance. Accessed 06/15/22. http://www.ihi.org/resources/Pages/Measures/MeasuresPreventCentralLineInfection.aspx
8. Braner DA, Lai S, Eman S, Tegtmeyer K. Videos in clinical medicine. Central venous catheterization—subclavian vein. *N Engl J Med.* 2007;357(24):e26.
9. Kelly CR, Rabbani LE. Videos in clinical medicine. Pulmonary-artery catheterization. *N Engl J Med.* 2013;369(25):e35.
10. Kern M, Sorajja P, Lim M. *The Interventional Cardiac Catheterization Handbook.* 4th ed. Elsevier; 2018.
11. Jiang CY, Zhao LL, Wang JA, Mohammod B. Anticoagulation therapy in intra-aortic balloon counterpulsation: does IABP really need anti-coagulation? *J Zhejiang Univ Sci.* 2003;4(5):607-11.

Index

Page numbers followed by *f* refer to figures; page numbers followed by *t* refer to tables.